Management of High-Risk Pregnancy
A Practical Approach

SS Trivedi MS FICOG FIMSA
Director Professor and Head
Department of Obstetrics and Gynecology
Lady Hardinge Medical College and SSK Hospital
New Delhi, India

Manju Puri MD
Professor
Department of Obstetrics and Gynecology
Lady Hardinge Medical College and SSK Hospital
New Delhi, India

JAYPEE BROTHERS MEDICAL PUBLISHERS (P) LTD

New Delhi • St Louis (USA) • Panama City (Panama) • London (UK) • Ahmedabad
Bengaluru • Chennai • Hyderabad • Kochi • Kolkata • Lucknow • Mumbai • Nagpur

Published by

Jitendar P Vij

Jaypee Brothers Medical Publishers (P) Ltd

Corporate Office

4838/24 Ansari Road, Daryaganj, **New Delhi** - 110002, India, Phone: +91-11-43574357
Fax: +91-11-43574314

Registered Office

B-3 EMCA House, 23/23B Ansari Road, Daryaganj, **New Delhi** - 110 002, India
Phones: +91-11-23272143, +91-11-23272703, +91-11-23282021
+91-11-23245672, Rel: +91-11-32558559, Fax: +91-11-23276490, +91-11-23245683
e-mail: jaypee@jaypeebrothers.com, Website: www.jaypeebrothers.com

Offices in India

- **Ahmedabad,** Phone: Rel: +91-79-32988717, e-mail: ahmedabad@jaypeebrothers.com
- **Bengaluru,** Phone: Rel: +91-80-32714073, e-mail: bangalore@jaypeebrothers.com
- **Chennai,** Phone: Rel: +91-44-32972089, e-mail: chennai@jaypeebrothers.com
- **Hyderabad,** Phone: Rel:+91-40-32940929, e-mail: hyderabad@jaypeebrothers.com
- **Kochi,** Phone: +91-484-2395740, e-mail: kochi@jaypeebrothers.com
- **Kolkata,** Phone: +91-33-22276415, e-mail: kolkata@jaypeebrothers.com
- **Lucknow,** Phone: +91-522-3040554, e-mail: lucknow@jaypeebrothers.com
- **Mumbai,** Phone: Rel: +91-22-32926896, e-mail: mumbai@jaypeebrothers.com
- **Nagpur,** Phone: Rel: +91-712-3245220, e-mail: nagpur@jaypeebrothers.com

Overseas Offices

- **North America Office, USA,** Ph: 001-636-6279734
  e-mail: jaypee@jaypeebrothers.com, anjulav@jaypeebrothers.com
- **Central America Office, Panama City, Panama,** Ph: 001-507-317-0160
  e-mail: cservice@jphmedical.com
  Website: www.jphmedical.com
- **Europe Office, UK,** Ph: +44 (0) 2031708910, e-mail: info@jpmedpub.com

Management of High-Risk Pregnancy—A Practical Approach

© 2010, Jaypee Brothers Medical Publishers (P) Ltd.

First Edition: **2010**

ISBN 978-93-80704-73-9

Typeset at JPBMP typesetting unit
Printed at Sanat Printers, Kundli.

Contributors

Abha Singh MD
Professor
Department of Obstetrics and Gynecology
Lady Hardinge Medical College
and SSK Hospital
New Delhi, India

Amita Suneja MD FICOG FIMCH MNAMS
Professor
Department of Obstetrics and Gynecology
The University College of Medical
Sciences (UCMS) and Guru Teg Bahadur
(GTB) Hospital
Delhi, India

Aruna Nigam MS
Assistant Professor
Department of Obstetrics and Gynecology
Lady Hardinge Medical College
and SSK Hospital
New Delhi, India

Chitra Raghunandan MD
Director Professor
Department of Obstetrics and Gynecology
Lady Hardinge Medical College
and SSK Hospital
New Delhi, India

Deepika Deka MD FICOG
Professor
Department of Obstetrics and Gynecology
All India Institute of Medical Sciences
(AIIMS)
New Delhi, India

Evita Fernandez FRCOG
Consultant Obstetrician
Fernandez Hospital for Women
and the Newborn
Hyderabad, Andhra Pradesh, India

KK Gombar MD
Ex-Professor and Head
Department of Anesthesia
and Intensive Care
Government Medical College
and Hospital
Chandigarh, India

Kazila Bhutia MD
Ex-Senior Resident
Department of Obstetrics and Gynecology
Lady Hardinge Medical College
and SSK Hospital
New Delhi, India

Kiran Aggarwal MD
Professor
Department of Obstetrics and Gynecology
Lady Hardinge Medical College
and SSK Hospital
New Delhi, India

Lambhir Dhaliwal DGO MD
Professor and Head
Department of Obstetrics and Gynecology
Postgraduate Institute of Medical
Education and Research (PGIMER)
Chandigarh, India

Madhu Goel MD DNB MNAMS
Senior Obstetrician and Gynecologist
Rockland Hospital
Qutub Institutional Area
New Delhi, India

Mandakini Pradhan MD DNB
Head of Department
Material and Reproductive Health
Sanjay Gandhi Post Graduate Institute
of Medical Sciences
Lucknow, Uttar Pradesh, India

Manisha MS
Assistant Professor
Department of Obstetrics and Gynecology
Lady Hardinge Medical College
and SSK Hospital
New Delhi, India

Manju Puri MD
Professor
Department of Obstetrics and Gynecology
Lady Hardinge Medical College
and SSK Hospital
New Delhi, India

Monika Madaan MD
Assistant Professor
Department of Obstetrics and Gynecology
Lady Hardinge Medical College
and SSK Hospital
New Delhi, India

Monika B Nagpal DCH MS
Senior Resident
Department of Obstetrics and Gynecology
Lady Hardinge Medical College
and SSK Hospital
New Delhi, India

Nidhi Bhatia MD DNB
Assistant Professor
Department of Anesthesiology
Government Medical College and Hospital
Chandigarh, India

Nidhi Malhotra MBBS
Postgraduate Student
Department of Obstetrics and Gynecology
Lady Hardinge Medical College
and SSK Hospital
New Delhi, India

Pakhee Aggarwal MD
Senior Resident
Department of Obstetrics and Gynecology
All India Institute of Medical
Sciences (AIIMS)
New Delhi, India

Pikee Saxena MD PGCHM PGDCR
Assistant Professor
Department of Obstetrics and Gynecology
Lady Hardinge Medical College
and SSK Hospital
New Delhi, India

Prabha Lal MD
Assistant Professor
Department of Obstetrics and Gynecology
Lady Hardinge Medical College
and SSK Hospital
New Delhi, India

Ratna Biswas MD
Professor
Department of Obstetrics and Gynecology
Lady Hardinge Medical College
and SSK Hospital
New Delhi, India

Reena Yadav MD DGO FICOG
Professor
Department of Obstetrics and Gynecology
Lady Hardinge Medical College
and SSK Hospital
New Delhi, India

Ritu Rana MD DNB MRCOG
Specialist Registrar
Department of Obstetrics and Gynecology
Princess Alexandra Hospital
Harlow, United Kingdom

SS Trivedi MS FICOG FIMSA
Director Professor and Head
Department of Obstetrics and Gynecology
Lady Hardinge Medical College
and SSK Hospital
New Delhi, India

Sandhya Jain MD DNB MNAMS
Assistant Professor
Department of Obstetrics and Gynecology
The University College of Medical
Sciences (UCMS) and Guru Teg Bahadur
(GTB) Hospital
New Delhi, India

Sarita Malhotra MD
Senior Resident
Department of Obstetrics and Gynecology
Maulana Azad Medical College
and Lok Nayak Jai Prakash Hospital
New Delhi, India

Satinder Gombar MD
Professor and Head
Department of Anesthesia
and Intensive Care
Government Medical College
and Hospital
Chandigarh, India

Seema Singhal MS
Assistant Professor
Department of Obstetrics and Gynecology
Lady Hardinge Medical College
and SSK Hospital
New Delhi, India

Shalini Malhotra MD DNB MNAMS
Ex-Senior Resident
Department of Obstetrics and Gynecology
Lady Hardinge Medical College
and SSK Hospital
New Delhi, India

Sharda Patra MD DNB
Assistant Professor
Department of Obstetrics and Gynecology
Lady Hardinge Medical
and SSK Hospital
New Delhi, India

Smiti Nanda MD
Senior Professor and Head
Department of Obstetrics and Gynecology
Pt Bhagwat Dayal Sharma Postgraduate
Institute of Medical Sciences
Rohtak, Haryana, India

Sudha Salhan MD
Professor, Consultant and Head
Department of Obstetrics and Gynecology
Vardhman Mahavir Medical College and
Safdarjung Hospital
New Delhi, India

Suneeta Mittal
MD FRCOG (Anesthesia) FICOG FAMS FICMCH FIMSA
Professor and Head
Department of Obstetrics and Gynecology
Director Incharge WHO-CCR in Human
Reproduction
All India Institute of Medical Sciences
(AIIMS)
New Delhi, India

Swaraj Batra MS FICOG
Director Professor and Head
Department of Obstetrics and Gynecology
Maulana Azad Medical College and
Lok Nayak Jai Prakash Hospital
New Delhi, India

Usha Gupta MD MNAMS FICOG FIMSA
Professor and Head of Unit
Department of Obstetrics and Gynecology
Lady Hardinge Medical College
and SSK Hospital
New Delhi, India

Contributors

Foreword

I would like to congratulate Dr SS Trivedi, Director, Professor and Head of the Department of Obstetrics and Gynecology from Lady Hardinge Medical College and Smt. SK Hospital, New Delhi for producing this magnificent book on the *Management of High-risk Pregnancy – A Practical Approach*. The topics have been highly selected and there are 29 chapters which cover the entire spectrum of high-risk pregnancy. The chapters are well laid down starting from prenatal diagnosis through to obstetric and medical disorders in pregnancy and labor and ending with a chapter on Drugs in Obstetrics. The individual chapters provide extensive knowledge needed in that particular topic. The scan pictures, photographs of actual patients and that using models to illustrate the mechanism of labor and the technical procedures of labor and delivery are very clear and worth commending. The latest information available in the literature from various clinical guidelines, cochrane data base and meta-analysis has been incorporated into each chapter. The summary, recommendations and key points which are given at the end of each chapter are commendable and make reading and remembering the important facts easy compared to standard textbooks. The references are up-to-date and the latest references up to the time of publication are provided.

The authors are well known for their expertise in high-risk pregnancy and have contributed to the literature in obstetric medicine. Navigating through each chapter has been made easy as every chapter has the same layout. The contents are of a high standard, which is applicable for those who are training to be specialists in obstetrics and gynecology as well as practicing clinicians. I would highly commend this book and this book should be with in the libraries of the hospitals and medical schools and the clinicians office.

Sir Sabaratnam Arulkumaran
Professor and Head of Obstetrics and Gynecology
St George's University of London

Preface

Management of high-risk pregnancy is a challenge for all practicing obstetricians. True to its title, *Management of High-Risk Pregnancy—A Practical Approach*, this book focuses mainly on the practical aspects of the management of high-risk pregnancies. The various chapters have been contributed by clinicians with vast academic and clinical experience. The text is presented in an easy-to-read and user-friendly manner. The material is essentially evidence based and derived from the personal experience of the contributors. A number of flow charts have been included to serve as ready reckoners. This book includes most of the high-risk pregnancy situations and will be valuable to practicing clinicians, residents and faculty. A dedicated Chapter on critical care in obstetrics—what an obstetrician should know, provides useful information which needs to be known to clinicians taking care of critically-ill obstetric patients. Topics like prenatal screening and diagnosis, diagnosis and management of congenital malformations and antepartum fetal surveillance have been included to guide the clinicians in screening and monitoring of high-risk pregnancy situations. We have also included a Chapter on drugs in pregnancy which discusses the safety profile of drugs used in the management of at-risk pregnancies. This is not a complete textbook of obstetrics, but will serve as a useful complement to the already existing textbooks with special emphasis on the management of high-risk pregnancies.

We are thankful to our Director, GK Sharma who encouraged us to take up the task of writing this book and gave his constant support. Our thanks are due to all the contributors who spared their valuable time to write the various chapters of this book. Efforts of Dr Shalini Singh deserve special mention as she tirelessly assisted us in giving the final shape to the book. Finally, this book would not have been possible without the expert and organized support and cooperation of our publishers M/s Jaypee Brothers Medical Publishers (P) Ltd.

We hope that all practicing obstetricians, residents and teachers will benefit from this book and we would welcome any comments and suggestions from them.

SS Trivedi
Manju Puri

Contents

1. Prenatal Diagnosis 1
   Ratna Biswas, Mandakini Pradhan

2. Screening and Management of Congenital Anomalies 27
   Manisha

3. Antepartum Fetal Surveillance 57
   Seema Singhal

4. Preterm Labor 72
   Monika B Nagpal

5. Premature Rupture of Membranes 98
   Sharda Patra

6. Prolonged Pregnancy 112
   Amita Suneja, Sandhya Jain

7. Polyhydramnios Oligohydramnios 120
   Prabha Lal

8. Antepartum Hemorrhage 132
   SS Trivedi, Madhu Goel, Monika B Nagpal

9. Multifetal Pregnancy 152
   Reena

10. Intrauterine Growth Restriction (IUGR) 176
    Abha Singh

11. Malpresentations 199
    Usha Gupta

12. Pregnancy with Previous Cesarean Section 230
    Ritu Rana

13. Rh Negative Pregnancy 255
    Aruna Nigam

14. Anemia in Pregnancy 273
    Manju Puri, Nidhi Malhotra

15. Hypertensive Disorders of Pregnancy 296
    SS Trivedi, Monika B Nagpal

16. Diabetes Mellitus with Pregnancy 322
    Manju Puri, Kazila Bhutia

17. Jaundice in Pregnancy 348
    Chitra Raghunandan

18. Heart Disease in Pregnancy 369
    Monika B Nagpal, Shalini Malhotra

19. Thromboembolism in Pregnancy 389
    Swaraj Batra, Sarita Malhotra

20. Thyroid Disorders with Pregnancy 405
    Kiran Aggarwal

21. Renal Disease in Pregnancy 426
    Pakhee Aggarwal, Suneeta Mittal

22. Tuberculosis in Pregnancy 441
    Lakhbir Dhaliwal

23. Epilepsy with Pregnancy 454
    Monika Madaan

24. TORCH Infections in Pregnancy 460
    Deepika Deka

25. HIV in Pregnancy 470
    Sudha Salhan

26. Obesity and Pregnancy 487
    Evita Fernandez

27. Gynecological Diseases in Pregnancy 499
    Smiti Nanda

28. Critical Care Issues in High-Risk Obstetric Patient 515
    Satinder Gombar, KK Gombar, Nidhi Bhatia

29. Drugs in Pregnancy 544
    Pikee Saxena

Index 567

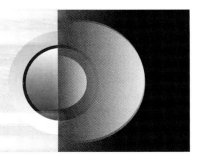

Prenatal Diagnosis 1

Ratna Biswas, Mandakini Pradhan

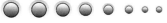

INTRODUCTION

Congenital disorder is one of the leading cause of mortality and morbidity in the fetus. The magnitude of problem is particularly significant in the developing world where congenital disorders are common because of consanguineous marriages and high birth rate. In India, half a million children born annually have congenital malformations and 21000 babies have Down syndrome.[1] In the absence of curative treatment the financial and social burden on the family and country is enormous. Herein lies the importance of early prenatal diagnosis.

Prenatal diagnosis involves initial screening to detect at risk couples followed by definite diagnosis. The prenatal diagnostic procedures are aimed at diagnosing the disease of the fetus. It could be chromosomal abnormalities, genetic diseases or structural defects. These procedures can be invasive or noninvasive. The diagnostic tests involve chromosomal, molecular or enzyme assays on fetal samples. The aim of the diagnostic procedures is to provide an accurate and early diagnosis of the fetal disease, so as to enable the couple to make an informative choice on the management options. The modalities of management are either termination of pregnancy, fetal therapy wherever applicable or to prepare for birth of an affected child. Preimplantation diagnosis, too, is a management option whereby an unaffected embryo is chosen for implantation. Thorough genetic counseling is essential and ethical issues need's to be considered when opting for this method.

Screening Methods

These are methods which can identify fetus at high risk of having malformations, genetic disorders, chromosomal abnormalities, etc. Though the screening methods widely discussed are for detection of fetal chromosomal aneuploidy, other fetal conditions which can affect the pregnancy outcome need to be kept in mind. For a screening method to be effective it needs to have a high detection rate with an acceptable false-positive rate. Following given methods can be used to detect couples at high risk of fetal disorder.

1. History:
   • During present pregnancy
   • Previous pregnancy
   • Past medical or surgical disorder
   • Family history.
2. Examination
3. Investigations:
   • Serum screening
   • Ultrasound
   • Other specific tests.

History

1. *History during present pregnancy*: Certain history during ongoing pregnancy may indicate a high-risk fetus.
   a. Exposure to teratogens like anticancer drugs, antiepileptics especially sodium valproate, anticoagulant like warfarin and radioactive iodine therapy for thyroid cancer etc.
   b. Contact with patients of infectious diseases like rubella.
   c. History of infectious diseases like chickenpox or fever with rash may indicate likelihood of fetus being infected.
   d. Anemia in the women (not due to iron deficiency or not improving after iron therapy) may need further evaluation to detect carrier of hemoglobinopathies. Such woman may be at risk of having an affected fetus.
2. *Past history*: Previous history of fetus being affected with a specific disease should warrant a prenatal diagnosis in subsequent pregnancy. The method of prenatal diagnosis differs depending upon the diagnosis in the previous child. Table 1.1 delineates few of the common disorders, their risk of recurrence and method of prenatal diagnosis.

Family history: A minimum three generation pedigree should be drawn to find out any significant risk to the couple of having an affected baby. For example, a history of maternal brother being affected with Duchenne muscular dystrophy may indicate a possibility of the woman being carrier and hence having 25% risk of affected child. A history of consanguinity may indicate towards investigating parents for carrier of a common autosomal recessive

Table 1.1: Some common disorders, their risk of recurrence and method of prenatal diagnosis				
Disorder	Mode of inheritance	Recurrence risk	Method of Prenatal diagnosis
Single gene disorder			
β-thalassemia	Autosomal recessive	25%	Mutation detection in both parents and subsequently in the fetal sample obtained after invasive method
Cystic fibrosis	Autosomal recessive	25%	Mutation detection in both parents and subsequently in the fetal sample obtained after invasive method
Sickle cell disease	Autosomal recessive	25%	Direct detection of mutation by molecular method in the fetal sample obtained after invasive method
Duchenne muscular dystrophy (DMD)	X- linked recessive	25% of all children or 50% of male children	Mutation detection in the previous affected child
Spinal muscular atrophy (SMA) the	Autosomal recessive	25%	If diagnosis is confirmed in previous affected child, mutation detection can be done in fetal sample obtained after invasive method
Achondroplasia	Autosomal dominant	50% if one of the parent is affected; 1% if both parents are normal as it is usually due to new mutation	Mutation detection in the fetal sample if couple is willing after counseling.
Multifactorial disease neural tube defect (NTD)	Unknown	3-5% after one affected pregnancy; 10% after two affected pregnancies	Ultrasound

disease like β-thalassemia. Some common disorders, their risk of recurrence and method of prenatal diagnosis are listed in Table 1.1.

Examination

As in any clinical setting, detail examination of a pregnant woman is important. It is more so because many of them visit a doctor for the first time and asymptomatic conditions can be picked-up, e.g. this woman with history of previous two pregnancies affected with polyhydramnios and club foot, on examination was found to have myotonia and thus clinching the diagnosis of myotonic dystrophy in the family which is a triple repeat disorder (Fig. 1.1).

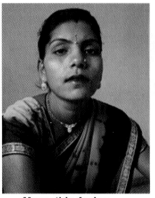
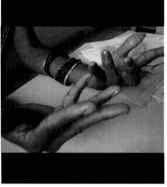

Myopathic facies   **Myotonia**

Figure 1.1: Myotonic dystrophy

Investigations

Various screening and diagnostic procedures for prenatal diagnosis are tabulated in Table 1.2.

Table 1.2: Screening and diagnostic procedures for prenatal diagnosis

Noninvasive Screening Procedures

a. Maternal serum screening
   1. First trimester screening
   2. Triple test
   3. Quadruple test
   4. Integrated screening
   5. Sequential screening and contingent screening
b. Fetal imaging
   1. Ultrasonography – 2D, 3D, 4D
   2. Doppler sonography
   3. Magnetic resonance imaging

Noninvasive Diagnostic Procedure

Detection of fetal DNA and fetal cells in maternal circulation

Invasive Diagnostic Procedures

a. Amniocentesis
   1. Early amniocentesis
   2. Second trimester amniocentesis
b. Chorionic villous sampling (CVS)
   1. Transcervical CVS
   2. Transabdominal CVS
c. Fetal blood sampling
   1. Percutaneous umbilical blood sampling or cordocentesis
   2. Fetal intrahepatic vessel sampling
   3. Fetal cardiac sampling.
d. Fetal tissue biopsy
e. Fetoscopy

Preimplantation Diagnosis

The noninvasive procedures are generally used for screening whereas the invasive procedures give a definite diagnosis.

Fetal aneuploidy is the commonest indication for prenatal diagnostic test. Aneuploidy is defined as an abnormal number of chromosomes in place of the usual diploid complement. Down syndrome (Trisomy 21), Edward syndrome (Trisomy 18), Patau syndrome (Trisomy 13) are the most common trisomies. Down syndrome occurs in 1: 800 to 1 :900 live births. It is compatible with life. Edward syndrome occurs in 1:3000 live births and Patau syndrome occurs in 1: 5000 live births. Both are lethal anomalies.[2] The age-related risk of Down syndrome in a pregnant woman at midtrimester is, 1: 417 at 33 years, 1: 250 at 35 years, 1:149 at 37 years, 1: 69 at 40 years and 1:19 at 45 years.[3]

The hallmark of screening Down syndrome till few years back was Triple test which is performed in the second trimester. Now screening procedures are available in the first trimester also. Awareness amongst women regarding these procedures is lacking, hence it is important to counsel and offer screening procedures to all pregnant women.

Recent guidelines from American College of Obstetrics and Gynecology (ACOG) 2007 and American College of Medical Genetics (ACMG) recommends screening of all pregnant women regardless of maternal age.[4,5]

ACOG 2007 guidelines also state that integrated or sequential screening be offered to all pregnant women who seek prenatal care in the first trimester and for those who come later than 14 weeks, the second trimester serum screening should be offered.

The screening strategy chosen depends on availability of chorionic villus sampling (CVS) and expertise for nuchal translucency (NT). In the absence of expertise in NT measurement the first trimester screening is incomplete and therefore the integrated and sequential and contingent screening too, cannot be done. However the integrated serum screening is an option if expertise in NT measurement is lacking. On the other hand when CVS facilities are unavailable, the sequential and contingent screening cannot be done because in these methods if screen is positive in the first trimester then directly CVS is to be done. However integrated screening is possible even in absence of CVS facilities because here results are declared only after the second trimester tests, and an amniocentesis is performed in case of positive result.

Screening Methods

First Trimester Screening

The methods used are:
a. Nuchal translucency (NT) sonography
b. Nasal bone sonography
c. Doppler sonography of ductus venosus
d. Pregnancy associated plasma protein A (PAPP-A) in maternal serum
e. Free β–subunit of hCG in maternal serum

It refers to the space between spine and overlying skin at the back of fetal neck. Measurement is done between 10 weeks + 3 days to 13 weeks + 6 days of gestation. Increased NT is a strong marker of Down syndrome.[6] Possible mechanisms leading to increased nuchal translucency are fluid accumulation secondary to heart failure caused by structural anomalies of heart, abnormal extracellular matrix or abnormal lymphatic development.[7]

NT can be obtained by transabdominal or transvaginal route. By trans-abdominal route it is possible to obtain 95% of NT measurements and combining the two routes results in 100% chance of obtaining the NT measurement. Correct technique for measurement of NT is to obtain a view of the midsagittal plane with the fetal head in neutral position and fetal image occupying 75% of viewable screen. The fetal image to be obtained consists of fetal head, neck and upper part of thorax. Crown-rump length (CRL) measurement is mandatory to accurately estimate the period of gestation since NT varies with gestational age. Distinction between amnion and overlying fetal skin should be confirmed on fetal movement. Calipers are placed at inner borders of the NT space.[6,8,9] Three to five NT measurements are obtained and the largest value taken.

NT measurement requires considerable skill which can be acquired with training. The accuracy of NT measurement is said to be reached when the difference in intra and interobserver variation is less than 0.5 in 95% of the measurements. Approximately 100 scans have to be performed to attain such level of perfection. A good quality ultrasound machine with video loop function and an ability to measure upto a 10th of a millimeter is needed for measuring NT.[9] Adequate time should be spared for proper measurement and at least 20 minutes time should be given before labeling an attempt unsuccessful.[2] In such a situation a rescan should be scheduled after a week's time or earlier depending on the period of gestation. Quality control measures need to be instituted for maintaining high standards of performance.

The rate of detection of Down syndrome based on NT in high-risk women ranges from 46-62%, whereas the detection rate in low-risk women varies from 29-91%.[8] The average detection rate with NT is 77% at false-positive rate of 5%.[8]

Specific cutoff values (2.5 or 3 mm) are inappropriate because of gestational age dependant variation in NT. Gestational age specific thresholds are available for NT measurement which is combined with maternal age to arrive at a risk estimate.[9] Alternatively it can be expressed as MoM and combined with PAPP-A and β hCG to give a risk estimate.

Detection of cystic hygroma during first trimester sonography for evaluation of NT is the most powerful predictor for trisomy 21 with 50% risk of fetal aneuploidy. This finding is an indication for a CVS.[6]

Nasal Bone Sonography

To obtain accurate measurement, the midsagittal plane is viewed with the neck in slight flexion position and the fetal profile facing upwards. In normal pregnancy two echogenic lines, one representing the fetal skin and the other the fetal nasal bone is visualized. Failure to visualize the nasal bone is an independent risk factor for Down syndrome.[6] However accurate imaging of fetal nasal bone in first trimester is technically challenging with a significant intra and interobserver variation.

The ultrasound beam should strike at right angles to the nasal skin for visualization of the nasal bone. The normal ossification of nasal bone develops on both sides of the cartilaginous septum from 10 weeks onwards. New ossification appears as less echogenic lines on both sides of bone. Only the echogenic part should be measured. Difference in timing of appearance and ossification of both nasal bones may cause technical difficulty in measurement leading to intra- and interobserver variation.[10,11] Hence its routine use in clinical setting is not recommended.

Ductus Venosus Sonography

The blood flow in the fetal ductus venosus in first trimester by Doppler ultrasound shows triphasic flow pattern with forward flow reaching peak during ventricular systole, early ventricular diastole and during atrial contraction. Absence or reversal of flow at atrial systole is a marker for trisomy 21.[6] Difficulty in measuring flow through ductus venosus limits its use in routine clinical practice.[10]

Biochemical Markers in Maternal Serum

PAPP-A is 50% lower in trisomy 21 as compared to normal pregnancy when measured between 10-13 weeks of gestation, whereas maternal serum levels of free β hCG is twice as high in trisomy 21 as compared to normal pregnancy.[6]

Combined First Trimester Screening

Combined NT, PAPP-A, β hCG in association with maternal age detects 85% of trisomy 21 with the false-positive rate of 5%. The earlier in first trimester the measurements are taken the higher is the detection rate, 87% at 11 weeks as compared to 82% at 13 weeks.[6]

A National Institute of Health (NIH) sponsored study called the Blood, Ultrasound and Nuchal Translucency (BUN) trial evaluating the results of first trimester screening in 8500 high-risk cases detected 79% of all Down syndrome cases with 5% false-positive rate.[12] The FASTER study with 36000 pregnancies detected 85% of Down syndrome with 5% of false-positive.[13]

The one stop clinic to assess risk (OSCAR) study involving 12000 pregnancies had a 90% detection rate at a false-positive rate of 5%.[14] The Serum, Urine and Ultrasound (SURUSS) study involving 48000 pregnancies had a 86% detection rate for a 5% false-positive rate.[15] The average derived from these 4 large trials is 85% which is better than quadruple screening in second trimester. Both BUN and FASTER study support the efficacy of free β hCG over total β hCG. However the recent guidelines from the American College of Medical Genetics state that free β hCG, total hCG or hyperglycosoylated hCG should be interchangeable.[5] As individual marker NT is most informative followed by PAPP-A.

Second Trimester Screening

It is indicated in pregnant women who present for the first time in second trimester or when expertise in first trimester screening, like measurement of NT is not available. Methods of second trimester screening are:
1. Biochemical serum markers
2. Sonographic detection of major structural malformation
3. Sonographic evaluation of minor markers.

Biochemical Serum Markers

a. Maternal serum alpha fetoprotein (MSAFP)
b. β hCG
c. Unconjugated estriol (uE3)
d. Inhibin A.

Maternal Serum Assay in Second Trimester

MSAFP screening is most accurate when performed between 16-18 weeks of gestation.[14] Low MSAFP has been associated with Down syndrome. One-third to one-fifth of Down syndrome pregnancies present with low MSAFP levels with the median MSAFP level of 0.7.[16] MSAFP values need correction for weight, race, diabetes and multiple gestation.[3] In insulin dependent diabetics MSAFP levels are 60% of nondiabetics.[16] In twin pregnancy the median MSAFP levels from 16-20 weeks of gestation is 2.5 MoM for single pregnancy. Combined biochemical screening procedures are:

Triple Test

MSAFP, unconjugated estriol and hCG are the components of triple test. Maternal serum levels of AFP and unconjugated estriol are 25% lower in Down syndrome as compared to normal pregnancy. Serum hCG is twice as high in Down syndrome as compared to normal pregnancy. It is usually performed between 15-18 weeks of gestation. The serum levels of each of the proteins is expressed as multiple of median (MoM) for women with gestational age same as patients. The composite estimate of the risk of trisomy 21 is calculated. Standard cut off is 1/270 which is equal to the second trimester risk of Down syndrome in a 35-year-old woman.[3,12] Triple test identifies around 60% of the pregnancies at risk of Down syndrome with 5% screen positive rate in women younger than 35 years. In women older than 35 years it detects 75% or more pregnancies affected with Down syndrome or other aneuploidies.[17]

Quadruple Test

Maternal serum inhibin A levels are increased to 2.1 times the median value of control in Down syndrome. Quadruple test is done between 14-21 weeks. It combines measurement of MSAFP, serum estriol, free β hCG and inhibin A together with maternal age.[3,18] It has a 67 to 76% detection rate of trisomy 21 in women younger than 35 years.[17] Some studies have quoted a detection rate of 80%.

Combined First and Second Trimester Screening

It maximizes the performance of these screening modalities. It is of two types—Integrated screening and sequential or contingent screening.

Integrated screening: It is a two step approach with the results announced at the time of the second test. In the first trimester, between 10-14 weeks of gestation NT and PAPP-A are measured. In the second trimester, between 15-16 weeks of gestation, MSAFP, hCG, estriol and inhibin A levels are measured. The results are analysed only at the end of second test and the probability of trisomy 21 is calculated using a computerized algorithm. The detection rate is 95% with a false-positive of 5%.[2,19]

Sequential and contingent screening: In sequential screening NT and PAPP-A or NT, PAPP-A and β-hCG are analysed to detect an interim risk in the first trimester. If interim risk is sufficiently high (e.g. >1 in 25 or > 1 in 50) then the pregnant women are informed of their screen positive result and offered early diagnostic intervention. All women who are below high-risk level subsequently go for second trimester screening with either a screen positive or negative result and advised for a diagnostic test according to the results of the second trimester screening. In the contingent screening the first trimester screening with NT and PAPP-A or NT, PAPP-A and β hCG is analysed to assess an interim risk. But instead of just a high interim risk group, a low interim risk group is also identified for e.g. < 1 in 2000. The high interim risk group is informed of their screen positive status like in sequential screening and advised diagnostic test while the low interim risk group do not need any further testing thereby reducing the cost incurred. The intermediate risk group which fall between the high- and low-risk group are advised for a second trimester screening with the four biochemical markers to receive a fully integrated report and accordingly advised diagnostic invasive testing based on the report.[2,19] The advantage of this screening is that if the first trimester screening is positive then chorionic villus sampling is offered to the pregnant women leading to early diagnosis and an early termination of pregnancy if needed.

The first trimester serum markers are also abnormal in trisomy 18. Levels of PAPP-A and βhCG are low and NT is increased. In the second trimester, alfa-fetoprotein, βhCG and estriol are all low in trisomy 18. Algorithms are available to detect risk of trisomy 18 based on first trimester and integrated screening.

Fetal Imaging

Sonographic Detection of Major Fetal Structural Malformation

This is done between 17-18 weeks of gestation to maximize fetal anatomic evaluation. The major structural malformations associated with aneuploidy are:[3,6,10]

1. Cardiac defects: Atrial septal defect, ventricular septal defects, teratology of Fallot, double outlet right ventricle, hypoplastic left heart, septal and endocardial cushion defects, valvular defects, coarctation of aorta.
2. Gastrointestinal malformations: Duodenal atresia, esophageal atresia, omphalocele, tracheoesophageal fistula, annular pancreas, imperforate anus, diaphragmatic hernia.
3. Central nervous system malformations: Meningomyelocele, holo-prosencephaly, agenesis of corpus callosum, ventriculomegaly (Fig. 1.2), microcephaly, posterior fossa defects, etc.

Ventriculomegaly

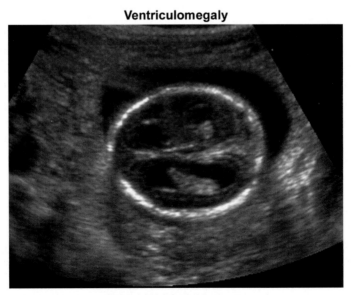

Figure 1.2: Venticulomegaly

4. Skeletal malformations: Club feet, rocker bottom feet, polydactyly.
5. Renal malformations: Horseshoe kidney, polycystic kidney, hydronephrosis.
6. Facial anomalies: Cleft lip and palate, microphthalmia, anophthalmia, macroglossia, cyclopia.

Sonographic Evaluation of Minor Markers

These are specific ultrasound findings that have been associated with increased risk of fetal aneuploidy. The minor markers are:

1. *Nuchal fold:* This measures the area between the outer aspect of occipital bone and outer aspect of skin in the axial plane passing through the posterior fossa. It is measured between 15-21 weeks. In normal pregnancy it is less than 5 mm, if it is more than 5 mm then the risk of Down syndrome increases by 11 fold.[6] It is also increased in Noonan's syndrome and in congenital cardiac defects. It is considered to be the single most sensitive and specific marker for aneuploidies in the second trimester sonography.[10]

2. *Echogenic bowel:* A very bright bowel in the fetal abdomen is associated with a 6.7 fold increased risk of Down syndrome. While performing ultrasound it is important to check the gain settings as false-positive results will occur if the gain settings are high. The echogenicity of bowel should be comparable to that of fetal bone.[6] It is also seen in association with disorders like cystic fibrosis, cytomegalovirus infection and other aneuploidies. Structural malformations like small bowel obstruction, malrotation of gut, meconium ileus and peritonitis are also associated with this observation.[10] In it's presence a maternal screening for cystic fibrosis, CMV infection and aneuploidy should be done. On the other hand amniocentesis can be done for fetal karyotyping, detection of cystic fibrosis mutation, and DNA analysis of CMV infection.

3. *Echogenic intracardiac focus:* This is caused by calcification of papillary muscles of ventricle. It is mainly seen in the left ventricle. To prevent overdiagnosis multiple angles are visualized to rule out specular reflections. The presence of echogenic intracardiac focus increases the risk of Down syndrome by 1.8 fold. However the point to be noted is that it may be present in 30% of normal Asian fetuses and hence it is not a sensitive or specific marker for aneuploidies. Therefore, other ultrasound findings or positive serum screening should be present to justify invasive testing.[6,10]

4. *Short humerus and femur:* In normal fetus the ratio of expected to observed length of these two bones should not be less than 0.90. The presence of short humerus increases the risk of Down syndrome by five fold, whereas short femur increases the risk by 1.5 fold. However racial difference in biometry exists and Asian fetuses have shorter biometric measurements. Hence normogram for individual population should be available to prevent overdiagnosis. The sensitivity and specificity of this marker is not high and hence it's isolated presence does not justify an invasive diagnosis.[6]

Prenatal Diagnosis

5. *Pyelectasis:* A renal pelvis measurement in the anteroposterior diameter of more than 4 mm is abnormal when measured between 14-20 weeks. Bilateral pyelectasis is associated with 1.5 fold increased risk of Down syndrome.[6]

6. *Nasal bones:* Hypoplastic or absent nasal bones on second trimester sonography is associated with increased risk of Down syndrome. The data available till now is limited to assess the strength of this association.[6]

7. *Choroid plexus cyst:* The presence of cyst in the choroid plexus in an axial view through the upper portion of fetal head has been correlated with the increased risk of trisomy 18. However isolated choroid plexus cyst in low risk woman is not clinically relevant[6,10] (Fig. 1.3). It disappears in 2% fetuses by 20 weeks and resolves in more than 90% by 26 weeks. It is a soft marker of aneuploidy.

Choroid plexus cyst

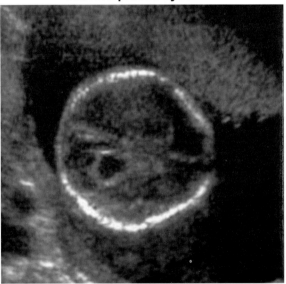

Figure 1.3: Choroid plexus cyst

Nicolaides and colleagues observed that detection of aneuploidy on sonography was related to the number of defects identified.[10,20] They assigned points to specific markers. Structural malformation and thickened nuchal fold were assigned two points each and shortened femur, shortened humerus, echogenic intracardiac focus, hyperechoic bowel and pylectasis were given one point each. An invasive test is recommended in high-risk women with one or more points or in low-risk women with two or more points based on his scoring system.

It is a targeted sonography which is done for fetal aneuploidy. It is done between 18 to 20 weeks of gestation and special attention is given to detect abnormal fetal biometry, fetal structural anomalies and minor (soft) markers of fetal aneuploidy.[17]

In Down syndrome the following sonographic findings should be looked for:

Skeletal abnormalities like sandal gap toes, 11 pairs of ribs, short fingers, brachymesophalangia, etc. Facial abnormalities like flattened face and occiput, oblique palpebral fissure, high arch palate, low nasal bridge, low set ears, nasal hypoplasia, macroglossia, epicanthic fold. CNS abnormalities which are frequently associated with Down syndrome are ventriculomegaly, microcephaly and brachycephaly. Cardiovascular defects include ASD, VSD, TOF, endocardial cushion defects, echogenic cardiac focus and pericardial effusion. Gastrointestinal and genitourinary abnormalities like duodenal atresia, tracheoesophageal fistula, omphalocele, annular pancreas, imperforate anus, hyperechogenic bowel and mild pylectasis. Hypotonia and goiter are other findings seen in trisomy 21. IUGR may or may not be an associated finding.[10]

In trisomy 18, growth is usually restricted. CNS abnormalities associated with Edward syndrome are choroid plexus cyst, abnormal cisterna magna, absent corpus callosum, cerebellar hypoplasia, ventriculomegaly, strawberry-shaped calvarium, and neural tube defects. Skeletal abnormalities include, limb reduction defects, overlapping index finger, clubbed feet, rocker bottom feet and polydactyly. Facial defects seen are, cleft lip and palate, micrognathia, low set ears, and microphthalmos. Cardiovascular abnormalities like septal and valvular defects may be present. Gastrointestinal and genitourinary anomalies associated with this syndrome are omphalocele, diaphragmatic hernia, hydronephrosis and horseshoe kidney. Umbilical cord cysts and double vessel umbilical cord may also be observed.[10]

Trisomy 13 is associated with growth restriction. CNS malformations like alobar holoprosencephaly, posterior fossa abnormalities, corpus callosum agenesis, ventriculomegaly and neural tube defects may be seen. Skeletal abnormalities like polydactyly and facial malformations like cyclopia, midline facial clefts, anophthalmia, hypoplastic nose are associated with Patau syndrome. CVS abnormalities like septal defects, tetralogy of Fallot, hypoplastic left ventricle, coarctation of aorta, echogenic intracardiac focus, gastrointestinal malformations like omphalocele and genitourinary abnormalities like polycystic kidneys, horseshoe kidney, enlarged echogenic kidney and nuchal thickening may be observed.[10]

1. *3D Ultrasound*: Other than the standard 2D ultrasound, 3D ultrasound allows multiplanar imaging and is an adjunct to the 2D ultrasound. In special situations such as fetal echocardiography, detection of cleft lip and cleft palate and in skeletal abnormalities, it's role is more certain.[2] Because of multiplanar imaging and rapid acquisition of volume data, more accurate information is possible like for example, in the evaluation of the extent and size of anomaly.[17] It provides better comprehension of fetal anatomy specially for the patient. It is semimanual and dependent on operator skill partly, hence adequate training is required.

2. *Magnetic resonance imaging (MRI)*: It was first used in obstetrics in 1983. It's advantage lies in it's ability to use multiple planes for reconstruction and a large field of view making the visualization of complicated anomalies easier. The development of single shot rapid acquisition sequence with refocused echoes and high quality T_2 weighted image provides excellent fetal imaging. This has obviated the need to sedate the mother or fetus. It is specially useful when ultrasound findings are inconclusive as in oligohydramnios, maternal obesity or when posterior cranial fossa is to be visualized where bone calcification hampers the ultrasonographic study. MRI has been used extensively in the diagnosis of ventriculomegaly, corpus callosum agenesis, posterior fossa abnormalities, cortical gyral malformations, hemorrhage, holo-prosencephaly, arachnoid cyst, neural tube defects and vascular malformations.[2]

Summary of Recommendations and Conclusions of ACOG Practice Bulletin No. 77 (2007)

Screening for Fetal Chromosomal Abnormalities

The following recommendations are based on good and consistent scientific evidence (Level A):

• First trimester screening using both nuchal translucency measurement and biochemical markers is an effective screening test for Down syndrome in the general population. At the same false-positive rates, this screening strategy results in a higher Down syndrome detection rate than does the second trimester maternal serum triple screen and is comparable to the quadruple screen.

• Measurement of nuchal translucency alone is less effective for first trimester screening than is the combined test (nuchal translucency measurement and biochemical markers).

• Women found to have increased risk of aneuploidy with first trimester screening should be offered genetic counseling and the option of CVS or second trimester amniocentesis.

- Specific training, standardization, use of appropriate ultrasound equipment, and ongoing quality assessment are important to achieve optimal nuchal translucency measurement for Down syndrome risk assessment and this procedure should be limited to centers and individuals meeting these criteria.
- Neural tube defect screening should be offered in the second trimester to women who elect only first-trimester screening for aneuploidy.[4]

The following recommendations are based on limited or inconsistent scientific evidence (Level B):
- Screening and invasive diagnostic testing for aneuploidy should be available to all women who present for prenatal care before 20 weeks of gestation regardless of maternal age. Women should be counseled regarding the differences between screening and invasive diagnostic testing.
- Integrated first and second trimester screening is more sensitive with lower false-positive rate than first trimester screening alone.
- Serum integrated screening is a useful option in pregnancies where nuchal translucency measurement is not available or cannot be obtained.
- An abnormal finding on second trimester ultrasound examination identifying a major congenital anomaly significantly increases the risk of aneuploidy and warrants further counseling and the offer of a diagnostic procedure.
- Patient who have a fetal nuchal translucency measurement of 3.5 mm or higher in the first trimester, despite a negative aneuploidy screen or normal fetal chromosomes, should be offered a targeted ultrasound examination, fetal echocardiogram or both.
- Down syndrome risk assessment in multiple gestation using first or second trimester serum analysis is less accurate than in singleton pregnancies.[4]

The following recommendations are based primarily on consensus and expert opinion (Level C).
- After first trimester screening, subsequent second trimester Down syndrome screening is not indicated unless it is being performed as a component of the integrated test, stepwise sequential, or contingent sequential test.
- Subtle second trimester ultrasonographic markers should be interpreted in the context of a patient's age, history and serum screening results.[4]

NonInvasive Diagnostic Method

Detection of Fetal DNA and Fetal Cells in Maternal Circulation

Presence of cell free fetal DNA in maternal plasma was first discovered in 1997. At present the circulating fetal DNA detected in maternal plasma can be analysed for noninvasive diagnosis of RhD status of the fetus, sex-linked disorders, single gene disorder like congenital adrenal hyperplasia, beta-thalassemia and achondroplasia.[22] Karyotyping is also possible.

The different fetal cells which can be isolated are nucleated erythrocytes, CD-34 positive hematogenic progenitors and syncytiotrophoblast. These cells can be detected as early as 6 weeks of gestation.[14] The fetal cells are differentiated from maternal cells by various cell sorting techniques like density gradient or protein separation, fluorescence activated cell sorting and magnetic activated cell sorting.[3] But there are certain limitations of fetal cell detection. These are—nucleated RBC cannot be expanded in cultures hence metaphase chromosomes are not available for prenatal diagnosis, CD-34 cells from previous pregnancies may persist and cause error in diagnosis and trophoblasts are not always present in maternal circulation. Hence none of these cells are ideal for analysis of fetal disease. Also the sorting methods are not consistently reliable for fetal cell detection.[23]

Fetal DNA is detected by real time PCR techniques. Recently plasma epigenetic markers have been used for differentiating maternal and fetal DNA. DNA methylation techniques is one such epigenetic method. Search is on for techniques which are superior to the methylation specific PCR assays like the mass spectrometric-based methods.[24,25]

Invasive Prenatal Diagnostic Procedures

These are techniques to obtain sample which are of fetal origin and can be used for analysis to make a definite fetal diagnosis.

In presence of indications patients have to be counseled for an invasive test such as amniocentesis. Counseling has to encompass all aspects of the procedure like the technique, the rate of complications especially that of pregnancy loss, the timing of results and the management options available. The decision of going for the procedure is absolutely voluntary and written consent mandatory. All the forms, i.e. Form D,E,F and G need to be filled up duely as per PNTD act.

Amniocentesis

It is an invasive procedure where a needle is introduced into the amniotic cavity under a sonographic guidance and amniotic fluid is withdrawn for analysis. The indications for amniocentesis are:[3]

I. Mother at high risk of fetal aneuploidy:
   1. Maternal age 35 years or more at the time of delivery in singleton pregnancy
   2. Maternal age 31 years or more at the time of delivery in twin gestation
   3. Increased risk on first or second trimester screening for Down syndrome
   4. Ultrasound finding suggestive of major structural malformation.[3]
   5. One of the parents is a carrier of balanced chromosomal translocation.
II. Fetus at high risk of metabolic disorder:
   1. A definite diagnosis was made in previous affected child.
   2. Previous affected child may have a typical clinical presentation/ investigations without a definite diagnosis.

III. Fetus at risk of single gene disorder (autosomal recessive, autosomal dominant and X-linked recessive disorder) where amniotic fluid can also be used for extracting DNA for diagnosis.

IV. RhD isoimmunized pregnancy management by spectrophotometric analysis of bilirubin in amniotic fluid and plotting of Liley's curve.

Amniocentesis is done between 15-20 weeks of gestation. Technically the procedure is easier to perform at this period of gestation since the uterus is accessible per abdomen and sufficient amount of amniotic fluid is available for withdrawing.

It is performed under aseptic precaution using a 22 G needle. A preliminary sonography is performed to document the number of fetuses, the viability of the fetus, gestational age, placental localization and liquor volume. A site which has sufficient liquor volume and which is free of placenta or cord is chosen for needle insertion. Local anesthesia at puncture site is optional. A sterile glove is put over the transducer and under sonographic vision, 22G needle is inserted into the amniotic cavity. The stilette is removed and fluid is aspirated (Fig. 1.4).[3,18]

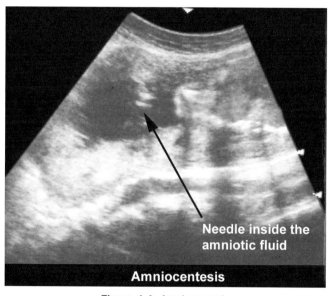

Figure 1.4: Amniocentesis

Dry tap during amniocentesis is due to tenting of membranes. In such a situation needle should be withdrawn into the myometrium and reinserted with a forceful thrust to penetrate the membranes. Another method for successful entry is to penetrate the needle into the posterior myometrium under sonographic guidance and then gradually withdraw the needle into the amniotic fluid pocket. The use of stylet with needle also helps to overcome the problem of tenting of membranes. The stylet is longer than the needle and by advancing the stylet 10 mm beyond the needle tip the membranes can

Prenatal Diagnosis

be entered.[26] Initial 3-4 ml of fluid is discarded to prevent contamination of maternal cells. Approximately 20 ml of fluid is aspirated and transferred into centrifugation tubes. Following the procedure the fetal heart rate is checked and anti-D is given to Rh negative mothers. Postprocedure amniotic fluid leakage occurs in 2% cases but is usually self-limiting. Chorioamnionitis occurs in 1 in 1000 procedures. The rate of pregnancy loss is as low as 0.3% in experienced hands.[16]

Early amniocentesis is performed between 11-14 weeks of gestation. The incidence of limb deformities, like talipes equinovarus is significantly high in early amniocentesis. It is seen in 0.75-1.7 % cases. The miscarriage rate is 1.5%.[3] Hence this procedure is not preferred. The Canadian Early and Midtrimester Amniocentesis Trial (CEMAT) randomized 4000 pregnant women for early and midtrimester amniocentesis. The success rate of culture was 97.7% with accuracy of 99.8% for early amniocentesis but there was higher rate of complications in form of fetal loss, increased incidence of talipes equinovarus and postprocedural amniotic fluid leakage.[27-29]

Amniotic fluid is analysed routinely for alfa fetoprotein levels. Fetal cells obtained from amniotic fluid or chorionic villus sampling are cultured for karyotype determination and DNA study. In recent times rapid diagnosis of common fetal aneuploidies like trisomy 13, 18, 21 and sex chromosomes is possible. The techniques of rapid diagnosis is fluorescent *in situ* hybridization(FISH) and quantitative fluorescent-PCR(QF-PCR). Specific probes for fluorescent *in situ* hybridization technique has been developed to detect numerical aberrations of metaphase chromosomes and interphase nuclei of nonmitotic cell.[18,30]

The limitations of rapid diagnostic techniques are that they fail to detect structural chromosomal aberrations like translocation and inversion and in addition they miss out nearly half (47.4%) of the aneuploidies when compared to karyotyping.[31]However in more recent studies involving more than 2000 women both the sensitivity and specificity of FISH on uncultured amniocytes for detecting these chromosomal abnormalities was > 99%. But there were both false-positive and negative reports. Further maternal cell contamination on uncultured cells remains a problem. Mosaicism and confined placental mosaicism(CPM) in CVS samples is not identified accurately by FISH. The American College of Medical Genetics does not recommend management on basis of result of FISH alone.

QF-PCR amplifies highly polymorphic short tandem repeats on chromosomes 13, 18, 21, X and Y using fluorescent primers and PCR. This method is comparable to FISH in sensitivity but maternal cell contamination is more easily identified. Hence it has replaced FISH for rapid aneuploidy screening in European countries.[30]

Newer technologies are being developed like the array-based comparative genome hybridization (aCGH). It has a high resolution, genome wide screening strategy for obtaining DNA copy number information in a single measurement. It is readily amendable to automation and is less labor intensive. But it's role in detection of submicroscopic chromosome imbalances is unclear. It fails to detect balanced chromosome rearrangements, alteration in ploidy levels like triploidy and tetraploidy, and mosaicism necessitating further diagnostic tests like karyotyping.[30] Role of aCGH in prenatal diagnosis needs further evaluation.

Chorionic Villus Sampling

This procedure is carried out between 10-13 weeks of gestation. It can be performed by transabdominal or transvaginal route. The indication of CVS is essentially the same as amniocentesis except for a few conditions which require either amniotic fluid or placental tissue for analysis.[3] The advantage of CVS is that the results are available earlier hence providing enough time for medical termination of pregnancy if needed. The complications of these two procedures are similar.

Transcervical Chorionic Villus Sampling

This procedure is performed using a polyethylene catheter of 5.7 F diameter and 27 cm length. The cervix and placenta are visualized by transabdominal sonography and the catheter is introduced through the cervix along the uterine wall to reach the placental tissue till it's distal end. The stylet is removed and 20 cc syringe containing 5 ml tissue culture fluid is attached to the catheter. Suction is applied as the catheter is gradually withdrawn.[32] This allows placental tissue aspiration into the syringe. If material obtained is inadequate then another two attempts are permitted with fresh catheters.[33] This route is rarely used because of higher miscarriage rate of 3.7% compared to midtrimester amniocentesis.[18]

Transabdominal Chorionic Villus Sampling

There are two techniques of transabdominal CVS. The two needle method recommended by Smidt Jensen and Hahnemann utilizes an outer needle as trocar to pierce the maternal skin, uterine myometrium and the placenta. A thinner needle is passed through it into the placental tissue. This technique allows reinsertion in case the tissue sample is inadequate and also prevents maternal contamination.[34]

The single needle technique proposed by Brambati[35] is the commonly preferred method for chorionic villus sampling. A 20 G spinal needle is inserted percutaneously into the placenta under sonographic vision. The stylet is removed and contents are aspirated into a 20 ml syringe containing 5 ml of media. The needle is moved backwards and forwards in the placental tissue for a few times to obtain adequate amount of tissue (Fig. 1.5).

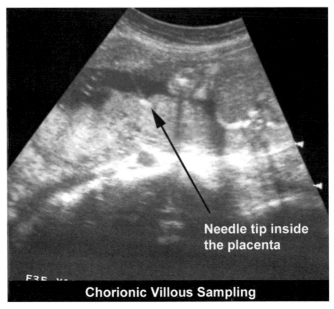

Figure 1.5: Chorionic villus sampling

The cytogenetic analysis is similar to amniocentesis. Chorionic villus has four different type of tissues—cytotrophoblast, mesenchyme, fetal blood vessels and fetal blood. Cytotrophoblast can be analysed by "rapid prep" between 24-48 hours because of presence of spontaneous mitosis in these cells. Mesenchymal cells need culturing and hence tissue analysis takes five to ten days time. But the result is more reliable. Sometimes there is a discrepancy between the placental and fetal tissue which could be either due to contamination by maternal cells or due to confined placental mosaicism. In confined placental mosaicism, the normal euploid chromosome is found along with abnormal cell line in the placental tissue, although the fetus may have normal karyotype. In such a situation amniocentesis is done to confirm fetal karyotype. Mosaicism is identified in 1% of CVS samples and the abnormal cell line is confirmed in 10-40% of these fetuses.[32] The complication of these procedures is vaginal spotting, bleeding or leakage of fluid which occurs in 7-10% of cases performed transvaginally and 1% of cases performed transabdominally. Miscarriage rate is 2.5%. Procedure related fetal malformations like limb reduction defects and oromandibular hypoplasia is seen if CVS is performed below 9 weeks hence early CVS has been abandoned now.[32]

Fetal Blood Sampling

1. Percutaneous umbilical blood sampling or cordocentesis.
2. Intrahepatic vessel sampling.
3. Fetal cardiac sampling.

Percutaneous Umbilical Blood Sampling or Cordocentesis

This procedure is done under real time ultrasonographic guidance. Pre-procedure antibiotics prophylaxis may be given and antenatal corticosteroid is administered in preterm fetuses 24 hours prior to the procedure. The free-hand technique of sampling uses a 20-22 G spinal needle of length around 15 cm to pierce the umbilical vein at relatively fixed segment of the cord near its insertion into the placenta. In this method the needle is free to move in all directions and hence the chances of injury to cord and other structures are more. In the other technique a fixed needle guide is attached to the ultrasound transducer through which a 22 to 25G needle is introduced. The predicted path of needle appears on screen and allows prior selection of sample site. Lateral movement of the needle is not possible.[36,37] The most accessible cord loop is selected for puncture. In both methods umbilical vein is punctured and the blood obtained is tested for its fetal origin. The acid dilution test of Londersloot distinguishes maternal from fetal blood. When fetal blood is added to 0.1 M potassium hydroxide it turns pink, while if maternal blood is added it turns brown. In addition the mean corpuscular volume of fetal blood can be measured which is larger than maternal RBC.[36] After confirming the fetal origin of blood the sample are put in tubes containing EDTA or heparin and sent for karyotyping. Postprocedure the puncture site is monitored for bleeding.

Fetal Intrahepatic Vessel Sampling

In this procedure intrahepatic vessels are sampled. This procedure is opted when cordocentesis is difficult to perform or is unsuccessful. It is rarely used nowadays. Fetal hepatic necrosis is a known complication.[38]

Fetal Cardiac Sampling

Fetal blood sampling by cardiac puncture is used when other methods fail to provide a sample. It is an easy procedure and is quite safe. This route can also be utilized for emergency fetal blood transfusion like in case of post procedural fetal bleed or for performing feticide.[38]

The results of karyotype analysis is available within a few days. Blood obtained from cordocentesis can also be analysed for fetal infection, fetal Rh D analysis, for assessment of fetal anemia and need for transfusion in Rh incompatibility, immunologic thrombocytopenias and coagulopathies.[37,38] The complications are cord vessel bleeding (50%), cord hematoma (17%), feto-maternal hemorrhage (66%), intrauterine death (1.4%).[3,37,38] Fetal loss is more when concurrent fetal pathology like growth restriction and hydrop fetalis is present.

Fetal Tissue Biopsy

Biopsy of fetal skin, liver and muscle is performed under sonographic or fetoscopic visualization. Tissue is analysed by electron microscopy or for biochemical analysis. Condition like muscular dystrophy, mitochondrial myopathy and skin disorders like epidermolysis bullosa can be diagnosed by this procedure.[3,38]

Fetoscopy

It is done through an endoscope which allows fetal inspection for structural anomalies and allows fetal blood sampling and tissue biopsy.

It is a technique of direct visualization of the fetus using a small bore fiberoptic endoscope. The trocar of the fetoscope measures 2.2 mm in diameter and the scope measures 1.7 mm in diameter.[16] In the first trimester embryofetoscopy, a 0.8 mm fiberoptic endoscope and a 27G needle are passed through a 16G double barrel instrument sheath. It is passed transabdominally into the extracelomic or amniotic cavity. Study of morphology of the embryo-fetus and fetal blood sampling are it's major clinical applications.[39] The drawback of fetoscopy is narrow field of vision and limited view of the small parts of the fetus because of short focal length. Scopes small enough to go through the shaft of a 20G needle have been developed but vision is hampered because of diminished intensity of light.[16]

Summary of Recommendations and Conclusions of ACOG Practice Bulletin No. 88 (2007)[40]

Invasive prenatal testing for aneuploidy

The following recommendation is based on good and consistent scientific evidence (Level A):
• Early amniocentesis (at less than 15 weeks of gestation) should not be performed because of the higher risk of pregnancy loss and complications compared with traditional amniocentesis (15 weeks of gestation or later).

The following conclusions are based on limited or inconsistent scientific evidence (Level B):
• Amniocentesis at 15 weeeks of gestation or later is safe procedure. The procedure-related loss rate after midtrimester amniocentesis is less than 1 in 300-500.
• In experienced individuals and centers, CVS procedure-related loss rates may be the same as those for amniocentesis.

The following recommendations and conclusions are based primarily on consensus and expert opinion (Level C):
• Invasive diagnostic testing for aneuploidy should be available to all women, regardless of maternal age.
• Patients with an increased risk of fetal aneuploidy include women with a previous fetus or child with an autosomal trisomy or sex chromosome abnormality, one major or at least two minor fetal structural defects

identified by ultrasonography, either parent with a chromosomal translocation or chromosomal inversion or parental aneuploidy.

• Nondirective counseling before prenatal diagnostic testing does not require a patient to commit to pregnancy termination if the result is abnormal.[39]

Preimplantation Diagnosis

It is a technique of diagnosing genetic abnormalities before the pregnancy is formally established. It has been used in couples who have an age-related risk of aneuploidies or who are carriers of balanced translocations. It has also been used for diagnosis of X-linked disorder or single gene disorder.[2,23]

Preimplantation diagnosis is done during *in vitro* fertilization procedures wherein the gametes or the cells from an embryo are biopsied for genetic analysis. The oocyte is tested indirectly by analyzing the first polar body. It is removed by micromanipulation technique and subjected to DNA analysis or chromosomal study. If the first polar body is tested abnormal then the oocyte is presumed to be normal and *vice versa*. The disadvantage of this procedure is that it is an indirect analysis and it can be used only for maternal carriers. Furthermore recombination will occur if defective gene lies away from the centromere making result indeterminate. Contamination with the cumulus cells can lead to error in diagnosis.

Sperm sorting techniques using molecular probes tagged with laser activated dye has been used followed by separation techniques like flow cytometry. But this method can cause considerable damage to the sperm.[16]

The most successful method of preimplantation diagnosis is biopsy of single cell from embryo at the eight cell stage or blastocyst stage. The eight cell stage embryo have independent cells and a single cell can be removed without damage to the neighboring cells because at this stage, cells do not develop gap junctions and are less adherent. But the drawback of this technique is that the cells are large hence difficult to remove, contamination can occur by sperm or cumulus cells and there is short time for analysis of results since successful implantation depends on early transfer of embryo.[16]

Blastomere biopsy is performed 5 days following fertilization at the 120 cell stage. It contains mainly trophoblastic cells but the inner cell mass that forms the embryo is clearly demarcated at this stage. The cells are biopsied after mechanical disruption of the zona or after spontaneous hatching. The advantages are that more number of cells are available for analysis and they are well-differentiated. The disadvantage is that there is increased risk of damage to the inner cell mass due to greater adherence of the cells to each other and there is limited incubation time. The trophoectoderm may not always be similar to the fetus in karyotype and biochemical status. The role of pre-implantation diagnosis at present is limited.[16]

- Prenatal screening procedures are non-invasive methods whereas the diagnostic procedures are usually invasive, except for the detection of fetal DNA and fetal cells which is a noninvasive diagnostic procedure. The ACOG 2007 and ACMG 2007 guidelines recommends screening for all pregnant women.
- The noninvasive prenatal screening procedures are a combination of maternal serum assays and fetal sonographic evaluation.
- The first trimester combined screening measures fetal nuchal translucency and maternal serum markers PAPP-A and β hCG and in association with maternal age provides a risk estimate for trisomy 18 and 21.
- The second trimester screening traditionally called the triple screening measures maternal serum alfa-fetoprotein, hCG, and unconjugated estriol and predicts relative risk of trisomy 18 and 21 in relation to the maternal age. Quadruple screening incorporates serum inhibin A levels in addition to the above three serum markers and has a better detection rate than triple screening.
- Combined first and second trimester screening has higher detection rate than individual screening. A positive result has to be confirmed by a diagnostic invasive procedure. If a pregnant woman presents early in pregnancy for antenatal care, that is before 14 weeks of gestation than integrated or sequential or contingent screening should be offered while if she presents after 14 weeks than a second trimester screening procedures should be recommended.
- Detection of fetal cells or DNA in maternal circulation can revolutionize the noninvasive methods of prenatal diagnosis but is still in the infancy stage.
- Invasive methods of prenatal diagnosis like chorionic villus sampling, amniocentesis, percutaneous umbilical blood sampling, etc. provide embryonic or extraembryonic tissue for chromosomal, genetic, or biochemical analysis. The techniques used for analysis of fetal material are PCR, FISH, aCGH or karyotyping of cultured fetal cells. Mutation study on DNA and biochemical analysis is also possible. While rapid aneuploidy tests like FISH and QF-PCR provide an early report, they have higher rate of false-positive and negative results. Traditional karyotyping gives more accurate results.
- Preimplantation diagnosis is an invasive method of diagnosis of fetal disease before the formal establishment of pregnancy. Hence it offers a choice to differentiate the healthy embryos from unhealthy ones and pick up the healthy embryos for embryo transfer.

Management of High-Risk Pregnancy—A Practical Approach

REFERENCES

1. Verma IC. Burden of genetic disorder in India. Indian J Pediatr 2000;67(12):893-98.
2. Goldman IC, Melon E. Advances in prenatal diagnosis. Appl Radiol 2005;34(9):8-18.
3. Cunningham GF, Gant FN, Levino KJ, Gillstrap LC, Hauth GC, Welstrom KD (Eds). Prenatal diagnosis and fetal therapy. In: William's Obstetrics. 22nd edn. Mcgraw Hill 2005;313-39.
4. ACOG Practice Bulletin No.77 Screening for Fetal Chromosomal Abnormalities Obstetrics and Gynecology 2007;109(1):217-26.
5. Palomaki GE, Lee J, Canick JA, et al. American College of Medical Genetics (ACMG). Laboratory Quality Assurance Committee: Technical standards and guidelines, 2007.
6. Melon FD. Sonographic and first trimester detection of aneuploidy. Queenan JT, Hopkins JC, Spong CY (Eds). In: Protocol for High Risk Pregnancy. 4th edn: Blackwell publishing, 2005; 75-88.
7. Nicolaides KH. Nuchal translucency and other first trimester sonographic markers of chromosomal abnormalities. Am J Obstet Gynecol 2004;191:45-67.
8. Said S, Malone FD. The use of Nuchal translucency in contemporary obstetric practice. Clinical Obstetrics and Gynaecology 2008;51(1):37-47.
9. Robyr R, Ville Y. First- Trimester Screening for Fetal Abnormalities. James DK, Weiner CP, Steer PJ, Gonik B (Eds). In: High Risk Pregnancy—Management Options. 3rd edn. Elsiever 2006;138-56.
10. Holmgreen C, Lacoursiere DY. The use of prenatal ultrasound in the detection of fetal aneuploidy. Clinical Obstetrics and gynaecology 2008;51(1):48-61.
11. Bekker M, Twist J, Vugt J. Reproducibility of fetal nasal bone length measurement. J Ultrasound Med 2004;23:1613-18.
12. Wapner R, Thom E, Simpson JL. First trimester screening of trisomy 21 and 18. N Engl J Med 2003;349:1405-13.
13. Malone F, Wald J, Canick J, et al. First and second trimester evaluation of risk (FASTER) trial principle result of the NICHD multicentric Down syndrome screening study. Am J Obstet Gynecol 2003;189:S56.
14. Spencer K, Spencer CE, Power M, et al. Screening for chromosomal abnormalities in the first trimester using ultrasound and maternal serum biochemistry in a one- stop clinic: A review of three years prospective experience. Br J Obstet Gynaecol 2003;110:281-86.
15. Wald NJ, Rodeck C, Hackshaw AK, et al. First and second trimester antenatal screening for Down syndrome: The result of Serum, Urine, Ultrasound screening study (SURUSS). J Med Screen 2003;10:56-104.
16. Ward K. Genetics and Prenatal diognosis. Scott JR, Gibbs RS, Karlan BY, Haney AF (Eds). In: Danforth's obstetrics and gynaecology. 9th edn. Lippincott Williams and Wilkins, 2003;105-28.
17. Yeo L, Vintzileous AM. Second trimester screening for fetal abnormalities. James PK, Weiner CP, Steer PJ, Gonik B (Eds). In: High Risk Pregnancy—Management Options. 3 edn. Elseiver 2006;157-89.
18. Wimalasundera RC. Fetal medicine in clinical practice. Edmonds KD (Ed). In: Dewhurst's Textbook of Obstetrics and Gynaecology. 7th edn. Blackwell publishing, 2007;132-44.
19. Saller DN, Canick JA. Current methods of prenatal screening for Down syndrome and other fetal abnormalities. Clinical Obstetrics and Gynaecology 2008;51(4):24-36.
20. Nicolaides KH, Snijders RJ, Gosden C, et al. Ultrasonographically detectable markers of fetal chromosomal abnormalities. Lancet 1992;340:704-07.
21. Malone FD, D'Alton ME. First trimester sonographic screening for Down syndrome. Obstet Gynecol 2003;102 (5pt1):1066-79.
22. Xian-hu F, Han-ping C. Advances on circulating fetal DNA in maternal plasma.Chin Med J 2007;120(14):1256-59.
23. Kumar S. Prenatal diagnosis and genetics. Edmonds KD (Ed). In: Dewhurst's Textbook of Obstetrics and Gynaecology. 7th edn. Blackwell Publishing 2007;125-31.
24. Yang I, Park IY, Jang SM, et al. Rapid quantification of DNA methylation through dNMP analysis following bisulfite-PCR. Nucleic Acids Research 2006;34:78.
25. Ogino S, Kawasaki T, Brahmandam M, et al. Precision and performance characteristics of bisulfite conversion real-time PCR (Methylight) For Quantitative DNA methylation analysis JMD 2006;8:209-17.

1

26. Perni CS, Chervenak FA. Amniocentesis. Apuzzio JJ, Vintzeleous AM, Iffy L. Taylor Francis (Eds). In: Operative Obstetrics 3edn 2006;57-63.
27. The Canadian Early and Midtrimester Amniocentesis Trial Group (CEMAT). Randomised trial to assess safety and fetal outcome of early and midtrimester amniocentesis. Lancet 1998;351:242-47.
28. Winsor EJF, Tomkins DJ, Kalousek D, et al. Cytogenetic aspects of The Canadian Early and Midtrimester Amniocentesis Trial (CEMAT). Prenat Diagn1999;19:629-37.
29. Johnson JM, Wilson RD, Singer J, et al. Technical factors in amniocentesis predict worse outcome. Results of the Canadian Early and Midtrimester Amniocentesis Trial (CEMAT) Prenat Diagn 1999;19:732-38.
30. South ST, Chen Z, Brothman AR. Genomic medicine in prenatal diagnosis. Clinical Obstetrics and Gynaecology 2008;51(1):62-73.
31. Leung WC, Lau ET, Lau WL, et al. Rapid aneuploidy testing (knowing less) versus traditional karyotyping (knowing more) for advanced maternal age: What would be missed, who should decide? Hong Kong Med J 2008;14:6-13.
32. Wapner RJ. Chorionic villus sampling. Queenan JT, Hopkins JC, Spong CY (Eds). In: Protocol for High Risk Pregnancy. 4th edn. Blackwell Publishing, 2005:119-24.
33. Trauffer PML, Silverman NS, Wapner RJ. Chorionic Villus Sampling. Apuzzio JJ, Vintzeleous AM, Iffy L (Eds). In: Operative Obstetrics. 3rd edn. Taylor Francis 2006;41-45.
34. Smidt Jensen S, Hahnemann N, Jensen PU, et al. Experience with the needle biopsy in first trimester-An alternative to amniocentesis. Clin Genet 1994;26;272.
35. Brambati B, Oldrini A, Lanzati A. Transabdominal chorionic villus sampling: A free hand ultrasound guided technique. Am J Obstet Gynecol 1987;157:134.
36. Ghidini A, Locatelli A. Fetal blood sampling. Queenan JT, Hopkins JC, Spong CY (Eds). In: Protocol for high risk pregnancy. 4th edn. Blackwell Publishing 2005:134-39.
37. Weiner CP. Cordocentesis. Apuzzio JJ, Vintzeleous AM, Iffy L (Eds). In: Operative Obstetrics. 3edn. Taylor Francis 2006;121-35.
38. Hunter A, Soothill P. Invasive procedure for antenatal diagnosis. James PK, Weiner CP, Steer PJ, Gonik B (Eds). In: High Risk Pregnancy—Management Options. 3rd edn. Elseiver 2006;209-24.
39. Reece EA, Vintzileous AM. First trimester embryofetoscopy. Apuzzio JJ, Vintzeleous AM, Iffy L (Eds). In: Operative Obstetrics. 3rd edn. Taylor Francis 2006;33-39.
40. ACOG Practice Bulletin No. 88. Invasive Prenatal Testing for Aneuploidy Obstetrics and Gynecology. 2007;110(6):1459-67.

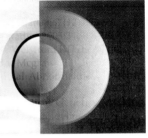

Screening and Management of Congenital Anomalies

2

Manisha

INTRODUCTION

An expecting mother always expects a normal child at birth, however 15% of conceptuses abort spontaneously, 1% are stillborn, 3% of neonates have a major congenital malformation, about 10% have minor defects and 0.7% of neonates have multiple congenital malformations. Cardiovascular defects are the most common birth defects with an incidence of 10/1000 births. Central nervous system defects are also common and seen in 8-10/1000 births. Gastrointestinal and renal anomalies are seen in 4/1000 births each. The causes of congenital malformation are genetic in 30-40% cases and environmental in 5-10% cases. The cause remains unknown in 50% cases. Among genetic causes, the cause could be multifactorial, chromosomal defect or single gene disorder.

PRENATAL SCREENING

Majority of birth defects occur in families with no prior history of birth defect. Prenatal diagnosis for only high-risk women fails to recognize most of the affected fetuses. Therefore antenatal screening tests are done to identify women at risk.

First Trimester Screening

Ultrasonography (USG)

Most fetal structures can be visualized at 12-13 weeks and this gestation age offers earliest opportunity to screen for fetal anomaly.

Objectives of First Trimester Screening

- *Identification of Viable Pregnancy:* Chances of miscarriage are around 2% after 14 weeks if a viable pregnancy is identified at this stage.[1]
- *Dating:* Gestational sac is always visible by 5 weeks by transvaginal sonography. Fetal heart is present by 7 weeks. Gestational age should not be altered if discrepancy between the last menstrual period and crown rump length (CRL) measurement is less than 7 days.
- *Detecting multiple pregnancy and determining chorionicity:* Twin pregnancy comprises 2% of all pregnancies. The first trimester is the best time to determine chorionicity. Characteristic USG finding in dichorionic twin is lambda sign.[2] In monochorionic twin pregnancy there is no layer of chorion between the two layers of amnion therefore the lambda sign is absent (Fig. 2.1).
- *Assessment of General Fetal Anatomy*

Central nervous system: From 9 weeks onwards the falx, lateral ventricles, and echogenic choroid plexus are visible (Fig. 2.2). From 14 weeks cerebellum

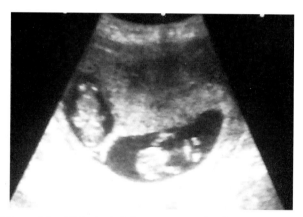

Figure 2.1: Dichorionic twin pregnancy showing lambda sign

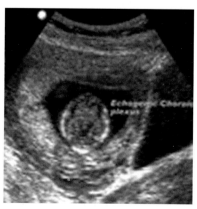

Figure 2.2: Transcerebral view showing echogenic choroid plexus and falx in 12 week fetus

and thalami are seen. Choroid plexus cysts, if present in isolation are not known to be associated with fetal chromosomal anomalies.[2]

Heart: The position, axis and four chamber view can be appreciated at 12 to 14 weeks. Women with increased nuchal translucency are at increased risk for cardiac anomaly.[3] Hypoplastic left heart can be diagnosed in the 1st trimester.

Stomach: Stomach bubble can be seen in all cases by 12-13 weeks.

Abdominal wall: Physiologic hernia of midgut into umbilical cord is a normal feature in early pregnancy but is not normal after 12 weeks.

Kidneys and bladder: In sagittal section the long axis of bladder is less than 6 mm in the 1st trimester. Kidneys appear as echogenic structure in the 1st trimester.

Skeleton: All long bones are similar in size at 11-14 weeks, ranging from 6 mm at 11 weeks to 13 mm at 14 weeks. Lethal defects can be diagnosed in the 1st trimester (Fig. 2.3).

Nuchal translucency (NT): It is the USG visualization of physiologic collection of fluid in the skin behind the fetal neck at 11-14 weeks (Fig. 2.4). Nuchal

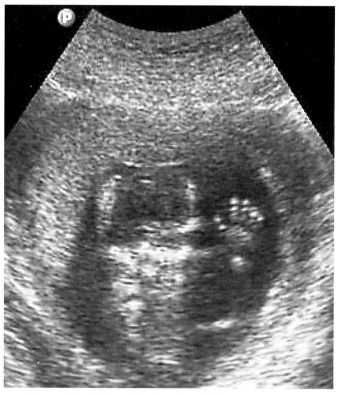

Figure 2.3: All five digits clearly visible in 12 weeks fetus

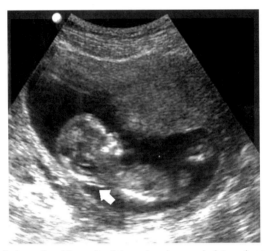

Figure 2.4: Saggital view of a 12 weeks fetus, showing nuchal translucency and nasal bone

thickness normally increases with CRL.[4] It is important to consider gestational age while deciding whether nuchal translucency is normal or increased. The chance of cardiac defects increases with increase in NT (see Chapter 1 for details of NT measurement).

Fetal nasal bone: Nasal bone is not visualized on USG between 11 to 14 weeks in 60% of fetuses with trisomy 21 and in only 3% of chromosomally normal fetus.[6]

Three Dimensional USG

It has the advantage of minimizing the actual scanning time for diagnosing anomalies in the first trimester. As it is easy to get the sagittal view, therefore NT can be measured easily.

Second Trimester Screening

Biochemical Screening

Maternal serum alpha fetoprotein for neural tube defects (NTD)
It was recognized in 1972 that in many pregnancies the open neural tube defects could be detected at 16 weeks gestation by assay of a protein in maternal serum known as α fetoprotein (AFP). The AFP is the fetal equivalent of albumin and is the major protein in fetal blood. If the fetus has an open NTD, the level of AFP is elevated in both amniotic fluid and maternal serum as a result of leakage from the open defect.

Unfortunately, maternal serum AFP is neither 100% sensitive nor specific. The curves for the levels of AFP in normal and affected pregnancies overlap so. that in practice an arbitrary cut off level is introduced below which no further action needs to be taken. This is usually either 95th centile or 2.5

Table 2.1: Conditions other than NTD associated with increased levels of AFP	
Multifetal gestation	Abdominal wall defects
Oligohydramnios	Underestimated gestational age
Chorioangioma of placenta	Urinary obstruction
Renal anomalies – polycystic kidney	Cystic hygroma
Sacrococcygeal teratoma	Chromosomal trisomies
Fetal death	
Conditions associated with decreased levels of AFP	
Gestational trophoblastic disease	
Increased maternal weight	

multiples of median and as a result 75% of screened open spina bifida cases are detected. The pregnant women with AFP level above this arbitrary cut off levels are offered detailed ultrasonography. AFP levels might be raised in conditions other than NTD; which are enumerated in Table 2.1.

Despite these limitations prenatal maternal serum AFP screening has been implemented widely and is one of the main factors which has led to striking decline in incidence of open NTD.

Second Trimester USG Scan

The sensitivity and detection of the anomaly depends upon the skill of the observer and the gestational age at the time of scan as many abnormalities appears later in the gestational age and some disappear with advancing gestation. In the low-risk women the USG helps in excluding anomaly and detecting normal features. Genetic sonography is offered to high-risk women and has a sensitivity of 50 to 93%. The examination starts with the examination of fetal head.

Intracranial Anatomy
1. *Transthalamic view*: Biparietal diameter is taken at this level, measured from outer margin to inner margin. Head circumference is measured at the outer margin. Observation about mineralization is made whether adequate or not, and about the shape whether elliptical or otherwise. Cavum septum pellucidum is seen in the midline anteriorly. Cerebral ventricle is measured through the atrium in axial plane, it is normally < 10 cm.
2. *Transcerebellar view*: Cerebellum is visualized and measured, its measurement is not affected by fetal growth restriction and can be used to assess the exact gestational age. Cisterna magna is seen behind the cerebellum (Fig. 2.5).

Nuchal fold: It is the skin thickness in the posterior aspect of fetal neck. A nuchal fold is measured in transverse section of fetal head at the level of

Screening and Management of Congenital Anomalies

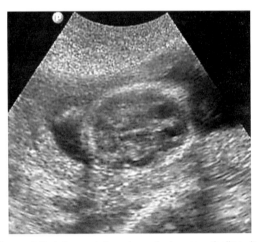
Figure 2.5: Intracranial anatomy in transcerebellar view

cavum septum pellucidum and thalami and angled posterior to include the cerebellum. The measurement is taken from outer edge of occipital bone to outer skin limit directly in the midline. The nuchal fold thickness more than 6 mm be considered significant between 18-24 weeks and a measurement of more than 5 mm considered significant at 16-18 weeks. A thickened nuchal fold should be distinguished from cystic hygroma in which the skin in this area is filled with fluid-filled locculations. A thickened nuchal fold should not be confused with nuchal translucency which is specific measurement of fluid in the posterior aspect of neck at 11 to 14 weeks of gestation. Increased nuchal fold thickness signifies increased risk of aneuploidy, single gene disorders and congenital cardiac defects in the fetus.

Face: It is important in the diagnosis of genetic disorders and syndromes. Important structures visualized are the orbits, its diameter and distance between them, nose, lips, palate, chin and the ears (Figs 2.6 and 2.7).

Spine: It is imaged in coronal, transverse and sagittal views. In transverse view, the vertebral segment normally consists of 3 echogenic ossification centers, two posterolateral and one in midline anteriorly. Normally they lie in symmetrical triangular configuration. Splaying of these ossification centers indicate neural tube defects.

Heart: Cardiac rate and rhythm is observed in M mode. The size of heart normally is one-third of fetal thorax. The axis of heart is said to be normal if the apex points towards left with angle of $45 \pm 20°$ to midline (Fig. 2.8). Demonstration of four chamber view allows detection of 40% of congenital heart defects and with visualization of outflow tracts the anomaly detection rate reaches 70%. Echogenic focus if seen in the ventricle is a soft marker for detection of Down syndrome. Doppler sonography assists in visualization and confirmation of heart abnormality. Indications for fetal echocardiography are enumerated in Table 2.2.

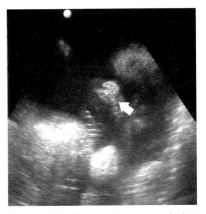

Figure 2.6: Showing the coronal view of face, upper lip appears as curved line

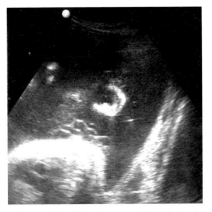

Figure 2.7: Showing ear of the fetus in sagittal view

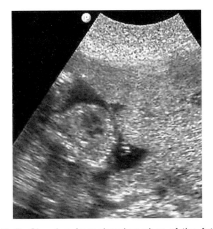

Figure 2. 8: Showing four chamber view of the fetal heart

Table 2.2: Indications for fetal echocardiography

Indications for fetal echocardiography are:

- Family history of congenital heart disease
- Maternal diabetes
- Maternal drug exposure or infections during pregnancy
- Maternal systemic lupus erythematosus
- Maternal phenylketonuria
- Polyhydramnios
- Nonimmune hydrops
- Fetal dysarrhythmia
- Fetal extracardiac abnormalities
- Fetal chromosomal abnormalities
- Symmetrical intrauterine growth restriction

Echogenic intracardiac focus (ECIF): It is defined as focus of echogenecity comparable to bone in the region of papillary muscle in either or both ventricles of the fetal heart. Studies suggest that the less frequent right sided, biventricular or particularly conspicuous echogenic intracardiac focus are associated with higher risk of fetal aneuploidy.

Abdomen: Abdominal circumference is measured at the transverse level where the umbilical vein joins the portal vein. It is the most sensitive indicator of intrauterine growth restriction. Stomach bubble is visualized in the transverse plane, located to the left above the diaphragm (Fig. 2.9). Normally bowel appears as midlevel echogenecity filling the abdomen.

Genitourinary tract: Kidneys are bilaterally hypoechoic paraspinal structures. Renal pelvis is measured in anteroposterior diameter. Abnormal findings are presence of cysts and dilatation of calyces. Doppler imaging is useful in identifying the renal artery especially when kidneys cannot be visualized on USG. Gender is assigned by the visualization of genitalia and not by lack of the image.

Fetal extremity: Survey of all long bones provides diagnostic information. Digits are visualized and counted in extension. Movement and tone of the extremities is observed. Absence, fractures, contractures and bowing of long bones is abnormal (Fig. 2.10).

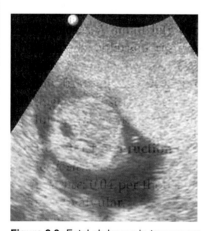

Figure 2.9: Fetal abdomen in transverse plane showing stomach bubble

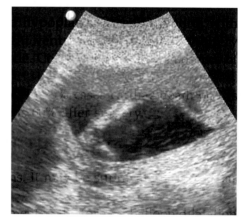

Figure 2.10: The longitudinal scan of normal leg and foot showing two bones and heel indicating there is no tallipes

INDIVIDUAL CONGENITAL MALFORMATIONS

CARDIAC DEFECTS

A. Fetal Cardiac Arrhythmia

Normal fetal heart rate is 100-160/min. Frequency of arrhythmia is 1-3% of all pregnancies.[7] Tachycardia is twice more common than bradycardia.

Maternal causes of arrhythmia are connective tissue disease, drugs, hyperthyroidism, infections and heritable diseases such as prolonged QT interval syndrome and tuberous sclerosis. The fetal causes leading to arrhythmia are hydrops fetalis, fetal compromise and structural cardiac disease.

Fetal echocardiography and Doppler are indicated to rule out structural cardiac disease.

Irregular heart rate
- *Premature atrial contractions*: It is the most common cause of dysrhythmia. It generally requires no treatment. Patient is asked to avoid caffeine. Investigations regarding illicit drug use, hyperthyroidism should be done.
- *Premature ventricular contractions*: This also does not require any treatment.

Tachycardia
It is diagnosed when the fetal heart beat is >160/minute.
- *Supraventricular tachycardia*: It is the most common cause of fetal tachycardia. Supraventricular tachycardia is diagnosed if there is 1:1 atrioventricular conduction. As it is difficult to predict which fetus with tachycardia will eventually develop hydrops most centers initiate treatment as soon as the diagnosis of fetal tachycardia is established.[8]

  The primary form of pharmacological intervention is maternal transplacental therapy. Other routes of treatment are intravascular and intramuscular treatment of fetus, which is mainly used in refractory cases. Digoxin is the most common drug used to treat fetal tachycardia.[8] Transplacental digoxin has been found to be effective in treating SVT complicated by fetal hydrops in a small percentage, but there has been no consensus regarding antiarrhythmic treatment if digoxin therapy fails. Flecainide and amiodarone both have been used with varying success.[9]
- *Atrial flutter*: It is associated with atrial rates 400-450 beats per minute. Most common form is 2:1 AV block. Structural heart defect is ruled out in all cases. Common structural defects causing flutter are Ebstein anomaly, atrial septal defect; hypoplastic left heart syndrome and cardiomyopathy.

Bradycardia: Fetal bradycardia is defined as persistent heart rate below 100 beats per minute not associated with uterine contractions or periodic decelerations. Bradycardia once detected, extrinsic causes are ruled out. These are drugs, maternal hypothermia and cord compression. Type of bradycardia is determined whether it is sinus bradycardia or partial or complete AV block. Maternal testing for connective tissue disorders, screening for anti-Ro, anti-La antibodies is done. Family history of arrhythmia or structural cardiac defect is also inquired.

B. Structural Cardiac Defects

Cardiac malformations are the most common birth defect. Incidence of structural cardiac defects is 4-5 per 1000 live births. It can be present in the form of septal defects, outflow tract obstruction or conotruncal malformation.

Septal defects

- *Atrial septal defect (ASD)*

  Incidence: 1 per 1000 live births.

  Diagnosis: Demonstration of either the absence or reduction in the dimension of foramen ovale flap.

  Prognosis: ASD does not impair cardiac function in utero. Associated defects, chromosomal abnormality or syndrome may be present and has to be ruled out.

- *Ventricular septal defect*

  Incidence: 2.5 per 1000 live births.

  Diagnosis: Classified by the location of septum, may be perimembranous, inlet, trabecular and outlet VSD. Diagnosis is made only when demonstrated while the USG beam is perpendicular to the septum.

  Prognosis: It is good but the extracardiac anomaly and karyotypic abnormality has to be ruled out.

- *Hypoplastic left ventricle*

  Incidence: 0.16 per 1000 live births.

  Diagnosis: A small left ventricle and hypoplastic ascending aorta with relatively enlarged right atrium, right ventricle and pulmonary artery point towards hypoplastic left ventricle. Color Doppler shows absence of flow from left atrium to ventricle.

  Prognosis: Postnatal prognosis is poor. In 25% cases cardiac death occurs during 1st week of life. Survival rate is 60% after surgery.

Outflow tract obstruction

- *Aortic stenosis*

  Incidence: 0.04 per thousand live births. It may be supravalvular, valvular or subvalvular.

  Prognosis and treatment: In utero treatment in the form of balloon dilatation of stenotic aortic valve by transverse puncture has been tried with technical success.[10] None of the babies survived past neonatal period.

- *Coarctation of aorta*

  There is narrowing of the portion of ascending aorta between subclavian artery and ductus arteriosus. Echocardiographic findings are an enlarged right ventricle and hypoplastic aortic arch.

  Incidence: 0.18 per 1000 live births. It is frequently associated with other cardiac anomalies such as VSD (in 90% cases), aortic stenosis, and transposition of great vessels. Extracardiac anomalies are also common.

Prognosis: There is no significant impact on intrauterine hemodynamics. Surgery is required after birth.

- *Pulmonary stenosis*
  Incidence: 0.9 per 1000 live births.
  Associated anomalies are ASD, Noonan syndrome and tricuspid regurgitation.
  Prognosis is good. Postnatal balloon valvoplasty is required.

Conotruncal malformation

These anomalies are commonly missed when the routine USG of heart only involves the 4 chamber view. It includes malformations like:

- Transposition of great vessels
- Tetralogy of Fallot
- Double outlet right ventricle
- Truncus arteriosus.
- *Transposition of great vessels*
  Incidence: 0.2 per 1000 live births.
  Prognosis: Rarely associated with other cardiac malformations or abnormal karyotype. In utero the fetus shows no signs of compromise but becomes cyanotic at birth and deteriorates rapidly. Survival after neonatal surgery is 85-90%.
- *Tetralogy of Fallot*
  It includes stenosis of pulmonary artery, ventricular septal defect, overriding of aorta and hypertrophy of right ventricle.
  Incidence: It is 0.4 per 1000 live births.
  Prognosis: Other cardiac defects should be ruled out. Karyotypic abnormalities are common. Survival rate after corrective surgery is 95%.

HEAD, NECK AND SPINE

A. Open Neural Tube Defect

Neural tube defect comprises of anencephaly, spina bifida and encephalocele.

Incidence: The incidence of neural tube defect is 4/1000 live births. They are most commonly multifactorial but can occur as a Mendelian syndrome, chromosomal abnormality or might result from teratogenic exposure. Only 5% of the children with NTD are born in the families with other affected members. So screening is required for all pregnant women.

Anencephaly

Diagnosis: Can be made as early as 10 weeks. It is diagnosed by ultrasound finding of absence of calvarium.

Prognosis: Pregnancy can be terminated after diagnosis at any period of gestation as it is lethal.

Encephalocele

Prognosis: Additional congenital anomalies are present in 50-65% of cases. Mortality rate is high, only 50% survive after surgery. Prognosis is better if encephalocele is frontal, microcephaly secondary to brain herniation shows poor prognosis (Fig. 2.11).

Spina Bifida

Diagnosis: It appears on USG as splaying of the posterior ossification centers (Fig. 2.12). The intracranial signs which aid in diagnosis are:
* Frontal notching (Lemon Sign) (Fig. 2.13)
* Ventriculomegaly (> 10 mm)
* Obliteration of cisterna magna

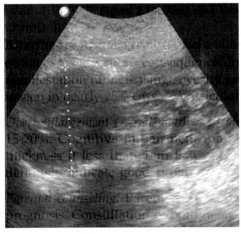

Figure 2.11: Transcerebral view showing microcephaly with encephalocele

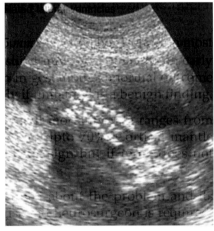

Figure 2.12: Showing splaying of lateral vertebral lamina in coronal view suggesting spina bifida

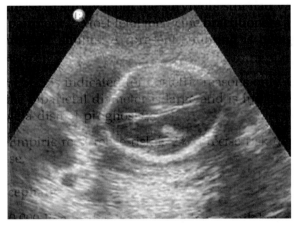

Figure 2.13: Transcerebral view showing 'lemon sign', ventriculomegaly and dangling choroid plexus

- Small BPD
- Banana sign (banana sign disappears after 24 weeks).

Ninety nine percent of fetuses with NTD have one of the above-mentioned 5 specific cranial abnormalities.

Prognosis: The entire anatomical survey should be done to exclude other anomalies; ventriculomegaly is present in majority of them. Fetal karyotype is recommended in all instances.

Prognosis depends upon the extent of defect. Lower extremity paralysis and incontinence of bowel and bladder are common. 75% of the fetuses have a long-term survival.[11] Neurologic state varies from normal to severe disability, late deterioration is common. On the whole about 75% will have mild to severe paralysis with only 17% having normal continence on late follow up.

It is difficult to predict the prognosis in the first half of pregnancy, option for termination is to be given if diagnosis is made before 20 weeks.

In utero treatment: The in utero closure of spinal defect has been tried on experimental basis.[12] If the diagnosis is made after viability, monitoring of fetal growth, head size and enlargement of ventricles is noted. Delivery is done at term. There is no clear evidence that the lower segment cesarean section (LSCS) improves the outcome thus LSCS for fetal indication is avoided.

Examination of fetus after delivery is advised.

Recurrence risk: The risk in the next pregnancy is 4% if it is due to a multifactorial cause. If it occurs as a part of genetic syndrome it depends upon the mode of inheritance of the syndrome associated, for example there is 25% recurrence risk in Meckle Grubber syndrome and Robert syndrome both of which show autosomal recessive inheritance.

Periconceptional administration of folic acid after birth of one affected child can reduce recurrence of the disease in the next baby in up to 70% cases.

B. Hydrocephalous

Diagnosis: It is a pathological increase in CSF usually within the lateral ventricles. The mean value of atrial diameter is 7 mm; it remains constant from 14 -38 weeks. Hydrocephalous is diagnosed when the atrial diameter is >10 mm. Choroid plexus appears as a dangling structure as it assumes a dependent posture (Fig. 2.14).

Prognosis: If hydrocephalous is detected, general structural survey to look for other anomaly is done as other abnormalities are associated in 90% of the cases. Fetal echocardiography is advised and possible causes need to be investigated. Amniocentesis for karyotyping is done as abnormal karyotype may be associated in up to 10% of the affected fetus. Pregnancy termination is offered if diagnosis is made before viability. If pregnancy is continued serial ultrasound to identify progressive ventricular enlargement is done.

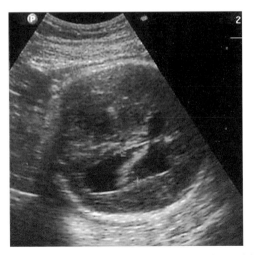

Figure 2.14: Axial scan showing dilated lateral ventricles

Borderline ventriculomegaly (Atrial width 10-15 mm): Isolated borderline–In most of the cases it is of no consequence. In a distinct minority it may be an early manifestation of increasing severity later on in gestation. Abnormal outcome is seen in nearly 25% cases. Ventriculomegaly if unilateral is a benign finding.

Overt enlargement (Atrial width > 15 mm): Overall mortality rate ranges from 15-70%. Cognitive impairment may be seen in upto 70%. Cortical mantle thickness if less than 1cm is a poor prognostic sign but if more does not definitely indicate good prognosis.

Parental counseling: Parents need to be informed about the problem and its prognosis. Consultation of both neonatologist and neurosurgeon is required. If the abnormality is detected before viability, option for termination should be offered.

In utero treatment: In utero placement of shunt did not yield encouraging results as there was increase in survival but the survivors still had varying degree of neurological impairment.[13] Most fetal medicine practitioners are not routinely placing intra-amniotic shunts. At present shunting is being done only on experimental basis.[14]

Mode of delivery: LSCS is indicated for obstetric reasons only. Cephalocentesis can be done if the biparietal diameter is large and is indicated only in those cases which have a dismal prognosis.

Recurrence risk: Empiric recurrence risk is 2%. Precise risk depends upon the underlying cause.

C. Holoprosencephaly

Incidence: 1 in 10,000 live births. It can be alobar, semilobar and lobar. These categories are based on degree of separation of cerebral hemispheres. Alobar is most severe with no evidence of cerebrocortical division. On ultrasound examination falx cerebri and interhemispheric fissure is absent and the thalami appear fused. Examination of face is necessary whenever we suspect holoprosencephaly.

Prognosis: Prognosis is uniformly poor. Most die shortly after birth. Survivors have profound mental retardation.[15] Karyotyping should be offered. Maternal diabetes is to be ruled out. A close look at the parents for minor signs should be done as it can be familial with autosomal recessive or dominant inheritance.

Labor and delivery: Option for termination before viability should be given. Macrocephaly may obstruct labor and cephalocentesis can be done.

Recurrence risk: In the absence of chromosomal abnormality empiric recurrence risk is 6-14%.

D. Facial Cleft

Careful search for other anomalies is done if facial cleft is suspected. Fetal karyotype should be offered.

Prognosis: It depends upon presence of associated anomalies and the severity of the defect. Prior to surgery there is difficulty in feeding. Diagnosis of cleft lip helps parents to prepare for a visibly disturbing deformity which is correctable.

E. Dandy-Walker Malformation

Incidence: 1in 30, 000 live births.

Diagnosis: It is characterized by complete or partial absence of cerebellar vermis with enlarged posterior fossa cyst (Fig. 2.15). There is associated

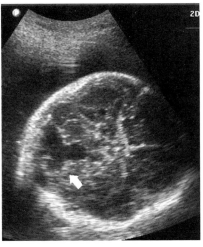

Figure 2.15: Showing Dandy-Walker syndrome with a large posterior fossa cyst and widely separated cerebellar hemispheres

hydrocephalus. In Dandy-Walker variant there is variable hypoplasia of cerebellar vermis with or without enlargement of posterior fossa. After diagnosis is made, we must look for other anomalies, which are seen in up to 85% of cases. There is increased risk of chromosomal abnormality also.

Prognosis: Prognosis is not good, especially when associated with other anomalies. Autosomal recessive inheritance is also seen. Recurrence risk in the absence of chromosomal anomaly is 1-5%.

F. Cystic Hygroma

Diagnosis: They appear as simple loculated fluid-filled cavities located postero-laterally in neck region. It is often associated with hydrops. Therefore whenever cystic hygroma is detected careful search for fluid accumulation in other cavities is noted. Fetal karyotype is essential (Figs 2.16 and 2.17).

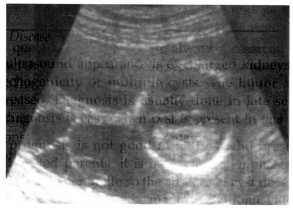

Figure 2.16: Axial scan at the level of BPD shows soft tissue swelling behind the neck with septae suggestive of cystic hygroma

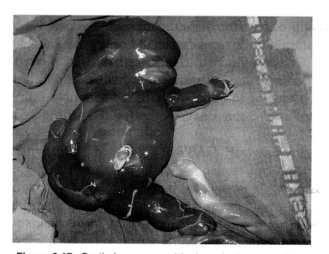

Figure 2.17: Cystic hygroma and hydrops in the same fetus

Prognosis: It depends upon associated anomalies. Prognosis is poor when there is associated hydrops. Careful postmortem examination is required.

GENITOURINARY SYSTEM

A. Kidney Abnormalities

Renal Agenesis

Bilateral renal agenesis is found in 1in 5000 live births and unilateral agenesis is seen in 1in 2000 live births. It is usually sporadic in occurrence but may be associated with chromosomal abnormality or with some syndrome like Fraser syndrome.

Diagnosis: The condition is suspected by presence of oligohydramnios and nonvisualization of kidneys on ultrasound usually around 16-18 weeks. Failure to visualize renal arteries on Doppler is another important clue.

Prognosis: Bilateral renal agenesis is lethal however unilateral agenesis has good prognosis. Oligohydramnios leads to pulmonary hypoplasia.

Recurrence risk: In nonsyndromic cases the risk of recurrence is 3%.

Multicystic Dysplasia

Incidence: 1 in 1000 live births.

Diagnosis: Appears antenatally as kidneys that have lost the normal shape and appears as collection of cysts that are of variable size (0.5-3 cm) not connected to the urinary tract (Figs 2.18 and 2.19). It is usually a sporadic abnormality but chromosomal defect or other abnormality may be associated in 50% cases.

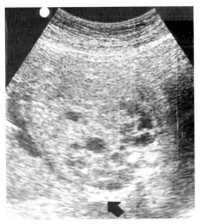

Figure 2.18: Transverse scan of the fetus with multicystic kidney disease involving right and left kidneys (RK & LK). Note the multiple cystic structures (C)

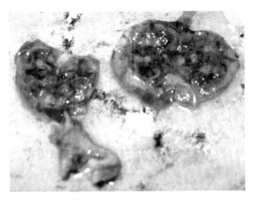

Figure 2.19: Bilateral multicystic kidney at autopsy

Screening and Management of Congenital Anomalies

Prognosis: It is good when unilateral but is uniformly bad in bilateral affection and when associated oligohydramnios is present.

Infantile Polycystic Kidney Disease (IPKD)

Diagnosis: It appears as bilaterally enlarged, homogenously hyperechoic kidneys that retain their shape. There is often associated oligohydramnios. The dilated cysts are dilated collecting ducts. The liver is always involved with portal fibrosis and proliferation of bile ducts.

Prognosis: The prognosis depends upon clinical variety of disease. The perinatal type has severe renal involvement and leads to stillbirth. The gene of IPKD has been mapped. Fetal blood can be saved for genetic analysis (Figs 2.20 and 2.21).

Recurrence risk: Since the disease is autosomal recessive the risk of recurrence is 25%.

Adult Polycystic Disease

Diagnosis: The ultrasound appearance is of enlarged kidneys with increased parenchymal echogenicity or multiple cysts. The liquor amount may be normal or decreased. Diagnosis is usually done in late second and third trimester. The diagnosis is easy when cyst is present in one of the parents.

Prognosis: The prognosis is not good in fetuses who present in utero. In counseling the affected parents, it is necessary to emphasize that in many cases the cysts develop later in life so the absence of cyst does not rule out the disease. The prenatal diagnosis can be made by chorionic villous sampling as the gene responsible has been identified.

Recurrence risk: It is 50% as the disease is autosomal dominant.

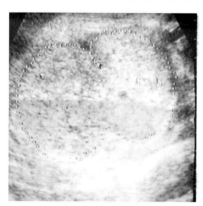

Figure 2.20: Transverse scan of fetus with infantile polycystic kidney disease. Multiple small cysts are visualized

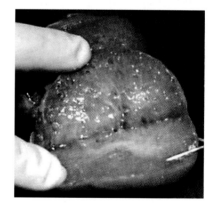

Figure 2.21: Cut section of same kidney showing multiple tiny cysts

B. Obstructive Uropathies

Pylectasis

Pylectasis is said to be present when anteroposterior diameter of the renal pelvis is more than 4-6 mm in second trimester and more than 10 mm in the third trimester.[16] It can be physiologic.

Incidence: 1-3% of pregnancies.

Hydronephrosis

Diagnosis: It is diagnosed when the anteroposterior diameter of renal pelvis is > 1.5 cm with calyceal dilatation. Fetal uropathies are classified by the level of dilatation. In upper obstruction only the kidneys are dilated. In midlevel obstructions ureters are also dilated. Upper and midlevel dilatation can be unilateral and bilateral. It may be due to obstruction of ureteropelvic junction, ureterovesical junction or due to ureteropelvic reflux.

Prognosis: It is good in unilateral dilatation. Corticomedullary differentiation is more important than cortical thickness in deciding the prognosis.

Lower Urinary Tract Obstruction

Posterior urethral valve is seen almost exclusively in males. In females may be due to complex pelvic floor malformations.

Abdominal Wall and Gastrointestinal System

Omphalocele

Incidence: 1 in 4000 births.

Diagnosis: The diagnosis is made after 11 weeks when on ultrasonography an anterior extraabdominal mass is detected upon which the umbilical cord inserts (Figs 2.22 and 2.23).

Prognosis: Other malformations are associated in 60% of the cases. Karyotypic abnormality is seen in up to 50%. We must look for other abnormalities on USG. Fetal echocardiography and karyotyping is advised. The survival rate in absence of any other abnormality is 75%.[20]

Labor and delivery: Elective cesarean section does not offer any benefit over vaginal delivery. Care of fetus immediately after delivery is required. Long-term prognosis is usually good.

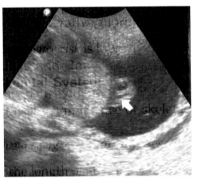

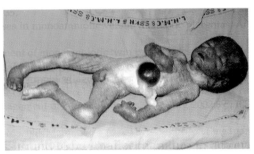

Figure 2.22: Transverse scan of fetal abdomen at the level of umbilicus demonstrating omphalocele

Figure 2.23: Typical omphalocele with lesion in midline covered by membrane

Recurrence risk: It is low in subsequent pregnancy.

Gastroschisis

It is an anterior abdominal wall defect. It occurs usually on the right side.

Incidence: 1 in 3000 live births.

Diagnosis: The loops of bowel appear floating freely in the amniotic fluid on USG giving appearance of a bunch of grapes.

Prognosis: The chance of presence of associated anomaly is less than 10%. The probability of associated chromosomal abnormality is < 1%. The prognosis of affected fetus is good with over 80% survival after surgical treatment. There is no evidence that cesarean delivery improves outcome. Primary surgical closure can be achieved in 52 to 85% cases.[21]

Recurrence risk: It is very low. Very few cases with familial occurrence have been noted.

Congenital Diaphragmatic Hernia

It is the herniation of the gastrointestinal contents into the thoracic cavity.

Incidence: 1 in 3500 live births.[22]

Diagnosis: Antenatal sonographic diagnosis is done by presence of abnormal position of heart or visualization of bowel or stomach beside the heart.

Prognosis: Prognosis is not good in the presence of additional anomalies, when diagnosis is made early in gestation, when liver is in the thorax and when the size of lung is small.

Fetal surgery is offered on experimental basis in the form of plugging of trachea which will prevent egress of lung fluid required for stimulating lung growth.[23]

Labor and delivery: Vaginal delivery is not contraindicated. Immediate intubation after delivery is required.

Esophageal Atresia with or without Tracheoesophageal Fistula

Incidence: 3 in 10,000 live births.[24]

Diagnosis: The most common antenatal presentation is polyhydramnios and failure to visualize the fetal stomach more so if noted after 20 weeks. A repeat examination within a few days should be done. Careful search for other anomalies is done, fetal karyotyping should be offered as abnormality is seen in 10% of the cases. It is also associated with syndromes such as VATER and DiGeorge sequence.

Prognosis: Termination of pregnancy can be offered if diagnosis is done before viability especially if associated abnormalities are present. Continuing pregnancies are managed by providing normal obstetric care. Therapeutic amniocentesis can be done.

Labor and delivery are not influenced by malformation. Immediate postdelivery care is given. Surgery is done after the condition of the infant is stable. The outcome of surgery is generally good.

Recurrence risk: Generally sporadic but may be familial.

Duodenal Atresia

Incidence: 1 in 6000 live births.

Diagnosis: Sonographic diagnosis is made by appearance of "double bubble" and presence of hydramnios (Fig. 2.24).

Prognosis and management: Associated anomalies are present in 50% cases; chromosomal abnormality is seen in 30% cases. Detailed ultrasonographic assessment is required. As there is high risk of heart abnormality fetal

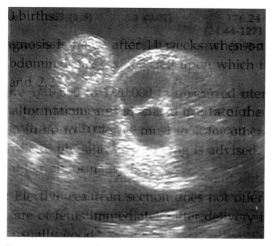

Figure 2.24: Transverse scan of upper abdomen of fetus with duodenal atresia. A typical double bubble is seen

echocardiography is also advised. Prognosis for the condition if isolated is good. Operative mortality rate is 4% with long-term survival as 86%.

Recurrence risk is low.

Skeletal System

Incidence: Prevalence of skeletal dysplasia is 1 in 5000 stillbirths.

Bone Length Abnormalities

If the length of any of the long bones is found to be smaller than the gestational age we must clarify the gestational age, measure all long bones and compare the measurement with nomograms available for limb biometry. The value less than 4 SD below mean definitely indicates skeletal dysplasia. The values between -2 to -4 SD can be due to syndromic causes, chromosomal cause or due to intrauterine growth restriction.

Short limbs can be micromelic (shortening of whole limb), rhizomelic (shortening of proximal part), mesomelic (shortening of middle part) or acromelic (shortening of distal part of limb). The various conditions associated with different types of shortening of limbs are described in Table 2.3.

After detection of abnormal length of bone, evaluation of density, bending, presence or absence of fractures is done (Fig. 2.25). Density of long bones is

Table 2.3: Types of shortening of limbs		
Rhizomelia	Mesomelia	Micromelia
Thanatophoric dysplasia	Ellis van Crevald (chondroectodermal dysplasia)	Achondrogenesis
Chondrodysplasia punctata	Robert syndrome	Short rib polydactyly
Congenital short femur		Osteogenesis imperfecta
Achondroplasia		

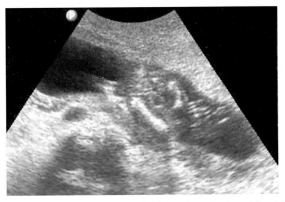

Figure 2.25: Scan showing normal right femur but short and bent left femur

adjudged by presence or absence of acoustic shadow behind the bone, intracranial visibility and whether the skull is compressed by the transducer.

Detailed examination of the skull, its shape and size, face for clefting, thorax for length and breadth, spine for kyphosis and scoliosis, digits for its number and foot for clubbing is noted to aid in diagnosis. Systemic examination especially cardiac and renal should be done.

Postnatal examination: Infantogram is done which should include antero-posterior and lateral view—thoracic and lumbar spine, lateral view—cervical spine and skull, anteroposterior view of pelvis, chest, long bones and hands.

Other studies like chromosomal analysis is advised in all cases, DNA testing may be done for some cases.

Counseling: It is to be provided after gathering all information. Counseling is to be provided by obstetrician and the geneticist both. The parents are informed about the recurrence risk in future pregnancies. Management plans for antenatal diagnosis in future pregnancy should also be explained.

Hydrops Fetalis

Definition

It is the presence of excessive extracellular fluid in the interestitial compartment secondary to disruption of normal intravascular and interstitial homeostatic mechanisms. Sonographic diagnosis of hydrops requires accumulation of fluid in two or more uterine cavities (Figs 2.26 and 2.27).

Incidence: The prevalence of 1:1000 has been reported. Fetal hydrops has been classified into immune (IH) and nonimmune hydrops (NIH). The ratio of

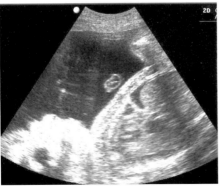

Figure 2.26: Longitudinal scan of the fetus showing pleural effusion (P), ascitis (A), and skin edema (E)

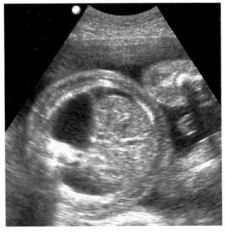

Figure 2.27: Transverse scan of the fetal abdomen showing ascitis (A)

Table 2.4: Etiology of nonimmune hydrops	
Causes	*Incidence (%)*
Cardiovascular	21.7
Hematologic	10.4
Chromosomal	13.4
Syndrome	4.4
Lymphatic dysplasia	5.7
Inborn errors of metabolism	1.1
Infections	6.7
Thoracic	6.0
Urinary tract malformations	2.3
Extra thoracic tumors	0.7
Twin-twin in transfusion syndrome-placental	5.6
Gastrointestinal	0.5
Miscellaneous	3.7
Idiopathic	17.8

NIH to IH has been reported to be 9:1. The etiology of nonimmune hydrops according to a recent meta-analysis is given in Table 2.4.

Prognosis

Although few cases of spontaneous remission of nonimmune hydrops have been reported the prognosis in majority of the infants is universally poor with perinatal mortality rate ranging from 70-90%.

Management and Treatment

Identification of the hydropic infant is easy but the real difficulty lies in identifying the underlying cause, determining the appropriate therapy and optimal time of delivery. After identification of a hydropic infant the first step is to rule out isoimmunization as the possible cause. Whether due to rhesus or any other antibody, this can be done by performing an indirect Coomb's test. A detailed ultrasound examination along with fetal echocardiography is the next step to exclude congenital anomalies in fetus and placenta. Other blood tests and amniotic fluid test as given in the Table 2.5 are also done to reach at a diagnosis. In most of the cases this diagnostic workup fails to give a definitive diagnosis. Management decision at this point depends upon gestational age. Before viability the option of pregnancy termination should be given. The prognosis before viability is poor. If decision for continuation is taken the dilemma is when to deliver. The risk of an intrauterine death has to be weighed against the risk of premature delivery with increased total

Table 2.5: Laboratory investigations in hydrops fetalis

Blood tests

- Complete blood count
- ABO type and rhesus antigen status
- Indirect Coomb's test
- Kleinhauer Betke stain
- Acute phase titers
- Toxoplasmosis
- Cytomegalovirus
- Serological test of syphilis(VDRL)
- G6 PD deficiency screen

Amniotic fluid tests

- Karyotyping
- L:S ratio after viability

lung water in the baby which would compound the problem of treating respiratory distress.

The approach for expectant management is to follow the fetus with frequent ultrasound examinations and biophysical profile until the clinical picture deteriorates or lung maturity is determined by L:S ratio of amniotic fluid. If preeclampsia is associated delivery is indicated. A chance of cesarean section is increased due to soft tissue dystocia and associated polyhydramnios. Patients are to be explained that chances of survival of fetus postdelivery are minimal.

The prognosis of nonimmune hydrops is good in selected groups such as cardiac dysarrhythmias amenable to transplacental medical therapy, in fetomaternal hemorrhage intrauterine transfusion can be done, in rare cause such as G6PD deficiency, removal of offending agent followed by intrauterine transfusion or delivery depending upon the gestational age can be done successfully.

NEED FOR EXAMINING FETUS, STILLBIRTH OR NEONATE

If a malformation is severe enough to terminate a pregnancy or if it is not treatable then generally no further investigations are carried out. However the information sufficient to take decision for termination of pregnancy may be totally inadequate to provide genetic counseling for the next pregnancy. The grieving family members may not be interested in knowing the cause of such mishap at that moment, but soon they may be concerned whether it can happen again in next pregnancy. To be prepared to answer this question appropriate investigations and autopsy must be carried out when a malformed baby is born.

Every fetus terminated due to prenatal ultrasonographic diagnosis of malformations needs to be examined after termination. It is essential not only for audit of ultrasonographer's skill but also for providing correct genetic counseling to the family. This is because even with best ultrasonographic setup autopsy shows additional findings in about 44 to 49% of cases.[26] These findings may be missed or may not be detectable by USG and may change in about 25-30% of the cases. Thus, genetic counseling based on ultrasonographic diagnosis may be erroneous.

Clinical Examination

The clinical examination includes careful observation and measurements. A photograph is much better than lengthy description and also provides opportunity to get second opinion especially from clinical geneticist.

Chromosomal Study

Chromosomal study is indicated in presence of malformations, fetal hydrops, intrauterine growth restriction and oligohydramnios or previous fetal loss. The sample can be aseptically collected from cord or fetal heart in a heparinized syringe.

Radiographic Study

Anterior and lateral radiographs are mandatory especially if skeletal dysplasia is suspected (Fig. 2.28).

Fetal Autopsy

Gross autopsy is extremely useful for separating subjects into normal and abnormal. If autopsy is not possible immediately, fetus can be stored in 10% formalin for transportation (Figs 2.29 and 2.30).

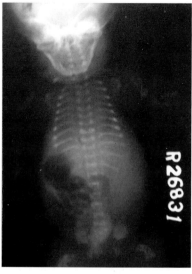

Figure 2.28: Radiograph of the infant with Thanatophoric dysplasia

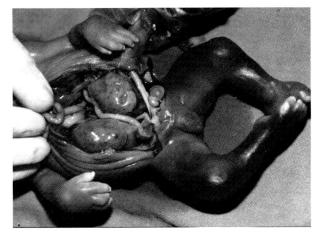

Figure 2.29: Autopsy of fetus showing polycystic kidney, ambiguous genitalia

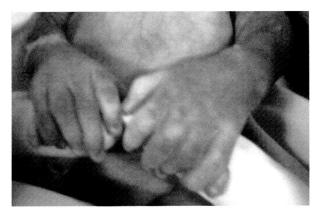

Figure 2.30: Polydactyly in the same fetus suggesting the diagnosis of Meckle-Gruber syndrome which has 25% recurrence risk in next pregnancy

Histopathology

Directed histopathological examination is required if gross abnormality is detected. For example it is useful in the diagnosis of polycystic kidney disease (Fig. 2.13)

Examination of Placenta and Cord

Fetal death can be attributable to placenta or cord abnormality in 15% cases. In cases of intrauterine infection placental histology may provide important information.

The uptake of perinatal autopsy services totally depends upon awareness among obstetricians regarding its use and utility.

- Approximately 3% of neonates have a major congenital malformation.
- Majority of birth defects occur in families with no prior history of birth defect.
- Most fetal structures can be visualized at 12-13 weeks.
- For measurement of nuchal translucency the optimal gestational age should be 11-13 weeks 6 days.
- Biochemical screening for neural tube defects (NTD) is done by maternal serum alfa fetoprotein estimation.
- Genetic sonography is offered to high-risk patients and has a sensitivity of 50-93% for detecting fetal aneuploidy.
- Cardiac malformations are most common birth defects.
- Associated malformations with cardiologic malformations are seen in 10% of cases of congenital malformation. Chromosomal abnormality is seen in 10-40%, Hence a detailed ultrasound evaluation and karyotyping is advised.
- After diagnosis multidisciplinary approach involving pediatric cardiologist, cardiac surgeon, obstetrician and geneticist is required.
- Counseling of the patient after diagnosis should involve the description of malformation, possibility of surgical correction, chances of short- and long-term survival, quality of life expected after correction and hazards of surgery.
- Follow up with echocardiography is done every 2-4 weeks.
- The delivery of fetuses with heart defect is to be done at a tertiary care center, most fetuses tolerate labor well and can be allowed vaginal delivery.
- Baby is to be assessed by pediatric cardiologist at birth and managed accordingly.
- If one child is affected the risk of recurrence in second child is 2-5%. The chance of heart disease in child if father is affected is 2% and if mother is affected is 6%.
- In anencephaly, pregnancy can be terminated at any period of gestation as it is lethal.
- In spina bifida on the whole about 75% will have mild to severe paralysis with only 17% have normal continence on late follow up.
- The risk in the next pregnancy is 4% if neural tube defect (NTD) is due to a multifactorial cause.
- After birth of one affected child periconceptional administration of folic acid can reduce recurrence risk of NTD in the next baby in up to 70% cases.
- In hydrocephalus amniocentesis for karyotyping is done as abnormal karyotype may be associated in up to 10% of the affected fetus.
- Parents are to be counseled that the overall mortality rate ranges from 15-70% in severe hydrocephalus. Cognitive impairment may be seen in up to 70%.

- The prognosis of unilateral hydronephrosis is good but is uniformly bad if bilateral affection and when associated oligohydramnios is present.
- Infantile polycystic kidney disease (IPKD) appears as bilaterally enlarged, homogenously hyperechoic kidneys that retain their shape. It is autosomal recessive and the risk of recurrence is 25%.
- The fetal prognosis depends on presence of pulmonary hypoplasia, if the mean vertical pocket of amniotic fluid on ultrasound is 10 mm, pulmonary hypoplasia is unlikely to occur.[18]
- For prediction of postnatal renal function, fetal urinalysis can be done with invasive testing and look for levels of sodium, α_2 microglobulin calcium, phosphorus and glucose.
- There is lack of high quality evidence to guide clinical practice regarding prenatal bladder drainage.[19] *In utero* drainage may improve survival in severely affected fetuses by improving renal function but in the long-term chronic renal failure is a rule. Many may require renal transplant.
- Fetal intervention is not done in unilateral cases, or when there is isolated uropathy with normal renal parenchyma or normal renal function.
- In case of fetal death. Examination after delivery must be done. Renal tissue is to be sent for histopathological examination.
- Fetal DNA must be stored if the termination is done for suspected genetic renal abnormality such as polycystic kidney disease.
- In omphalocele, karyotypic abnormality is seen in up to 50% cases.
- In gastroschisis, the probability of associated chromosomal abnormality is < 1%.
- The measurement of long bone less than 4 SD below mean definitely indicates skeletal dysplasia.
- Although few cases of spontaneous remission of nonimmune hydrops have been reported, the prognosis in majority of the infants is universally poor with perinatal mortality rate ranging from 70-90%.
- There is need for examining fetus, stillbirth or neonate to arrive at etiological diagnosis for counseling regarding risk in next pregnancy.
- A photograph, infantogram, chromosomal study is indicated in presence of malformations, tissue directed histopathological examination is also required.

REFERENCES

1. Sepulveda W, Sebire NJ, Hughes K, et al. The lambda sign at 10–14 weeks of gestation as a predictor of chorionicity in twin pregnancies. Ultrasound Obstet Gynecol 1996;7: 421-23.
2. Goldstein SR. Embryonic death in early pregnancy: A new look at first trimester. Obstet Gynecol 1994;83:738-40.
3. Carvalho JS, Senat MV, Schwarzler P, Ville Y. Increased nuchal translucency and ventricular septal defect in the fetus. Circulation 1999;99:E10.

4. Snijders RJM, Noble P, Sebire N, et al. UK multicentre project on assessment of risk of trisomy 21 by maternal age and nuchal translucency thickness at 10-14 weeks of gestation. Lancet 1998;351:343-46.
5. Sauka AP, Kramp E, Bakalis S, et al. Outcome of pregnancy in chromosomally normal fetuses with increased nuchal translucency in the first trimester. Ultrasound Obstet Gynecol 2001;18:9-17.
6. Circero S, Curcio P, Papageorghiou A, et al. Absence of nasal bone in fetuses with trisomy 21 at 11-14 weeks of gestation: An observational study. Lancet 2001;358: 1665-67.
7. Cameron A, Nimrod C, Nicholson S, et al. Evaluation of fetal cardiac dysarrhythmias with two dimensional, M mode, and pulsed Doppler ultrasonography. Am J Obstet Gynacol 1998;158:286.
8. Oudijk MA, Ruskamp JM, Ambachsheer BE, Ververs TF, Stoutenbeek P, Visser GH, Meijboom EJ. Drug treatment of fetal tachycardias. Pediatr Drugs 2002;4(1):49-63.
9. Mandakini P, Manisha, Renu S, Aditya K. Amiodarone in treatment of fetal supraventricular tachycardia—A case report and review of literature. Fetal Diagn and Ther 2006;21:72-76.
10. Khol, Shaland G, Allan LD, et al. World experience of percutaneous ultrasound guided balloon valvuloplasty in human fetuses with severe aortic valve obstruction. Am J Cardiol 2000;85:1230-33.
11. Bowman RM, McLone DG, Grant JA, et al. Spina bifida outcome: A 25-year prospective. Pediatr Neurosurg 2001;34:114-20.
12. Brunner JP, Tulipan N, Paschall RL, et al. Fetal surgery for myelomeningocele and incidence of shunt dependent hydrocephalus. JAMA 1999;282:1819-25.
13. Holzgreve W, Evans MI. Non-vascular needle and shunt placement for fetal therapy.
14. Cavalheiro S, Moron AF, Zymberg ST, Dastoli P. Fetal hydrocephalus—Prenatal treatment. Childs Nerv Syst 2003;19:561-73.
15. Cohen MM Jr, Shoita K. Teratogenesis of holoprosencephaly. Am J Med Genetics 2002;109:1-15.
16. Ouzounian JG, Castro MA, Fresquez M, et al. Prognostic significance of antenatally detected fetal pylectasis. Ultrasound Obstet Gynacol 1995;7(6):424-28.
17. Nicolaides KH, Cheng HH, Abbas A, et al. Fetal renal defects. Associated malformations and chromosomal defects. Fetal Diagn Ther 1992;7:1-11.
18. Kilbride HW, Yeast J, Thibeault DW. Defining limit of survival: Lethal pulmonary hypoplasia after midtrimester premature rupture of membranes. Am J Obstet Gynacol 1996;175(3pt 1): 675-81.
19. Clark TJ, Martin WL, Diwakaran TG, et al. Prenatal bladder drainage in management of fetal lower urinary tract obstruction: A systematic review and meta-analysis. Obstet Gynecol 2003;102(2):367-82.
20. Salihu HM, Boos R, Schmidt W. Omphalocele and gastroschisis. J Obstet Gynecol 2002; 22:489-83,738-40.
21. Babcook C, Hedrick MH, Goldstein RB, et al. Gastroschisis: Can sonography of fetal bowel accurately predict postnatal outcome? J Ultrasound Med 1994;13:701-6.
22. Blakelock R, Upadhyay V, Kimble R, et al. Is a normally functioning gastrointestinal tract necessary for normal growth in late gestation? Pediatr Surg Int 1998;13:17-20.
23. Quinn TM, Adzick NS, Fetal Surgery. Obstet Gynecol Clin of North Am 1997;24:143-57.
24. Shulman A, Mazkareth R, Zalel Y, et al. Prenatal identification of esophageal atresia: The role of ultrasonography for evaluation of functional anatomy. Prenat Diagn 2002;22: 669-74.
25. Carlo Bellini, Raoul CM Hennekam, Ezio Fulcheri, Mariangela Rutigliani, Guido Morcaldi, Francesco Boccardo, and Eugenio Bonial. Etiology of Nonimmune Hydrops Fetalis: A systematic review. Am J Med Genet 2009;Part A 149A: 844-51.
26. Snowdon C, Elbourne DR, Garcia J. Perinatal pathology in the context of a clinical trial: A review of the literature. Arch Dis Child Fetal Neonatal edn. 2004;89(3):F200-3.

Antepartum Fetal Surveillance 3

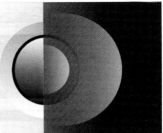

Seema Singhal

INTRODUCTION

The assessment of fetus in uterus still remains a challenge to the obstetrician because of the inability to perform a direct examination. With the evolution of technology more specific assessment of the fetus is possible now. As fetal compromise has varied etiology, tests which are developed for fetal surveillance should be able to assess both acute fetal asphyxia and chronic disease states.

OBJECTIVES OF FETAL SURVEILLANCE

The objectives of fetal surveillance are to assess fetal well-being to
1. Identify fetus at risk of intrauterine death or neonatal morbidity or mortality.
2. Identify potential threats early enough to allow timely interventions and improve neonatal outcomes.

INDICATIONS OF FETAL SURVEILLANCE

Currently, there are multiple maternal and fetal indications to perform antepartum fetal surveillance. Some conditions which require surveillance are:
- Diabetes mellitus
- Hypertensive disorders of pregnancy (chronic hypertension, preeclampsia)
- Renal disease
- Collagen vascular disorders
- Maternal thyrotoxicosis
- Severe anemia or maternal hemoglobin disorders
- Isoimmunization

- Prior unexplained fetal death
- Third-trimester vaginal bleeding
- Decreased fetal movements
- Prolonged pregnancy
- Abnormal or irregular fetal heart rate on auscultation
- Selected fetal anomalies, e.g. gastroschisis
- Multiple gestation
- Intrauterine growth restriction
- Amniotic fluid abnormalities (oligohydramnios/polyhydramnios).

WHEN TO START?

Usually recommended between 30 to 34 weeks, may be done earlier depending on severity of disease. Timing of fetal surveillance depends on:
1. prognosis for neonatal survival and
2. severity of maternal disease.

Frequency recommended is once a week but more frequent testing can be done. Condition specific antenatal testing is recommended because a form of surveillance that is ideal for one condition may be totally inappropriate for another.

ANTEPARTUM FETAL SURVEILLANCE TECHNIQUES

Several techniques are used which include:
1. Fetal movement assessment
2. Contraction stress test/oxytocin challenge test (CST/OCT)
3. Nonstress test (NST)
4. Biophysical profile (BPP)
5. Modified biophysical profile (MMPP)
6. Amniotic fluid volume
7. Doppler velocimetry.

Fetal Movement Assessment (Fetal Kick Count)

- Most women are aware of fetal movements around 16-18 weeks gestation, but perception of fetal movements is maximum at around 28-32 weeks. It is advantageous because it has no contraindications and is simple, inexpensive, noninvasive and understandable to patients. Presence of good fetal movements is a sign of fetal well-being and an indirect measure of normal fetal acid-base status. A decrease in fetal movements is often followed by fetal death, in some cases by several days.[1] Women perceive about 80% of ultrasonographically visualized fetal movements.[2]

The relationship between decreased fetal activity and poor perinatal outcome has been well-established. It is found that women with inactive fetus are more likely to have a stillborn or do poorly during labor and immediate neonatal period.[3]

There are many factors which influence maternally perceived fetal movements, some of which are as follows:

- *Maternal factors* like activity, obesity, ingestion of medications or drugs that depress or increase fetal movements. Methadone depresses fetal movements whereas cocaine increases fetal movements.
- *Fetal factors* like behavioral states, gestational age, congenital anomalies (e.g. neuromuscular disorders and fetal akinesia syndrome).
- *Uterine factors* like placental location, amniotic fluid volume, etc.

The ideal duration for counting movements has not been determined. Many approaches have been formulated but the most popular is to have the patient lie on her left side and count distinct fetal movements.[4] Counting 10 movements in a period of up to 12 hours is felt to be reassuring. Another reliable method is to count fetal movements for one hour after each of three main meals in left lateral position, and total of movements perceived should be more than or equal to ten. If the count is not reassuring further evaluation is recommended.

Contraction Stress Test/Oxytocin Challenge Test (CST/OCT)

The CST evaluates the response of the fetal heart rate to uterine contractions. It relies on the assumption that if fetal oxygenation is only marginally adequate with the uterus at rest, it will worsen when uterine contractions occur. The intermittent fetal hypoxemia during contractions leads to late decelerations of the fetal heart rate in suboptimally oxygenated fetus.[5] Uterine contractions may also produce variable decelerations due to cord compression, suggesting oligohydramnios.

Technique of Contraction Stress Test

- Lying in lateral recumbent position, the patient has an external fetal monitor to record both the FHR and uterine contractions simultaneously for a 20-30 minutes interval. The fetal heart rate and contraction activity is monitored and a baseline tracing is obtained. The contraction is considered satisfactory if at least 3 contractions of 40 seconds duration or more are present in a 10-minute period. If fewer, then contractions are induced with either nipple stimulation or intravenous oxytocin. Nipple stimulation is usually successful in inducing an adequate contraction pattern. Patient is instructed to rub one nipple gently, through her clothing for 2 minutes or until a contraction begins. She is instructed to restart after 5 minutes if the first nipple stimulation does not induce 3 contractions in 10 minutes. Oxytocin may also be used to stimulate contractions by infusing it at 0.5-1.0 mU/min, doubled every 15-20 minutes until an adequate contraction pattern establishes.

The contraction stress test is interpreted by the presence or absence of late fetal heart rate decelerations, defined as decelerations that reach their nadir after the peak of the contraction and persist beyond the end of the contraction. The results of the contraction stress test are categorized as follows:[6]

- *Negative*: No late or significant variable decelerations.
- *Positive*: Late decelerations following 50% or more of contractions (even if the contraction frequency is fewer than three in 10 minutes).
- *Equivocal-suspicious*: Intermittent late decelerations or significant variable decelerations.
- *Equivocal-hyperstimulation*: Fetal heart rate decelerations in the presence of contractions that are more frequent than every two minutes or last longer than 90 seconds.
- *Unsatisfactory:* Fewer than three contractions in 10 minutes or a tracing that is not interpretable.
  Relative contraindications to the contraction stress test usually include conditions that are associated with an increased risk of preterm labor and delivery, uterine rupture or history of vaginal bleeding. According to ACOG, these conditions include the following:
- Preterm labor or high risk of preterm labor.
- Preterm rupture of membranes.
- History of uterine surgery, previous myomectomy or classical cesarean section scar.
- Known placenta previa.

The most common result is a negative CST, which indicates adequate fetal oxygenation in the presence of contractions and is associated consistently with good fetal outcome. The literature suggests that there is a low incidence (1%) of antepartum fetal death within 1 week of a negative test. However, this test will not predict acute fetal compromise unrelated to placental insufficiency, such as in cord prolapse.[7,8] Fetal deaths after a negative CST are often due to abruption, congenital malformations and poor glucose control in diabetics. A positive CST means uteroplacental insufficiency and has been associated with adverse perinatal outcome and increased chances of intrauterine deaths.[6] The most important limitation of CST in predicting fetal outcome is its high false positivity, which has been reported to be as high as 50%.

Nonstress Test (NST)

In the nonstress test, the heart rate of a fetus who is not acidotic or neurologically depressed will temporarily accelerate with fetal movement. Heart rate reactivity is believed to be a good indicator of normal fetal autonomic function. Loss of reactivity is commonly associated with a fetal sleep cycle but may result from any cause of central nervous system depression, including fetal acidosis.

The FHR is monitored with a Doppler ultrasound transducer, while a tocodynamometer may be used to record uterine contractions, if any. Fetal activity is also recorded with the results displayed on the strip; however, the patient need not document fetal movement for the test to be interpreted.

The purpose of NST is to identify both a normal fetus and those with asphyxia/hypoxia. The NST (compared with CST) has the advantage of time, easier interpretability and lack of contraindications.[9]

The tracing is categorized as reactive (normal) or nonreactive. While various definitions of reactivity have been used, the most common is presence of ≥ 2 FHR accelerations [which peak, but do not necessarily remain, at least 15 bpm in amplitude above the baseline and last 15 seconds from baseline-to-baseline] within a 10 to 20 minutes period, with or without fetal movement.[10] It may be necessary to continue the tracing for 40 minutes to account for variations in the fetal sleep-wake cycle, because it may take this long for a healthy term fetus to display two FHR accelerations. If, after 40 minutes (from the start of testing), the criteria are still not met, the test is considered nonreactive. On initial testing, almost 85% of high- risk patients show a reactive NST and the remaining 15% are nonreactive.[11]

Factors which lead to nonreactive NST are fetal hypoxia, asphyxia, behavioral states, gestational age, depressants (narcotics, phenobarbital,) beta blockers and smoking.[12] Transient fetal heart decelerations can be seen in upto 50% of NSTs but they are of no obstetric significance if they are transient and brief but if they are repetitive (at least 3 in 20 minutes) they are associated with an increased risk of cesarean delivery.[13]

Routine NST interpretation does not take gestation age into account, but gestational age is an important consideration.[14] Preterm fetuses are less likely to have accelerations with fetal movements. The frequency and amplitude of accelerations increase as gestation advances. Preterm fetuses may also normally exhibit decelerations between 20-30 weeks.The nonstress test of the neurologically healthy preterm fetus is frequently nonreactive; from 24-28 weeks of gestation, up to 50% of nonstress tests may not be reactive and from 28-32 weeks of gestation, 15% of nonstress test are not reactive.

ACOG recommends that NST is typically repeated at weekly intervals, although certain high-risk conditions may warrant twice weekly testing.[5]

Fetal movements commonly produce heart rate decelerations. Variable fetal heart rate decelerations during nonstress test are not a sign of fetal compromise. ACOG (1999) has concluded that variable decelerations, if nonrepetitive and brief, i.e. less than 30 seconds, do not indicate fetal compromise or need for obstetrical evaluation. In contrast repetitive variable decelerations that is at least three in 20 minutes, even if mild, have been associated with an increased risk of cesarean delivery for fetal distress. Decelerations lasting 1 minute or longer are associated with even worse prognosis.[15]

NST is not considered an ideal test for primary fetal surveillance because of its inability to recognize early stages of fetal distress. The false-negative rate of the test (reactive NST in a fetus who is actually in distress) is 3.2/1000, indicating that the likelihood of fetal death or serious fetal morbidity following a negative (reactive) test is extremely low.[16] The false-positive rate (nonreactive results in normal patients) is very high: 50% for morbidity and 80% for mortality, indicating that the probability of serious fetal problems when the test is positive (nonreactive) is low. Therefore when a nonreactive NST is seen either we extend the time of NST or proceed with other forms of testings like biophysical profile. A reactive FHR even after extended NST is found to be associated with good fetal outcome, however persistent absence of reactivity may be associated fetal compromise in most cases.[17]

Vibroacoustic Stimulation (VAS)

VAS is a test of fetal well-being in which the fetus is stimulated *in utero* by using an artificial larynx which elicits a startle response and the effect of this response on fetal heart is studied. It has an advantage of differentiating normal fetal sleep from asphyxia.

Method

Artificial larynx can be positioned on the maternal abdomen over the fetal vertex with a stimulus of 1-2 second being applied. This may be repeated up to three times at 1 minute intervals for progressively longer durations of up to 3 seconds to elicit fetal heart accelerations.

The normal fetal response of VAS include accelerations in FHR, increase in long-term variability and gross body movements. Test offers the advantage of safely reducing testing time without compromising detection of acidemic fetus.[18] It is safe and harmless to the fetus. A combination of VAS and NST have a higher sensitivity in detecting abnormal outcomes (66% vs 39%) compared to NST alone.[19]

Biophysical Profile

Electronic fetal heart rate monitoring in the form of the nonstress test (NST) is the most frequently used method for antepartum detection of fetal asphyxia. However, this method has its limitations because it relies solely on the fetal heart rate for determining the state of fetal health. Although a reactive NST is effective in determining that the fetus is not asphyxiated at the time of testing, it is associated with high false-positive rates (50-75%).

The BPP is performed using real time ultrasonography to assess multiple fetal biophysical activities and amniotic fluid volume. The BPP assesses both acute and chronic markers of fetal well being. The acute markers of fetal well-being are FHR reactivity, fetal breathing movements and tone whereas amniotic fluid volume is a chronic marker. The first step in BPP is performing an NST following which a real time sonography is performed to assess other parameters. The observation is continued until either normal activity is seen or 30 consecutive minutes of scanning have elapsed.

The fetus responds to central hypoxemia or acidemia by altering its movement, tone, breathing and heart rate pattern. The presence of normal biophysical activities implies that CNS of fetus is functional and that fetus is not significantly hypoxic.

Biophysical score was introduced by Manning et al in 1980.[20] It provides a fair assessment of the risk of intrauterine fetal death in near future. Scoring system assigns a numeric value (usually 0 or 2) to each of the biophysical components (Table 3.1).

The original score which was given by Manning,[20] each of the five parameters (FHR, breathing, tone, movements and AFV were either given a score of 2 when normal and 0 when abnormal with no scores in between. As a result of which there was no intermediate score for the fetus who had some movements and tone but did not fit into criteria for score 2. To deal with this limitation Vintzileos, et al. in 1983 proposed another scoring system which gave intermediate scores and also included placental grading as one of biophysical variables. A normal score (of > 8) is predictive of a nonacidotic fetus.[21]

Physiologic Basis for the BPP

Each BPP parameter represents a normally functioning area of CNS, which develops *in utero* at a predictable gestational age. Vintzileos, et al. proposed the gradual hypoxia concept, which states that the biophysical activity developed last *in utero* is the first to become abnormal in the presence of fetal acidemia or infection.[21]

1. The CNS center controlling fetal tone, located in subcortical area is the first to develop at around 7.5 weeks.

Table 3.1: Biophysical profile scoring		
Variable	*Normal (score = 2)*	*Abnormal (score = 0)*
Fetal breathing movements	≥ 1 episode of ≥ 30 s in 30 min	Absent or no episode of ≥ 30s in 30 min
Gross body movements	≥ 3 discrete body limb movements in 30 min (Simultaneous limb and trunk movements are counted as a single movement)	≤ 2 episodes of gross body movements in 30 min
Fetal tone	≥ 1 episode of active extension with return to flexion of fetal limb(s) or trunk. Opening and closing of hand considered normal tone	Either slow extension with return to partial flexion movement of limb in full extension or absent fetal movement
Reactive fetal heart rate	≥ 2 episodes of acceleration of ≥ 15 bpm lasting for ≥ 15 s associated with fetal movement in 20 min	< 2 episodes of acceleration of fetal heart rate of or acceleration of < 15 bpm in 20 min
Qualitative amniotic fluid volume	≥ 1 pocket of fluid measuring 2 cm in vertical axis	Either no pocket or largest ≤ 2 cm in vertical axis

2. The CNS center controlling body movements develop at 8.5-9.5 weeks in cortex nuclei.
3. The CNS center controlling breathing movements develops after 20-21 weeks in ventral surface of the fourth ventricle.
4. The CNS center controlling FHR reactivity functions by the end of the second/ beginning of third trimester.
   Therefore in early stages of fetal compromise there are FHR reactivity and breathing abnormalities, the tone is abolished last of all.

Interpretation of Biophysical Profile and Pregnancy Management

1. A score of 10 is interpreted as normal, nonasphyxiated fetus; and no intervention is indicated. Recommended management is to repeat the test weekly except in diabetic women and post-term pregnancy, where it has to be done twice weekly.
2. A score of 8 with normal fluid also indicates a normal nonasphyxiated fetus and no intervention is indicated and repeat testing is recommended as per protocol.
3. Score of 8 with oligohydramnios is suspicious of chronic fetal hypoxia and delivery is recommended if > 37 weeks, otherwise repeat testing is recommended.
4. Score of 6 indicates possible fetal asphyxia and the recommended management is:
   - If abnormal AFV: Delivery
   - If normal AFV and period of gestation > 36 weeks with favorable cervix: Delivery
   - If normal AFV and period of gestation < 36 weeks then test should be repeated.
   - If repeat test < 6: Delivery
   - If repeat test > 6: Observe and repeat per protocol.
   In immature fetus repeat testing or Doppler velocimetry may also be advised before any intervention is recommended.
5. Score of 4 is considered probable fetal asphyxia and test should be repeated same day; if repeat BPP score is < 6, deliver.
6. A score of 0 to 2 is almost certain of fetal asphyxia and immediate delivery is recommended.

The data strongly suggest that the application of BPP to the high-risk pregnant population results in a dramatic improvement in perinatal mortality rates.[22] Absence of fetal breathing movement was most predictive of fetal distress in labor, even more so than a nonreactive NST. Lack of fetal movement was most predictive of fetal demise.[23] A normal BPP indicates a low risk of stillbirth. The false-negative rate of the BPP (fetal death within 1 week of normal test) ranges from 0.645 to 7.000 per 1000.[23,24]

The frequency of BPP testing (1-2/week) is arbitrary, but more frequent testing can be done depending on individual judgement, training, preferences and experience.

A variety of medications especially magnesium sulfate and corticosteroids that are commonly used in obstetric practice have significant effects on the BPP. If one is not aware of the effects of medications on the BPP, inappropriate interpretation of the results may occur resulting in the possibility of iatrogenic and unnecessary premature delivery. Corticosteroids and magnesium sulfate decrease the FHR variability and fetal breathing movements but have no effects on fetal tone or amniotic fluid volume.[25,26]

Modified Biophysical Profile

The modified BPP is composed of NST which is an acute indicator of fetal acid-base status and AFV which indicates chronic uteroplacental function. It is used by many centers as a primary mode of surveillance. The amniotic fluid index (AFI) is the sum of measurements (cm) of the deepest cord-free amniotic fluid pocket in each of the four maternal uterine quadrants. AFI > 5 cm is generally considered to be an adequate amniotic fluid.[27] The modified BPP score is normal when the NST is reactive and the AFI is more than 5 cm.[5] An abnormal test occurs if either NST is nonreactive or the AFI is 5 cm or less.

A protocol is suggested[28] for the interpretation of modified BPP:
1. If NST is reactive and AFV is normal—Twice weekly testing is recommended.
2. If NST is reactive with oligohydramnios—Delivery is recommended if gestation is greater than 36 weeks. But if gestation is less than 36 weeks then Doppler with increased frequency of testing should be done.
3. If NST is nonreactive then real-time ultrasound is done and management is done according to findings.
   • If fetal breathing movements are present—Manage according to AFV.
   • If fetal breathing movements are absent and fetal movements and tone are normal—Extend NST (120 min) or repeat BPP or Doppler.
   • If all biophysical activities are absent—Deliver promptly.

Amniotic Fluid Volume Assessment

Amniotic fluid (AF) essentially provides a compartment for normal development, growth and movement of the fetus. AFV is a chronic marker of fetal well-being. Normal AFV also protects the fetus from cord compression during fetal activity or uterine contractions.

Various techniques have been developed to assess AFV:
1. 2 cm rule: Single largest vertical pocket is measuring > 2 cm is considered as normal AFV.[29]
2. AFI (Amniotic fluid index): Uterus is divided into four quadrants (Linea nigra and umbilicus divide the uterus into right/left halves and upper/lower halves respectively), the vertical diameter of largest umbilical cord free pocket is measured. The summation of the values in all the quadrants is AFI.[30]

3

Antepartum Fetal Surveillance

AFI ≤ 5 cm suggests oligohydromnios while
AFI > 25 cm indicates polyhydramnios
Out of the two techniques AFI is found to be superior as compared to determination of a single vertical pocket.[27,29]

Doppler Ultrasonography

Doppler ultrasonography is a noninvasive technique used to assess the hemodynamic components of vascular impedance.

Commonly measured flow indices based on the characteristics of peak systolic frequency shift (S), end-diastolic frequency shift (D) and mean peak frequency shift over the cardiac cycle (A), include the following:
- Systolic to diastolic ratio (S/D)
- Resistance index (S-D/S)
- Pulsatility index (S-D/A).

Fetal Arterial Doppler

Umbilical artery: The normal Doppler flow pattern of umbilical artery is a low impedance circulation, with an increase in amount of end diastolic flow with advancing gestation.[31,32] Thus the S/D ratio decreases from about 4.0 at 20 weeks to 2.0 at term. The S/D ratio is generally less than 3.0 after 30 weeks[33] Umbilical arterial Doppler waveforms reflect the status of the placental circulation and the increase in end diastolic flow seen with advancing gestation is a direct result of an increase in the number of tertiary stem villi. Diseases that obliterate small muscular arteries in placental tertiary stem villi result in a progressive decrease in end diastolic flow in umbilical arterial Doppler waveforms until absent and then the flow reverses during diastole.[34] Reversed diastolic flow represents an advanced stage of placental compromise.[35] Absent or reversed flow is commonly associated with severe IUGR and oligohydramnios.[36]

Middle cerebral artery: The normal Doppler flow pattern of middle cerebral artery is a high impedance circulation with continuous forward flow throughout the cardiac cycle. In the presence of fetal hypoxemia, central redistribution of blood flow occurs which results in an increase in blood flow to the brain, heart and adrenals and reduction in flow to the peripheral and placental circulations. This is known as brain sparing reflex and has a major role to play in fetal adaptation to hypoxemia.[37] Often used to asses fetal well- being in suspected IUGR. An increase in flow in MCA indicates fetal compromise. Although the MCA indices of resistance are low in association with fetal compromise, the values overlap with the lower part of normal range in many small fetuses. To differentiate and recognize a deteriorating situation, cerebroplacental ratio has been suggested. It is defined as middle cerebral artery pulsatility index value divided by umbilical artery pulsatility index value and is used to identify the fetuses in whom the placental insufficiency is associated with altered cerebral blood flow.[38] Ratio of less than 1.0 indicates severe neonatal morbidity. The measurement of peak systolic velocity in the middle cerebral artery has become the standard method for assessment of fetal anemia in rhesus alloimmunization. In cases of fetal anemia values are increased because of increased cardiac output and decreased blood viscosity.[39]

Fetal Venous Doppler

The flow velocity waveforms in great veins like ductus venosus, inferior vena cava (IVC) and umbilical vein have been studied. The flow velocity waveform in the central fetal veins are influenced by the central venous pressure which is a reflection of cardiac function. In cases of fetal growth restriction, the changes in arterial circulation have a major effect on afterload, preload and cardiac contractility. High resistance in umbilical circulation leads to increased right ventricular afterload. In the most compromised fetuses low resistance in cerebral circulation reduces the left ventricular afterload. With further hypoxemia myocardial contractility and cardiac output fall.[40]

Fetal Ductus Venosus and Inferior Vena Cava

They reflect the physiologic status of the right ventricle. Specific information with regard to right ventricular preload, myocardial compliance and right ventricular end diastolic pressure can be derived from Doppler flow studies of the IVC and ductus venosus in the fetus. A large number of parameters have been calculated from the doppler waveform of these vessels. These parameters are related to fetal blood gas status and especially fetal hypoxemia.[41] Ductus venosus is used more widely because of its unique pattern.

Maternal Uterine Circulation

With advancing gestation a progressive decrease in impedance is noted in uterine circulation. The presence of notch in the waveforms and an increase in resistance index after 22 weeks is characteristic of abnormal uterine circulation. Pregnancies that show abnormal uterine circulation in late second and third trimester have an increased risk of complications like IUGR, pre-eclampsia, preterm delivery.[42]

Clinical Implications of Doppler in Fetal Compromise

Doppler studies can be used at two points in the evaluation of fetal compromise in high-risk pregnancy.[43]
1. Umbilical Doppler studies are used to identify high-risk pregnancy and confirm the potential for fetal compromise.
2. Direct fetal Doppler test are used to quantify the fetal risk.

Antepartum Fetal Surveillance

Use of umbilical artery Doppler assumes that placental vascular lesions underlie all fetal compromise except in cases of acute fetal deterioration, e.g. placental abruption. The use of umbilical artery Doppler flow studies have been evaluated by several randomized control trials. Metaanalysis[44] has established that women with high-risk pregnancies with a compromised fetus should have access to Doppler studies of the umbilical artery. Metaanalysis of these trials demonstrated a reduction in the perinatal deaths by 38%.

Direct fetal Doppler is used to quantify fetal condition and determine the time of delivery. Of the non-Doppler flow test, FHR monitoring relates to CNS control of cardioregulation and BPP to CNS behavior determination. Cerebral Doppler defines the redistribution of cardiac output. Central venous Doppler defines changes in cardiac load and contractility. But more evaluation is needed particularly with long-term neurological performance as an end point.[45]

CONDITION SPECIFIC ANTEPARTUM FETAL TESTING

Evidence-based observations have shown that there are different pathophysiologic processes that can place the fetus at risk; thus, the efficacy of the various fetal tests depend on the underlying pathophysiologic condition. It also follows that no one test is ideal for all high-risk fetuses. Therefore, multiple parameter assessment of combinations of different tests may often be the optimal surveillance strategy depending on the testing indication.[46]

KEY POINTS

- Antepartum surveillance of the fetus helps in detecting fetal compromise (acidemia), so that timely intervention can be done. It is able to detect both acute and chronic disease states.
- Fetal movement monitoring is a simple, inexpensive, noninvasive method of antepartum surveillance. The relationship between decreased fetal activity and poor perinatal outcome has been well-established.
- A negative contraction stress test indicates fetal ability to tolerate uterine contractions. A positive test implies potential uteroplacental insufficiency and has been associated with adverse perinatal outcome and an increased incidence of intrauterine death.
- Fetal heart rate reactivity is a good indicator of normal fetal autonomic function and well-being.
- Preterm fetuses are less likely to have FHR accelerations in association with fetal movements.
- The predictive value of a negative nonstress test (NST) is very high. The reactive NST predicts good perinatal outcome in about 95% of cases but the false-positive rate of a nonreactive NST is also very high.
- The normal fetal response to vibroacoustic stimulation (VAS) includes FHR reactivity along with increase in long-term FHR variability and gross

body movements. VAS also offers the advantage of safely reducing testing time without compromising detection of the acidemic fetus.

- The biophysical profile (BPP) is unique in that it assesses both acute and chronic markers of fetal condition.
- The "gradual hypoxia concept" implies that the biophysical activities developed last *in utero* are the first to become abnormal in the presence of fetal acidemia or infection. In accordance with this concept, early stages of fetal compromise are manifested by abnormalities in FHR reactivity and breathing, while movement and tone are generally not abolished until much later stages of compromise.
- Oligohydramnios is associated with adverse pregnancy outcome, such as umbilical cord occlusion, fetal distress in labor, meconium aspiration, operative deliveries and stillbirth.
- The interpretation of FHR patterns should incorporate knowledge of gestational age, maternal condition, medications and other factors that could influence FHR components.
- The use of umbilical artery Doppler flow velocity waveforms to study high-risk pregnancy is associated with a 32% reduction in perinatal mortality.
- Throughout pregnancy, there is a progressive decrease in resistance to blood flow to the placenta in the umbilical arteries as the placenta grows and this is reflected by changing pattern of the umbilical artery flow velocity waveforms.
- The presence of a high-resistance pattern in the umbilical artery flow velocity waveforms is manifested as increased S/D ratio, absent or reversed end diastolic flow and is associated with an increased risk of intrauterine growth restriction, fetal distress *in utero*, fetal distress in labor and need for early delivery.
- In the middle cerebral artery, a pattern of low resistance predicts fetal hypoxia. In fetal anemia, the peak velocity of the MCA flow velocity waveforms can be used as an index of the degree of anemia and requirement of fetal intravascular transfusion.
- The central fetal veins like ductus venosus, IVC show changes in flow velocity waveforms in condition of fetal compromise. Retardation of flow velocity in the ductus venosus waveform at the time of atrial systole indicates developing fetal hypoxemia.
- A high-resistance pattern in the uterine artery flow velocity waveform is signaled by low diastolic flow velocities and the nondisappearance of diastolic notch by late second trimester. This predicts pregnancy at risk of pre-eclampsia and fetal growth restriction.
- Abnormality in the umbilical artery flow velocity waveform signals developing placental vascular pathology, which may lead to fetal hypoxemia and acidosis. Changes in the fetal aortic, middle cerebral artery and ductus venosus waveform correlate with the degree of hypoxemia and fetal condition.

3

1. Pearson JF, Weaver JB. Fetal activity and fetal well being: An evaluation. Br Med J 1976; 1:1305.
2. Rayburn WF. Clinical significance of perceptible fetal motion. Am J Obstet Gynecol 1980; 138:210.
3. Rayburn WF. Antepartum fetal assessment: Monitoring fetal activity. Clin Perinatol 1982; 9:231.
4. Moore TR, Piacquadio K. A prospective evaluation of fetal movement screening to reduce the incidence of antepartum fetal death. Am J Obstet Gynecol 1989; 160: 1075.
5. ACOG Practice Bulletin no. 9. Antepartum fetal surveillance. Washington: American College of Obstetricians and Gynecologists; 1999; 911.
6. Freeman RK, Anderson G, Dorchester W. A prospective multi-institutional study of antepartum fetal heart rate monitoring: Risk of perinatal mortality according to antepartum fetal heart rate test results. Am J Obstet Gynaecol 1982; 143: 771.
7. Evertson LR, Gauthier RJ, Collea JV. Fetal demise following negative contraction stress tests. Obstet Gynecol 1978;51:671-673.
8. Lagrew DC. The contraction stress test. Clin Obstet Gynecol 1995;38:11.
9. Keegan KA. Jr, Paul RH, Broussard PM, et al. Antepartum fetal heart testing. V. The nonstress test. Am J Obstet Gynecol 1980;136:81.
10. Evertson LR, Gauthier RJ, Schifrin BS, Paul RH. Antepartum fetal heart rate testing. I. Evolution of the nonstress test. Am J Obstet Gynecol 1979;133:2.
11. Phelan JP. The nonstress test: A review of 3000 tests. Am J Obstet Gynecol 1981;139:7.
12. Margulis E, Binder D, Cohen AW. The effect of propanolol on the nonstress test. Am J Obstet Gynecol 1984;148:340.
13. Anyaegbunam A, Brustman L, Divon M, Langer O. The significance of antepartum variable decelerations. Am J Obstet Gynecol 1986;155:707.
14. Navot D, Yaffe H, Sadovsky E. The ratio of fetal heart rate accelerations to fetal movements according to gestational age. Am J Obstet Gynecol 1984;149:92.
15. Bourgeois FJ, Thiagrajah S, Harbert GN Jr: The significance of fetal heart rate decelerations during nonstress testing. Am J Obstet Gynecol 2004;150:138.
16. Devoe LD, Castillo RA, Sherline DM. The nonstress test as a diagnostic test: A critical reappraisal. Am J Obstet Gynecol 1985; 152:1047-53.
17. Devoe LD, McKenzie j, Searle NS, Sherline DM. Clinical sequelae of the extended nonstress test. Am J Obstet Gynecol 1985; 151: 1074.
18. Smith CV, Phelan JP, Platt LD, et al. Fetal acoustic stimulation testing. 11. A randomized clinical comparison with the nonstress test. Am J Obstet Gynecol 1986; 155:131.
19. Trudinger BJ, Boylan P. Antepartum fetal heart rate monitoring: Value of sound stimulation. Obstet Gynecol 1980;55:265.
20. Manning FA, Platt LD, Sipos L. Antepartum fetal evaluation: Development of a fetal biophysical profile. Am J Obstet Gynecol 1980; 136: 787.
21. Vintzileos AM, Campbell WA Ingardia CJ, Nochimson DJ. The fetal biophysical profile and its predictive value. Obstet Gynecol 1983; 62:271.
22. Manning FA, Harman CR, Morrison I, et al. Fetal assessment based on fetal biophysical profile scoring. 1V. An analysis of perinatal morbidity and mortality. Am J Obstet Gynecol 1990; 162:703.
23. Manning FA, Morrison I, Lange IR, et al. Fetal assessment based on fetal biophysical profile scoring: Experience in 12620 referred high risk pregnancies.I.Perinatal mortality by frequency and etiology. Am J Obstet Gynecol 1985; 151:343.
24. Platt LD, Eglinton GS, Sipos L, et al. Further experience with the fetal biophysical profile Obstet Gynecol 1983; 61: 480.
25. Deren O, Karaer C, Onderoglu L, et al. The effects of steroids on the biophyisical profile and Doppler indices of umbilical and middle cerebral arteries in healthy preterm fetuses. EurJ Obstet Gynecol Reprod Biol 2001; 99:72.
26. Carlan SJ, O"Brien WF. The effects of magnesium sulfate on the biophyisical profile of normal term fetus. Obstet Gynecol 1991; 77:681.

27. Rutherford SE, Phelan JP, Smith CV, Jacobs N. The four quadrant assessment of amniotic fluid volume: an adjunct to antepartum fetal heart rate testing. Obstet Gynecol 1987; 70: 353.

28. Vintzileos AM, Knuppel RA. Multiple parameter biophysical testing in the prediction of fetal acid base status. Clin Perinatol 1994; 21:823.

29. Chamberlain PF, Manning FA, Morrison I, et al. Ultrasound evaluation of amniotic fluid volume. I. The relationship of marginal and decreased amniotic fluid volumes to perinatal outcome. Am J Obstet Gynecol 1984; 150:245.

30. Phelan JP, Smith CV, Broussard P, Small M. Amniotic fluid assessment with the four quadrant technique at 36- 42 weeks gestation. J Reprod Med 1987; 32:540.

31. Fleischer A, Schulman H, Farmakides G, et al. Umbilical artery waveforms and intrauterine growth retardation. Am J Obstet Gynecol 1985; 151:502.

32. Ott WJ. The diagnosis of altered fetal growth. Obstet Gynecol Clin North Am 1988; 15: 237.

33. Fleischer A, Schulman H, Farmakides G, et al. Uterine artery Doppler velocimetry in pregnant women with hypertension. Am J Obstet Gynecol 1986;154:806.

34. Trudinger BJ, Stevens D, Connelly A, et al. Umbilical artery flow velocity waveforms and placental resistance: The effects of embolizations of the umbilical circulation. Am J Obstet Gynecol 1987;157:1443.

35. Kingdom JC, Burrell SJ, Kaufmann P. Pathology and clinical implications of abnormal umbilical artery Doppler waveforms. Ultrasound Obstet Gynecol 1997; 9: 271.

36. Copel JA, Reed KL. Doppler Ultrasound in Obstetrics and Gynecology. New York, Raven Press, 1995, pp 187-198.

37. Mari G, Deter RL. Middle cerebral artery flow velocity waveforms in normal and small for gestational age fetuses. Am J Obstet Gynecol 1992;166:1262.

38. Arias F. Accuracy of the middle cerebral to umbilical artery resistance index ratio in the production of neonatal outcome in patients at high risk for fetal and neonatal complications. Am J Obstet Gynecol 1994;171:1541.

39. Segeta M, Mari G, Fetal anemia: New technologies. Curr Opin Ogstet Gynecol 2004; 16:153.

40. Reece, John C. Hobbins, Norman F. Gant Jr. (Ed). Doppler Ultrasonography and Fetal Well-Being. In: Handbook The of Clinical Obstetrics: Fetus & Mother 3rd edn, Blackwell Publishing Ltd 2008;575-76.

41. Rizzo G, Capponi A, Arduini D, Romanini C. The value of fetal arterial cardiac and venous flow in predicting pH and blood gases in umbilical blood at cordocentesis in growth retarded fetuses. Br J Obstet Gynecol 1995;102:963.

42. Hernandez- Andrade E, Brodszki j, Lingman G, et al. Uterine artery score and perinatal outcome. Ultrasound Obstet Gynecol 2002; 19: 438.

43. Reece, John C. Hobbins, Norman F, Gant Jr. (Eds). Doppler Ultrasonography and Fetal Well-Being. In: The Handbook of Clinical Obstetrics: Fetus & Mother 3rd edn, Blackwell Publishing Ltd; 2008: 577.

44. Laudy JA, Gaillard JL, van der Anker JN, et al. Doppler ultrasound imaging: A new technique detect lung hypoplasia before birth? Ultrasound Obstet Gynecol 1996;7:189.

45. Thornton JG, Hornbuckle J, Vail A, et al. The GRIT study group. Infant well being at 2 years of age in the growth restricted intervention trial (GRIT): Multicentered randomized controlled trial. Lancet 2004;364:513.

46. Kontopoulos EV, Vintzileos AM. Condition- specific antepartum fetal testing. Am J Obstet Gynecol 2004;191:1546.

3

Preterm Labor

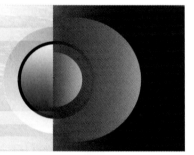

4

Monika B Nagpal

INTRODUCTION

Preterm birth complicates 10-15% of all pregnancies and is a leading cause of neonatal morbidity and mortality. Idiopathic preterm labor accounts for about 40% of all preterm births, 35% of preterm births follow preterm prelabor rupture of membranes and around 25% are iatrogenic because of obstetric or medical complications of pregnancy. Preterm birth besides being serious, is also a very costly problem as there is often need for neonatal intensive care. It is well-known that preterm babies are at increased risk for morbidity and mortality which is inversely related to the gestational age. Respiratory distress syndrome, intraventricular hemorrhage, apnea, necrotizing enterocolitis, retinopathy of prematurity as well as long-term disabilities including mental retardation, cerebral palsy, chronic lung disease, gastrointestinal problems, vision and hearing loss and poor neurodevelopment outcomes are much higher in babies born preterm as compared to those born at term.

Clinically it is difficult to distinguish true preterm labor from Braxton Hicks contractions. In order to improve the accuracy of diagnosis standard criteria are used. Preterm labor is defined as onset of labor after the period of viability but prior to completed 37 weeks of pregnancy. Onset of preterm labor may be determined according to ACOG and AAP 1997 criteria which include:

- Frequency of contractions—Four in 20 minutes or eight in 60 minutes and progressive change in cervix.
- Cervical dilatation greater than 1 cm.
- Cervical effacement of 80% or greater.

Threatened preterm labor may be diagnosed when there are documented uterine contractions but no evidence of cervical change. Though the survival rates for preterm babies have improved over last decade because of better neonatal facilities, every effort should be made to inhibit preterm labor after careful patient selection, which may allow time for in-utero transfer of a pregnancy at risk to an appropriate tertiary referral center, administration of glucocorticosteroids and antibiotics prophylaxis to reduce the risk of neonatal sepsis where required.

ETIOPATHOGENESIS

The etiopathogenesis of preterm labor is not well-understood, it is often not clear whether preterm labor represents early idiopathic activation of the normal labor process or results from a pathologic mechanism. The underlying biochemical and hormonal mechanisms of parturition are quite complex and intricate. The process is heralded by an increase in myometrial gap junctions, oxytocin receptors, enhanced myometrial contractile efficiency and changes in cervical collagens and matrix. This complex cascade results in contractions, effacement of the cervix and ultimately expulsion of the fetus. Several theories are proposed regarding the initiation of labor including:[1]

Activation of Hypothalamopituitary Axis

As parturition nears, the fetal-adrenal axis becomes more sensitive to adrenocorticotropic hormone, increasing the secretion of cortisol. Both fetal and maternal stress can lead to early activation of the axis. Maternal stress could be due to environmental factors and medical conditions like hypertension, renal disease, heart disease, etc. Fetal stress may be associated with growth restriction and abnormal placentation. Cortisol stimulates corticotropin releasing hormone (CRH) release in the decidua, trophoblast and membranes which in turn drives the maternal and fetal HPA activation. Cortisol then stimulates trophoblast 17 [alpha]-hydroxylase activity, which decreases progesterone secretion and leads to a subsequent increase in estrogen production. This reversal in the estrogen/progesterone ratio results in increased prostaglandin formation, initiating a cascade of events that culminate in labor and subsequent delivery. Although this mechanism is well-documented in sheep, its role in humans has not been confirmed.

Pathologic Uterine Overdistention

The stretching of myometrium as in multiple gestation and polyhydramnios causes formation of gap junctions leading to upregulation of oxytocin receptors[2] and production of prostaglandins which leads to cervical ripening and uterine contractions.

Decidual Hemorrhage

Vaginal bleeding in placenta previa and abruptio placentae can predispose to preterm birth. Following decidual hemorrhage tissue factor is released which interacts with various hemostatic factors to generate thrombin which in turn binds to the decidual membrane receptors upregulating the expression of proteases and metalloproteinases leading to cervical ripening and uterine contractions.

Inflammation/Infection

Both systemic and ascending genital tract infection has been linked with preterm labor.[3] Clinical and subclinical chorioamnionitis has been found to be more common in preterm than in term pregnancies. It has been shown that there is overgrowth of potential pathogens in the vagina or cervix associated with bacterial vaginosis and the most commonly isolated organisms include Ureaplasma urealyticum, fusibacterium and *Mycoplasma hominis*. Following amniochorionic decidual infection, activated macrophages and granulocytes release proinflammatory substances such as cytokines and matrix metalloproteinases. These in turn stimulate prostaglandin production and ripen the cervix triggering preterm labor. In addition some organisms directly produce proteases, collagenases, elastases and phospholipase A2 which can degrade the fetal membranes and stimulate uterine contractions.This mechanism has been proposed to cause increased risk of preterm birth after ART.

Abnormal Cervical Function

The function of the cervix is to retain the pregnancy within the uterus and to prevent ascent of potential bacterial pathogens from vagina. It has been shown that cervical length,[4] strength and quality of cervical mucus contribute towards this function. Conditions like diethylstilbesterol exposure *in utero*,[5] congenital anomalies in the genital tract (bicornuate, subseptate or unicornuate uterus),[6] previous cervical surgery (conization of cervix) and cervical incompetence[7] lead to cervical weakness hampering normal functioning.

PREDICTION

Prediction is the first step toward prevention. Hence, prediction of preterm labor is important. Any method used to predict labor should be safe, sensitive, specific and preferably inexpensive. While such an ideal method still eludes the medical community, the various methods that are being used presently are discussed below:

Risk Scoring

To identify the women who are at high risk of preterm labor 'risk score' is calculated. The demographic profile of preterm labor has been used as a basis for the evolution of various scoring systems. Various parameters like maternal age, race, educational status, social status, marital status, smoking, cocaine use, prepregnancy weight, weight gain during pregnancy are taken into account for predicting preterm labor. The more important factors responsible for preterm labor can be identified in previous obstetric history. History of one preterm birth is associated with a recurrence risk of 17-40%. The risk of preterm labor is also increased in women who have experienced one or more second trimester abortions. Not surprisingly, the risk of preterm labor decreases with the number of prior term deliveries. Certain current pregnancy problems like multiple gestation, polyhydramnios, APH, fetal abnormalities, etc. also predispose the patient to preterm labor. In addition, factors like uterine malformation, previous abdominal surgical procedure, cervical biopsy, DES exposure, etc. influence onset of preterm labor. While the clinical validity of risk scoring systems is still debatable, it is important to recognize that some of these factors like smoking are preventable and also alerts the obstetrician to the possibility of preterm labor. A commonly used scoring system is the Papernik scoring system. A patient with a score of 10 or more is considered being at high risk.

Cervical Assessment

Various studies have shown that frequent serial cervical examination by the same obstetrician is helpful in predicting preterm labor. The position, length, consistency of cervix, development of lower uterine segment at each antenatal visit during the late second and third trimester has been practiced to identify women at high risk of preterm labor. Ultrasound screening has now almost replaced the clinical cervical examination. It is proposed that full bladder may falsely elongate the cervix and precise anatomic landmarks of internal and external os are difficult to visualize, so some authorities recommend scanning the patient with both full and empty bladder. Endovaginal ultrasound is a better option as compared to transabdominal examination. Shortening of the cervix < 30 mm, widening of endocervical canal, thinning of lower uterine segment, bulging of membranes in the endocervical canal are predictive of preterm labor. Gomez introduced the cervical index (tunnel length + 1/endocervical length) for prediction of preterm labor. A cervical index > 00.52 was associated with a sensitivity of 76% and specificity of 94% for prediction of preterm labor. Transperineal cervical sonography has recently been advocated and has the advantage of avoiding vaginal instrumentation.

Home Uterine Activity Monitoring

It has been shown that women destined to develop preterm labor show an increase in the frequency of uterine contractions at least a week in advance.

This increased frequency, however, is not perceived by the women. Ambulatory home uterine activity monitoring was introduced with the intention of recording this increased frequency and initiating therapeutic intervention before the actual onset of preterm labor.

This system provides for the recording of uterine activity. It consists of a patient unit and a practitioner unit. The patient unit consists of light weight external pressure device or sensor based on the guard ring principle, a transmission device and a recorder. The recorder can store uterine activity data up to 3 hours. Transmission occurs through a telephone to the obstetrician's unit.

The baseline tone is 0 mm Hg and the peak deviation from the baseline tone is considered proportional to intensity. Contractions with duration of 35 seconds or longer and with an amplitude of greater than 5 mm Hg are considered significant.

Until the 30th week of pregnancy one contraction/hour in primi and 2 contractions/hour in multigravida are accepted as normal. Beyond 30th week usually 2 contractions/hour are normal. More than 3 contractions between 26-28 weeks and > 5 contractions between 30-32 weeks are considered to be predictive of preterm labor and an indication for therapeutic intervention.

As with all other predictors of preterm labor the clinical validity of this method is also open to debate while some authorities strongly advocate it and show improved neonatal outcomes when therapeutic interventions are initiated on the basis of home uterine monitoring, others argue that there has been no significant decrease in the incidence of preterm births and the benefit is mainly due to close nursing supervision and remarkable patient education and there is no real need for such an expensive form of screening.

Cervicovaginal Fibronectin

A relatively new method proposed for the screening of preterm labor is the assessment of fetal fibronectin in the cervicovaginal secretions. Fibronectin is a glycoprotein produced by fetal amnion, hepatocytes, malignant cells, fibroblasts and endothelial cells. It is present in high concentration in maternal blood and amniotic fluid. Fetal fibronectin can be detected in vaginal secretions just prior to onset of labor and appears to reflect stromal remodeling of cervix prior to labor. It is detected by ELISA and a value of > 50 ng/ ml is considered to be a positive result.

However, contamination of the sample by amniotic fluid and maternal blood should be avoided.

Biochemical Markers

Various biochemical markers have been advocated to predict preterm labor. These are currently under study:
- Salivary estriol to progesterone ratio
- Salivary estriol
- Serum collagenase
- Neutrophil collagenase
- Tissue inhibitor of metalloproteinase (TIMP)
- Serum relaxin
- Corticotropin releasing hormone.

Mediators of Inflammation and Infection

It has been postulated that infection predisposes to preterm labor. Hence, an attempt has been made to detect the mediators of inflammation and infection and their association with preterm labor. Cervical IL-6 and TNF (tumor necrosis factor) levels have been correlated with the risk of preterm delivery. However, most of these mediators have been shown to be of no practical help in predicting preterm labor.

PREVENTION OF PRETERM LABOR

As discussed, there is hardly any test that reliably predicts preterm labor. Even categorization of patients into low and high risk is not very beneficial. Hence, prevention of preterm labor is an important component of antenatal care.

Prepregnancy Initiative

Ideally, prepregnancy counseling should be done in all women. Not only preterm labor but a variety of other obstetrical problems can be markedly reduced by prepregnancy counseling. Childbearing at right age, adequate spacing between pregnancies, avoidance of multiple MTP's, and to avoid smoking are some of the measures that can be initiated.

Patient Education

Education of patient is of utmost importance. All women should be adequately counseled regarding the risk of preterm labor and to seek early medical care if warning signs and symptoms of preterm labor in the form of low dull backache, menstrual like cramps, increase in vaginal discharge or uterine contractions develop.

Education of Nursing Personnel

Uterine contractions prior to term are generally dismissed as Braxton Hicks contractions. In order to document preterm labor Herron and associates (1982) recommended the following criteria—regular uterine contractions after 20 weeks and before 37 weeks which are 5-8 minutes apart or less and accompanied by one or more of the following:

A. Progressive change in the cervix
B. Cervical dilation of 2 cm or more
C. Cervical effacement of 80% or more.

Behavioral Alteration

In patients who are at high risk for preterm labor some of the following measures would be highly beneficial:

- Bed rest
- Limitation of physical activity
- Coital abstinence
- Cessation of smoking.

Treatment of Infection

Concurrent UTI and bacterial vaginosis should be treated.

Cervical Cerclage

This form of treatment is mainly helpful for patients with cervical incompetence. It has also been used by some authorities for preterm labor. However, different studies revealed conflicting results as regards its benefits.

DIAGNOSIS OF PRETERM LABOR

Although the diagnosis is straightforward in advanced preterm labor, it is difficult to make the diagnosis accurately with lesser degrees of dilatation and effacement. The pregnant women may initially present with nonspecific features like sense of pelvic pressure, backache, menstrual like cramps and periodic painless or painful tightening of the abdomen with mucoid discharge on per-speculum examination which may or may not be mixed with blood. These women need to be thoroughly evaluated for any underlying predisposing factors. A complete history including accurate estimation of period of gestation is recorded. Additionally, any associated   medical or obstetric conditions should be evaluated which might contraindicate tocolytic therapy. This is followed by a complete clinical examination particularly the gestational age, presentation, fetal weight and perspeculum examination to rule out any evidence of infection, leaking and to collect vaginal and cervical swabs and cultures as required. The diagnosis is based on clinical criteria of regular uterine contractions associated with cervical change and supplemented with laboratory evaluation.

The lab evaluation of these women is aimed at etiological work up, discrimination of false and true labor and establishing fetal well-being. It includes the following:

- Complete blood count with differential count—To look for evidence of infection.
- Urine routine, microscopy and culture—To exclude urinary tract infection.
- Vaginal wet mount preparation for bacterial vaginosis and trichomonasis.
- Cervical cultures for Neisseria and Chlamydia.
- Amniocentesis—for Gram stain, glucose, white cell count. This information can be used to identify those women who are higher risk of chorioamnionitis and neonatal sepsis in order to maximize care.
- Fetal fibronectin assay—It is a glycoprotein present in amniotic fluid, placenta, extracellular substance of the decidua and the placenta. It is normally present in vaginal secretions before 20 weeks and after 36 weeks, if present between 20-36 weeks in a symptomatic woman then there is a chance of preterm birth within 7 days in 40% of these women. But if it is negative the risk of preterm delivery is less than 1%. It has been shown to be a better predictor than clinical indices and such discrimination can allow better targeting of therapy and resources.
- Ultrasound is done for gestational age, number of fetuses, fetal size and biometry, gross congenital anomaly, placental localization, any subchorionic hemorrhage and grading, amniotic fluid index and cervical length. Cervical length estimation by ultrasound along with fetal fibronectin testing have been used to differentiate true from false preterm labor. A negative fibronectin and a long cervix > 1.5 cm are strong negative predictors of imminent preterm birth.
- Cardiotocography is useful for confirming fetal well-being.

TREATMENT

The goals of treatment in women admitted with preterm labor include the following:
- Antibiotic administration in those with evidence of infection.
- Delay in delivery where beneficial, so that:
  - Corticosteroids can be administered.
  - *In utero* transfer to a tertiary care center be arranged.
  - Neonatal morbidity can be decreased.

Decisions regarding further management (immediate or delayed delivery) are based on gestational age, estimated fetal weight and contraindications to labor suppression.

Pregnancies between 24 to 34 weeks of gestation or estimated fetal weight between 600-2500 gm, with no evidence of infection benefit from tocolysis.

Pregnancies between 20-24 weeks of gestation may be allowed to deliver as these fetuses are not generally considered viable.

Once a pregnancy has continued beyond 34 weeks fetal survival rate is within 1% of the term survival and long-term sequelae are rare. Hence steroids and tocolysis may not provide additional benefit.

Contraindications to tocolytic therapy are shown in Table 4.1.

Table 4.1: Contraindications to tocolytic therapy	
Maternal	*Fetal*
• Severe hypertensive disease	o Period of gestation ≥ 34 weeks
• Uncontrolled diabetes	o IUD
• Cardiac arrhythmias/valvular heart disease	o Fetal distress
• Antepartum hemorrhage	o IUGR
• Chorioamnionitis	o Rh-incompatibility
• ARDS/pulmonary edema	o Congenital anomalies incompatible with life
• Cervical dilatation > 4 cm	o Ruptured membranes
• Hyperthyroidism	

The interventions for the management of pregnancies with preterm labor between 24-34 weeks gestation include the following:

Bed Rest

Bed rest is one of the most commonly prescribed interventions used for the prevention and/or treatment of threatened preterm labor. However, there are no prospective randomized studies that have independently evaluated the effectiveness of bed rest for the prevention of preterm labor. Although a reduction of physical activity may seem appropriate for some women at risk of preterm birth, a Cochrane review has confirmed that there is insufficient evidence to support or refute the usefulness of this intervention, especially when extended to full bed rest.

Hydration/Sedation

Another common practice used for the initial treatment of preterm labor is oral or intravenous hydration. This is based on physiologic evidence that hypovolemia may be associated with increased uterine activity and women in preterm labor may have plasma volumes below normal. A Cochrane review has recently reported that there is no evidence that intravenous hydration is effective in decreasing uterine activity. Intravenous hydration is not without risk, especially because administration of tocolytics after intravenous hydration may place the patient at increased risk for pulmonary edema.

Sedation is also a commonly used intervention in women with premature contractions. There are limited data documenting the efficacy of sedation in preterm labor and current literature does not support the use of hydration and/or sedation as the initial treatment of preterm labor.

Corticosteroids

Antenatal glucocorticoid therapy results in a significant decrease in the incidence of respiratory distress syndrome associated with a decrease in perinatal mortality in newborns born before 34 weeks and has become the standard of care. The incidence of intraventricular hemorrhage and necrotizing enterocolitis is also lower. The optimal benefits appeared more than 24 hours after the start of treatment, peak at 48 hours and last for 7 days. There has been controversy regarding the safety of multiple doses of corticosteroids if the pregnancy continues beyond 7 days. It was previously reported that there was no added benefit with repeated courses and that multiple courses may be associated with growth abnormalities and delayed psychomotor development in the infant. However, a recent Cochrane review has reported that repeated weekly doses decrease the incidence of respiratory difficulties and serious health problems if the pregnancy lasts more than 7 days.[8] Long-term follow-up of infants exposed *in utero* to a single course of antenatal corticosteroid therapy has not demonstrated any adverse effect on growth, physical development, motor or cognitive skills, or school progress at 3 and 6 years. The commonly utilized steroids for the enhancement of fetal maturity are betamethasone (12 mg intramuscularly every 24 hours, two doses) and dexamethasone (6 mg intravenously every 12 hours, four doses). These two glucocorticoids have been identified as the most appropriate for antenatal use as they readily cross the placenta and have long half-lives and limited mineralocorticoid activity with no significant difference in efficacy between the two.

Antibiotics

Preterm labor, especially at less than 30 weeks' gestation, has been associated with occult upper genital tract infection. Many, if not all, of the bacterial species involved in this occult infection are capable of inciting an inflammatory response, which ultimately may culminate in preterm labor and delivery. Antibiotics therefore have the potential to prevent and/or treat spontaneous preterm labor. This use has been extensively studied with mixed results. A recent Cochrane metaanalysis compared antibiotic therapy (mostly penicillin derivatives) with a placebo for the treatment of documented preterm labor. Overall the use of antibiotics was not associated with reduction in neonatal morbidity or mortality or prolongation of pregnancy. The only positive health benefit was significantly decreased risk for maternal infection in women who had received antibiotics. Thus antibiotic therapy for women in preterm labor should be limited to GBS prophylaxis, women with preterm PROM or treatment of a specific infection and not for the sole purpose of preventing preterm delivery.

Tocolysis

Tocolytic agents aimed at inhibiting contractions of the uterus have been used to prolong pregnancy. This may improve perinatal outcomes by allowing the fetus to mature more before being born, enhance lung maturation by antenatal corticosteroid administration and allow time for in utero transfer to a tertiary care center with neonatal intensive care facilities. The ideal tocolytic agent is one which is effective in prolonging pregnancy but has no side effects for the mother or the infant. When considering whether or not to use tocolytic agents in preterm labor, consideration needs to be given to the risks and benefits for both mother and infant, including the side effects of medication used. Several tocolytic agents have been used including betamimetics, calcium channel blockers, prostaglandin synthase inhibitors, magnesium sulfate, nitric oxide donor and oxytocin receptor antagonists.

Betamimetics

Like the endogenous catecholamines epinephrine and norepinephrine, this class of drugs stimulate all beta-adrenergic receptors present throughout the body. Betamimetics include ritodrine, terbutaline, albuterol, fenoterol, hexoprenaline, isoxsuprine, metaproterenol, nylidrin, orciprenaline, and salbutamol, they have been used extensively as tocolytic agents over last 20 years. Ritodrine, isoxsuprine and terbutaline are the beta-2 receptor agonists most commonly used.

Mechanism of Action

Three types of beta-adrenergic receptors have been described in humans: beta-1 receptors are prevalent in the heart, small intestine, and adipose tissue; beta-2 receptors predominate in the smooth muscle of blood vessels, uterus, bronchioles, diaphragm and in the liver; whereas beta-3 receptors are found predominantly on white and brown adipocytes. Stimulation of the beta-2 receptors results in uterine smooth muscle relaxation as well as hepatic glycogen production and insulin secretion from pancreatic islet cells. Although some beta-sympathomimetic agents have been proposed as beta-2 receptor selective agents, at the dosages used pharmacologically, stimulation of all receptor types often occurs. Such stimulation results in many of the side effects associated with the beta-sympathomimetic agents. Beta-adrenergic agonists activate adenyl cyclase to form cyclic adenosine 3',5' monophosphate (cAMP). The increased cellular levels of cAMP decrease myosin light-chain kinase activity, both by phosphorylation of the myosin light-chain kinase itself and by reducing intracellular calcium through increasing calcium uptake by sarcoplasmic reticulum and results in decreased myocyte contractility.

Dosage and Administration

Ritodrine: Ritodrine is the only medication among betamimetics approved by the United States Food and Drug Administration for the treatment of preterm labor. Ritodrine is a rapid acting drug, it is metabolized in the liver and excreted in the urine. It can be administered intravenously, intramuscularly, or orally.

Treatment usually begins with intravenous infusion to allow maximal bioavailability. Serum levels reach 75% of maximum within 20 minutes of infusion. There is an initial half-life of 6 to 9 minutes followed by a second half-life of 2 to 3 hours and elimination time of 2.5 hours. For intravenous administration, the infusion is begun at 50-100 µg/min and increased every 20 minutes till either uterine quiescence is achieved or unacceptable side effects occur, or a maximum infusion rate of 350 µg/min is reached. Once labor is inhibited, the labor inhibiting infusion rate is maintained for 60 minutes and then decreased by 50 µg/min every 30 minutes until the lowest effective rate is achieved (but not less than 50 µg/min). The lowest effective infusion rate is then arbitrarily maintained for 12 hours. If labor recurs within this 12-hour period, the process is repeated.[9] Tachyphylaxis may occur after prolonged exposure, therefore, the myometrium may remain quiescent longer with pulsatile administration of lower doses. The patient should be closely monitored for pulse, blood pressure, fluid balance, cardiac status, and electrolytes, including potassium and glucose. Oral ritodrine is used for maintenance tocolysis with approximately 30% of an oral dose absorbed.[10]

Terbutaline: Terbutaline is used as off-label betamimetic as it is not approved by the Food and Drug Administration for specific use in preterm labor, but there exists significant evidence for its safety and efficacy. It can be administered by intravenous, subcutaneous and oral routes. The intravenous infusion rate of terbutaline is generally started at 2.5 to 5 µg/min and increased every 20 minutes by increments of 5 µg/min to a maximum of 25 µg/min. Once labor is inhibited, the labor inhibiting rate is sustained for 60 minutes and thereafter reduced by 2.5 µg/min every 30 minutes until the lowest effective dose is established. This rate is maintained for 12 hours. Subcutaneous administration is also used for acute tocolysis with a typical dose of 0.25 mg subcutaneously every 1 to 6 hours with repeated dosing titrated to uterine activity and maternal side effects, stopping the dose at a pulse rate greater than 120 bpm. A rapid onset of action is seen in 3 to 5 minutes after subcutaneous administration. Orally administered terbutaline has mostly been used to prevent recurrence of already inhibited contractions. Generally, a dose of 2.5 to 5 mg every 4-6 hours, titrated by patient response and maternal pulse is used, it has been shown to be superior to oral ritodrine in preventing recurrent preterm labor and prolonging pregnancy.[11]

Maternal Side Effects
The limiting factor in the use of betamimetics is the maternal side effects. The clinical side effects reported are due to stimulation of beta-receptors throughout the body, they are often dose-related and consequently most apparent with intravenous administration. Serious maternal cardiopulmonary side effects seen with beta-adrenergic agents include hypotension, tachycardia, pulmonary edema, myocardial ischemia, arrhythmia and even maternal death. Although

Preterm Labor

83

the overall incidence of cardiac arrhythmias is low, supraventricular tachycardia without hemodynamic compromise is the most commonly seen arrhythmia. Rarely atrial fibrillation, premature atrial contractions and ventricular ectopy may occur. Electrocardiographic changes suggestive of ischemia have been noted.[12] However, these electrocardiographic changes are likely to be associated with beta–agonist induced tachycardia and hypokalemia and are not associated with elevations in cardiac isoenzymes and usually resolve when therapy is stopped. Patients may also have tremor (10–15%), palpitations (33%), nervousness (5–10%), or restlessness (5–10%).[13] Nausea, vomiting, headache, chest pain and shortness of breath have also been noted.[14] These symptoms are greatest when the infusion rate is increasing or at its maximum.

One of the most serious complications of beta-agonist therapy is pulmonary edema. Pulmonary edema may occur in about 3-5% of patients receiving parenteral ritodrine and has been associated with maternal death. The etiology may be multifactorial, including tachycardia, elevated cardiac output, excessive volume expansion, decreased plasma oncotic pressure and increased vascular permeability secondary to infection. Cardiogenic dysfunction does not appear to be responsible. Predisposing factors associated with this complication include multiple gestation, excessive fluid administration, blood transfusion, anemia, hypertension, polyhydramnios, and underlying cardiac disease.[15,16] More than 90% of reported cases occur after 24 hours of treatment. Pulse, blood pressure and respiratory status should be closely monitored and discontinuation of therapy be strongly considered with any respiratory distress or a heart rate greater than 120 beats per minute.

Metabolic complications seen with beta agonists include hyperglycemia and hypokalemia. Ketoacidosis can occur, especially with insulin-dependent diabetes and unrecognized gestational diabetes. A relative hypokalemia results from shift of potassium from the extracellular space to the intracellular space resulting from an increase in insulin and glucose concentrations, which drives potassium intracellularly. Potassium replacement is not required unless serum potassium decreases to less than 2.5 mEq/l. This condition generally resolves within 6–12 hours of discontinuing therapy.[17]

Fetal Side Effects

Beta-agonists cross the placenta and may cause beta-adrenergic responses in the fetus and neonate similar to those seen in the mother. During ritodrine infusion, the average fetal heart rate increase was from 0 to 9 beats per minute. Supraventricular tachycardia and atrial flutter have also been seen but these usually resolve within a few days to 2 weeks after cessation of therapy. Fetal cardiac septal hypertrophy has been described, the degree of which correlates with the duration of therapy and usually resolves within 3 months of age. Other, more serious fetal complications include hydrops, pulmonary edema, myocardial ischemia and cardiac failure. Neonatal hypoglycemia due to hyperinsulinism induced by beta-stimulation of the fetal pancreas has been associated with beta-adrenergic agents and it usually develops when delivery occurs within 2 days of treatment, it is usually transient. Neonatal hyperbilirubinemia and hypocalcemia have also been reported. Neonatal periventricular and intraventricular hemorrhage may be increased with beta-sympathomimetic therapy.[18]

Contraindications

Beta-agonists should be used with great caution. They should be avoided in patients with cardiac arrhythmias, poorly controlled thyrotoxicosis, poorly controlled diabetes mellitus, severe anemia, hypertension and those on digitalis treatment. In women with controlled diabetes serial evaluations of glucose, potassium and urine ketones should be done. Parenteral insulin infusion may be necessary in these women.

Efficacy

According to a recently published Cochrane review,[19] betamimetics are effective in delaying birth for 48 hours which is sufficient to allow the transfer of a woman to a higher level of care and to allow the administration of antenatal corticosteroids to facilitate fetal lung maturation. However, this benefit is balanced by more frequent unpleasant and sometimes potential life-threatening adverse effects. There is not enough evidence to suggest that one betamimetic agent is superior to another. Therefore, the choice of tocolysis should be based on maternal conditions, potential adverse effects, gestational age, and hospital facilities.

Magnesium Sulfate

Mechanism of Action

The exact mechanism by which magnesium sulfate acts is not well-known. The mechanism appears to be via the competitive inhibition of calcium at the voltage operated calcium channels at the plasma membrane of the myocytes leading to hyperpolarization of the membrane. Magnesium may directly compete with intracellular calcium by decreasing the calcium-calmodulin binding affinity to MLCK (myosin light chain kinase), thereby inhibiting myometrial contractility.[20-22]

Pharmacology/Dosage and Administration

Magnesium sulfate must be administered intravenously to achieve therapeutic levels, it is excreted primarily by the kidneys. The recommended dosing consists of an initial loading dose of 4-6 g intravenously over 20 minutes in

4

Preterm Labor

100 ml fluid followed by continuous maintenance infusion of 1-3 g per hour. Individual titration to uterine quiescence and maternal side effects is recommended. Maternal toxicity can be assessed clinically by monitoring the respiratory rate, deep tendon reflexes and urine output or by evaluation of serum magnesium concentrations which should be maintained in the range of 5-8 mg/dl which is considered therapeutic for inhibiting myometrial activity. Once uterine quiescence is achieved, the patient is generally maintained at the lowest effective infusion rate for 12–24 hours and then tapered and stopped.

Maternal Side Effects

Magnesium is relatively well-tolerated when compared with other tocolytic agents, especially betamimetics. Maternal side effects secondary to magnesium sulfate are typically dose-related. Symptoms commonly experienced with magnesium sulfate infusion include flushing, perception of warmth, nausea, emesis, dizziness, blurry vision, nystagmus and muscle weakness, diplopia, dryness of the mouth, lethargy and shortness of breath. Pulmonary edema has been reported in approximately 1% of women treated with magnesium sulfate and the risk is increased in patients with multifetal gestations and those receiving combined tocolytic therapy. These symptoms are maximal during the magnesium sulfate bolus infusion, but may persist for the duration of therapy. Serious toxic maternal side effects may occur at serum levels just slightly greater than therapeutic levels. Loss of patellar reflexes are seen at serum levels of 8 to 12 mg/dl, but respiratory difficulty and cardiac arrest are not seen until serum levels are 15 to 17 mg/dl and 30 to 35 mg/dl, respectively. Adverse effects may be minimized by closely monitoring urinary output, deep tendon reflexes, pulse rate, respiratory rate and pulmonary auscultation. On rare occasions, hypotension and loss of responsiveness can be seen with normal doses and nontoxic serum magnesium concentrations. The toxic effects of high magnesium levels can be rapidly reversed with the administration of 1 g of calcium gluconate slow intravenously.

Fetal/Neonatal Effects

Magnesium readily crosses the placenta, achieving fetal steady state levels within hours of the start of treatment and at delivery, neonatal concentrations are 10% lower than maternal concentrations. The transplacental transfer of magnesium sulfate may result in a nonreactive heart rate in 50% of the fetuses and decreased fetal breathing movements, but no effect was seen on fetal tone, movement and amniotic fluid volume.[23] Prolonged magnesium sulfate infusion to the mother may be associated with demineralization of bones, which was reported in 50% of infants whose mothers were treated with magnesium for more than 7 days.[24] Several observational reports have suggested a possible fetal neuroprotective effect and decreased incidence of cerebral palsy with antenatal magnesium sulfate treatment for preterm labor or preeclampsia in very low birth weight infants which needs to be confirmed.

Contraindications

Due to the risk of cardiorespiratory depression, magnesium sulfate infusion should be avoided in patients with myasthenia gravis, heart block and myocardial damage. Caution should be taken when administering magnesium sulfate to women with renal disease and recent myocardial infarction. Concurrent use of calcium channel blockers and magnesium sulfate can theoretically result in profound hypotension and probably should be avoided, especially because there is no evidence of greater efficacy for combination treatment relative to either treatment used alone.[25]

Efficacy

Though magnesium sulfate has been widely used as a tocolytic for many years, systematic review by Cochrane revealed the surprising fact that the evidence to support it's use was sparse and generally of poor quality. The currently available evidence shows magnesium sulfate to be ineffective in delaying preterm birth and thus it cannot be recommended as a tocolytic agent for women in preterm labor. However, it was less likely than betamimetics to cause maternal side effects, although compared with other tocolytics it was more likely to cause maternal side effects. Moreover, there was no evidence of any substantial improvements in neonatal morbidity. A nonsignificant reduction in the risk of cerebral palsy was reported at follow up at 18 months corrected age.[26]

Prostaglandin Synthetase Inhibitors

Mechanism of Action

Prostaglandins are 20-carbon cyclopentane carboxylic acids derived from membrane phospholipids (primarily arachidonic acid) via the enzymatic action of phospholipase A and cyclooxygenase (prostaglandin synthetase). Prostaglandins have been shown to have a significant role in the labor process. Prostaglandins stimulate myometrial gap junction formation and raise intracellular calcium levels by increasing calcium influx across the cell membrane and stimulating calcium release from the sarcoplasmic reticulum. Prostaglandin synthetase inhibitors are reversible competitive inhibitors of cyclooxygenase, blocking the conversion of free arachidonic acid to prostaglandin. Because prostaglandin E and F series are mediators of uterine contractions, a decrease in production results in decreased contractile activity therefore, this pathway represents a key target for pharmacological intervention. Indomethacin is the most commonly used agent in this class, but other agents such as sulindac and ketorolac are also undergoing investigation.

Indomethacin: Indomethacin is usually administered orally or rectally. A loading dose of 50-100 mg is followed by 25 mg orally every 4-6 hours for 48 hours, a total 24-hour dose not greater than 200 mg.[27,28] Indomethacin is rapidly absorbed after oral administration. Indomethacin is metabolized extensively by the liver and 10% is excreted unchanged in the urine.

Ketorolac: Ketorolac may be administered intramuscularly as an initial dose of 60 mg, followed-up by subsequent doses of 30 mg every 6 hours as needed to result in uterine quiescence up to 48 hours.

Sulindac: Sulindac is a prodrug that is converted to an active metabolite in the liver and has a half-life as long as 16 hours. It is excreted in the urine in an inactive form and is reported to be relatively renal sparing. Sulindac is administered 200 mg orally every 12 hours for 48 hours. Peak plasma concentrations are attained within 2 hours after oral dosage.

Maternal Side Effects

The maternal side effects seen with indomethacin are minimal and are generally well-tolerated. The most common side effects are mild nausea, vomiting and heartburn, seen in approximately 4% of treated women and these can usually be relieved by taking the medication with meals or using an antacid. The maternal cardiovascular system is not affected.

Neonatal Side Effects

The potential for fetal and neonatal side effects is the source of concern for this class of tocolytics. Indomethacin readily crosses the placenta, appearing in the fetal bloodstream within 15 minutes with fetal levels equilibrating with maternal concentrations about 5 hours after administration.[29] Indomethacin has been associated with potentially serious side effects such as constriction of the fetal ductus arteriosus which can lead to pulmonary hypertension, reversible decrease in renal function with oligohydramnios, intraventricular hemorrhage, necrotizing enterocolitis and hyper-bilirubinemia. However, these complications have been reported when exposure to indomethacin exceeds 48 hours. The sensitivity of the ductus arteriosus to these agents increases after 32 weeks, with more than 50% of fetuses showing ductal constriction as compared with 5–10% before 32 weeks, therefore, indomethacin is not recommended after 32 week gestation. Fetal echocardiographic evaluation should be considered if the duration of therapy exceeds 48-72 hours to monitor the patency of the ductus arteriosus.[30]

Fetal urine output has been shown to decrease in 5–10% of patients treated with indomethacin, an effect mediated by antidiuretic hormone. Long-term therapy may result in the development of oligohydramnios, although the timing of the onset is unpredictable. Oligohydramnios is reversible when the dose is decreased or discontinued, resolution usually occurs within 48-96 hours of discontinuation of treatment.[31] Therefore the amniotic fluid index should be followed while the patient is receiving long-term therapy and if the amniotic fluid index falls below 5 cm, therapy is usually discontinued. However, persistent anuria, renal microcystic lesions and neonatal death have been reported with prenatal indomethacin exposure to doses greater than 200 mg per day for more than 48 hours without adequate amniotic fluid assessment. Bedside ultrasonography to rule out oligohydramnios should be considered before initiation of therapy with these agents.

Some reports have suggested that *in utero* exposure to indomethacin is a risk factor for necrotizing enterocolitis and intraventricular hemorrhage, grades III to IV, which has not been proved in other trials.[32,33]

Contraindications

Maternal contraindications to indomethacin use include patients with significant renal or hepatic impairment, active peptic ulcer disease, nonsteroidal anti inflammatory drug sensitive asthma, coagulation disorders, thrombocytopenia or other sensitivity to nonsteroidal agents. Fetal contraindications include pre-existing oligohydramnios and congenital fetal heart disease in which the fetal circulation is dependent on the ductus arteriosus.

Efficacy

According to a systematic review cyclooxygenase (COX) inhibitors inhibit uterine contractions, are easily administered and have fewer maternal side effects compared to conventional tocolytics. However, adverse effects have been reported on the fetus and newborn as a result of exposure to COX inhibitors. The results of this review show that, COX inhibitors were not associated with improvements in neonatal mortality or any markers of neonatal morbidity. There is insufficient information on which to base decisions about the value of cyclooxygenase (COX) inhibition for women in preterm labor.[34]

Calcium Channel Antagonists

Mechanism of Action

Nifedipine is the most common calcium channel blocker used for tocolysis. These agents inhibit the influx of calcium ions through the voltage-dependent calcium channels in the muscle cell membrane and reduce uterine vascular resistance. They may also inhibit release of intracellular calcium from sarcolemmal stores and increase calcium efflux from the cell. The resultant decrease in intracellular-free calcium leads to inhibition of calcium-dependent MLCK phosphorylation and results in decreased myometrial activity.

Nifedipine is administered orally and sublingually and is nearly completely absorbed from the gastrointestinal tract after ingestion. Onset of action after oral nifedipine is less than 20 minutes and maximum plasma concentrations occur within 15-90 minutes after oral administration.[35,36] Onset appears somewhat faster with sublingual dosing. Nifedipine is almost completely metabolized in the liver and 70-80% is excreted by the kidneys and 30% through bowel. An appropriate dosing regimen of nifedipine for the treatment of preterm labor has not been demonstrated and different dosing regimens were used in various study protocols. One recommended regimen is to administer 10 mg orally every 20 minutes for up to four doses followed by 20 mg orally every 4-8 hours.[37] Others have administered an initial loading dose of 30 mg, followed-up by 10 to 20 mg doses every 4-6 hours.

Maternal Side Effects

Nifedipine is a peripheral vasodilator and can result in symptoms of dizziness, light-headedness, flushing, nausea, headache, peripheral edema and palpitations. Nifedipine is also associated with transient hypotension, because of arteriolar smooth muscle relaxation with a reflex increase in maternal pulse of 10 beats per minute . The incidence of these side effects is approximately 17%, with severe effects resulting in the discontinuation of therapy in 2-5% of patients.[38] Close monitoring of maternal vital signs is recommended, as well as assuring adequate maternal hydration is important.

Fetal/Neonatal Effects

Calcium channel blockers can cross the placenta. One concern is the potential adverse effect calcium channel blockers may have on uteroplacental blood flow, as has been reported in animal studies, but it has not been demonstrated in human studies.[39]

Contraindications

Contraindications to the use of nifedipine or any of the calcium channel blockers include hypotension, congestive heart failure and aortic stenosis. Concomitant use with magnesium sulfate should be avoided because of reports of neuromuscular blockade and profound hypotension.

Efficacy

According to a systematic review comparing the effects of calcium channel blockers (mainly nifedipine) with other tocolytic agents (mainly betamimetics), calcium channel blockers were reported to be more effective tocolytic agents (less births within seven days of initation of treatment and before 34 weeks gestation) with improvement in some clinically important neonatal outcomes (less respiratory distress syndrome, intraventricular hemorrhage, necrotizing enterocolitis and jaundice) and a marked reduction in adverse maternal side effects. Also, there is the advantage of oral formulation. They concluded that when tocolysis is indicated for women in preterm labor, calcium channel blockers are preferable to other tocolytic agents compared, mainly betamimetics.[40]

Oxytocin Antagonists

Mechanism of Action

Atosiban is a selective oxytocin-vasopressin receptor antagonist capable of inhibiting oxytocin induced myometrial contractions. The mechanism appears to be competitive inhibition of oxytocin receptors in the myometrium and decidua. Oxytocin stimulates contractions by stimulating the conversion of phosphatidylinositol to inositol triphosphate. This binds to a protein in the sarcoplasmic reticulum leading to calcium release into the cytoplasm. Thus, oxytocin antagonists result in a decrease in intracellular free calcium that results in decreased myometrial contractility.

Dosage and Administration

Atosiban is a nonapeptide. Atosiban has not been approved by the Food and Drug Administration, but is licensed in the UK for treatment of threatened preterm labor. Atosiban is typically administered intravenously, beginning with a single bolus of 6.75 mg over one minute, followed immediately by a 300 μg/min intravenous infusion for 3 hours and then 100 μg/min for up to 45 hours.[41] Atosiban is not active orally.

Maternal Side Effects

A potential advantage of atosiban is it being highly organ specific for the myometrium and fetal membranes, thus minimizing side effects. Infusion of atosiban for 12 hours has been well tolerated. Side effects include nausea, vomiting, headache, chest pain, and dysgeusia.[42] Discontinuation because of side effects was not required in any patients. No clinically observable antidiuretic effects have been noted.

Fetal Side Effects

Atosiban crosses the placenta. There is only a small data pool to examine neonatal outcomes, but so far, no effect on umbilical cord gases and no observable antidiuretic effects on the newborn have been seen.

Nitric Oxide Donors

Nitric oxide is a potent endogenous hormone that facilitates smooth muscle relaxation in the vasculature, the gut and the uterus. Nitric oxide donors which have been used for tocolysis include nitroglycerin and glycerol trinitrate.

Nitric oxide donors, activate the cyclic guanosine monophosphate pathway involved in smooth muscle relaxation. The activation of cyclic guanosine monophosphate results in decreased intracellular free calcium that leads to decreased activation of MLCK and decreased myometrial contractility.

Pharmacology/Dosage and Administration

Nitric oxide donors have been administered intravenously and by transdermal patch. The dosing and administration have varied in studies, but are primarily titrated to cessation of contractions while maintaining adequate blood pressure. The transdermal regimen used is an initial 10 mg transdermal glyceryl trinitrate patch applied to the skin of the abdomen. If after 1 hour, there was no reduction in contraction frequency or strength, an additional patch was applied. No more than two patches were administered simultaneously and these were left in place for 24 hours after which they were removed and patient reassessed.

Maternal Side Effects

The primary side effect is maternal hypotension related to smooth muscle relaxation of blood vessels. Symptoms included headache, light-headedness, nausea and vomiting. Clinical use of these agents for the treatment of preterm labor remains experimental.

Fetal/Neonatal Effects

There are no clear data indicating that nitric oxide donor therapy adversely affects the infant.

Contraindications

Preexisting maternal hypotension.

Combination Tocolytic Therapy

Few studies have assessed the concomitant use of two labor inhibiting agents. While there was a suggestion of improved efficacy in one trial[43] this has not been supported by other trials.[44] Side effects with combined regimen were found to be significantly increased. Given the limited and conflicting data on efficacy and safety, it is not recommended to use combined therapy for labor inhibition.

Maintenance Tocolytic Therapy

Patients who are successfully treated for an acute episode of preterm labor remain at risk for having recurrent episodes of preterm labor. Maintenance tocolytic therapy has been used in these patients with the hope that the risk of recurrence will decrease. But a meta analysis has shown that maintenance tocolytic therapy was not associated with a significant reduction in the rates of recurrent preterm labor or preterm delivery.[45]

Summary of Tocolytics

Thus to summarize, although treatment with tocolytics can significantly reduce the rate of delivery within 48 hours and 7 days, they have not been shown to improve perinatal outcomes, but do have adverse health effects on women.[46] However, they do appear to delay delivery long enough for successful administration of corticosteroids. Therefore, as a general rule, if tocolytics are given, they should be given concomitantly with corticosteroids. Candidates for labor inhibition must be evaluated and chosen carefully with the goals of labor inhibition clearly defined in each situation. Though the ideal tocolytic agent has not yet been discovered, the choice of pharmacologic agent must be tailored to the individual patient with particular attention to side effects of and contraindications to these potent medications so as to choose the tocolytic most suitable to the individual patient. Maternal and fetal status should be closely monitored with frequent reassessment during therapy to identify the evolution of contraindications to labor inhibition, such as infection and specific side effects and toxicities. Labor inhibition therapy should be stopped if the risks outweigh the benefits of continuing therapy. A recent metaanalysis has performed a quantitative analysis of randomized controlled trials of tocolysis and concluded that prostaglandin inhibitors were superior to the other agents and may be considered the optimal first-line agent before 32 weeks of gestation to delay delivery.[47]

Conduct of Labor and Delivery

These women should deliver in a tertiary care setting equipped with neonatal intensive care unit. These babies are at an increased risk of intrapartum asphyxia and there should be relatively low threshold for delivery by cesarean in presence of fetal heart rate abnormalities. Apgar scores are often low in these babies due to physiologically immature nervous system. This needs to be differentiated from asphyxia by routine cord blood pH. The route of delivery of very low birth weight infants is debatable and there is no conclusive evidence of a benefit of routine cesarean delivery. A recent Cochrane review infers that the limited evidence available suggests that cesarean section may have beneficial effects for the baby.[48] However, this needs to be weighed against the higher morbidity in the mother for which the evidence was not sufficient. During cesarean section it is important to ascertain that the uterine incision is adequate for extracting the fetus without delay to avoid unnecessary trauma. This often requires a vertical incision especially when the lower uterine segment is incompletely developed. During vaginal delivery a generous episiotomy should be considered, especially if the perineum is rigid to reduce the risk of injury. There is no evidence supporting elective forceps delivery for protecting the fetal head.

NEONATAL OUTCOME

The prognosis for the preterm infant depends on the level of neonatal care in the delivery room and nursery. The gestational age is a more important predictor of neonatal outcome as compared to the weight. The babies require to be monitored for side effects due to tocolytic agents. Even in babies who survive, there is a risk of short-term and long-term morbidity. Some associated conditions are acute and amenable to treatment but others such as cerebral palsy, neurodevelopmental delay and pulmonary disorders can result in long-term severe disability.

Neonatal morbidity and survival varies widely across centers depending on facilities making generalization difficult. However a rough guide is presented below to facilitate decision making and counseling.

Gestational age (weeks)	Birth weight (grams)	Survivors (%)	Intact survivors* (%)
24-25	500-750	60	35
25-27	751-1000	75	60
28-29	1001-1250	90	80
30-31	1251-1500	96	90
32-33	1501-1750	99	98
>34	1751-2000	100	99

*Intact defined as not blind, deaf, retarded, or with cerebral palsy.

The problems of prematurity which are related to difficulty in extrauterine adaptation due to immaturity of organ systems include the following:

Respiratory: Apnea, hyaline membrane disease, bronchopulmonary dysplasia

Neurologic: Perinatal depression, intracranial hemorrhage

Cardiovascular: Hypotension, patent ductus arteriosus, congestive heart failure

Hematologic: Anemia, hyperbilirubinemia

Gastrointestinal: Necrotizing enterocolitis

Metabolic: Hypoglycemia, hypocalcemia

Renal: Acid base and electrolyte imbalance due to low glomerular filtration rate

Temperature regulation: Hypothermia, hyperthermia

Immunologic: Increased risk of infection

Ophthalmologic: Retinopathy of prematurity.

KEY POINTS

- Preterm birth is defined as delivery of the baby after the period of viability and before 37 weeks of pregnancy.
- Preterm birth complicates 10-15% of all pregnancies and is a leading cause of neonatal morbidity and mortality.
- Idiopathic preterm labor accounts for about 40% of all preterm births.
- Assessment of risk of preterm delivery should be done at each antenatal visit concentrating on identification of modifiable risk factors.
- Five etiopathogenic mechanisms identified include—premature activation of HPA axis, uterine overdistention, infection, decidual hemorrhage and cervical factors.
- Clinical criteria of diagnosis include—
  1. Four contractions in 20 minutes or eight in 60 minutes and progressive change in cervix.
  2. Cervical dilatation greater than 1 cm.
  3. Cervical effacement of 80% or greater.
- Diagnostic goals are to identify etiology and to differentiate true from false preterm labor.
- Cervical length estimation by ultrasound along with fetal fibronectin testing have been used to differentiate true from false preterm labor. A negative fibronectin and a long cervix > 1.5 cm are strong negative predictors of imminent preterm birth.
- Therapeutic goal is to identify the subgroup of women who will benefit from tocolysis and corticosteroids.
- Pregnancies between 24 to 34 weeks of gestation or estimated fetal weight between 600 to 2500 gms with no evidence of infection, benefit from tocolysis.
- Once a pregnancy has continued beyond 34 weeks fetal survival rate is within 1% of the term survival and long-term sequelae are rare. Hence steroids and tocolysis may not provide additional benefit.
- Acute tocolysis should be used to allow enough time for the effect of steroids after ruling out contraindications.
- There is limited role of bed rest, hydration and sedation in these women.
- Antibiotics are indicated only for those with documented infection, for GBS prophylaxis and in women with preterm PROM.
- These women should deliver in a tertiary care setting equipped with neonatal intensive care unit.
- The route of delivery of very low birth weight infants is debatable and there is no conclusive evidence of a benefit of routine cesarean delivery.

4

Preterm Labor

1. Iams JD. Early detection of preterm birth in Protocols for High Risk Pregnancies Queenan JT, Hobbins JC, Spong CY 2005 (4 Eds), Blackwell Publishing Limited Oxford UK 467-74.
2. Ou CW, Chen ZQ, Qi S,Lye SJ: Increased expression of the rat myometrial oxytocin receptor messenger ribonucleic acid during labor requires both mechanical and hormonal signals. Biol Reprod 1998;59:1055.
3. Iams JD, Roberto Romero. Preterm Birth, Obstetrics Normal and Problem Pregnancies 5th (Eds) Gabbe SG, Niebyl JR, Simpron JL, Churchill Living-stone Elseivier: Philadelphia, 2007.
4. Anderson HF, Nugent CE, Wanty SE, et al. Prediction of risk for preterm delivery by ultrasonographic measurement of cervical length. Am J Obstet Gynaecol 1990;163:859.
5. Kaufman RH, Adam ERVI, Hatch EE, et al. Continued follow up of pregnancy outcome in DES- exposed offspring. Obstet Gynaeco 2000;l96:483.
6. Raga Faiz, Bauset C, Remohi J, et al. Reproductive impact of congenital Mullerian anomalies. Hum Reproduction 1997;12,2277.
7. Iams JD, Johnson FF, Sonek J, et al. Cervical competence as a continuum: A study of ultrasonographic cervical length and obstetric performance. Am J Obstet Gynaecol 1995;172:1097.
8. Crowther CA, Harding JE. Repeat doses of prenatal corticosteroids for women at risk of preterm birth for preventing neonatal respiratory disease.Cochrane Database of Systematic Reviews 2007, Issue 3. Art. No.: CD003935. DOI: 10.1002/14651858.CD003935.pub2.
9. Caritis SN, Venkataramanan R, Darby MJ, et al. Pharmacokinetics of ritodrine administered intravenously. Recommendations for changes in the current regimen. Am J Obstet Gynecol. 1990;162:429–37.
10. The Canadian Preterm Labor Investigators' Group. The treatment of preterm labor with beta-adrenergic agonist ritodrine. N Engl J Med 1992;327:308–12.
11. Caritis S, Toig G, Heddinger L, et al. A double-blind study comparing ritodrine and terbutaline in the treatment of preterm labor. Am J Obstet Gynecol 1984;150:7–14.
12. Benedetti T. Maternal complications of parenteral beta sympathomimetic therapy for preterm labor. Am J Obstet Gynecol 1983;145:1–6.
13. Barden TP, Peter JB, Merkatz IR. Ritodrine hydrochloride: A betamimetic agent for use in preterm labor I. Obstet Gynecol 1980;56:1–6.
14. Hearne, Amy E. Nagey, David A. Therapeutic agents in preterm labor: Tocolytic Agents.Clinical Obs and Gynae 2000;787-801.
15. Lam F, Elliot J, Jones JS, et al. Clinical issues surrounding the use of terbutaline sulfate for preterm labor. Obstet Gynecol Surv 1998;53(11):S85–S95.
16. Benedetti TJ. Maternal complications of parenteral sympathomimetic therapy for premature labor. Am J Obstet Gynecol 1983;145(1):1–6.
17. Kirkpatrick C, Qeunon M, Desir D. Blood anions and electrolytes during ritodrine infusion in preterm labor. Am J Obstet Gynecol 1980;138:523.
18. Groome LJ, Goldenberg RL, Cliver SP,et al. Neonatal periventricular-intraventricular hemorrhage after maternal beta-sympathomimetic tocolysis. The March of Dimes Multicenter Study Group. Am J Obstet Gynecol 1992;167:873.
19. Anotayanonth S, Subhedar NV, Neilson JP, Harigopal S. Betamimetics for inhibiting preterm labor. Cochrane Database of Systematic Reviews 2004, Issue 4. Art. No.: CD004352. DOI: 10.1002/14651858.CD004352.pub2.
20. Monga M, Creasy RK. Pharmacologic management of preterm labor. Semin Perinatol 1995; 19:84–96.
21. Sanborn BM. Ion channels and the control of myometrial electrical activity. Semin Perinatol. 1995; 19:31.
22. Ohki S, Ikura M, Zhang M. Identification of magnesium binding sites and the role of magnesium on target recognition by calmodulin. Biochemistry 1997;36:4309–16.
23. Peaceman AM, Meyer BA, Thorp JA,et al. The effect of magnesium tocolysis on the fetal biophysical profile. Am J Obstet Gynecol 1989;161:771-74.
24. Holcomb WL Jr, Shackelford GD, Petrie RH. Magnesium tocolysis and neonatal bone abnormalities: A controlled study. Obstet Gynecol 1991;78:611.
25. Ben-Ami M, Giladi Y, Shalev E. The combination of magnesium sulfate and nifedipine: A cause of neuromuscular blockade. Br J Obstet Gynaecol 1994;101:262–63.

26. Crowther CA, Hiller JE, Doyle LW. Magnesium sulphate for preventing preterm birth in threatened preterm labor. Cochrane Database of Systematic Reviews 2002, Issue 4. Art. No.: CD001060. DOI:
27. Niebyl JR, Blake DA, White RD, et al. The inhibition of premature labor with indomethacin. Am J Obstet Gynecol 1980; 44:787–90.
28. Zuckerman H, Shalev E, Gilad G, et al. Further study of the inhibition of premature labor by indomethacin. Part II double-blind study. J Perinat Med 1984;12:25–30.
29. Neibyl JR. Prostaglandin synthetase inhibitors. Semin Perinatol 1981;5:274.
30. Jeyabalan and Arun, Caritis, Steve N.Pharmacologic Inhibition of Preterm Labor. Clinical Obstetrics and Gynae 2002;45(1):99–113.
31. Walker MP, Moore TR, Cheung CY, et al. Indomethacin-induced urinary flow rate reduction in the ovine fetus is associated with reduced free water clearance and elevated plasma arginine vasopressin levels. Am J Obstet Gynecol 1992;167:1723–31.
32. Souter D, Harding J, McCowan L, et al. Antenatal indomethacin-adverse fetal effects confirmed. Aust N Z J Obstet Gynaecol 1998;38:11–16.
33. Gardner M, Owen J, Skelly S, et al. Preterm delivery after indomethacin: A risk factor for neonatal complications? J Reprod Med 1996;41:903–6.
34. King J, Flenady V, Cole S, Thornton S. Cyclo-oxygenase (COX) inhibitors for treating preterm labor.Cochrane Database of Systematic Reviews 2005, Issue 2. Art. No.: CD001992. DOI.
35. Garcia-Velasco JA, Gonzalez GA. A prospective randomized trial of nifedipine vs. ritodrine in threatened preterm labor. Int J Gynaecol Obstet 1998;61: 239–44.
36. Ferguson JE, Schutz T, Pershe R,et al. Nifedipine pharmacokinetics in preterm labor tocolysis. Am J Obstet Gynecol 1989;161(1):1485–90.
37. Papatsonis DN, Van Geijn HP, Ader HJ, et al. Nifedipine and ritodrine in the management of preterm labor: A randomized multicenter trial. Obstet Gynecol 1997;90:230–34.
38. Goldenberg, Robert L.The Management of Preterm Labor. Obstet Gynaecol. November 2002;100 (5, Part 1), 1020–37.
39. Mari G, Kirshon B, Moise KJ, et al. Doppler assessment of the fetal and uteroplacental circulation during nifedipine therapy for preterm labor. Am J Obstet Gynecol 1989; 161: 1514–18.
40. King JF, Flenady VJ, Papatsonis DNM, Dekker GA, Carbonne B. Calcium channel blockers for inhibiting preterm labor. Cochrane Database of Systematic Reviews 2003, Issue 1. Art. No.: CD002255. DOI: 10.1002/14651858.CD002255.
41. Romero R, Sibai BM, Sanchez-Ramos L, et al. An oxytocin receptor antagonist (atosiban) in the treatment of preterm labor: A randomized, double-blind, placebo-controlled trial with tocolytic rescue. Am J Obstet Gynecol. 2000; 182:1173–83.
42. Goodwin TM, Valenzuela G, Silver H,et al. Treatment of preterm labor with the oxytocin antagonist atosiban. Am J Perinatol 1996;13:143–46.
43. Hatjis C, Swain M, Nelson L, et al. Efficacy of combined administration of magnesium sulfate and ritodrine in the treatment of preterm labor. Obstet Gynecol 1987;69:317–22.
44. Ferguson J, Hensleigh P, Kredenster D. Adjunctive use of magnesium sulfate with ritodrine for preterm labor tocolysis. Am J Obstet Gynecol. 1984; 148:166–71.
45. Sanchez-Ramos L, Kaunitz AM, Gaudier FL,et al. Efficacy of maintenance therapy after acute tocolysis: A meta-analysis. Am J Obstet Gynecol. 1999; 181 (2): 484–90.
46. Gyetvai K, Hannah ME, Hodnett ED, Ohlsson A. Tocolytics for preterm labor: A systematic review. Obstet Gynecol 1999;94:869–77.
47. Haas, David, Imperiale, Thomas, Kirkpatrick, Page, Klein, Robert, Zollinger, Terrell, Golichowski, Alan, Tocolytic Therapy: A Meta-Analysis and Decision Analysis. Obstet and Gynecol. 2009;113(3):585-94.
48. Grant A, Glazener CMA. Elective caesarean section versus expectant management for delivery of the small baby. Cochrane Database of Systematic Reviews2001, Issue 2. Art. No.: CD000078. DOI: 10.1002/14651858.CD000078.

4

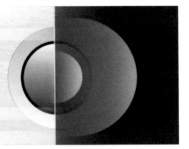

Premature Rupture of Membranes

5

Sharda Patra

DEFINITION AND INCIDENCE

Premature rupture of membranes or prelabor rupture of membrane (PROM) is rupture of fetal membranes in the absence of uterine contractions regardless of gestational age.[1,2] PROM occurring after 37 completed weeks of gestation is known as term PROM and that occurring before 37 weeks is preterm PROM (PPROM). The overall incidence of premature rupture of the fetal membranes (PROM) is 5-10% of all pregnancies.[2] The incidence of term PROM is 8% and preterm PROM is 2-4%. Preterm PROM is the leading cause of premature birth and accounts for approximately 18 to 20% of perinatal deaths.[2]

ETIOPATHOGENESIS

A number of mechanisms have been proposed for PROM. These are intrinsic membrane weakness due to defect in collagen synthesis, increased collagen degradation, ascending infection and mechanical stress due to distention.

The tensile strength of fetal membranes is maintained by a balance between the synthesis and degradation of the various components of the extracellular matrix. The degradation of collagen is mediated primarily by matrix metalloproteinases (MMP) which are inhibited by a specific tissue inhibitor of metalloproteinase-1 (TIMP-1) and other protease inhibitors. When there is an imbalance between the activities of matrix metalloproteinases predominantly MMP-9 and their tissue inhibitors, there is degradation of extracellular matrix of the membrane causing rupture.[4] Conditions which cause weakening of the fetal membranes are local infection and inflammation, poor maternal nutrition, deficiency of copper and vitamin C, maternal smoking and collagen deficiency syndromes like Ehlers–Danlos syndrome.[3]

Choriodecidual inflammation has an important role in preterm PROM, particularly when membranes rupture remote from term. Certain strains of bacteria predominantly hemolytic streptococci, *Chlamydia trachomatis*, *Neisseria gonorrheae*, *Trichomonas vaginalis*, *Gardnerella vaginalis*, *Mobiluncus* species and genital mycoplasma harbored in the lower genital tract, ascend through the cervical canal and cause localized inflammation with production of proteolytic enzymes like collagenase, elastase and gelatinase. These enzymes cause local weakening of the membranes. This is subsequently followed by release of prostaglandins which lead to occult contractions and increased shearing stress at the internal cervical os.[3]

Mechanical distention of the membranes near the internal os as seen in polyhydramnios, twin gestation, trauma and incompetent cervix causes stretching of the fetal membranes which in turn up-regulates the production of prostaglandin E_2. Prostaglandin E_2 increases uterine irritability, decreases synthesis of fetal membrane collagen and increases production of matrix metalloproteinases (MMP-1 and MMP-3) and interleukin-8 which stimulate collagenase activity. Stretch also increases MMP-1 activity within the membranes.[4]

FACTORS PREDISPOSING TO PROM

The various factors which can predispose a woman to PROM are listed in Table 5.1.[2,5] However, most often preterm PROM occurs in otherwise healthy women without an identifiable risk factor.[2] Of the various predisposing factors, women with previous history of preterm PROM have a 14-fold increased risk of developing preterm PROM and three-fold increased risk of preterm birth in subsequent pregnancy. There is a three to seven-fold risk of PROM in

Table 5.1: Predisposing factors for premature rupture of membranes[2,5]		
Obstetric history		*Medical /surgical factors*
Past pregnancy	*Present pregnancy*	
• Preterm premature rupture of membranes (PROM) • Preterm labor	• Vaginal infections • Antepartum vaginal bleeding 2nd, 3rd trimester • Placental abruption • Advanced cervical dilatation (cervical insufficiency) • Cervical shortening in the 2nd trimester (< 2.5 cm) • Uterine overdistention (polyhydramnios, multiple pregnancy) • Procedures—amniocentesis, chorinic villus sampling	• Collagen vascular disorders (such as Ehlers-Danlos syndrome, systemic lupus erythematosus) • Cigarette smoking • Nutritional deficiencies of copper and ascorbic acid • Prior cervical conization

women with history of second or third-trimester bleeding in index pregnancy.[2] A short cervix (< 25 mm) on transvaginal ultrasonography with a positive fetal fibronectin is also associated with preterm PROM in both nulliparous and multiparous women.[6] There is a strong link between hypertension, diabetes mellitus, amnionitis and abruption in current pregnancy and PROM.[7] Women with Ehlers-Danlos syndrome are highly susceptible to PROM, but interestingly there is no correlation between Marfan syndrome and PROM despite the fact that both are collagen deficiency syndromes.[2,7] Presence of trichomoniasis and group B streptococcal infection strongly predisposes to PROM. However, a weaker link between PROM and bacterial vaginosis has been reported.[7-9] The risk of PROM increases to two- to four-fold among smokers compared to non-smokers. Certain procedures like amniocentesis and chorionic villus sampling also cause PROM in 1.2 percent and 0.7 percent of pregnant women respectively.[10] Factors like sexual intercourse, speculum examination, maternal exercise and parity are not known to be associated with preterm PROM.[11]

CLINICAL PRESENTATION AND DIAGNOSIS

Women with PROM present with a typical history of sudden gush of clear or pale yellow fluid from the vagina. However, many women may present with history of intermittent or constant leaking of small amounts of fluid or just a sensation of wetness within the vagina or on the perineum. In the initial evaluation it is essential to note the duration, amount and persistence of fluid leakage. Conditions like urinary incontinence, recent vaginal or cervical infection, recent sexual activity and douching should be ruled out for a correct diagnosis. Timely and accurate diagnosis of PROM allows for gestational age-specific obstetric intervention and is critical to optimize pregnancy outcome. A false positive diagnosis of PROM especially preterm PROM may lead to unnecessary obstetric intervention, including hospitalization, administration of antibiotics and corticosteroids and even induction of labor.

Per Speculum Examination

The next step in the diagnosis of PROM includes a sterile per speculum examination to demonstrate leaking. Pooling of fluid in the posterior fornix or leakage of fluid from the cervical os confirms the diagnosis of PROM. If no amniotic fluid is immediately visible, the woman is asked to push or do valsalva maneuver or cough to express amniotic fluid from the cervical os. A sterile speculum examination not only helps in the diagnosis of PROM but also allows for inspection of the cervix for any local cervical lesion like cervicitis, cord prolapse, cervical dilatation and effacement and also to take sample for cultures. A per vaginum examination should not be done as it increases the risk of intrauterine infection and preterm labor.[12] Moreover, per vaginum examination adds little to the information obtained by the speculum examination unless the patient is in active labor or immediate delivery is planned. At times the findings at speculum examination are doubtful or equivocal. In these women two simple and practical bed side tests, nitrazine test and fern test can help to diagnose PROM.

Nitrazine Test

This is based on the principle of differentiating amniotic fluid from the vaginal secretions by the pH. Amniotic fluid has a pH ranging from 7.0 to 7.7 compared to the acidic vaginal pH in pregnancy of 3.8 to 4.2. Nitrazine test is positive when a yellow nitrazine paper turns blue by coming in contact with amniotic fluid. However, in 5% of cases the result can be either false positive or false negative. It is false positive in the presence of alkaline fluids in the vagina, such as blood, seminal fluid, soap or bacterial vaginosis whereas with intermittent prolonged leakage or if the amniotic fluid is diluted by other vaginal fluids it is false negative. Hence the sensitivity and specificity of this test in diagnosing PROM ranges from 90 to 97% and 16 to 70%, respectively.[13]

Fern Test (Fig. 5.1)

This is another test to confirm presence of amniotic fluid in the vagina. Fluid from the posterior vaginal fornix is swabbed onto a glass slide and allowed to dry for at least 10 minutes. Amniotic fluid produces a delicate ferning pattern in contrast to the thick and wide arborization pattern of dried cervical mucus. This method, however, is not sufficiently accurate. It may produce false results in as many as 30 percent of the cases. False positive fern test may result from well estrogenized cervical mucus or a fingerprint on the microscope slide. False negative result can be due to inadequate amniotic fluid on the swab or heavy contamination with vaginal discharge or blood.

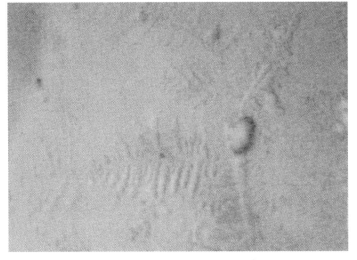

Figure 5.1: Ferning pattern in PROM

Though these two tests are very simple and easy to perform, the main drawback with these two tests is their high rate of inaccuracy which increases progressively when more than one hour has elapsed since membranes rupture and the tests become inconclusive after 24 hours.[14] In cases where PROM is prolonged or associated with oligohydramnios, examination by ultrasound may be of value in supporting the diagnosis of PROM.

Ultrasonography

Evidence of diminished amniotic fluid volume either by clinical examination or by ultrasound alone cannot confirm the diagnosis, but may help to suggest PROM in an appropriate clinical setting. Approximately 50 to 70% of women with PROM have low amniotic fluid volume on initial ultrasonography. The presence of anhydramnios or severe oligohydramnios combined with a characteristic history of leaking per vaginum is highly suggestive of rupture of membranes. However, conditions causing anhydramnios or oligohydramnios, for example renal agenesis, obstructive uropathy, or severe utero-placental insufficiency should be excluded before the diagnosis of PROM is made on the basis of ultrasonography.[15]

Indigo Carmine Test

Another method of confirming PROM is instillation of 1 ml indigo carmine diluted in 9 ml of sterile saline into the amniotic cavity transabdominally under ultrasound guidance. Blue staining of a tampon kept vaginally after one and half hour indicates leakage of amniotic fluid.

Newer Tests

Owing to the limitations of the conventional tests for diagnosis of PROM newer and more objective tests have been emerging. These tests are based primarily on the identification of one or more biochemical markers in the cervicovaginal discharge. Several such markers like alpha-fetoprotein, fetal fibronectin, insulin-like growth factor binding protein-1 (IGFBP-1), prolactin, subunit of human chorionic gonadotropin, creatinine, urea, lactate, placental alpha microglobulin-1 (PAMG-1) can be identified. As a general rule, these tests are either too invasive or too cumbersome or too expensive to have a routine application in clinical practice. However, the tests based on detection of proteomic markers like placental alpha microglobulin-1 have come up with very convincing results.

Amnisure test is a FDA approved, new immunoassay slide test for detection of placental alpha microglobulin-1. This test is simple, easy to perform, rapid (takes about 5-10 minutes), noninvasive and does not require a speculum examination. In this test sterile swab is inserted into the vagina for one minute and placed into a vial containing a solvent for one minute. An Amnisure test strip is dipped into the vial and the test result is revealed by the presence of one or two lines within the next 5 to 10 minutes. One visible line indicates a negative result for amniotic fluid, two visible lines a positive result and no visible lines indicate an invalid result. Placental alpha microglobulin-1 (PAMG-1) is a placental protein that is abundant in amniotic fluid (2,000-25,000 ng/mL) but is present in far lower concentrations in maternal blood (5-25 ng/mL). The protein is present in even lower concentrations in cervicovaginal secretions (0.05-0.2 ng/mL). This 10,000-fold difference in concentration between amniotic fluid and cervicovaginal secretions makes PAMG-1 a very attractive marker for preterm PROM. The minimum detection threshold of Amnisure immunoassay is 5 ng/mL, which is sufficiently sensitive to detect preterm PROM with an accuracy of approximately 99%. The test has a very high sensitivity of 98.9%, specificity of 100%, positive predictive value of 100%, and a negative predictive value of 99.1%.[5,16,17]

CLINICAL COURSE IN PROM

The clinical course of PROM is latency followed by labor and delivery. The interval from ruptured membranes to delivery is the latent period. The risk of infection to both mother and fetus increases with prolongation of latency period. Factors affecting latency are gestational age, degree of oligo-hydramnios, etc. An inverse relation exists between the gestational age at the time of PROM and latent period. At term in the absence of any obstetric intervention, 50% of women with PROM will go into labor spontaneously within 12 hours, 70% within 24 hours, 85% within 48 hours, and 95% within 72 hours.[5] In women with preterm PROM remote from term, 50% will go into labor within 24 to 48 hours and 70 to 90% within 7 days.[5] Furthermore, women with preterm PROM at 24 to 28 weeks of gestation are likely to have a longer latency period than those with preterm PROM closer to term. This was observed in a study that the latency at 20 to 26 weeks' gestation was 12 days and at 32 to 34 weeks' gestation, it was only 4 days.[4] The latent period is shorter in women who have severe oligohydramnios.[18] Evidence of excessive thinning of the myometrium at the fundal region of the uterus in a patient who is not in labor with preterm PROM (< 12 mm) as measured by transabdominal ultrasound has been associated with a shorter latency interval. A fundal myometrial thickness less than 12.1 mm was 93.7% sensitive and 63.6% specific for the identification of women whose latency period was less than 120 hours.[19] Twin pregnancies complicated by preterm PROM have a shorter latency period than singleton pregnancies.

MATERNAL AND PERINATAL COMPLICATIONS

PROM is associated with a high risk of maternal and perinatal complications (Table 5.2).

Table 5.2: Maternal and fetal risks of preterm PROM	
Maternal risks	*Fetal risks*
• Chorioamnionitis	Prematurity
• Placental abruption	Infection
• Malpresentation	Cord prolapse
• Dysfunctional labor	Cord compression
• Cesarean section	Pulmonary hypoplasia
• Postpartum endometritis	Skeletal compression deformities

Maternal complications include chorioamnionitis which occurs in 13 to 60% of women with preterm PROM as compared to 1% in term PROM.[1,2] The risk of chorioamnionitis increases with prolonged leaking, presence of severe oligohydramnios and multiple per vaginal examinations.[5] There is an increased risk of cord prolapse and abruptio placentae.[2,5] The risk of cesarean delivery with its attendant surgical complications also increases in preterm PROM as compared to term PROM. This mainly occurs because of increased incidence of malpresentation, especially in multiple pregnancies. Severe oligohydramnios leading to cord compression and nonreassuring fetal testing (fetal distress) in labor further adds to the increased risk of cesarean section.[1,2] Postpartum complications include postpartum hemorrhage, retained placenta, endometritis (2 to 13%) and puerperal sepsis (1%).

The perinatal complications are more common with preterm PROM as compared to term PROM. There is an increased risk of respiratory distress syndrome (RDS), intraventricular hemorrhage (IVH) and neonatal sepsis leading to a 4-fold increase in perinatal mortality and a 3-fold increase in neonatal morbidity in preterm PROM.[2,20] Other neonatal complications related to severity and duration of preterm PROM include pulmonary hypoplasia, skeletal deformities and neurodevelopmental impairment.[5] Infection, cord prolapse and other factors contribute to the 1 to 2% of intrauterine fetal demise after preterm PROM.[2] Prolongation of pregnancy by as little as one week in preterm PROM prior to 28 weeks of gestation has profound benefit on neonatal morbidity and mortality.[21]

MANAGEMENT OF PROM

Management of PROM depends on factors like gestational age, duration of leaking, whether patient is in labor or not, fetal presentation, fetal heart rate (FHR) tracing pattern and presence or absence of chorioamnionitis. In addition, the level of available neonatal care also plays an important role in deciding the course of management. Initially all pregnant women presenting with a history of watery discharge per vaginum should be hospitalized and subjected to a detailed clinical examination and laboratory tests to confirm the diagnosis of PROM.

Management Options: The management can be broadly classified into:

- Management of term PROM
- Management of preterm PROM.

Management of Term PROM

Active vs Expectant management: At term mostly patients go in spontaneous labor within 24 hours of rupture of membranes. The major question regarding management of these patients is whether to allow them to enter labor spontaneously or to induce labor. The major risk at this gestational age is of intrauterine infection which increases with the duration of rupture of membrane. The risk of chorioamnionitis with term PROM has been reported to be less than 10% and increases to 24% after 24 hours of PROM. Evidence supports that induction of labor as opposed to expectant management decreases the risk of chorioamnionitis without increasing the cesarean delivery rate.[2] Proper counseling should be followed by an informed consent regarding the risks and benefits of termination of pregnancy from the woman and her relatives. The next step in clinical management is to determine whether the cervix is favorable for induction of labor or not. If the cervix is favorable, induction of labor with oxytocin infusion is recommended.[2] However, if the cervix is unfavorable labor may be induced with prostaglandins either intracervical PGE_2 gel 0.5 mg every 6 hours for two doses or intravaginal misoprostol 25 µgm every 6 hours for 5 doses.[2]

Once a decision for termination of pregnancy is taken, this is followed by a careful fetomaternal monitoring till delivery which includes measurement of maternal pulse and temperature every 4 hourly. A complete blood count should be done for a baseline total leucocyte count (TLC) and differential leucocyte count (DLC). High vaginal swab should be sent on admission for any vaginal infection.

The routine use of prophylactic antibiotics in women with term PROM has not been proved to reduce the incidence of infectious morbidity. Prophylactic antibiotics should be started preferably in women with prolonged leaking (>18 hours) or with any evidence of chorioamnionitis (Flow Chart 5.1).

Management of Preterm PROM

The management options in patients with preterm PROM include immediate delivery and expectant management. The factors that need to be considered in formulating a management plan are the risk of prematurity and risk of infection to the neonate and availability of neonatal intensive care. Taking the above facts into consideration women with preterm PROM can be further subdivided into those more than 34 weeks of gestation and those below 34 weeks. In absence of intensive neonatal care unit women with preterm

PROM (less than 34 weeks) should be transferred to a tertiary care facility with sufficient support from neonatology unit.

Immediate delivery: Termination of pregnancy is indicated in women with:
- Gestational age more than 34 weeks
- Signs/symptoms suggestive of chorioamnionitis
- Signs of fetal distress as evidenced by meconium stained liquor with/without abnormal fetal heart rate patterns
- Abruptio placentae
- Severe oligohydramnios.

Expectant management: An expectant approach should be the option in women with preterm PROM at a period of gestation less than 34 weeks and in the absence of an indication for immediate delivery. The major aim of the expectant management is to prolong pregnancy so as to achieve fetal lung maturity and to identify when clinically significant chorioamnionitis is evolving and deliver the fetus at the right time. Once this is opted the risks and potential benefits of expectant management should be discussed with the patient and her family and an informed consent should be obtained.

The decision to continue pregnancy with expectant management in preterm PROM should only be made following a complete maternal and fetal evaluation on admission including a per speculum examination to collect discharge or swabs either from the cervix or from posterior fornix for bacteriological culture to diagnose any subclinical infection. Electronic fetal heart rate monitoring and uterine activity monitoring is carried out to identify occult umbilical cord compression and presence of any uterine contractions. It is important to remember that NST at less than 32 weeks of gestation may be false non-reactive in an immature but otherwise healthy fetus. However, after a reactive baseline test, a subsequent nonreactive test should be considered to be abnormal or suspicious.[2]

COMPONENTS OF EXPECTANT MANAGEMENT

The basic components of expectant management are:
- Maternal fetal monitoring
- Drug treatment.

Maternal-Fetal Monitoring

The woman is advised adequate bed rest and subjected to close monitoring of vital parameters four times a day including pulse and temperature. Though these are crude late indicators of evolving chorioamnionitis but are easily performed and are non-invasive. The woman is daily assessed for leaking as regards its amount, color and odor. Daily per abdomen examination is done to look for amount of liquor, any uterine tenderness, uterine contractions and fetal heart rate.

Table 5.3: Investigations in preterm PROM

- Amniotic fluid collected per speculum for microbiological culture
- Ferning to confirm liquor
- Swabs
    - High vaginal swabs for Gram's staining and culture and sensitivity
    - Endocervical swab for *Neisseria gonorrhea* and *Chlamydia*
    - Urethral and anorectal swab culture in women suspicious of genital infection
- Urine for microscopy and culture

Table 5.4: Signs and symptoms of chorioamnionitis

- Maternal fever > 38° C
- Increased white cell count (>15,000/cmm)
- Maternal tachycardia (> 100 bpm)
- Fetal tachycardia (>160 bpm)
- Uterine tenderness
- Offensive smelling vaginal discharge
- C-Reactive protein > 40 mg/l

All baseline investigations including complete blood count (CBC) with peripheral smear examination, urine routine and microscopy examination, high vaginal swab for culture and sensitivity and estimation of C-reactive protein (CRP) should be done (Table 5.3). This is to be followed by daily TLC/ DLC if leaking persists or every 72 hours if leaking stops. White blood cell count and level of C-reactive protein (CRP) are possibly better predictors of evolving chorioamnionitis. The patient should be closely observed for signs and symptoms of chorioamnionitis as detailed in Table 5.4. In the absence of other preexisting infections, the presence of fever exceeding 38°C or 100.4°F with or without uterine tenderness and/or maternal or fetal tachycardia is suggestive of chorioamnionitis. It is important to remember that a rising maternal blood leukocyte count may be consequent to administration of antenatal corticosteroids and may persist for 5-7 days.[2,11]

Fetal monitoring should be performed at least once a day. Daily fetal movement count (DFMC) and intermittent fetal heart rate auscultation should be done. USG is usually performed once or twice weekly to assess fetal growth and liquor volume. A scan will provide information on gestational age, presentation, placental position and fetal weight to decide further planning for delivery and counseling on neonatal outcome. While oligohydramnios has been associated with shorter latency and chorioamnionitis, it alone is not an indication for delivery when other tests of surveillance are reassuring. Digital cervical examination is to be avoided as far as possible throughout expectant management. It should only be done to decide the mode of delivery and not the timing of delivery.

Drug Treatment

This includes administration of antibiotics to prevent chorioamnionitis and steroids to enhance fetal lung maturity.

Prophylactic antibiotic therapy: Once a decision to manage a patient expectantly has been made prophylactic antibiotics should be given. Prophylactic antibiotics are beneficial to women with preterm PROM as these are seen to prolong pregnancy and reduce neonatal morbidity. However, the choice as to which antibiotic should be preferred is less clear. A number of antibiotic regimens are being used in patients with preterm PROM. Co-amoxiclav has been seen to be associated with an increased risk of neonatal necrotising enterocolitis and should be avoided.[22] The regime recommended by ACOG is a combination of ampicillin 2 gm and erythromycin 250 mg intravenously every six hours for 48 hours, followed by oral amoxicillin 250 mg and erythromycin 333 mg every eight hours for five days.[2] Women receiving this combination showed increased latency of up to three weeks despite discontinuation of the antibiotics after seven days.

Antenatal corticosteroid treatment: A single course of corticosteroids should be administered to reduce the risk of neonatal respiratory distress syndrome (RDS), intraventricular hemorrhage (IVH) and necrotizing enterocolitis (NEC). Corticosteroids decrease perinatal morbidity and mortality after preterm PROM.[2] The recommended schedule of antenatal corticosteroid is two doses of 12 mg of betamethasone given intramuscularly (IM) at 24-hour intervals or four doses of dexamethasone 6 mg given intramuscularly (IM) at 12-hour intervals.[23] The National Institute of Health recommends administration of corticosteroids before 32 weeks of gestation, assuming fetal viability and no evidence of intra-amniotic infection. RCOG recommends steroid administration even upto 34 weeks.[24] Multiple courses are not recommended because studies have shown that two or more courses can result in decreased infant birth weight, head circumference, and body length.[25]

Tocolytics: The use of tocolytic drugs in patients of preterm PROM is controversial. Tocolytic therapy may prolong the latent period for a short time but does not appear to improve neonatal outcome.[26] In the absence of adequate data, a short course of tocolysis after preterm PROM to allow initiation of antibiotics, administration of corticosteroid and maternal transport may be considered; however, long-term therapy in patients with PROM is not recommended.[2]

Timing of Delivery

Traditionally in the absence of fetal or maternal compromise, delivery should be accomplished at 34 weeks. The rationale is that at this gestation the risk of infection is thought to be greater than the neonatal complications due to prematurity.[2]

Mode of Delivery

In the absence of any fetal or maternal compromise and cephalic presentation, vaginal delivery is usually indicated. Where the presentation is breech, decision

Flow chart 5.1: Management of premature rupture of membranes

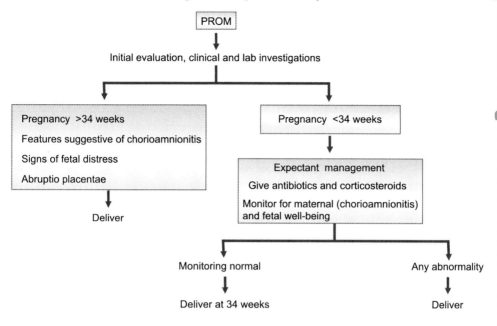

needs to be individualized as there is no evidence to suggest that cesarean section improves neonatal outcome.

KEY POINTS

- Premature rupture of membranes (PROM) complicates 5-10% of all pregnancies. Preterm PROM occurs in 2 to 4% of all pregnancies.
- The etiopathogenesis of PROM is still unknown, however, infection remains the major contributor in its genesis.
- The fetal membranes serve as a barrier to ascending infection. Once the membranes rupture, both the mother and fetus are at risk of infection and of other complications.
- The hallmark of diagnosis of PROM is history of leaking and direct visualization of pooling of amniotic fluid in the vagina or leakage of fluid from the cervical os on per speculum examination.
- Management of a woman presenting with suspected PROM includes confirming the diagnosis, documenting correct gestational age, assessing fetal well-being and deciding on the plan of management.
- Immediate termination of pregnancy irrespective of the gestational age should be the option in women with signs/symptoms suggestive of chorioamnionitis, signs of fetal distress and abruptio placentae.
- The management of term PROM includes administration of antibiotics and induction of labor.
- Expectant management should be the option in women with preterm PROM less than 34 weeks with no evidence of chorioamnionitis.

- The components of expectant management includes admission to hospital, feto maternal monitoring, administration of antenatal corticosteroids and prophylactic antibiotics (Flow chart 5.1). In the absence of fetal or maternal compromise, termination of pregnancy should be accomplished if pregnancy is more than 34 weeks.

REFERENCES

1. American College of Obstetricians and Gynecologists, authors. Premature Rupture of Membranes. Washington, DC: American College of Obstetricians and Gynecologists; 1998. (ACOG Practice Bulletin No. 1).
2. ACOG Committee on Practice Bulletins-Obstetrics, authors. Clinical management guidelines for obstetricians-gynecologists. (ACOG Practice Bulletin No. 80: Premature rupture of membranes). Obstet Gynecol 2007;109:1007-19.
3. Samuel Parry, Jerome F. Strauss Premature Rupture of the Fetal Membranes.New England Journal of Medicine 1998;338(10):663-70.
4. Gillian D, Bryant-Greenwood, Lynnae K Millar. Human Fetal Membranes: Their Preterm Premature Rupture Biology of Reproduction. 2000;63:1575B-79.
5. Aaron B Caughey, Julian N Robinson. Contemporary Diagnosis and Management of Preterm Premature Rupture of Membranes. Rev Obstet Gynecol 2008;1(1):11-22.
6. Mercer BM, Goldenberg RL, Meis PJ, et al. The NICHD Maternal-Fetal Medicine Units Network, authors. The Preterm Prediction Study: Prediction of preterm premature rupture of membranes through clinical findings and ancillary testing. Am J Obstet Gynecol 2000;183:738-7.
7. Tanya M, Medina D, Ashley Hill. Preterm premature rupture of membranes: Diagnosis and management. Am Fam Physician 2006;73:659-64.
8. Romero R, Chaiworapongsa T, Kuivaniemi H, Tromp G. Bacterial vaginosis, the inflammatory response and the risk of preterm birth: A role for genetic epidemiology in the prevention of preterm birth. Am J Obstet Gynecol 2004;190:1509-19.
9. Hillier SL, Nugent RP, Eschenbach DA, et al. Association between bacterial vaginosis and preterm delivery of a low-birth-weight infant. The Vaginal Infections and Prematurity. Study Group. N Engl J Med 1995;333:1737-42.
10. Allen SR. Epidemiology of premature rupture of the fetal membranes. Clin Obstet Gynecol 1991;34:685-93.
11. Royal College of Obstetricians and Gynaecologists (RCOG). Preterm prelabour rupture of membranes. London (UK): Royal College of Obstetricians and Gynaecologists (RCOG); 2006 (Guideline; no. 44).
12. Lewis DF, Major CA, Towers CV, et al. Effects of digital vaginal examinations on latency period in preterm premature rupture of membranes. Obstet Gynecol 1992;80:630-34.
13. Gorodeski IG, Haimovitz L, Bahari CM. Reevaluation of the pH, ferning and Nile blue sulphate staining methods in pregnant women with premature rupture of the fetal membranes. J Perinat Med 1982;10:286-92.
14. De Haan HH, Offermans PM, Smits F, et al. Value of the fern test to confirm or reject the diagnosis of ruptured membranes in modest in nonlaboring women presenting with nonspecific vaginal fluid loss. Am J Perinatol 1994;11:46-50.
15. Naylor CS, Gregory K, Hobel C. Premature rupture of the membranes: an evidence-based approach to clinical care. Am J Perinatol 2001;18:397-413.
16. Cousins LM, Smok DP, Lovett SM, Poeltler DM. Amnisure placental alpha macroglobulin-1 rapid immunoassay versus standard diagnostic methods for detection of rupture of membranes. Am J Perinatol 2005;22:317-20.
17. Lee SE, Park JS, Norwitz ER, et al. Measurement of placental alpha-microglobulin-1 in cervicovaginal discharge to diagnose rupture of membranes. Obstet Gynecol 2007; 109: 634-40.
18. Park JS, Yoon BH, Romero R, et al. The relationship between oligohydramnios and the onset of preterm labor in preterm premature rupture of membranes. Am J Obstet Gynecol 2001;184:459-62.

19. Buhimschi CS, Buhimschi IA, Norwitz ER, et al. Sonographic myometrial thickness predicts the latency interval of women with preterm premature rupture of the membranes and oligohydramnios. Am J Obstet Gynecol 2005;193:762-70.
20. Greenwald JL. Premature rupture of the membranes: Diagnostic and management strategies. Am Fam Physician 1993;48(2):293-306.
21. Mercer B, Milluzzi C, Collin M. Periviable birth at 20 to 26 weeks of gestation: Proximate causes, previous obstetric history and recurrence risk. Am J Obstet Gynecol 2005;193 (3 Pt 2):1175-80.
22. Sara Kenyon, Michel Boulvain, James P Neilson. Antibiotics for preterm rupture of membranes Cochrane Database of Systematic Reviews 2009 Issue 4.
23. Harding JE, Pang J, Knight DB, Liggins GC. Do antenatal corticosteroids help in the setting of preterm rupture of membranes? Am J Obstet Gynecol 2001;184:131-39.
24. Royal College of Obstetricians and Gynaecologists (RCOG). Antenatal corticosteroid to prevent respiratory distress syndrome London (UK): Royal College of Obstetricians and Gynaecologists (RCOG); 2004 (Guideline; no. 7).
25. Vidaeff AC, Doyle NM, Gilstrap LC III. Antenatal corticosteroids for fetal maturation in women at risk for preterm delivery. Clin Perinatol 2003;30:825-40,vii.
26. Weiner CP, Renk K, Klugman M. The therapeutic efficacy and cost-effectiveness of aggressive tocolysis for premature labor associated with premature rupture of the membranes. Am J Obstet Gynecol 1991;165:785.

5

Premature Rupture of Membranes

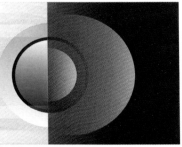

Prolonged Pregnancy 6

Amita Suneja, Sandhya Jain

INTRODUCTION

Prolonged pregnancy is a common clinical situation and causes considerable anxiety to women and the treating obstetrician. Because of the associated perinatal morbidity and mortality it demands accurate diagnosis, antenatal fetal surveillance and timely intervention.

The terms postterm, prolonged, postdates and postmature are often loosely used interchangeably to signify pregnancies that have exceeded a duration considered to be the upper limit of normal. Postmature should be used to describe an infant with recognizable clinical features indicating a pathologically prolonged pregnancy. Postdates probably should be abandoned because the real issue in many postterm pregnancies is "post-what dates?" Therefore, postterm or prolonged pregnancy is the preferred expression for an extended pregnancy.

DEFINITION

The standard internationally recommended definition of prolonged pregnancy, endorsed by the American College of Obstetricians and Gynecologists (2004)[1] is 42 completed weeks (294 days) or more from the first day of last menstrual period. Pregnancies between 41 weeks 1 day and 41 weeks 6 days, although in the 42nd week, do not complete 42 weeks until the seventh day has elapsed.

INCIDENCE

The estimated date of confinement or delivery (EDD) is calculated as 40 weeks after the first day of last menstrual period (LMP), assuming normal 28 days cycle (Naegle's formula). About 1% of women deliver on the day of EDD. The incidence of pregnancy continuing beyond 41 weeks is about 18% and 10% beyond 42 weeks.

DIAGNOSIS

The management of pregnancy beyond 40 weeks' gestation relies on an accurate assessment of the gestational age. Dating gestational age with LMP alone assumes both accurate recall by the patient and ovulation on 14th day of the menstrual cycle. The duration of follicular phase may vary from 7 to 21 days; also, delayed ovulation is an important cause of perceived prolonged pregnancy. A Cochrane review[2] found that, compared with selective ultrasonography, routine prenatal ultrasonography before 24 weeks' gestation provides better gestational age assessment and earlier detection of multiple pregnancies and fetal malformations. First trimester ultrasound should be offered, ideally between 11 and 14 weeks, to all women, as it is a more accurate assessment of gestational age than last menstrual period with fewer pregnancies prolonged past 41+0 weeks (I-A).

PREDISPOSING FACTORS

Certain *maternal demographic factors* have been related to prolonged pregnancy such as primiparity, prior postterm birth, higher socioeconomic class, BMI >35 kg/m^2, sedentary life style and elderly multiparae. A woman with single previous prolonged pregnancy has a 30% chance of recurrence. The tendency of some mothers to have repeated postterm births suggests that prolonged pregnancies are biologically determined.[3] One study has shown that this tendency also recurred across generations in Swedish women.[4] Increased fish consumption in first two trimesters has been reported to be associated with prolonged pregnancy.[5]

Fetoplacental factors have been seen to predispose to postterm pregnancy. These include anencephaly, adrenal hypoplasia, and X-linked placental sulfatase deficiency. These cause a lack of the usually high estrogen levels of normal pregnancy. Estrogen helps in initiation of labor by increasing the release of oxytocin from posterior pituitary, stimulates oxytocin receptor synthesis in myometrium and decidua, accelerates prostaglandin, myometrial contractile protein synthesis and also increases excitability of myometrial cell membranes. A relative fetal adrenocortical deficiency may contribute to delay in onset of labor and an increased risk of intrapartum hypoxia and even death in postterm pregnancy. Infants born postterm may have an inherent biological defect, since it has been found that there is increased risk of demise up to 2 years of age; sudden infant death syndrome is also more common in them.

In term laboring women cervical nitric acid release helps in cervical ripening. Reduced cervical nitric oxide release may be a factor for prolonged pregnancy.[6]

Postmaturity Syndrome

The postmature infant has wrinkled, patchy, peeling skin and body wasting; nails are long and neonate looks old and worrisome. These changes are due to loss of vernix caseosa. Most of them are not growth restricted. The syndrome is present in about 10% of pregnancies between 41 and 43 weeks. The incidence increases to 33% at 44 weeks.[7]

Placental Dysfunction

The concept that postmaturity is due to placental insufficiency has persisted despite an absence of morphological or significant qualitative findings. It has been reported that placental apoptosis—programed cell death—was significantly increased at 41 to 42 completed weeks. The post-term placenta shows a decrease in length and diameter of chorionic villi, fibrinoid necrosis, and accelerated atherosis of vessels. There are foci of hemorrhagic infarcts and calcium deposition.

The postterm fetus may continue to gain weight, though at a slower rate between 38 and 42 weeks. This at least suggests that placental function is not compromised.

Amniotic Fluid Changes

There are quantitative and qualitative changes with prolongation of pregnancy. The amniotic fluid volume reaches a peak of 1000 ml at 38 weeks and 800 ml at 40 weeks. It further decreases with prolonged gestation; the mechanism seems to be diminished production of urine by the fetus. Fetal heart tracing shows variable decelerations and saltatory baseline pattern consistent with cord occlusion due to oligohydramnios. At term, the fluid becomes milky and cloudy due to abundant flakes of vernix caseosa. It becomes greenish-yellow with passage of meconium. Meconium also makes it thick and viscous increasing the chances of 'meconium aspiration syndrome'.

Fetal Macrosomia

The incidence of fetal macrosomia (defined as birth weight greater than 4500 gm) increases from 1.4% at 37 to 41 weeks to 2.2% at 42 weeks or more.[8] The ACOG guidelines do not support a policy of early labor induction in women at term who have suspected macrosomia.[9] Moreover, vaginal delivery is not contraindicated for women with estimated fetal weight upto 5000 gm. Cesarean delivery is recommended for estimated fetal weight greater than 4500 gm in the presence of prolonged second stage of labor or arrest of descent.

Advances in obstetric and neonatal care have lowered the absolute mortality; however, retrospective studies of postterm pregnancies have found an increased risk to the mother and fetus. The most significant increase occurs intrapartum. Risks associated with postterm pregnancy include increased chances of cephalopelvic disproportion, instrumental and operative delivery, macrosomia, birth asphyxia, meconium aspiration, bone fracture, peripheral nerve paralysis, stillbirth, and intrauterine death.[10]

The perinatal mortality rate (i.e. stillbirths plus neonatal deaths) of two to three deaths per 1,000 deliveries at 40 weeks gestation approximately doubles by 42 weeks and is four to six times greater at 44 weeks.[11,12] The major causes of death include chemical pneumonitis due to meconium aspiration, prolonged labor with cephalopelvic disproportion, unexplained anoxia and malformations.

There is increased maternal morbidity due to hazards of induction, instrumental and operative delivery. There is considerable maternal anxiety once they go beyond the estimated date of confinement; moreover many women find the physical burden of pregnancy at or near term to be intolerable.

MANAGEMENT OF PREGNANCY BEYOND 40 WEEKS GESTATION

Pregnancies complicated by gestational diabetes, hypertension, or other high-risk conditions should be managed according to guidelines for those conditions and should not be allowed to go postdated. An algorithm for the management of low-risk, post-term pregnancies is given in Fig. 6.1.[13] Low risk patients should be offered induction of labor at 41 weeks. The risks and benefits of labor induction versus expectant management should be discussed with the patient at 41 weeks gestation. With appropriate obstetric and neonatal care, the absolute mortality rate is low with either management option.

Recommendations for Induction of Labor

Current obstetric guidelines from Canada[14] and UK[15] recommend offering induction of labor at 41 weeks. An American College of Obstetricians and Gynecologists news release in May 2003 claimed that labor induction at 41 weeks lowers cesarean section rates.[16,17] According to a latest Cochrane review involving 19 trials,[18] labor induction at 41 completed weeks should be offered to low-risk women. The message from this review is that such a policy is associated with fewer deaths although the absolute risk is small. There does not seem to be any increased risk of operative vaginal or abdominal delivery. It would be prudent to discuss the pros and cons with women at 41 weeks or more, who are at low risk of pregnancy complications, so that an informed decision is made. If the woman chooses to wait for spontaneous labor onset it would be prudent to have regular fetal monitoring as

6

Prolonged Pregnancy

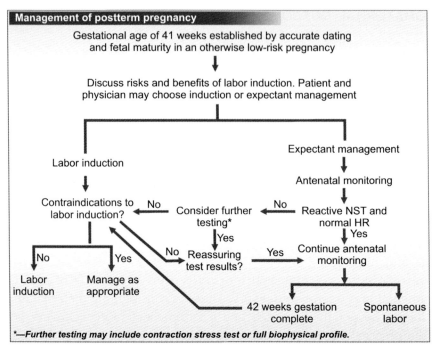

Management of postterm pregnancy

Gestational age of 41 weeks established by accurate dating and fetal maturity in an otherwise low-risk pregnancy

Discuss risks and benefits of labor induction. Patient and physician may choose induction or expectant management

Labor induction

Expectant management

Antenatal monitoring

Contraindications to labor induction? ← No — Consider further testing* ← No — Reactive NST and normal HR

No | Yes

No — Reassuring test results? — Yes — Continue antenatal monitoring

Labor induction | Manage as appropriate

42 weeks gestation complete | Spontaneous labor

*—Further testing may include contraction stress test or full biophysical profile.

Figure 6.1: Algorithm for management of low-risk postterm pregnancy[13]

longitudinal epidemiological studies suggest increased risk of perinatal death with increasing gestational age. During labor it is recommended to do early rupture of membranes to detect meconium stained liquor. Fetal heart rate monitoring should preferably be continuous where facilities are available.

Fetal Monitoring

When the physician and patient choose expectant management of a low-risk prolonged pregnancy, fetal monitoring must be performed. This often includes daily fetal movement count, twice-weekly nonstress test, biophysical profile (BPP), modified BPP (a combination of NST and AFI), and Doppler velocimetry of umbilical and middle cerebral artery.

Evidence of benefit from antenatal surveillance is lacking[19] and no single antenatal test is superior to another.[12] Normal antenatal monitoring results usually are reassuring. For the outcome of stillbirth, a reactive NST has a negative predictive value of 99.8%, and a modified BPP or full BPP has a negative predictive value greater than 99.9%.[19] The efficacies of the tests do not relate to acute compromising events such as abruption or prolapsed umbilical cord. The positive predictive values of abnormal antenatal monitoring are more difficult to estimate but generally are lower. Using surrogate markers of fetal distress as an outcome, a nonreactive NST has a positive predictive value of approximately 10%, and an abnormal modified BPP has a positive predictive value of 40%. An abnormal antenatal test should be investigated according to the clinical scenario. Umbilical artery Doppler velocimetry may be of benefit only in pregnancies complicated by intrauterine growth restriction; middle cerebral artery Doppler velocimetry is still investigational.[18] *The American College of Obstetricians and Gynecologists has given a Level C recommendation (consensus and expert opinion) for initiation of fetal surveillance between 41 and 42 weeks because of evidence that perinatal morbidity and mortality increase as gestational age advances and that a twice weekly assessment of amniotic fluid and a NST should be adequate.*[20] *The Royal College of Obstetricians and Gynaecologists recommends the same from 42 weeks onwards in women who decline labor induction.*[21] For amniotic fluid assessment, measurement of the single deepest vertical pocket (at least 2 cm) seems a better choice since the use of the amniotic fluid index is associated with overdiagnosis of oligohydramnios, with resultant increase in the rate of induction of labor without improvement in peripartum outcomes.[22]

PREVENTION OF POST-TERM PREGNANCY

Sweeping (or stripping) of membranes of the lower uterine segment has been reported to stimulate the onset of labor. During a vaginal examination, the fetal membranes are separated from the cervix and lower uterine segment as far as possible, sweeping a finger inserted through the cervical os to 360° if possible. This procedure necessitates a sufficiently dilated cervix, usually representing a favorable Bishop score. When the cervix is closed, some clinicians attempt to stretch the cervix open or perform cervical massage. Sweeping results in the release of endogenous prostaglandins, softening the cervix and augmenting oxytocin-induced uterine contractions. Membrane sweeping is generally most efficacious in nulliparous women with unfavorable Bishop scores. In a study by Berghella, et al. 45 patients were randomized to weekly sweeping of membranes or gentle examination starting at 38 weeks. Time to delivery was significantly decreased with membrane stripping, and fewer pregnancies reaching past 41 weeks.[23] A recent Cochrane review assessed 22 trials involving sweeping of membranes and recommended that women should be offered this option commencing at 38 to 41 weeks, following a discussion of risks and benefits (Level of evidence I-A).[24]

Nipple stimulation has been shown to be of no benefit in reducing the incidence of post-term pregnancy (Level of evidence I-A).[25]

KEY POINTS

- Prolonged pregnancy is defined as pregnancy beyond 42 completed weeks (294 days) calculating from the first day of last menstrual period.
- The perinatal mortality rate (i.e. stillbirths plus neonatal deaths) approximately doubles by 42 weeks gestation and is four to six times greater at 44 weeks.

- First trimester ultrasound should be offered, ideally between 11 and 14 weeks to all women, as it is a more accurate assessment of gestational age than last menstrual period with fewer pregnancies prolonged past 41+0 weeks (I-A).
- Low-risk women should be offered induction of labor at 41 weeks.
- Antenatal testing used in the monitoring of the 41 to 42 week pregnancy should include biweekly nonstress test and an assessment of amniotic fluid volume (I-A).
- Good communication between the physician and patient, along with a discussion of the risks and benefits involved, is critical to ensure that informed decisions are made.
- Women should be offered the option of weekly membrane sweeping, commencing at 38-41 weeks, following a discussion of risks and benefits to prevent postterm birth.

REFERENCES

1. American College of Obstetricians and Gynecologists: Management of post-term pregnancy. Practice Bulletin No. 55, September 2004.
2. Neilson JP. Ultrasound for fetal assessment in early pregnancy. Cochrane Database Syst Rev 2004;(3):CD000182.
3. Bakketeig LS, Bergsj P. Post-term pregnancy: Magnitude of the problem. In Chalmers I, Enkin M, Keirse M (Eds): Effective care in pregnancy and childbirth. Oxford, Oxford University Press, 1991;765.
4. Mogren I, Stenlund H, Hogberg U. Recurrence of prolonged pregnancy. Int J Epidemiol 1999; 28:253.
5. Slen SF, Osterdal ML, Salvig JD, et al. Duration of pregnancy in relation to seafood intake during early and mid pregnancy: Prospective cohort. Eur J Epidemiol 2006;21(10):749-58. Epub 2006 Nov 17 [abstract].
6. Vaisanen-Tommiska M, Nuutila M, Ylikorkala O. Cervical nitric oxide release in women post-term. Obstet Gynecol 2004;103:657.
7. Shime J, Gare DJ, Andrews J, et al. Prolonged pregnancy: Surveillance of the fetus and the neonate and the course of labor and delivery. Am J Obstet Gynecol 1984;148:547.
8. Martin JA, Hamilton BE, Ventura SJ, et al. Births: Final data for 2001. National Vital Statistics Reports, Vol 51, No. 2. Hyattsville, Md: National Center for Health Statistics, 2002.
9. American College of Obstetricians and Gynecologists: Fetal macrosomia. Practice Bulletin No. 22, November 2000.
10. Olesen AW, Westergaard JG, Olsen J. Perinatal and maternal complications related to post-term delivery: A national register-based study, 1978 -1993. Am J Obstet Gynecol 2003;189:224.
11. Hollis B. Prolonged pregnancy. Curr Opin Obstet Gynecol 2002;14:203-7.
12. Rand L, Robinson JN, Economy KE, Norwitz ER. Post-term induction of labor revisited. Obstet Gynecol 2000;96(5 pt 1):779-83.
13. Bricose D, Nguyen H, Mencer M, Gautam N, et al. Management of pregnancy beyond 40 weeks gestation. Am Fam Physician 2005;71:1935-41.
14. BC Reproductive 2005. British Columbia Reproductive Care Program. Post-term pregnancy: Obstetric guideline 7. http://www.rcp.gov.bc.ca/guidelines/Obstetrics/Post-term.
15. RCOG/NICE 2001 Royal College of Obstetricians and Gynaecologists. Induction of labour. London, UK: RCOG/NICE, 2001.
16. ACOG 2003 American College of Obstetricians and Gynecologists. Labor induction at 41 weeks lowers cesarean rate; ACOG News Release 2003.
17. Sanchez-Ramos L, Olivier F, Delke I, Kaunitz AM. Labor induction versus expectant management for post-term pregnancies: A systematic review with meta-analysis. Obstet Gynecol 2003;101:1312-18.

18. Induction of labor for improving birth outcomes for women at or beyond term (Review) Copyright © 2009 The Cochrane Collaboration. Published by John Wiley and Sons Ltd.
19. ACOG practice bulletin. Antepartum fetal surveillance. Number 9, October 1999. Clinical management guidelines for obstetrician-gynecologists. Int J Gynaecol Obstet 2000;68: 175-85.
20. American College of Obstetricians and Gynecologists. Practice Bulletin No. 55, 2004. Management of post-term pregnancy.
21. Royal College of Obstetricians and Gynecologists. Induction of labor. Evidence based clinical Guideline No. 9, June 2001. London: RCOG Press.
22. Nabhan AF, Abdelmoula YA. Amniotic fluid index versus single deepest vertical pocket as a screening test for preventing adverse pregnancy outcome. Cochrane Review 2008.
23. Berghella V, Rogers RA, Lescale K. Stripping of membranes as a safe method to reduce prolonged pregnancies. Obstet Gynecol 1996;87:927-31.
24. Boulvain M, Irion O. Stripping/sweeping the membranes for inducing or preventing post-term pregnancy. Cochrane Database Syst Rev 2004;(3):CD001328.
25. Allott HA, Palmer CR. Sweeping the membranes: A valid procedure in stimulating the onset of labor? Br J Obstet Gynaecol 1993;100:898-903.

6

Prolonged Pregnancy

Polyhydramnios Oligohydramnios

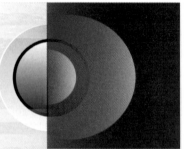

7

Prabha Lal

INTRODUCTION

Amniotic fluid is a faintly alkaline (pH 7.2) watery content of amniotic sac where fetus grows. It is the sum of inflow and outflow of fluid into amniotic sac and reflects fetal fluid balance. It is primarily of fetal origin with a small maternal contribution via extraplacental membranes. Exact site of origin differs according to the gestational age. In the first trimester it is mainly a transudate of plasma with transudation occurring across the maternal surface of uterine decidua–placental surface and directly through the skin of fetus. Later in gestation, it is the fetal urine and fetal lung secretions which contribute to its formation so that the components of amniotic fluid at term include urea and creatinine. Compositionally 98-99% is water and rest are solids such as proteins (0.25%), uric acid and creatinine (2%). Levels of electrolytes like sodium and potassium are low at term.

Amniotic fluid is not a static collection of fluid but rather one whose volume is maintained by a circulatory process of fetal lung and urine production being balanced by swallowing and absorption directly across the amnion into the fetal circulation. Earliest detection of amniotic fluid occurs at 8 weeks of gestation and its volume progressively increases with increasing age of gestation. Amniotic fluid is 30 ml at 10 weeks, 190 ml at 16 weeks and 800-1000 ml at 32-35 weeks gestation. Thereafter, it declines to 550 ml by 42 weeks.[1]

Amniotic fluid provides fetus a protective low resistance environment suitable for growth and development. It also reflects the maternal hydration because the fluid shifts freely across the placenta predominantly in response to osmotic gradient.

Direct measurement of amniotic fluid volume is cumbersome. Symphysio fundal height (SFH) is unreliable for estimation of amniotic fluid. Clinical assessment is done subjectively by bimanual palpation. Amniotic fluid volume may be better assessed by sonographic evaluation by estimating the deepest vertical pool (DVP) and amniotic fluid index (AFI). AFI is more sensitive and is calculated by dividing uterus into 4 quadrants by the midline and transverse axis and measuring the DVP free of fetal parts and umbilical cord. Measurements of all 4 quadrants are added to give AFI.[2] The normal AFI is 5-25 cm.

DISORDERS OF AMNIOTIC FLUID

Incidence

Amniotic fluid derangements are usually classified as hydramnios (polyhydramnios) and oligohydramnios. Hydramnios occurs in 1-3.5% of all pregnancies. However, it is severe in only 5%. The prevalence of oligohydramnios defined as AFI < 5 is 8%, but only 1% if criteria of DVP < 2 cm is considered.

POLYHYDRAMNIOS

Polyhydramnios is defined as excess of liquor amni in the amniotic cavity of a gravid uterus. It is suspected clinically and confirmed sonographically. It is defined as a DVP of 8 cm or more or an AFI of more than 25 cm.
Hydramnios is classified as follows:

	DVP	AFI
Mild hydramnios	8-10 cm	25-35 cm
Moderate hydramnios	11-12 cm	36-45 cm
Severe hydramnios	>12 cm	> 45 cm

Hydramnios may be acute or chronic in onset or a combination of both:

Acute polyhydramnios: Patients are usually symptomatic. It develops rapidly within a few days in midpregnancy (16-20 weeks) and is exclusively associated with monozygotic twin pregnancy with recipient twin-to-twin transfusion syndrome (RTTTS) and usually ends in premature labor (PTL) at around 28 weeks.[3]

Chronic polyhydramnios: It is more common than the acute form. Develops in late pregnancy mostly idiopathic in origin. Accumulation of fluid occurs gradually and patient may tolerate the excessive abdominal distention with relatively less discomfort and usually does not require intervention.

Etiology

Majority of cases of hydramnios are idiopathic. Hydramnios due to maternal or fetal causes is detected in only 20% cases. The likelihood of a fetal

7

121

Table 7.1: Causes of hydramnios	
Maternal causes	*Fetal and placental causes*
• Diabetes mellitus and diabetes insipidus: Diabetes causes fetal polyuria secondary to osmotic diuresis. It may arise in pregnancies with suboptimal glycemic control.[5] • Lithium therapy: An antidepressant drug used for bipolar affective disorders. It is associated with maternal nephrogenic diabetes insipidus leading to rapid filling of bladder and fetal polyuria as observed on sonography.[6] • Substance abuse: It has been observed that incidence of polyhydramnios is higher in patients resorting to substance abuse in some form or other.	• Congenital structural abnormalities of upper gastrointestinal tract, e.g. esophageal atresia, duodenal atresia and pyloric stenosis. In these conditions amniotic fluid cannot flow beyond the obstruction. • External compression of upper gastrointestinal tract of the fetus secondary to thoracic and mediastinal masses and diaphragmatic hernias. • Neurological conditions giving rise to lack of swallowing such as anencephaly, myotonic dystrophies and arthrogryposis. • Genetic conditions like trisomy 18 and Beckwith-Wiedemann syndrome with associated macroglossia. • Fetal hydrops of immune and nonimmune origin is associated with hydramnios in upto 50% of instances. • Recipient twin-to-twin transfusion syndrome. • Fetal anemia. • High output cardiac failure. • Congenital infections, e.g. syphilis and viral hepatitis. • Chorioangioma.

abnormality varies with degree of polyhydramnios, being 1%, 2% and 11%, respectively in cases of mild, moderate and severe hydramnios.[4] Among the fetal causes abnormal turnover of amniotic fluid is the main cause of polyhydramnios. It is due to lack of swallowing and absence of free flow into gut that interrupts the normal turnover of amniotic fluid causing imbalance and accumulation of excessive fluid in the amniotic sac. Inability of fetuses to swallow amniotic fluid may be due to various reasons. The causes of hydramnios are listed in Table 7.1.

Complications Associated with Hydramnios

Maternal Complications

During pregnancy: Maternal complications in hydramnios during pregnancy are usually due to over distention of uterus. Patients usually complain of discomfort and in severe cases she may complain of dyspnea for which she has to adopt an upright posture to get relief. Pressure effects on major venous system give rise to edema of lower extremities, vulva and lower abdominal wall. Very rarely pressure on ureters can give rise to oliguria. Intraamniotic pressure is markedly raised in women with severe hydramnios thus causing increased risk of prelabor rupture of membranes and preterm labor. Other maternal complications include malpresentations and unstable lie leading to increased risk of cesarean section.

During labor: There is increased risk of rupture of membranes leading to cord prolapse. Sudden decompression of uterine cavity can cause severe abruptio placentae.[7] There can be uterine inertia leading to dysfunctional labor. All these can result in increased incidence of cesarean section, atonic postpartum hemorrhage, retained placenta and shock.

Fetal Complications

Increased perinatal mortality associated with hydramnios is due to presence of congenital anomalies, preterm premature rupture of membranes or preterm delivery. It is directly related to the severity of hydramnios. Perinatal mortality is due to the following reasons:

- Spontaneous preterm labor responsible for about 22% of cases after exclusion of congenital anomalies.[8]
- Increased intraamniotic pressure due to hydramnios adversely affects uteroplacental perfusion resulting in hypoxia and acidemia. This hypothesis is supported by the observation of increased blood flow after amnioreduction. Hypoxia may be secondary to cord prolapse, abruptio placentae and uteroplacental dysfunction.

Diagnosis

The clinician must have a high index of suspicion in women with risk factors. Diagnosis is suspected on clinical findings of fundal height more than period of gestation (POG), difficulty in palpating fetal parts due to overdistended uterus and inability to hear fetal heart sounds. The diagnosis is confirmed on USG.

Differential Diagnosis

Clinical diagnosis may be confused with:
- Ascites
- Large ovarian cyst
- Multiple pregnancy
- Hydatidiform mole
- Macrosomia.

Investigations

Diagnostic evaluation of hydramnios is done to:
- Confirm diagnosis
- Assess degree of hydramnios
- Look for presence of multiple gestation
- Estimate the fetal weight
- Rule out congenital anomalies

- Fetal bladder dynamics
- Genetic amniocentesis for karyotyping and viral infections.

There are two methods of assessment of amniotic fluid volume: Direct and indirect.

Direct

Dye dilution method: A predetermined amount of dye is injected into the amniotic sac and after allowing time for its mixing and distribution it is retrieved and measured. It is a cumbersome method and not commonly used.

Indirect

- *Ultrasonography*: This can be done by estimation of deepest vertical pool (DVP) or measuring amniotic fluid index (AFI). AFI is reliable for both oligo and polyhydramnios. In addition to confirming diagnosis, ultrasound assessment helps to diagnose fetal abnormalities and to see recipient bladder fullness in monochorionic placenta in twin-to-twin transfusion syndrome (TTTS).
- *Karyotyping*: In the past it was recommended in all cases but now with the advent of sonography its utility has decreased.
- *GTT*: It is indicated to rule out maternal diabetes.
- *Serological studies*: For alloimmunization and for evidence of TORCH infection.
- *Doppler study*:
  1. For middle cerebral artery peak systolic velocity estimation in cases of suspected fetal anemia.
  2. For diagnosis and management of chorioangioma.
  3. For diagnosis of fetal placental insufficiency.

Treatment

Principles of treatment of polyhydramnios are to:
- Relieve symptoms
- Prolong the pregnancy till fetal maturity
- To give appropriate treatment in cases of known etiologies.

Mild Polyhydramnios

Expectant line of management with bedrest and monitoring is advocated.

Moderate to Severe Polyhydramnios

Treatment is usually required during mid or early third trimester in these patients. Criteria for treatment are AFI > 40 cm or DVP >12 cm. It may be in the form of amnioreduction, either by drugs or intervention.

Medical Amnioreduction

- **Indomethacin**: It is a prostaglandin synthetase inhibitor, given in a dose of 50-200 mg per day. It antagonizes the antidiuretic effect of vasopressin on the collecting tubules of kidney and enhances proximal tubular reabsorption of water and sodium. This leads to decrease in urine output in fetus. It is usually discontinued by 32 weeks because of the associated neonatal morbidity in later gestation. Morbidity includes premature closure of ductus arteriosus, cerebral vasoconstriction in the fetus and impaired renal function.[9]
- **Sulindac**: It is an alternative prostaglandin synthetase inhibitor, similar to indomethacin but with lesser side effects on prolonged therapy. It is given in a dose of 200 mg twice daily.

Invasive Amnioreduction

It is done in moderate to severe hydramnios where patient is symptomatic. Informed consent is taken after counseling the patient about the procedure and its merits and demerits.A risk of 0.3% fetal loss due to chorioamnionitis and preterm labor is explained.

Procedure

After due aseptic precautions, an 18 gauge needle is inserted through the locally anesthetized abdominal wall under USG guidance avoiding placenta and lateral wall. Mid anterior uterine wall is selected for entering the uterine cavity. Confirmation of intra-amniotic needle tip location and membrane tenting is done by aspiration of an aliquot of amniotic fluid. Diagnostic sample is collected and sent for karyotyping. Next a three-way canula is attached to the needle hub and aspiration of fluid started at the rate of 500 ml per hour with the help of a 50 ml syringe till the DVP is 5-8 cm or AFI of 10-20 cm. The removal of amniotic fluid is controlled with screw clamp. Anti-D is given to all pregnant women who are Rh-negative. NST is done after the procedure if POG is more than 26-28 weeks especially if it was complicated or the fetus was compromized. Serial amnioreduction is done if AFI rises > 40-45 cm or DVP goes >12 cm.

Cases where the etiology is obvious, treatment is given to correct the condition responsible for hydramnios, e.g.

- Hydramnios in cases of diabetes needs tight glycemic control.
- TTTS may be treated by therapeutic amniocentesis or fetoscopic laser ablation of the communicating vessels.
- Intrauterine interventions for various congenital anomalies are under study.

OLIGOHYDRAMNIOS

Definition

It would be appropriate to define oligohydramnios as amniotic fluid volume below the 5th percentile for gestational age. More commonly in clinical practice, sonographic assessment of amniotic fluid index (AFI), which is an integral part of biophysical profile, of less than 5 cm is used as a criteria to label patients as having oligohydramnios.

It is further classified on the basis of DVP[10] as:

Mild	< 3 cm
Moderate	< 2 cm
Severe	< 1 cm

Etiology

Oligohydramnios can be due to maternal or fetal causes listed in Table 7.2. Basic mechanism of amniotic fluid production in early gestation differs from that in the later period. In early gestation before the establishment of fetal urine production and fetal swallowing, the most important mechanism of amniotic fluid maintenance in the amniotic space is passive movement of water down the solute gradient. After 17-18 weeks, fetal urine production and later respiratory secretion of fluids are major sources of amniotic fluid. Therefore even in congenital absence of fetal kidneys, AFV may appear normal before 17 weeks.

Earlier studies were suggestive of chronic fetal hypoxia due to placental insufficiency to be the cause of oligohydramnios, consequent to reduced urine output and reduced renal perfusion with brain sparing effect. Recent studies by Brace show that placental insufficiency may be a cause of increased intramembranous absorption of water into fetal and maternal vascular compartment, rather than reduced fetal urinary output.[1]

Oligohydramnios can be early onset or late onset. Early onset oligohydramnios occur in early midtrimester and congenital anomalies are mainly responsible. Congenital renal anomalies account for 33-51% cases and include bilateral renal agenesis, bilateral multicystic kidneys, infantile polycystic kidney disease and lower urinary tract obstruction like posterior urethral valves. Chromosomal anomalies such as aneuploidy (4%) cause symmetrical early onset IUGR with severe oligohydramnios. Congenital toxoplasma, rubella and CMV infection also cause severe IUGR. PPROM before 25 weeks of pregnancy carries worse prognosis with over 90% mortality rate.[11]

Table 7.2: Causes of oligohydramnios	
Maternal causes	*Fetal causes*
• Conditions causing severe placental insufficiency, e.g. PIH • Twin pregnancy with donor TTTS • Maternal dehydration • Maternal medication such as ACE inhibitors, prostaglandin synthetase inhibitors, indomethacin, sulindac, etc.	• PPROM accounts for 50% of cases in second trimester • IUGR (20%) • Congenital anomalies (15%) • Chromosomal abnormalities usually aneuploidy (4%) • Idiopathic (5%) • Others, e.g. term PROM and IUD

Late onset oligohydramnios is due to term prelabor rupture of membranes and complicates 3-17% of term pregnancies. Other causes include late onset IUGR, post-maturity and prolonged use of maternal medications like indomethacin, sulindac, and ACE inhibitors.

Complications

Maternal

Oligohydramnios *per se* is asymptomatic in the mother. Underlying causes of oligohydramnios such as preeclampsia, PPROM and increased rate of cesarean deliveries and intrauterine deaths may adversely affect maternal health.

Fetal

Pulmonary hypoplasia and skeletal deformities are two important complications of oligohydramnios and are known as oligohydramnios deformation syndrome or oligohydramnios sequence.

Pulmonary hypoplasia occurs in upto 13-20% autopsies.[12,13] The crucial canalicular phase of lung development occurs around 16-25 weeks of pregnancy. Therefore the severity of development of pulmonary hypoplasia is related to the gestational age. Patients with earlier onset of oligohydramnios have more severe hypoplasia. Further, hypoplasia also depends upon severity and duration of oligohydramnios.[14]

It results from thoracic compression which may prevent chest wall excursion and lung expansion, loss of fetal breathing, reduced lung inflow, failure to retain amniotic fluid outflow by impaired lung growth.

Various skeletal deformities are seen secondary to oligohydramnios, e.g. talipes equinovarus, curved lower limbs, spinal deformity, etc. The severity depends upon the duration of oligohydramnios. It occurs as a result of adhesion of fetal surface with amniotic membrane following uterine pressure, less intrauterine space and lack of cushioning effect of amniotic fluid. Risk of low birth weight babies is upto 13%. Perinatal mortality is increased specially in cases of PPROM with gestational age less than 29 weeks. Newborn survival rate can be improved with better obstetric and neonatal care.

Diagnosis

History

Correct diagnosis of oligohydramnios is essential for optimal outcome.

History of passage of gush of clear fluid per vaginum followed by persistent leak is suggestive of PROM. Any history of infections (TORCH) in early pregnancy, drug intake, smoking, alcoholism, heart disease, type I diabetes with history of vascular involvement, lupus erythematosus, any past history of stillbirth, recurrent abortions or midtrimester loss should be elicited.

There may be no specific symptoms except those due to complicating features. On abdominal palpation uterine height may appear less than period of gestation. Uterus may feel full of fetus. Malpresentation is more common in these cases.

Investigations

Ultrasound is indicated to confirm the diagnosis and its severity, further investigations are done to find out the possible etiology. USG level II is indicated to diagnose various congenital anomalies like bilateral renal agenesis, lower urinary tract obstruction (LUTO) and infantile polycystic kidneys.[15]

Demonstration of early symmetrical IUGR indicates possibility of chromosomal abnormalities such as trisomy 18 and aneuploidy. Hourly filling and emptying of bladder excludes presence of renal agenesis.

The various tests done are maternal serology for toxoplasma, rubella, CMV and herpes simplex (TORCH) infections, antiphospholipid antibody (APA), lupus-anticoagulant antibody (LAC). Doppler study is done to diagnose placental insufficiency and visualize the fetal renal arteries. Karyotyping and diagnostic amniocentesis is done to rule out chromosomal anomalies and congenital infections.

Prognosis

The ultimate prognosis depends on the gestational age at onset, underlying etiology, severity and duration of oligohydramnios. Second trimester oligohydramnios has 50% chances of major anomalies with a poor survival rate of 10%.Oligohydramnios in third trimester have 22% chances of congenital anomalies and 85% survival rate. According to Chamberlain et al, in absence of anomalies, perinatal mortality rate is 10.9% when DVP < 1 cm and 3.8% and when DVP is < 2 cm.

Treatment

Bedrest and limited activity is the only established treatment. Treatment of underlying etiology with a definitive treatment option as in PIH is initiated. Patients with suspected IUGR are monitored with enhanced fetal surveillance in form of DFMR, BPP and umbilical artery Doppler flow studies. Glucocorticoids are administered where premature termination is anticipated as in severe IUGR.The recommended schedule is 2 doses of 12 mg betamethasone 24 hours apart. Elective induction at 36 weeks is recommended or earlier intervention is indicated if NST is not reassuring and when there is absent or reversal of end diastolic flow in umbilical artery.

In PPROM, a close watch is kept for early detection of signs and symptoms of chorioamnionitis. Prophylactic antibiotics are started in PPROM. Forced maternal hydration is suggested to improve amniotic fluid volume. Drinking of 2 liters of fluid before USG in patients with normal pregnancy and oligohydramnios, increases the AFI by 2.01 cm. This short-term improvement in AFI can continue long term if maternal hydration is continued at the rate of two liters per day for a week.[16] Serial amnioinfusion and vesicoamniotic shunting have been used to prevent pulmonary hypoplasia in selected euploid fetuses with functioning renal tissue to improve outcome. However, most patients with midtrimester PPROM are unsuitable as fluid leaks out immediately.[17]

Amnioinfusion: It is done under sonographic guidance. A 20 guage needle is introduced into the amniotic cavity through the mid-anterior uterine wall avoiding placenta and lateral myometrial wall. Infusion of 0.9% normal saline or Hartman's solution is done with 50 ml syringe till the AFI is 20 cm or DVP of 6 cm. Concomitant karyotyping can be done on the initial amniotic fluid aspirate. After the procedure, umbilical artery flow is checked by Doppler and pads are checked for leaking. Repeat amnioinfusion is done at weekly intervals. NST is performed if the fetus is beyond period of viability.

Other advances in treatment which are under trial with encouraging results include cervical occlusion with fibrin plug, intraamniotic sealing techniques, intraamniotic administration of gelatin sponge (gelfoam), application of aminopatch (platelet and cryoprecipitate injection) and maternal oxygen therapy.[18]

Fetal cystoscopy has been attempted to diagnose and destroy posterior urethral valve with laser.

KEY POINTS

- Earliest detection of amniotic fluid occurs by 8 weeks.
- Amniotic fluid volume is 30 ml at 10 weeks, 190 ml at 16 weeks and level gradually increases to peak volume of 800-1000 ml at 32-35 weeks. Thereafter, it declines to 550 ml by 42 weeks.
- Transudation from maternal plasma is the source during early gestation but beyond 17 weeks fetal urination and lung secretions are the main sources.
- Polyhydramnios is sonographically defined as AFI of >25 cm or DVP of > 8 cm.
- Severity is classified as:
  Mild   AFI 25-35 cm/DVP 8-10 cm.
  Moderate   AFI 36-45 cm/DVP 10-12 cm.
  Severe   AFI > 45 cm/DVP >12 cm.
- Hydramnios occurs in 1-3.5% of pregnancies and is severe in 5% of cases. Majority are idiopathic. In severe cases 80% have a known underlying etiology like congenital anomalies, diabetes, lithium therapy and substance abuse.

- Fetal abnormalities are associated in 1%, 2% and 11% of cases of mild, moderate and severe polyhydramnios respectively.
- Maternal complications are due to uterine over distention and major venous system compression.
- Fetal complications include spontaneous preterm labor in 22% of cases.
- Direct method of assessment like dye dilution methods are cumbersome and not routinely done. Ultrasonography is the main modality of investigation.
- In moderate to severe cases, amnioreduction by either drugs or invasive intervention is required.
- Oligohydramnios is sonographically defined as AFI of < 5 cm or DVP of < 1 cm.
- Early onset oligohydramnios is usually due to PPROM and congenital anomalies. Late onset is due to term PROM, late onset IUGR and postmaturity.
- Investigations include ultrasonography and serological studies.
- Ultrasonography helps to assess: degree of oligohydramnios, presence of IUGR, fetal and uterine blood flow studies and presence of fetal anomalies.
- Pulmonary hypoplasia and skeletal deformities are two important complications.
- Recent advances in management include cervical occlusion with fibrin plug, intraamniotic sealing techniques with gelfoam, amniopatch application, vesicoamniotic shunting, maternal hydration and oxygen therapy.

REFERENCES

1. Brace RA. Amniotic fluid dynamics. In Creasy RK, Rosnik R (Eds): Maternal Fetal Medicine: Principles and Practice. Philadelphia: Elsevier 2004;45-54.
2. Moor TR. Superiority of the four quadrant sum over the single deepest pocket technique in ultrasonographic identification of abnormal amniotic fluid volume. Am J Obstet Gynaecol 1990;163(3):762-67.
3. Duncan KR, Denbow M, Fisk NM. The etiology and management of twin to twin transfusion syndrome: Prenatal diagnosis 1997;17:1227-36.
4. Dashe JS, McIntiro DD Ramus RM. Hydramnios: Anomaly prevalence and sonographic detection. Obstet Gynaecol 2002;100:134-39.
5. Vink JY, Poggi SH, Ghidini A, et al. Amniotic fluid index and birth weight: Is there a relationship in diabetic with poor glycemic control? Am J Obstet Gynaecol 2006;195:848-50.
6. Ang MS, Thorp JA, Parisi VM. Maternal lithium therapy and polyhydramnios. Obstet Gynaecol 1990;76:517-19.
7. Pritchard JA, Mason R, Corley M, et al. Genesis of severe placental abruption. Am J Obstet Gynaecol 1970;108(1):22-27.
8. Hill LM, Brackle R, Thomas ML, et al. Polyhydramnios: Ultrasonographically detected prevalence and neonatal outcome. Obstet Gynaecol 1987;69(7):21-25.
9. Mamopaulos M, Assimakopoulos E, Reece EA, et al. Maternal indomethacin therapy in treatment of polyhydramnios. Am J Obstet Gynaecol 1990;162(5):1225-29.
10. Manning FA, Hill LM, Platt LD. Qualitative amniotic fluid volume determination by ultrasound: Antipartum detection of intrauterine growth retardation. Am J Obstet Gynaecol 1981;139(3):254-58.

11. Wigglesworth JS, Desai R. Is fetal respiratory function a major determinant of perinatal survival? Lancet 1982;1(8266):264-67.
12. Knox WF, Barson AJ. Pulmonary hypoplasia in a regional perinatal unit. Early human development 1986;14(1):33-42.
13. Kilbride HW, Yeast J, Thibeault DW. Defining limits of survival: Lethal pulmonary hypoplasia after midtrimester rupture of membrane. Am J Obstet Gynaecol 1996;175(3Pt 1):675-81.
14. Chauhan SP, Sanderson M, Hendrix NW, et al. Perinatal outcome and AFI in antepartum and intrapartum periods: A metaanalysis. Am J Obstet Gynaecol 1999;181(6):1473-78.
15. Moor TR, Longo J, Leopold GR, et al. The reliability and predictive value of an amniotic fluid scoring system in severe second trimester oligohydramnios. Obstet Gynaecol 1989; 73 (5 Pt 1):739-42.
16. Kilpatick SJ, Safford KL, Pomeroy T, et al. Maternal hydration increases amniotic fluid index. Obstet Gynaecol 1991;78(6):1098-1102.
17. Fisk NM, Ronderos-Dumit D, Soliani A, et al. Diagnostic and therapeutic transabdominal amnioinfusion in oligohydramnios. Obstet Gynaecol 1991;78(2):270-78.
18. Scisione AC, Manley JS, Pollock M, et al. Intracervical fibrin sealant: A potential treatment for early preterm premature of membranes. Am J Obstet Gynaecol 2001;184(3):368-73.

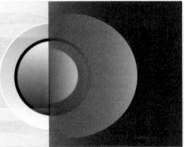

Antepartum Hemorrhage 8

SS Trivedi, Madhu Goel, Monika B Nagpal

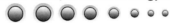

INTRODUCTION

Antepartum hemorrhage continues to be one of the most serious complications of pregnancy and is an important cause of maternal and perinatal morbidity and mortality. Antepartum hemorrhage occurs in 2-5% of all pregnancies[1] and is defined as bleeding from or into the genital tract after the gestational age of viability but before delivery of the baby. Many authorities consider 20 weeks to be the age of viability while defining antepartum hemorrhage (APH). Complete assessment and management of APH in a well-equipped hospital with facilities for resuscitation, replacement of blood and blood products and operative delivery improves the maternal and fetal outcome. Massive and uncontrollable hemorrhage can occur in this condition and prompt and aggressive management by expert team can save lives. This chapter focuses on the effective management of antepartum hemorrhage which at times presents as a life-threatening obstetric emergency.

CAUSES OF ANTEPARTUM HEMORRHAGE

Antepartum hemorrhage can occur due to a variety of causes (Flow chart 8.1). Most common causes are placenta previa and abruptio placentae. Abruptio placentae or accidental hemorrhage refers to premature separation of a normally situated placenta in the upper segment of the uterus, whereas placenta previa is defined as the presence of placenta in the lower uterine segment.

Extraplacental causes of APH include cervical or vaginal lesions like cervical polyp, varicose veins, cervicitis, trauma and neoplasms. Antepartum

Flow chart 8.1: Causes of antepartum hemorrhage

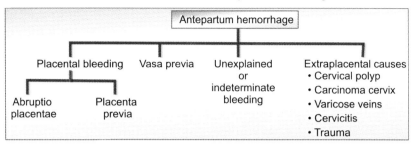

hemorrhage could be due to carcinoma of the cervix. Extraplacental causes are not very common but must be looked for and excluded in women with APH. Rarely, antepartum hemorrhage could be due to vasa previa where fetal vessels lie below the presenting part and blood loss in this situation is fetal. It is a rare but important cause of fetal loss in APH. Excessive show may also present as APH but can be diagnosed by the associated mucoid discharge. In about one-third cases of APH no definite cause is found and these are classified as indeterminate, unexplained or unclassified bleeding.

Rarely bleeding from hemorrhoids or urinary tract may be confused as vaginal bleeding.

PLACENTA PREVIA

Placenta previa is a condition in which the placenta is implanted wholly or partially in the lower segment of the uterus and is an important cause of antepartum hemorrhage. Stretching of the lower uterine segment during pregnancy and labor leads to separation of placenta causing antepartum hemorrhage.

Lower Uterine Segment—Definitions

Metric definition: Lower segment towards term, lies within 5 cm from the internal cervical os.[2] It approximately represents the distance over which the uterine cavity can be explored by the examining finger passed through the cervix during vaginal examination.

This definition is also useful in identifying placenta previa at ultrasonography.

Anatomical definition: Anatomically the lower uterine segment is the part of the uterus which lies below the level at which the peritoneum on the anterior surface of the uterus ceases to be intimately applied to the uterus. The loose peritoneum over the lower segment identifies it at cesarean section.

Physiological definition: Lower uterine segment passively stretches in labor and hardly takes any active contractile part in the expulsion of the fetus. This is in contrast to upper uterine segment which contracts and retracts during labor.

Incidence

Placenta previa occurs in about 0.4-0.8% of pregnancies. The frequency with which the zygote implants in the lower part of the uterus is much higher but many of these pregnancies end in abortions. In many others the placenta migrates and comes to lie in the upper uterine segment which is primarily due to differential growth of upper uterine segment as compared to lower segment. Anomaly scan at 18-20 weeks diagnoses placenta previa in about 25% cases. 34%, 49%, 62%, and 73% of placenta previa would persist as such if diagnosed at 20-23, 24-27, 28-31, and 32-35 weeks' gestation, respectively.[3]

Etiology

Placenta previa is caused by low implantation of the blastocyst in the uterine cavity but the cause of this low implantation is not known. Following factors predispose to placenta previa.

Multiparity: The incidence of placenta previa is much higher in parous women, 5% in grand multipara, as compared to 0.2% in nulliparous women.

Advanced maternal age: Placenta previa is 2-3 times more common in women after 35 years as compared to women less than 20 years of age.

Placental size: Incidence of placenta previa is higher in twin pregnancy, presumably because of large placental size.

Uterine scars and pathology: Placenta previa is found more commonly in cases with previous cesarean section, previous dilatation and curettage, myomectomy and endometritis.

Placental pathology: Marginal or velamentous cord insertion, succenturiate lobe, bipartite placenta and fenestrated placenta are more commonly associated with placenta previa.

Smoking: It increases the risk of placenta previa and may be due to compensatory placental enlargement.

Previous history of placenta previa: Incidence of placenta previa in a woman with previous history of placenta previa is 4-6% which is almost 8-12 times higher.

Associated Conditions

Abnormal placentation: Morbidly adherent placenta (placenta accreta, increta and percreta) may be associated with placenta previa especially if there is a previous cesarean scar.

Malpresentations: The low lying placenta prevents engagement of fetal head and may predispose to malpresentation. Therefore, it is often associated with high floating head, breech presentation, oblique or transverse lie.

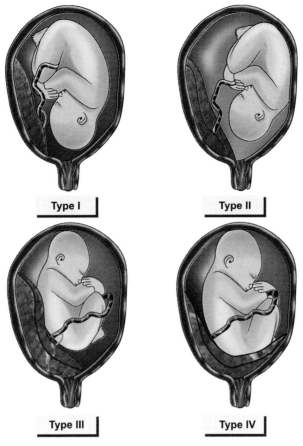

Type I

Type II

Type III

Type IV

Figure 8.1: Types of placenta previa

Congenital anomalies: Incidence of congenital anomalies is almost twice as high in women with placenta previa. The reason is not known.

Classification

Traditionally four types or grades of placenta previa have been identified, depending on the degree of extension of placenta into the lower uterine segment.[5] Since grade of placenta is used to describe maturity of placenta on ultrasonology, 'Type' is usually used to classify placenta previa (Fig. 8.1).

Type-I: (Low lying placenta) – Placenta encroaches on the lower segment. It lies within 5 cm of the internal os but does not extend to the internal os.

Type-II: (Marginal) – Placenta reaches the internal os but does not cover it.

Type-III: (Partial) – Placenta covers the os asymmetrically and ceases to do so as the cervix dilates.

Type-IV: (Total) – Placenta covers the internal os symmetrically and covers it even when the cervix is dilated.

Clinical Features

Placenta previa may be asymptomatic. A high head, oblique lie or transverse lie may be the only clinical feature of placenta previa or it may present as antepartum hemorrhage.

Painless, causeless and recurrent bleeding in late pregnancy is strongly suggestive of placenta previa. The onset of bleeding is usually sudden, it may follow intercourse, although in most cases there is no particular cause. The bleeding may vary from being slight to profuse; usually the first bout of bleeding is not alarming and stops spontaneously, only to recur later. Bleeding in some cases may not occur till the onset of labor.

The absence of abdominal pain and uterine contractions has classically been considered an important distinguishing feature between placenta previa and accidental hemorrhage. Painful labor may however precipitate bleeding from placenta previa, hence this diagnosis must be excluded by sonography in all cases of bleeding during second half of pregnancy.

The general condition of the woman corresponds to the amount of blood loss. If the bleeding has been profuse, the signs of hypovolemic shock will be present. There may be restlessness, agitation, syncope, anxiety or confusion. Woman may be dyspneic with cold and clammy skin and pallor, tachycardia, hypotension denote significant bleeding. Oliguria and anuria are signs of persistent hypovolemic shock.

On abdominal examination the size of the uterus corresponds to the period of gestation. The uterus is relaxed, soft without any area of tenderness. The fetal parts are easily palpable in contrast to the cases of placental abruption where fetal parts are difficult to palpate because of the tense and tender uterus. The presenting part is usually high and fetus may be in oblique or transverse lie. Fetal heart sounds are present unless there is a major degree of placental separation or hypovolemic shock. No per vaginum examination is done outside the operation theater to diagnose placenta previa in a case of APH.

Diagnosis

Placenta previa is usually diagnosed in a woman who presents with causeless, painless vaginal bleeding after 20 weeks of pregnancy and with clinical features of placenta previa as described above. Diagnosis is confirmed on ultrasonography.

Many of the cases of placenta previa are diagnosed on a routine trans-abdominal anomaly scan.

Ultrasonography

Ultrasonography is the method of choice for diagnosing placenta previa and most often the diagnosis of placenta previa is made on a routine anomaly scan. It is diagnosed in about 25% cases at 18-20 weeks but it persists only in about 3% at term. A false-negative rate of 7% is also reported at 20 weeks.[4] A posterior placenta may be missed at transabdominal ultrasound. Ultrasound is more accurate near term and transvaginal ultrasound has higher accuracy as compared to transabdominal scan. Placenta previa is diagnosed on transvaginal ultrasound scan when the placental edge is less than 2 cm from internal os and the placenta is said to be low lying if it lies within 2-5 cm from os. Transvaginal ultrasound is shown to be safe. The apprehension that it may provoke bleeding has not been found to be correct as the vaginal probe does not touch the cervix. For visualization of placenta, probe need not be inserted more than 3 cm into the vagina. Another alternative to TVS is transperineal or translabial scan. Translabial scan has been reported to have 100% sensitivity for detection of placenta previa.

The current RCOG recommendation is to perform a transvaginal scan (TVS) on all women in whom a low lying placenta is suspected on their transabdominal scan, in order to reduce the number of those for whom a follow up is needed.[5]

The distance between cervical internal os and placental edge on TVS after 35 wks gestation is valuable in planning route of delivery. Sonographers should report the actual distance from the placental edge to the internal cervical os in millimeters.[6] When the placental edge lies more than 20 mm away from the internal cervical os, women can be offered a trial of labor with a high success rate. When placental edge lies within 20 mm from the internal os, it is associated with a higher cesarean section rate, although vaginal delivery is still possible depending on the clinical circumstances. In general, if the placental edge is within 20 mm of internal os anteriorly and 30 mm of internal os posteriorly after 35 weeks, it is an indication for cesarean section as route of delivery.[7]

Doppler ultrasound is indicated in women with placenta previa and a prior cesarean section, as they are at high risk for morbidly adherent placenta. The current RCOG recommendation is to perform antenatal imaging by color flow Doppler ultrasound in patients with placenta previa particularly in those who are at high risk of placenta accreta. In settings where such facilities are not available, the woman should be treated as placenta accreta unless proved otherwise. If there is imaging evidence of pathological adherence of the placenta, delivery should be planned in appropriate setting with adequate resources.[7]

Magnetic Resonance Imaging (MRI)

MRI has been used in the diagnosis of placenta previa where transabdominal scans have been unsatisfactory. MRI has the advantage of being possible without a full bladder and it removes operator error. It is particularly useful in imaging posterior placenta and morbidly adherent placenta when the diagnosis is doubtful. However, it is very expensive and currently it is only recommended for research.

Antepartum Hemorrhage

Management

The management of placenta previa depends on whether it is asymptomatic or presents as antepartum hemorrhage.

Management of Asymptomatic Placenta Previa

With widespread use of ultrasonography during pregnancy many women diagnosed with placenta previa are asymptomatic but are at risk of hemorrhage which may be severe especially if it is a major placenta previa. In cases where midtrimester anomaly ultrasound scan reveals placenta previa but the woman is asymptomatic, the woman and her caregivers should be counseled and it must be ensured that they understand the risks associated with the condition and the possibility that the bleeding can occur at any time. Clear instructions should be given to them to report to hospital if slightest bleeding occurs. Anemia if present must be treated. The woman is followed up closely in the antenatal clinic.

In most of the cases placental migration occurs during the second trimester owing to the development of the lower uterine segment. In women with minor placenta previa, follow up imaging is done at 36 weeks, if the woman does not bleed in the interim.

If the follow up scan reveals a minor placenta previa, the woman can be left till 38 completed weeks, when a per vaginum examination is done in operation theater with all the facilities for cesarean section and labor is induced if findings confirm minor placenta previa. A constant watch should be kept during labor for any bleeding.

In cases of suspected major placenta previa on transabdominal scan, transvaginal sonography should be performed at 32 weeks to confirm the diagnosis and allow planning for third trimester management and delivery.

If the follow up scan at 32 weeks or later reveals a major placenta previa, the woman should be counseled regarding the diagnosis, home versus hospital management, the risk of sudden hemorrhage, the possibility of requiring blood transfusion and possibility of major surgical interventions like cesarean section, internal iliac artery ligation, hysterectomy, etc.

Traditionally such women are admitted in the hospital at 32-34 weeks. An anemic woman and those with no immediate access to transport should be kept admitted in a well-equipped center.

Women who are managed at home because of family circumstances and woman's desire should have proper safety precautions in place. Accessibility to the hospital is the most important criteria. The woman should be thoroughly counseled that if she experiences any bleeding, pains or contractions she should reach the hospital immediately. Although several studies have documented the safety, efficacy and cost saving of outpatient management in such patients,[7-9] the risks associated should be clearly understood by the woman.

Management of Symptomatic Placenta Previa

Prehospital management: A woman who starts bleeding at home must be instructed to remain in bed. Arrangements should be made to shift the woman to a well-equipped center. All APH cases must be admitted to the hospital, even if they stop bleeding. This is important because the initial bleeding may be small and may cease spontaneously but it can recur at any time and may be life-threatening.

Management in hospital: All women admitted with antepartum hemorrhage should have an immediate overall assessment especially the amount of blood loss. Resuscitation if required, is initiated.

A comprehensive history is taken followed by complete examination except a perspeculum or pervaginum examination. Gestational age is estimated by last menstrual period or previous ultrasonography (USG). Information about placental localization and its relationship to previous scars if any is evaluated.

Detailed physical examination is done to assess both maternal and fetal condition and includes:

- Assessment of general condition of patient and clinical evidence of pallor and shock.
- Recording maternal pulse, blood pressure and respiratory rate.
- Abdominal examination – It is important to exclude uterine tenderness or rigidity and contractions and to note whether fundal height is corresponding with gestational age. Lie and presentation should be noted and fetal heart is auscultated for any evidence of fetal distress.
- Vulva is inspected to assess the amount of blood loss and to determine whether bleeding has stopped or is continuing.
- Per vaginal examination is not done.

An intravenous line is established with wide bore cannula and blood sample is drawn for full blood count, blood grouping, cross matching and for coagulation studies. Routine urine examination for albumin and sugar is done. Intravenous fluids should be started if bleeding is continuing or is severe while cross matched blood is being awaited. If maternal and fetal condition is stable, an USG should be performed for placental localization. Depending on the maturity of fetus, amount of bleeding, maternal and fetal condition and whether the woman is in labor, the management can be expectant or active (Flow chart 8.2).

Expectant Management

Aim of the expectant management is to prolong the pregnancy till the fetus matures and is indicated if the fetus is preterm, alive with no serious malformations, bleeding is not excessive, mother is hemodynamically stable and is not in labor.

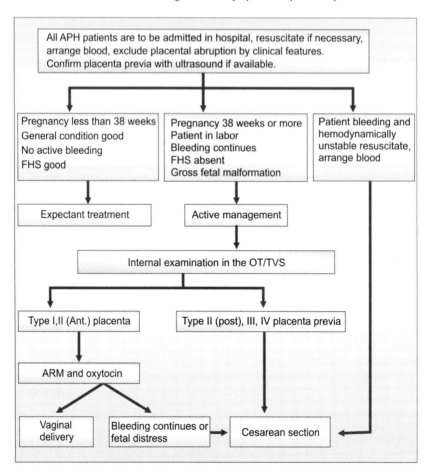

All APH patients are to be admitted in hospital, resuscitate if necessary, arrange blood, exclude placental abruption by clinical features. Confirm placenta previa with ultrasound if available.

| Pregnancy less than 38 weeks
General condition good
No active bleeding
FHS good | Pregnancy 38 weeks or more
Patient in labor
Bleeding continues
FHS absent
Gross fetal malformation | Patient bleeding and hemodynamically unstable resuscitate, arrange blood |

Expectant treatment — Active management

Internal examination in the OT/TVS

Type I,II (Ant.) placenta — Type II (post), III, IV placenta previa

ARM and oxytocin

Vaginal delivery — Bleeding continues or fetal distress → Cesarean section ←

Absolute bed rest is given for at least 72 hours after the bleeding stops. Careful monitoring of pulse, blood pressure, fundal height, fetal heart and vaginal bleeding is done. Antenatal steroids for fetal lung maturity should be administered in women with gestation between 24-34 weeks. Rh-negative woman should be given anti-D immunoglobulin. Ultrasound examination if not done earlier, is done to localize placenta and to exclude any fetal malformation. When bleeding stops, a gentle per speculum examination is done to exclude local causes. Hematinics are given and woman is kept in hospital under observation. Use of cervical cerclage to prevent bleeding and prolong pregnancy is not a recommended practice. Tocolytics have been tried with a view to prolong the pregnancy but are not advocated. Expectant management is continued till fetal maturity is attained or if bleeding continues or becomes excessive. In these conditions active management as described below is instituted. Despite expectant management 20% of women deliver before 32 weeks of pregnancy.

Active Management

Active management of placenta previa is directed at delivering the fetus and is indicated in the following conditions:
- In women who are admitted with severe bleeding and are hemo-dynamically unstable.
- In women with pregnancy more than 38 weeks.
- In women who are in labor.
- Where fetus is dead or congenitally malformed.
- Recurrent bouts of bleeding in women on expectant management.
- In women who have been on expectant treatment and reach 38 weeks of pregnancy.

Based on type of placenta previa, the amount of bleeding and presence of associated conditions an elective cesarean section or per vaginal examination in operation theater with facilities for immediate cesarean section is planned. Most of the cases with confirmed diagnosis of major degree placenta previa and those with profuse vaginal bleeding are taken up for cesarean section. Minor degree placenta previa and cases of antepartum hemorrhage with inconclusive or no ultrasound report are taken up for per vaginal examination in operation theater and allowed vaginal delivery after excluding major degree placenta previa.

Per Vaginal Examination in OT

In cases who have minimal bleeding or have minor placenta previa on ultra-sound, active management includes examination of the patient in operation theater with all preparation for an immediate cesarean section and blood transfusion (double set up examination). Examination is usually done without anesthesia but anesthetist should be ready. A gentle per speculum examination is done to exclude local causes in the cervix and vagina like polyps, varicose veins, etc.

Vaginal examination is carefully done, first through the fornices and if no bogginess is felt, then finger is introduced through the os to feel for placenta. If no placenta is felt, the finger is swept above the os in a concentric fashion till the whole of the lower segment is explored. If no placenta is felt or it is type I or type II anterior (minor placenta previa), rupture of membranes is done followed by oxytocin administration. Labor is carefully monitored. Excessive vaginal bleeding and appearance of fetal distress are indications for cesarean section.

Postpartum hemorrhage is a serious complication of placenta previa. Even a mild PPH may potentiate the effects of already depleted blood volume due to antepartum hemorrhage. Postpartum hemorrhage is also more common because placental site is in the lower uterine segment which does not contract

Antepartum Hemorrhage

and retract as efficiently as the upper segment. Active management of third stage and careful watch for postpartum hemorrhage should be done in all cases of placenta previa.

Cesarean Section in Placenta Previa

Cesarean section is indicated for type II posterior, type III or type IV placenta previa. It has been found that placental edge especially if thick (1 cm), within 2 cm from the internal os anteriorly or within 3 cm posteriorly is likely to need delivery by cesarean section. If there are associated indications like malpresentations, cesarean section is performed. In cases who are admitted with severe bleeding and are hemodynamically unstable, an emergency cesarean section is indicated.

The choice of anesthetic technique for cesarean section for placenta previa must be made by the anesthetist in consultation with obstetrician and the mother. General anesthesia had been advocated in the past but there is increasing evidence to support the safety of regional blockade.

Lower segment cesarean section is preferred and it must be performed by an experienced obstetrician. An ultrasound done prior to cesarean section may help in planning the incision on the uterus and reaching the membranes thus avoiding the placenta. Care should be taken while giving an incision on the lower segment as it is highly vascular in such cases. In cases where placenta is implanted anteriorly, the placenta is separated manually to reach the margin of the placenta and membranes are ruptured and baby delivered. Alternatively one may cut through the placenta and deliver the baby. In both these conditions the cord must be clamped promptly to prevent further fetal blood loss. Complete hemostasis should be achieved in all cases. Placental bed bleeding is controlled by figure of 8 stitches in the lower uterine segment.

Postpartum hemorrhage is common in cases of placenta previa and should be prevented with prophylactic oxytocics.

Postpartum hemorrhage should be managed diligently with manual uterine compression and oxytocics. Uterine packing may be tried. It can be particularly useful while awaiting expert obstetrician's arrival. Bilateral uterine artery and internal iliac artery ligation may be required to control PPH. If these fail, timely hysterectomy may be life saving in these cases and should not be delayed. Newborn must be monitored carefully and may require blood transfusion.

In case of placenta accreta, increta or percreta the risk of hemorrhage, blood transfusion and hysterectomy should be discussed with the woman as part of the consent procedure.

In women with major degree of placenta accreta (Fig. 8.2) hysterectomy is a safer option. Although successful conservative management has been described, there is currently insufficient data to recommend this approach to management routinely.[10]

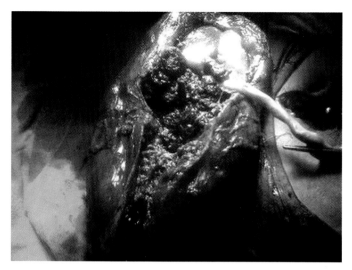
Figure 8.2: Placenta increta

ABRUPTIO PLACENTAE

Abruptio placentae, also known as ablatio placenta or accidental hemorrhage is a serious condition that despite the modern medical advances cannot be predicted or prevented and can lead to high fetal loss and maternal complications. Abruptio placentae, the premature separation of a normally situated placenta accounts for 30% of cases of antepartum hemorrhage. It occurs in about 0.5 to 1% of deliveries,[11] the severe form occurring in about 1 in 500 deliveries.

Etiology

The exact cause of separation of normally situated placenta is not always known.

Following are some of the conditions which lead to abruptio placentae[12]

- External trauma—Fall or blow on abdomen or rarely external cephalic version.
- Acute decompression of polyhydramnios—Sudden diminution of surface area of uterus where placenta is attached.
- Preterm rupture of membranes predisposes to placental abruption.
- Hypertension is the most commonly associated condition with placental abruption. In severe abruption, pregnancy induced or chronic hypertension was found in 50% of the cases. In milder form of abruption the incidence of hypertension is not high.
- Other predisposing factors include advanced maternal age, multiparity, uterine leiomyoma, smoking and previous history of abruption (10% risk of recurrence) and cocaine abuse.
- Folic acid deficiency though implicated has not been proved to be the cause of abruption.

- In many cases, no cause is found. Congenital or acquired thrombophila may be responsible in some cases.

Pathophysiology

Placental abruption is initiated by hemorrhage into the decidua basalis. As the decidual hematoma expands, it separates and compresses the placenta. The blood then separates the membranes and escapes giving rise to revealed type of abruptio placentae (Fig. 8.3). The placental detachment is usually incomplete and complications are fewer and less severe. The revealed form of abruptio placentae is more common and is found in approximately 80% of the cases. In early stages there may not be any clinical features suggestive of abruption. On inspection of the placenta after delivery a circumscribed depression with dark clotted blood is found. Abruption if recent, however may not show any evidence of separation on placental examination following delivery.

In concealed variety, the placental margins or the membranes remain adherent to the uterine wall and blood keeps collecting behind the placenta. This is a severe form of abruptio placentae and is seen in about 20% of the cases. Following the separation of the placenta, the blood does not escape out but is retained behind the placenta within the uterine cavity. Fetal death, coagulation disorders and other maternal complications are more common. Blood may enter the amniotic cavity after breaking through the membranes. In some cases the fetal head which is closely applied to the cervix may prevent the blood to escape.

In the more severe form of placental abruption widespread extravasation of blood occurs into the uterine musculature and beneath the serosa giving rise to couvelaire uterus which appears ecchymotic and purplish on laparotomy. These myometrial hematomas do not interfere with uterine contractility and do not warrant hysterectomy.

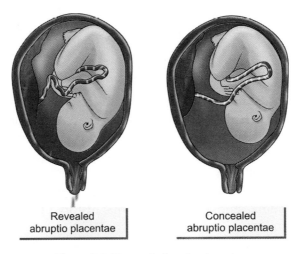

Revealed abruptio placentae

Concealed abruptio placentae

Figure 8.3: Types of abruptio placentae

Clinical Features

Clinical presentation may vary depending upon the severity and type of abruption whether concealed or revealed. In mild cases there may not be any symptoms or signs.

In majority of the cases, vaginal bleeding is the predominant feature and is found in about 70-80% of the cases. Bleeding is most often associated with abdominal pain. Back pain and uterine contractions may be observed in some cases. Uterine tenderness and rigidity is present in most of these cases and is an important sign of placental abruption. Depending on the severity of abruption fetal heart sounds may or may not be present. Fetal distress is found in about 50% of the cases and fetal death occurs in about 15% of the cases.

In mild cases of abruption, vaginal bleeding may not be associated with abdominal pain and may not produce any signs of abruption. Uterus may feel nontense, nontender. Diagnosis is made on examination of placenta after delivery, which reveals a retroplacental clot.

Typical signs of placental separation may be absent initially in a case of abruptio placentae. As the blood collects behind the placenta the uterus becomes tender and tense and the uterine height may rise. Hence every woman who presents with vaginal bleeding must be monitored carefully to detect this condition. Uterine tenderness and rigidity may be absent in abruption of a posteriorly situated placenta.

In severe forms of concealed hemorrhage, no vaginal bleeding may be observed but the uterus is found to be tense and tender and fetal heart sounds are usually absent. The woman may develop a hemorrhagic diathesis due to disseminated intravascular coagulation with depletion of fibrinogen as well as other clotting factors. This may lead to active bleeding from all the sites. Hypovolemic shock and renal failure may develop.

Diagnosis

Diagnosis of abruptio placentae is clinical and high index of suspicion is required to diagnose mild and atypical cases. All cases of vaginal bleeding or pain in latter half of pregnancy and those with history of trauma must be evaluated and observed carefully to diagnose or exclude abruption.

Ultrasound is not always helpful in diagnosing abruptio placentae, it may be normal in these cases but it helps to exclude placenta previa. There may be no findings in revealed abruption as there is no retroplacental clot. Retroplacental clot if present may take a variety of appearances from hypoechoic to isoechoic to hyperechoic and the diagnosis of abruption may be confused by the retroplacental complex which appears hyperechoic on ultrasound. The hyperechoic retroplacental complex which is usually no more than 2 cm in thickness demonstrates very high amounts of blood flow by color Doppler. When the retroplacental clot is large, ultrasound identifies

Antepartum Hemorrhage

it as hyperechoic or isoechoic compared with the placenta. This echogenicity may also be misinterpreted as a thick placenta. In women on expectant management with small retroplacental clot, resolution of the clot appears hyperechoic within one week and sonolucent within 2 weeks.

Depending upon the degree of abruption and its clinical effects the cases are graded as follows:

Grade 0

Clinical features suggestive of placental separation are absent, the diagnosis is made retrospectively when retroplacental clots are detected incidentally following delivery.

Grade 1

There is hemorrhage and uterine irritability and pain but there is no maternal or fetal compromise.

Grade II

In this grade antepartum hemorrhage is accompanied by classic features of abruptio placentae and the fetus is alive. The uterus is tense and tender and fetal heart abnormalities are present.

Grade III

Along with the features of grade II there is fetal death. It has associated maternal shock, coagulation failure or renal failure.

Management

Management of abruptio placentae depends on the severity of the case and on the condition of the mother and the fetus. All cases require intensive monitoring and individualized management (Flow chart 8.3).

In cases of mild abruption where the uterus is soft and not tender, the pregnancy should be terminated by induction of labor with low rupture of membranes and oxytocin. Many cases of abruption are already in established labor and may not require oxytocin.

Careful watch on progress of labor, condition of woman and fetus is important. Signs of hemorrhage, revealed or concealed should be looked for. Vital signs, uterine height, vaginal bleeding, urinary output and coagulation profile should be carefully monitored. Blood and fresh frozen plasma should be available. An early delivery with adequate replacement of fluid or blood and careful monitoring results in good outcome. If uterus becomes rigid and fetal distress develops cesarean section should be done. Coagulation profile, if found to be abnormal, should be promptly treated.

Flow chart 8.3: Management of abruptio placentae

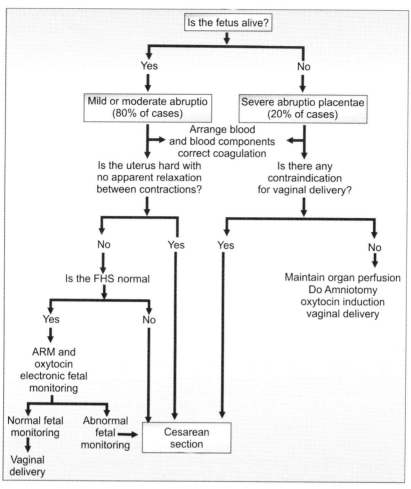

If the fetus is alive and the uterus is rigid, the abruption is large but is less than 50%, chances of fetal distress are high and therefore patient should be prepared for immediate cesarean section with blood and fluid replacement. Coagulation profile should be checked and corrected before taking the patient for cesarean section.

Women with fetal death should be delivered vaginally. Amniotomy should be done as soon as possible and if required oxytocin drip is started. Strict watch on uterine contractions is maintained as the uterus is hypertonic. Careful monitoring of vital signs, coagulation profile and urinary output is important. Women with severe preeclampsia may appear to be normotensive despite excessive blood loss.

The average intrapartum blood loss with severe abruptio placentae associated with fetal death has been shown to be about 2500 ml in a term pregnancy. These patients, therefore, require prompt and adequate transfusion of fluids and blood. Two wide bore intravenous lines should be established

Antepartum Hemorrhage

to allow rapid administration of fluids and blood. Hematocrit and coagulation studies should be done 4-8 hourly depending on the grade of placental abruption. Indwelling urinary catheter should be inserted and vital signs monitored. Hematocrit should be maintained at 30% or more, to sustain the oxygen carrying capacity of the blood. Urinary output of at least 30 ml per hour signifies effective intravascular volume and prevents acute tubular or cortical necrosis, the most common cause of maternal mortality in abruptio placentae. Central venous pressure may be monitored by putting a catheter in internal jugular vein and maintaining it at 10 cm of water. This helps in infusing correct volume of fluids. Lung bases must be auscultated for signs of overload along with other clinical signs.

Third stage of labor should be managed actively. Oxytocin drip and uterine massage is usually sufficient to prevent postpartum hemorrhage. Total blood loss should be estimated, retroplacental clots must be measured and recorded. Very often the blood loss is underestimated and woman may go into hypovolemic shock. Close monitoring must be continued after delivery with special watch for postpartum hemorrhage and urinary output.

Only in very mild cases of placental abruption with slight bleeding where fetus is preterm and maternal and fetal condition is stable, expectant treatment can be given in the hospital under very close supervision. Periodic ultrasound examinations are done to monitor fetal growth and the size of the clot. Although tocolysis to prolong pregnancy in selected cases has been reported to improve perinatal outcome in preterm pregnancies but is not advocated as it may mask the signs of abruption and blood loss.

In cases with incidental finding of a small retroplacental clot on ultrasound, conservative management with careful monitoring is advisable. Predisposing factors like smoking or hypertension should be looked for and managed.

Management of Coagulopathy

In severe abruption acute disseminated intravascular coagulation may occur leading to fall in fibrinogen levels, other coagulation factors and elevation of fibrin degradation products and D-dimers. Fibrinogen levels may fall below 140 mg/dl and there may be fall in platelet count along with prolongation of partial thromboplastin time (PTT) and prothrombin time (PT). In absence of facilities for coagulation studies a simple bedside clot observation test is invaluable in managing these cases. A venous blood sample is drawn and is placed in a clean dry test tube. It is observed for clot formation and clot lysis. Failure of clot formation within 5-10 minutes or dissolution of a firm clot when the tube is gently shaken at the end of an hour suggests clotting deficiency due to lack of fibrinogen, platelets and other coagulation factors. Aggressive blood and coagulation factors replacement should be carried out. Fresh frozen plasma and cryoprecipitates can be given as they contain all necessary coagulation factors. Fresh whole blood which is less than

3 days old can be used for replacing blood loss and treating clotting deficiency. Platelet transfusion in a bleeding patient is indicated if count is below 50,000/mm^3 and in all patients with a platelet count less than 20,000/mm^3 even if there is no bleeding. Coagulation defect has to be treated if cesarean section or episiotomy is carried out.

Management of Renal Failure

Acute renal failure is rare with lesser degrees of placental abruption but is seen in cases when there is delayed or incomplete treatment of hypovolemia. The possibility of renal cortical or tubular necrosis must be considered if oliguria persists after an adequate intravascular volume has been restored. An attempt should be made to improve renal circulation and promote diuresis by increasing fluid volume under close monitoring. If renal failure persists, dialysis is indicated.

PROGNOSIS

Maternal

Maternal mortality in abruptio placentae ranges from 0.5-5%. Hemorrhage, coagulation failure, hypovolemic shock and renal failure are responsible for high mortality. Early diagnosis and prompt and definitive therapy results in lowered maternal mortality and morbidity.

Fetal

Perinatal mortality rates of 4.4-68% have been reported and depend upon the severity of the abruption and the neonatal facilities available. Live born infants have a high morbidity due to hypoxia, birth trauma and prematurity. Neonatal anemia may be marked in these cases.

OTHER CAUSES OF ANTEPARTUM HEMORRHAGE

Besides placenta previa and abruptio placentae, antepartum hemorrhage is caused by incidental causes, marginal placenta and vasa previa.

Local Lesions of Cervix

These include cervicitis, cervical erosion, polyps, varicose veins in vagina or cervix and cancer cervix. Per speculum examination will reveal these lesions but they may coexist with other causes of antepartum hemorrhage like placenta previa, which should therefore be excluded.

Vasa Previa

This is a rare condition occurring in one in two thousand to three thousand deliveries. Clinically it presents as fetal distress and is confirmed by testing vaginal blood for presence of fetal hemoglobin in cases of APH. Cesarean section is indicated if fetal bleeding is detected. Fetal mortality is high if the condition is not diagnosed. Antenatal diagnosis with Doppler ultrasound has been advocated in high-risk cases, that is, those with low lying placenta, velamentous insertion of cord, multifetal pregnancies and those following IVF.[13]

Indeterminate Bleeding

Many cases of antepartum hemorrhage have no evidence of placenta previa, abruption or any local cause. The cause of bleeding in these cases is not known. It can be due to marginal separation of placenta in some cases. The bleeding is usually slight. Perinatal mortality is high in this group. The management of these patients is expectant if pregnancy is less than 38 weeks. At 38 weeks, vaginal examination in operation theatre to exclude placenta previa is followed by rupture of membranes and oxytocin drip. Close maternal and fetal monitoring is required.

KEY POINTS

- Antepartum hemorrhage is defined as bleeding from or into the genital tract after the period of viability of pregnancy but before delivery of the baby and occurs in 3-5% of all pregnancies.
- Antepartum hemorrhage can be due to placental, extraplacental and indeterminate causes.
- When the placenta is implanted wholly or partially in the lower uterine segment of the uterus it is called placenta previa and it occurs in about one in two hundred deliveries.
- Bleeding in placenta previa is painless, causeless and recurrent, the uterus is soft and nontender, usually the presenting part is high or there is a malpresentation. Diagnosis is confirmed by ultrasound.
- Expectant treatment is given if pregnancy is less than 38 weeks, fetus is live with no serious congenital malformation, bleeding is not excessive and patient is not in labor and is hemodynamically stable.
- Termination of pregnancy is indicated if pregnancy is more than 38 weeks, patient is in labor, bleeding is excessive or fetus is dead or malformed.
- Vaginal delivery is allowed in placenta previa type I and II anterior. Cesarean section is done in type II posterior, type III and IV placenta previa or if there are associated indications for cesarean section.
- Abruptio placentae is the premature separation of normally situated placenta and occurs in about 1% of deliveries.
- Bleeding in abruptio placentae is usually associated with pain. Uterus is tense and tender, fetal parts are not easily made out and fetal heart may be absent. In concealed variety of abruptio placentae there is no external bleeding but patient may be in shock with all the other signs of abruptio placentae.
- Severe hemorrhage, shock, coagulation failure and renal failure may be present in severe cases.

- Prompt and adequate administration of fluid, blood and fresh frozen plasma, early delivery with careful monitoring of vital signs, coagulation profile and urine output is included in the management.
- Vaginal delivery is preferred with careful fetal monitoring in mild cases with relaxed uterus and in cases with dead fetus.
- Cesarean section is indicated in severe cases with a live fetus and in cases with associated conditions requiring cesarean section.
- Coagulation disorder, if present, must be corrected before surgical procedure.
- All women with antepartum hemorrhage are at high risk for postpartum hemorrhage and should be managed appropriately.

REFERENCES

1. McShane PM, Heye PS, Epstein MF. Maternal and Perinatal mortality resulting from placenta praevia. Obstet Gynecol 1985:65:176-82.
2. Levery JP. Placenta previa. Clin Obstet Gynecol 1990;33:414.
3. Dashe JS, McIntire DD, Ramus RM, Santos-Ramos R, Twickler DM. Persistence of placenta previa according to gestational age at ultrasound detection. Obstet Gynecol 2002;99:692-7.
4. McClure N, Dornam JC. Early identification of placenta previa. BJOG 1990;97:959-61.
5. RCOG guidelines, Placenta Praevia and Placenta Praevia Accreta: Diagnosis and Management (Green-top 27).
6. Oppenheimer L, et al. Diagnosis and Management of Placenta Previa SOGC Clinical Practice Guideline no. 189, March 2007.
7. Mouer JR. Placenta Previa : Antepartum conservative management, inpatient versus outpatient. Am J Obstet Gynecol 1994;170:1683.
8. Wing DA, Paul RH, Miller LK. Management of the symptomatic Placenta previa: A randomized, controlled trial of inpatient versus outpatient expectant management. Am J Obstet Gynecol 1996;175:806.
9. D Angelo LJ, Irwin LF. Conservative management of placenta previa: A cost – benefit analysis. Am J Obstet Gynecol 1984;148:320.
10. Oyelese Y, Smulian JC. Obstet Gynecol 2006;107(4):927-41.
11. Clark SL. Placenta praevia, and abruption placentae. In Creasy RK, Resnik R (Eds): Maternal–fetal Medicine: Principles and Practice, 5th edn, Philadelphia: WB Saunders Company, 2004; 713.
12. Kyrklund–Blomberg NB, Gennser G, Cnattingius S. Placental abruption and perinatal death. Paediatr Perinat Epidemiol 2001;15:290-7.
13. Sinha P, Kaushik S, Kuruba N, Beweley S. Vasa previa: A missed diagnosis .J Obstet Gynecol 2008;28(6):600.

8

Antepartum Hemorrhage

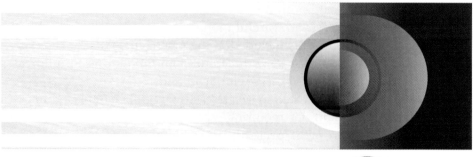

Multifetal Pregnancy 9

Reena

INTRODUCTION

Multifetal gestation is a high-risk pregnancy. The frequency of multifetal pregnancy varies worldwide. The rate of twins and other higher order multiple births have increased remarkably in the last two decades.[1] The increase is basically iatrogenic because of treatment of infertility using ovulation induction drugs and assisted reproductive techniques. These changes translate into significantly greater proportion of multiples among premature and low birth weight infants. Preterm birth and growth aberrations are indeed the most important adverse consequences of so-called epidemic of multiple gestations. The perinatal mortality rate associated with multiple pregnancy increases as the number of fetuses increase and relates to higher incidence of preterm delivery, fetal growth restriction, fetal anomaly, antepartum hemorrhage and preeclampsia in mother. Apart from major complications of pregnancy, the mother is more likely to suffer from minor ailments of pregnancy.

PREVALENCE

The incidence of monozygotic twins is relatively constant worldwide at 1 in 250 pregnancies and is not influenced by factors like maternal age, heredity, etc. except use of assisted reproductive techniques which are associated with an increased incidence.[2] The incidence of dizygotic twinning and higher order birth rates vary widely and is affected by maternal age, parity, family or personal history, racial background and use of assisted reproductive techniques

(ART). Twin pregnancy resulting from spontaneous conception accounts for 1:80 births. In our hospital, over the past two years the incidence of twins was 14/1000 and 0.49/1000 for higher order birth. Hoekstra et al reported an average incidence of 13/1000 maternities,[3] but much more with use of ovulation induction. Over the past few decades there is a 40% increase in rate of twinning and a three-to-four fold increase in higher order births. This increase is largely due to increased application of assisted reproductive techniques.[4] Advanced maternal age also accounts for a slight increase in spontaneously conceived multiple gestations.[5] The lowest prevalence of twin births is reported from Japan (6.7 per 1000 deliveries) and highest prevalence from Africa (40 per 1000 deliveries).[6] Majority of the twins after ART are dizygotic (85%) and only 15% are monozygotic.[5]

ETIOPATHOGENESIS

Multiple births can result either from fertilization of separate ova known as dizygotic or fraternal twins or from splitting of a single fertilized ovum known as monozygotic or identical twins. In multifetal pregnancies, about 70% are dizygotic and 30% are monozygotic.

Monozygotic Pregnancy

Delayed transfer of fertilized ovum through the fallopian tube increases the risk of its splitting into two. ART increases the risk of monozygotic twinning to 1 in 50 as compared to 1 in 250 following natural conceptions. Several mechanisms have been proposed to explain the increased risk associated with ART. Extended culture and blastocyst transfer with in vitro fertilization (IVF), micromanipulation of zona pellucida with intracytoplasmic sperm injection (ICSI) and minor trauma to the blastocyst during assisted reproductive techniques may lead to increased incidence of monozygotic twins.[7]

The type of monozygotic pregnancy is decided by timing of division (Fig. 9.1). In 30% of monozygotic twins the division occurs before the formation of inner cell mass that is in less than 72 hours of fertilization, resulting in monozygotic, diamniotic, dichorionic multifetal pregnancy with two embryos, two amnions, two chorions and a separate placenta for each fetus. In 70% cases division occurs when inner cell mass has already formed and cells destined to form chorion are differentiated, that is between four to eight days, resulting in two embryos of monozygotic, diamniotic, monochorionic type with a single placenta (Fig. 9.2). Rarely division occurs after 8 days when the chorion and amnion have already differentiated; two embryos of monozygotic, monoamniotic, monochorionic type develop. If division is delayed even further, when embryonic disk is formed, it will lead to incomplete cleavage resulting in conjoined twins.

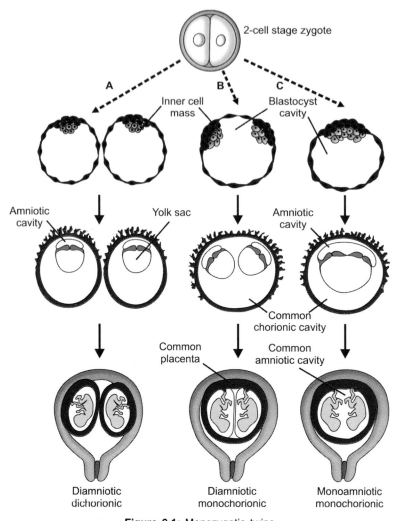

Figure 9.1: Monozygotic twins

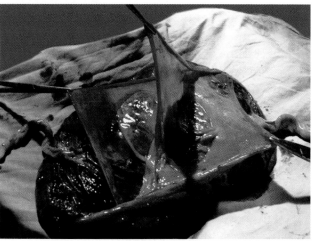

Figure 9.2: Monochorionic diamniotic placenta

Dizygotic Twins

Dizygotic twins result from fertilization of two different ova and each twin has its own placenta and amniotic sac. They are always diamniotic-dichorionic type.The frequency of dizygotic twins is influenced by a number of factors like race, heredity, maternal age parity, nutritional factors, ovulation induction drugs, assisted reproductive techniques, etc. Recent research confirmed that taller women and women with a body mass index >30 Kg /m^2 are at greater risk of dizygotic twinning.[3]

Race

Frequency of multifetal pregnancy is more in blacks as compared to whites. In some areas of Africa, it is found to be 1 in every 20 births. In white women it is 1 in 100 pregnancies as compared to nonwhite where it is 1 in 80. These differences may be because of the racial variations in the levels of follicular stimulating hormones.[2]

Maternal Age and Parity

Increasing maternal age and parity have been shown to increase the incidence of multifetal pregnancy. As the age advances, hormonal stimulation increases the rate of multiple ovulations especially around 35 years of age. The reported incidence at 35 years of age is 2%. Similarly in grand multipara with parity four or more, the frequency of multifetal pregnancy is almost doubled (2% after four pregnancies) as compared to first pregnancy.[4]

Heredity

Family history of multifetal pregnancy in mother or sister is much more important as compared to that in father and his family. One explanation given is that tendency to release multiple ova is inherited and dizygotic twinning may be influenced by an autosomal dominant gene.[8]

Ovulation Induction Drugs

Induction of ovulation by clomiphene citrate or by gonadotrophins with HCG markedly enhances the likelihood of multiple ovulations. With clomiphene, the frequency of multifetal pregnancy varies from 6-12%, while with gonadotropins it is 16-40%.[2]

Assisted Reproductive Technique (ART)

ART procedures which use superovulation and retrieval of multiple ova and subsequent transfer of two or more embryos into the uterine cavity after fertilization, results in multifetal pregnancy.

PHYSIOLOGICAL CHANGES

The degree of maternal physiological changes is greater with multifetal pregnancy compared to singleton pregnancy. Women with multifetal pregnancy have excessive nausea and vomiting. The maternal blood volume expansion is greater in multifetal pregnancy. It is about 50-60% in twin pregnancy. The increase in requirements of both iron and folic acid along with marked increase in blood volume predispose the woman to increased incidence of anemia.[11] Cardiac output is also increased by 20% as compared to that in singleton pregnancy predominantly because of increased stroke volume.[12] As far as arterial blood pressure change is concerned, the diastolic blood pressure is lower at 20 weeks of gestation as compared to singleton but increases is more towards term. The increase is at least 15 mm Hg in 95% of women with multifetal pregnancy as compared to 54% in singleton pregnancies.[13] Uterine growth in multifetal pregnancy increases during pregnancy. Uterus with its contents may achieve a volume of 10 liters or more. This extra weight carried with multiple gestations exaggerates the minor ailments of pregnancy like backache, breathlessness, pressure symptoms, difficulty in walking especially in third trimester. The average blood loss with vaginal delivery of twins is nearly 500 ml more than with the delivery of a singleton fetus.

MATERNAL AND FETAL RISKS

Higher order pregnancies confer significant risk to both mother and the fetuses and reduce the chance of both a live birth or birth of a child without significant handicap. Maternal morbidity is seven fold greater in multiple gestations than in singletons. Perinatal mortality rates are four-fold higher for twins and six- fold higher for triplets, and cerebral palsy rates are 1-1.5% in twins and 7.8% in triplets.[9] Mackay et al reported pregnancy related mortality among women with multifetal pregnancy. In their study, the risk of maternal death in twins and higher order pregnancies was 3.6 times that of women with singleton pregnancies. The leading causes of death were embolism, hypertensive disorders of pregnancy, hemorrhage and infection. They concluded that women with multifetal pregnancies have a significantly higher risk of pregnancy related death than their counterparts with singleton pregnancies and that holds true for all women regardless of their age, race, marital status and level of education.[10]

Maternal Risks

Hydramnios

Hydramnios may occur in one or both amniotic sacs. It is one of the important causes of preterm delivery. Acute hydramnios is more in monochorionic pregnancy. It may be caused by fetal anomalies. In some cases, there may not be any apparent cause. The reported incidence is 12%.[6]

Hypertension

The incidence of hypertensive disorders of pregnancy is higher in multiple pregnancy. It is 13-37% in twin pregnancy. Multifetal gestations have significantly higher rates of preeclampsia associated complications such as preterm delivery and abruptio placentae.[14] Primigravidae with multifetal pregnancy are at almost 5 times more risk of developing preeclampsia as compared to one with singleton pregnancy and for multigravidae risk is 10 times greater.[15] The rate of severe preeclampsia is significantly higher in women carrying triplets.[16] In a recent study, Bdolah et al reported a two to three times higher incidence of preeclampsia than singleton pregnancy. They demonstrated that excess placental secretion of circulating antiangiogenic molecule, soluble fms-like tyrosine kinase1 (sFlt1) may have pivotal role in the pathogenesis of preeclampsia. This molecule act by antagonizing placental growth factor (PlGF). The ratio of sFlt1/PlGF, a biologically more reliable index of the circulating angiogenic state rather than either marker alone and was found to be a better predictor for risk of preeclampsia. Circulating sFlt1 concentrations were 2.2 times higher in maternal serum samples from twin pregnancy compared to singleton pregnancy. PlGF concentrations did not differ significantly between twin and singleton pregnancy. But the mean sFlt1/PlGF ratio was 2.2 times higher in twin pregnancy than in singleton pregnancy. These findings suggest that increased placental mass with accompanying increase in circulating sFlt1 may contribute to increased susceptibility to preeclampsia in women with multifetal pregnancy.[14]

Antepartum Hemorrhage

Risk of placental abruption is more with twins especially after the delivery of first fetus. Increased size of placenta or multiple placentae may encroach upon lower uterine segment, thereby increasing the chances of placenta previa.[17]

Malpresentations

Most common presentation is both vertex. Others combinations are first vertex-second breech, both breech, first breech- second vertex, first transverse-second vertex and so on. Nonvertex presentations increase chances of operative intervention including both operative vaginal delivery and cesarean section.

Preterm Labor

Preterm birth is one of the major causes of neonatal morbidity and mortality. Spontaneous preterm birth accounts for a large proportion of preterm births associated with multifetal pregnancy. The rate of preterm birth varies from 30 to 50%[6] The mean duration of pregnancy decreases as the number of fetuses increase in utero. The mean gestational age in twins is 35 weeks.[1]

The mean gestational age for triplets at delivery is reported as is 32.2+/–3.2 weeks.[18] Strauss et al[19] reported the mean gestational age of 31.5, 29.5 and 28.4 weeks for triplets, quadruplets and quintuplets respectively. The risk of preterm birth to the mother is associated with need for the hospitalization and use of tocolysis with its harmful side effects. Preterm premature rupture of membranes occurs more frequently in multifetal pregnancy.

Postpartum Hemorrhage (PPH)

In multifetal pregnancies, overdistention of uterus may weaken the contraction and retraction of uterine muscles and cause increase risk for postpartum hemorrhage following delivery. A study by Shunj et al reported the risk of PPH in twin pregnancy as 24% and reported it to be more if gestation age is more than 39 weeks or when the labor was induced.[20] Large surface area of placenta is also responsible for increased risk for PPH.[21]

Fetal Risks

Abortion

The rate of abortion is more common in multifetal gestation than in singleton. Monochorionic abortuses greatly outnumber dichorionic abortuses implicating monozygosity as a risk factor for spontaneous abortion. The rate of missed abortion is approximately twice as compared to singleton at 10-14weeks of gestation.[22] Sometimes during the first trimester, one or more of the multifetal gestation sacs fails to develop and get absorbed. This is known as vanishing twin syndrome where pregnancy has been diagnosed initially by ultrasonography as multifetal but later on, one or more gestation sac disappears. Women with vanishing twin may present with slight vaginal bleeding in first trimester. The reported incidence ranges from 10-20% with most cases occurring prior to 12 weeks.[23] The prognosis of the remaining fetus at that early gestation is good.[24] Sometimes one of the twin fetus dies and gets compressed between uterine wall and other growing healthy twin and later presents as fetus papyraceus (Fig. 9.3).

Low Birth Weight

Chances of babies being born with low birth weight are more in multifetal gestations as compared to singletons. This is both because of increased incidence of prematurity as well as intrauterine growth restriction. Larger the number of fetuses, greater the degree of growth restriction and increased are the chances of premature onset of labor. The percentage of small for gestational age babies is about 27% in twins and 46% in triplets.[19,25] Growth abnormalities which include intrauterine growth restriction and weight discordancy between twins are common in multifetal pregnancy.[26] Accurate dating of pregnancy and knowledge of the chorionicity are essential and both can be reliably

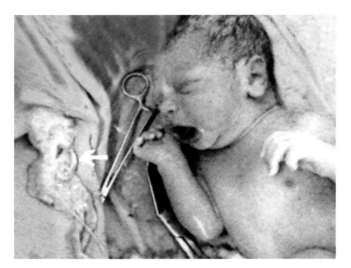

Figure 9.3: Fetus papyraceus

determined by first trimester ultrasonography.[27] The risk of low birth weight is much more in monochorionic twins.[28] A fetus is considered small for gestational age if both abdominal circumference and estimated fetal weight is below tenth percentile. The chance of both fetuses being low birth weight is twice as high in monochorionic gestations (17%) as compared to dichorionic twins (8%).[4] There can be growth discordancy between two fetuses. The parameters to detect growth discordancy are the abdominal circumference and birth weight. A difference of 20 mm in abdominal circumference after 24 weeks and birth weight difference of 20% are suggestive of discordant growth.The incidence of discordancy is 12% in twins and 34% in triplets.[29] Growth discordancy complicates both monochorionic as well as dichorionic multifetal gestations, however the growth pattern and underlying pathophysiology is different. The onset of discordancy is unpredictable in monochorionic twins and can present early or late in gestation. Whereas in dichorionic twins it is usually apparent late in pregnancy.[30]

The possible reasons for discordancy in monozygotic twins could be either unequal allocation of blastomeres between monochorionic embryos or vascular anastomoses within the placenta causing unequal distribution of nutrients and oxygen.

In dizygotic multiple gestations, unequal placentation may be responsible for size difference between fetuses with one placenta receiving better blood supply than the other. Difference in genetic growth potential may also be responsible for different sizes.

Fetal risks associated with growth restriction are intrauterine death, neurological morbidity due to chronic oxygen and nutrient deprivation. Growth discordancy and growth restriction together increase risk of adverse perinatal outcome. Growth discordant monochorionic twins are at a higher risk of adverse outcome than growth discordant dichorionic twins.[31]

Congenital Malformations

The prevalence of malformations is much more in multifetal pregnancy compared to singleton with a reported rate of 4% as compared to 2% in singletons.[32] In twins with known chorionicity the prevalence of congenital anomalies in monochorionic twins is reported as 6% compared to 3% in dichorionic twins.[32] The rate is increased for all major anomalies except chromosomal abnormalities. The increase is almost entirely due to high incidence of structural defects. Structural anomalies are 1.2-2 times more common in twins than in singletons. Most studies do not subgroup incidence of congenital anomalies by either zygosity or placentation. It seems rate of anomalies per fetus in dizygotic twin is same as singleton whereas for monozygotic twins rate is two to three times higher. Abnormalities associated with twins are neural tube defect, brain defects, facial clefts, gastrointestinal defects, anterior abdominal wall defects and cardiac defects.[4] Exact mechanism of structural anomalies in monozygotic twins is unknown. It is possible that the twinning process itself is teratogenic owing to unequal distribution of inner cell mass. Vascular events in early embryogenesis and later fetal life might account for part of the discordant brain and heart anomalies. The presence of cardiac anomalies in monozygotic twins is reported to be 2.3% as compared to 0.6% in general population.[4]

There are some problems specific to monochorionic multifetal pregnancy like conjoined twins, twin reversed arterial perfusion and twin-to-twin transfusion syndrome.

Monoamniotic Twins

The incidence is 1 in 10,000 pregnancies and constitutes 1% of monozygotic twins.[33] The umbilical cords insert close to each other with multiple deep and superficial anastomoses connecting placental stem vessels of the twins.[34] The diagnosis can reliably be made in first trimester by the presence of single yolk sac, one amniotic cavity containing two fetal poles and a single placenta. High fetal mortality is associated with this type of twins. The reported chance of fetal demise is 10%.[13] Monoamniotic twins are at increased risk of congenital anomalies and sudden intrauterine death.[35] Intertwinning of their umbilical cords, a common cause of death, is estimated to complicate at least half of the cases. Umbilical cord of twins frequently entangle, but the factors which lead to pathological umbilical vessel constriction during entanglement are unknown. Increased fetal surveillance and delivery by cesarean section as soon as fetal lung maturity is achieved can decrease the mortality rate.

Conjoined Twins (Fig. 9.4)

Conjoined twins should be excluded when ever there is monoamniotic twin pregnancy. Incidence of conjoined twin is 1 in 50,000 pregnancies. The diagnosis is possible as early as in first trimester by the close and fixed apposition of the

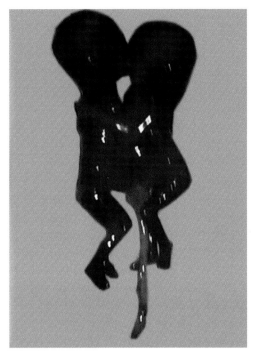

Figure 9.4: Conjoined twins

fetal bodies with fusion of the skin lines at some point.[36] Depending upon the part of the body involved in fusion, there are various types of conjoined twins, e.g. thoracopagus, pyopagus, ischiopagus, craniopagus. Diagnosis can be easily made later in pregnancy on USG when two heads or two breeches are always at same level. Intrauterine death occurs in 60% of conjoined twins and those who are live born, majority of them die because of severe anomalies or as a consequence of surgery to separate them.[37] Unless the conjoined twins are very small or macerated, delivery should be done by cesarean section.

Twin Reversed Arterial Perfusion (TRAP) Sequence/Acardiac Twin

It is one of the rare but serious complications of monochorionic monozygotic twins. The syndrome occurs in 1% of monochorionic multiple gestations. There is one normal donor twin and the other with absent heart and other structures. It is hypothesized that there is large artery-to-artery shunt in placenta and perfusion pressure is more in the donor twin so the recipient receives reverse blood flow from its sibling, this blood flow preferentially goes in the iliac vessels thus perfuse only the lower part of the body leading to disruption and deterioration of growth and development of upper part of body. This is also known as twin reversed arterial perfusion (TRAP) sequence. TRAP sequence in the recipient twin causes hypoxia particularly to the cephalic pole leading to acardia, acephaly and abnormalities of upper part of body. The pump twin is at high risk, due to hazards of congestive heart failure from a prolonged high output state and also the risk of prematurity. The mortality rate is reported to be between 50-70% for the pump twin.[38] At least 20% of monozygotic co-pump twin can be expected to have congenital anomalies and 55% of these die in neonatal period. Early ultrasound prenatal diagnosis is problematic because this condition only becomes pronounced in later pregnancy. Classically, the Doppler ultrasound finding demonstrate the absence of cardiac movement, a reverse or abnormal blood flow through the umbilical cord, a poorly defined head and trunk and abnormal upper limb.[4] The optimal management of acardiac twin is controversial because of the rarity of this condition and widely varied presentation but the objective is to achieve survival of pump twin. Since the mortality of pump twin is very high, therefore invasive procedures to occlude blood flow to acardiac twin have been practiced by most authors. Interruption of vascular communication between donor and recipient at around 20 weeks of gestation can improve the survival of the normal twin. Such procedures include endoscopic umbilical cord ligation, ultrasound guided thermocoagulation of the umbilical cord, endoscopic laser coagulation of umbilical artery and radiofrequency ablation.[39-41] These vessels can be ligated or ablated in utero. A systematic review of minimally invasive techniques, i.e. radiofrequency ablation and monopolar coagulation aiming to occlude vascular supply to acardiac twin has shown a overall pump twin survival rate as 76%.[42] A conservative approach has been described by Sullivan et al from 10 cases of acardiac twin in which the neonatal mortality of the pump twin was reported to be lower than that from invasive management. Nine of ten women delivered healthy pump twin. Their management included two weekly serial USG, fetal echocardiography, Doppler flow study, along with performing a nonstress test and a biophysical profile. It appears from their study that expectant management with close surveillance in a antenatally diagnosed TRAP sequence deserves consideration.[43]

Twin-to-Twin Transfusion Syndrome (TTTS)

Vascular anastomoses are present mostly in monochorionic twins. Most of these communications are hemodynamically balanced. In 10-15% of monochorionic twins, a chronic imbalance develops resulting in twin-twin transfusion syndrome.[4]

When significant shunts are present between fetuses, they can cause twin-to-twin transfusion syndrome, exact incidence of which is not known. In this syndrome, blood is transfused from donor to the recipient such that donor becomes anemic and growth restricted and the recipient becomes polycythemic and may develop circulatory overload and features of hydrops. Neurological damage like cerebral palsy, microcephaly and porencephaly are serious complications associated with vascular anastomoses in twin pregnancy. Damage is most likely by ischemic necrosis leading to cavitory brain damage.

In the donor twin, ischemia results from hypotension and anemia. In the recipient twin, ischemia is because of unstable blood pressure and episodes of severe hypotension.[44] Spontaneous abortion, preterm delivery and fetal death may occur from cardiac failure in recipient and from poor perfusion in donor. TTTS usually occurs between 15 and 26 weeks.The diagnosis of twin-to-twin transfusion is difficult. Antenatal criteria recommended for defining twin-to-twin transfusion syndrome include the following: same sex fetuses, monochorionicity with placental vascular anastomoses, weight difference of more than 20%, hydramnios in the larger twin and oligoamnios in the smaller twin and the hemoglobin difference greater than 5 gm/dl.[45]

The postnatal diagnosis is based on discordancy in weight of 15-20% and a hemoglobin difference of 5 gm% or more. But there can be a number of reasons like anomalies and infection for discordancy.

Pathophysiology of TTTS is explained by angioarchitectural basis. There are two types of vascular anastomoses, superficial and deep. Superficial anastomoses are arterioarterial or venovenous. They are bidirectional anastomoses. Arteriovenous anastomoses are usually referred as deep anastomoses. They occur at capillary level deep in a shared cotyledon receiving arterial supply from one twin and providing venous drainage to the other twin. The AV anastomoses allow flow in one direction only, thus create imbalance in the interfetal transfusion leading to TTTS.[46]

Discordant nuchal translucency of at least 20% can be used to screen early loss and twin-to-twin transfusion syndrome.[46] Recent Doppler based longitudinal study through arterio-venous anastomoses shows that it is their size rather than their number and direction that determines transfusional complications in monochorionic twins. In monochorionic diamniotic twin with transmitted pattern in umbilical artery there is increased risk of sudden death and abnormal cranial lesions in the larger co-twin.[46]

Several therapies are currently used for twin-to-twin transfusion including amnioreduction, septostomy, laser ablation of vascular anastomoses and selective feticides by cord occlusion. Selective reduction has generally been considered when severe amniotic fluid and growth disturbances develop early. Selection of the twin to be terminated is based on the evidence of damage to either fetus. Various techniques include injection of an occlusive substance into the umbilical vein, fetoscopic ligation, monopolar coagulation or bipolar cautery of umbilical cord.[47,48]

Cochrane review[49] of various interventions for twin-twin transfusion syndrome reported that laser coagulation resulted in less overall death as compared to amnioreduction (48% vs 59%), less perinatal death 26% vs 44% and neonatal death 8% vs 24%.There is no difference in perinatal outcome between amnioreduction and septostomy. Their results suggest that endoscopic laser coagulation should be considered in the treatment of all stages of TTTS to improve perinatal and neonatal outcome.

History

History of advanced maternal age, family history of twins, grandmultiparity, past history of twins and history of treatment of infertility in the form of ovulation induction drugs or pregnancy following ART should be elicited. History of hyperemesis gravidarum may be present. Features of anemia may be apparent.

Clinical Examination

The height of uterus is more than the period of amenorrhea evident especially in second trimester around 20 weeks. Between 20 and 30 weeks fundal height, on an average is about 5 cm greater than expected for singleton of same age.[55] On palpation of the abdomen, multiple fetal parts are palpable, two fetal heads may be appreciated in different quadrants. The palpation is difficult if hydramnios is present or the woman is obese. Two distinct fetal hearts can be heard with an area of silence in between the two, with a difference of minimum 10 beats per minute.

Ultrasonography

With the use of USG, multiple gestation sacs can be seen as early as 5 weeks after fertilization.Chorionicity should be determined by ultrasound as it is important for prognosis. If the scan is performed at 10-14 weeks of gestation, twin peak sign can be seen, which is an echogenic chorionic projection of tissue between the dividing membranes which is present in dichorionic twins[56] (Fig. 9.5) and a T-sign when there is only a thin line (two amnions) with no echogenic tissue in between, suggestive of monochorionic twins. As gestation age increases this sign disappears. The dividing membrane is thicker in dichorionic twins, the cut

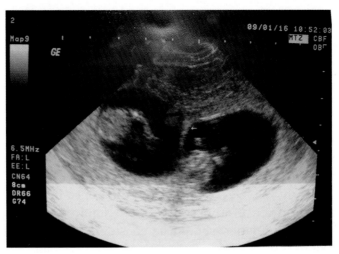

Figure 9.5: Twin peak sign

off of 2 mm is mentioned in literature.[57] For confirming diagnosis of twins, ideally two heads or two abdomens should be seen in same plane to avoid scanning the same fetus twice and interpreting it as twins. Routine midtrimester USG examination can detect almost all multifetal gestation (99%) before 26th week.[58] Higher order multiple gestations are difficult to evaluate. With detail midtrimester scan, structural congenital abnormalities can be identified.

MANAGEMENT

Antenatal Management

Following the diagnosis of multifetal pregnancy, it is important to explain the need for regular antenatal care to the pregnant woman. This allows the mother to make appropriate changes in her lifestyle. For multifetal pregnancies, there is a growing body of evidence linking good maternal nutrition and weight gain to positive perinatal outcomes including decrease in incidence of low birth weight and very low birth weight infants. Nutritional intervention appears to have important clinical implications for infant morbidity and mortality. Nutritional counseling can help women improve and maximize their intake of nutrients such as iron, folate, essential fatty acids and calcium. Calorie consumption should be increased by about 300 kcal/day.[59]

Frequent antenatal visits at every two weeks from second trimester onwards can lead to early detection of hypertension. Clinical assessment of fetal growth has poor correlation with fetal size in twin pregnancy. It is difficult to detect early discordant growth clinically. An overall clinical assessment should however include maternal weight gain, symphysiofundal height, and abdominal girth. Having established the correct gestational age of twin pregnancy by first and second trimester ultrasonography, it is helpful to commence serial USG measurements especially in third trimester every 3 weeks in dichorionic and every 2 weeks in monochorionic pregnancies. Assessment of amniotic fluid volume is also important. When discordant growth is identified, Doppler evaluation of vascular resistance may provide a measurement of fetal well-being. Increased resistance and diminished diastolic flow often accompanies growth restriction. Nonstress test or biophysical profile is commonly used in the management of multifetal pregnancy. Care must be taken to evaluate each fetus separately.

Preterm labor and subsequent birth present greatest risk to the fetus. It is difficult to predict which patient will go in preterm labor. Cervical assessment and fetal fibronectin levels predicted preterm labor. Cervical assessment by digital examination or by USG has been suggested as a useful way to evaluate the risk of preterm labor. At 24 weeks, a cervical length of 25 mm or less is the best predictor of birth before 32 weeks.[60] In multifetal gestations, a positive fibronectin test at 28-30 weeks is associated with preterm birth before 32 weeks.[61] Women with multifetal gestations at 24 weeks who had a closed internal os on digital cervical examination, a normal cervical length on USG and a normal fetal fibronectin test are at a low risk to deliver before 32 weeks.[62]

Several antenatal interventions have been tried to reduce the risk of preterm birth in multifetal gestations. These include bedrest in hospital, use of tocolysis and prophylactic cerclage. It has been shown by various studies that bedrest in hospital in an uncomplicated multifetal pregnancy neither reduces the risk of preterm birth nor lead to reduction in perinatal mortality. The Cochrane review of randomized trial of routine hospitalization for bedrest shows an increased likelihood of preterm birth.[63] The value of admission for rest in higher order multifetal gestations is uncertain. One study in triplets showed reduction in preterm birth after hospitalization.[64] Limited physical activity, early work leave, more frequent antenatal checkups and USG examination and maternal education on the risks of preterm delivery have been advocated to be effective in reducing preterm births in multifetal gestations.[2]

There is no evidence that tocolytic therapy improves neonatal outcome in multiple gestation. Tocolysis can have harmful effect in multifetal pregnancy. This is in part because of increased plasma volume and cardiovascular demands in the pregnant woman. Women with multiple gestations have significantly more cardiovascular complications with the use of betamimetic tocolytic agents. Their use is not recommended in multifetal gestations.[2]

Prophylactic cervical cerclage has not shown any benefit in various studies as regard to improvement in neonatal outcome.[65,66] Elective cerclage contributes little in prolongation of gestational age at the time of delivery in women with twin pregnancy.[67] It seems prudent to reserve cervical cerclage for cases with evidence of cervical incompetence.

Corticosteroids should be given in women with multifetal pregnancy who are at risk for preterm birth before 34 weeks or when there is a chance of preterm termination because of maternal indication.[68] Guidelines for use of corticosteroids are same as for singleton pregnancy, i.e. two doses of 12 mg of betamethasone intramuscularly 24 hours apart.

Intrapartum Management

Recommendations for intrapartum management of twins include:[2]
1. Delivery preferably in a tertiary level unit.
2. An expert obstetrician should be there throughout labor and preferably two obstetricians during delivery.
3. An intravenous line should be established early in labor.
4. Blood should be sent for cross matching. All blood transfusion products should be available.
5. Continuous electronic monitoring of both the fetuses should be done. Once the membrane rupture and cervix is dilated, internal electronic monitoring of the presenting fetus can be carried out.

6. An ultrasound machine should be readily available in labor ward to evaluate the position of the second fetus after the delivery of the first twin.
7. An experienced anesthesiologist should be available.
8. Two pediatricians, one of whom is skilled in neonatal resuscitation should be present at the time of birth.

Vaginal Delivery

When first twin is presenting as cephalic, with no other associated complications, mother is allowed to go in spontaneous labor. Continuous monitoring of labor and of both the fetuses is done. When the cervix is fully dilated, delivery of first twin is conducted as in singleton fetus. Following the delivery of first twin, cord is doubly clamped and cut, placental end of the cord remains clamped. The lie, presentation and size of the second twin are assessed by abdominal and vaginal examination. If lie is longitudinal and uterine contractions are good, let the presenting part enter the pelvis then rupture of membrane and conduct the delivery of second twin.

If uterine contractions subside after the delivery of first twin, start oxytocin drip for stimulation of uterine activity. Once contractions set in, do amniotomy and delivery proceeds with maternal efforts during contractions. Continuous monitoring of second twin is recommended as there are more chances of intrapartum asphyxia.

If the second twin is cephalic, deliver it in the same way as the first. If second twin is an average sized breech, with a flexed head and no fetopelvic disproportion, conduct assisted breech delivery.

If the second twin is in transverse lie, one can go for external cephalic version. Usually it is easy to do external cephalic version (ECV) for second twin because of laxity of abdominal wall and a short distance the head has to traverse in transverse lie. If it fails then internal podalic version with breech extraction can be carried out under anesthesia.

Controversial discussions have taken place on the importance of time interval between the birth of first and second twin. Stein et al analyzed 4110 twin pregnancies and studied the impact of twin-to-twin interval on neonatal outcome. Complications after the delivery of the first twin such as fetal distress, placental abruption and cord prolapse were related to increased time interval. Vaginal operative delivery and cesarean section rates were associated with increased time interval and a decline in mean umbilical arterial pH, base excess and fetal acidosis consequent to it. They concluded that twin-to-twin time interval seems to be an independent factor for adverse short-term outcome of the second twin.[69] The risk of fetal distress and acidosis is increased if twin – twin interval exceeds 30 minutes.[70]

At times there is need to hasten the delivery of second twin like cord prolapse or nonreassuring fetal heart pattern or when signs of abruptio placentae appear. In such cases if second twin is in cephalic presentation at

Multifetal Pregnancy

brim, high vacuum can be used for its delivery and if as breech, breech extraction or cesarean section is advocated. In case it is transverse lie, internal podalic version with breech extraction under anesthesia or cesarean section is indicated.

As far as induction of labor is concerned, if an uncomplicated twin pregnancy does not go in labor by expected date of delivery, then labor should be induced if there is no contraindication to it. Multifetal pregnancy should not be allowed to go beyond expected date of delivery because of increased chances of fetal distress and perinatal mortality. Other indications for induction are associated complications like preeclampsia and fetal growth restriction.[6]

As far as labor analgesia is concerned, epidural analgesia is recommended.[71] It provides excellent pain relief, but one should be cautious in multifetal pregnancy because of increased risk of supine hypotension during labor and delivery.

Active management of third stage should be done after the birth of second twin, as overdistention of uterus leads to increased risk of postpartum hemorrhage. To prevent PPH, intravenous infusion of 10-20 units of oxytocin in 500 ml of lactated Ringer solution should be started following the delivery of all the fetuses.

Indications of Cesarean in Multifetal Pregnancy

The various indications of cesarean section in multiple pregnancy are listed below:
1. Monoamniotic twins
2. Triplet and higher order births
3. Viable conjoined twins
4. When the first twin is noncephalic, cesarean section is often preferred.[72] Although no series suggests that vaginal delivery is inappropriate.
5. Cesarean delivery of second twin if:
   • Second twin is larger and cephalopelvic disproportion anticipated.
   • Second twin is transverse and obstetrician is not skilled in the performing internal podalic version.
   • When cervix contracts and thickens after delivery of first twin and does not dilate subsequently.
   • Nonreassuring fetal heart rate develops.
   • Abruption following delivery of first baby.

Postpartum Management

During postnatal period, taking care of two or more babies may be stressful for the mother. Breastfeeding should be encouraged, though at times it may be insufficient for two or more babies. There is an increased risk of infection and subinvolution of uterus. Maternal nutrition should be given special attention. Supplementation of iron and calcium should continue for a minimum of 3 months. A high percentage of depression is reported in mothers of twins, so additional support should be provided. Contraceptive advice is necessary.

Special Situations

Single Fetal Demise

Sometimes one fetus dies in utero and pregnancy continues with one living fetus. Risk of single fetal death in twin pregnancy as reported by Saito et al[50] is 6.2%. In general population scanned between 10-14 weeks of gestations, the prevalence of single fetal demise is reported as 4% in dichorionic twins and 1% in monochorionic twins, double intrauterine fetal death as 1.6% in dichorionic and 2% in monochorionic[51] twins. Gross unequal placental sharing and hemodynamic imbalance in monochorionic twins may cause single fetal demise. Whereas in dichorionic twins it may be because of discordant chromosomal or structural anomalies or suboptimal placentation. After 14 weeks onward, single fetal death occurs in 2% of dichorionic and 4% of monochorionic twin pregnancies.[4] The prognosis of surviving twin depends on the period of gestation at the time of death, chorionicity, length of time between the death and the delivery of the surviving twin. Early demise such as in first trimester does not appear to increase the risk of death in surviving twin. Later in gestation, demise of one of the fetuses could trigger coagulation abnormalities in the mother. Very few cases of maternal coagulopathy have been reported after single fetal demise. The surviving twin has an extremely high risk of cerebral palsy and cerebral impairment.[52] The management decision should be based on the cause of death and the risk to the surviving twin. Majority of the cases of fetal death in multifetal pregnancy involve monochorionic placentation. Evidence indicates that morbidity in the survivor is almost always due to vascular anastomoses. Pregnancy management depend on diagnosis and the status of both mother and the surviving fetus. When death of one dichorionic twin is due to congenital anomaly, it should not affect the other fetus. Santema et al studied 29 cases with single fetal demise. The cause of death was not clear in all. They recommended conservative management of the living fetus.[53] Lee et al studied twin chorionicity and risk of stillbirth. They compared overall survival in monochorionic–diamniotic twins with dichorionic–diamniotic twins without any other pregnancy complication. Stillbirth rate was 3.6% in monochorionic-diamniotic and 1.1% in dichorionic- diamniotic twin pair. They concluded that monochorionicity has a negative effect on the in utero survival of twins even among monochorionic–diamniotic twins without any abnormalities.[54]

Locked Twins (Fig. 9.6)

This is one of the very rare complications of twin pregnancy during labor. Incidence reported is 1 in 90,000 cases. The types of locking described are

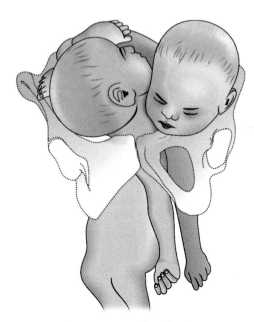

Figure 9.6: Locking of twins

vertex-vertex, breech-vertex, vertex-transverse. There is a chance of locking when two fetal sacs appear together and the twins are less than average in size. As for locking of two fore-coming heads, this seldom results in serious consequences, as the second head can nearly always be pushed out of the way. Much more serious variety is locking of after coming head of first child by the forecoming head of the second child. The risk of death of first twin is very high, as is the risk of fetal hypoxia for second twin. An attempt should be made to push up and hold up the head of second while delivering the first twin by breech extraction under anesthesia. If it is unsuccessful and baby is still alive, immediate cesarean section is indicated. But if because of prolonged asphyxia first twin is already dead, the usual course is to decapitate the first and deliver the second twin and finally remove the severed head. Cesarean section is indicated if obstetrician is not an expert in doing decapitation.

During cesarean section, the head of the first twin is maneuvered upwards, enabling birth of the second twin's head and body. The first twin may then be delivered.

Selective Reduction and Termination

Although most professional societies have issued guidelines to reduce the number of embryos to be transferred during assisted reproductive techniques, the incidence of multifetal pregnancies remains unacceptably high. The negative psychological, social and medical consequences for the patients and their offspring outweigh the benefits in term of increased success rate. Multifetal reduction is an ethically acceptable solution if and only if the physician has taken all reasonable steps to prevent the occurrence of multiple pregnancies.[73]

When there is higher order multiple gestation, reduction to two or three fetuses may improve the chances of survival of the remaining fetuses. Reduction is done early in pregnancy. It can be done transcervically, transvaginally or transabdominally. The easiest route is transabdominal. Reduction is performed between 10 and 13 weeks because at this gestation whatever chance of spontaneous abortion are there, it is already over and remaining fetuses can be evaluated ultrasonographically. The dead fetus is too small and will be absorbed and chances of affecting remaining fetuses is very less. The risk of aborting the entire pregnancy because of the procedure is minimal. The fetus which is the smallest or anomalous is selected for reduction. The method used for selective reduction involves intracardiac injection of potassium chloride. The pregnancy loss rate varies form 4.5% in triplets to 15% for six or more fetuses.[74] Cochrane review on selective reduction found that available nonrandomized studies provide limited insight into the benefits and risks associated with fetal reduction procedures.[75]

Selective termination is mostly done for an anomalous fetus or for a genetic abnormality in one of the twins or marked discordancy among twins. Since anomalies can be seen reliably by ultrasonography in second trimester, selective termination is done in second trimester. Termination at this time of gestation carries more risks. Therefore, this type of termination is considered only if continuation of pregnancy with such a fetus has more risks than the risk of the procedure. Prerequisites for selective termination include precise diagnosis of the anomalous fetus and absolute certainty of its location. Unless a special procedure such as umbilical cord interruption is used, selective termination should be performed only in dichorionic multiple gestations to avoid damaging the surviving fetus.[2]

Risks of selective reduction and termination include abortion of remaining fetuses, abortion of normal fetus, retention of genetic or structurally abnormal fetus after damage without death to fetus, preterm labor, development of discordancy or growth restricted fetuses, maternal infection and hemorrhage.[2]

The patient should be counseled about the risks and benefits of the procedure and an informed consent should be obtained before subjecting the patient to selective reduction or termination.

KEY POINTS

- Multifetal pregnancy is a high-risk pregnancy with increased maternal and perinatal risk.
- Women who are undergoing ART should be counseled regarding the risk of multifetal pregnancy.
- Early ultrasonography for dating and determining chorionicity is important and detailed USG at 18-20 weeks of gestation to rule out congenital anomalies is indicated.

- Two weekly antenatal checkups from second trimester onward should be carried out.
- Early signs and symptoms of preeclampsia, preterm labor, intrauterine growth restriction should be detected.
- Ultrasonographic assessment of cervical changes and fetal fibronectin may be used for screening for preterm labor.
- Regular assessment of fetal growth by ultrasonography at 2-3 week intervals is advocated.
- Hospitalization is indicated if any complications develop.
- Delivery should be done preferably at a tertiary level hospital.
- Watchful expectancy for the patient to go into spontaneous labour if there are no complications.
- Expert obstetrician, pediatrician and anesthesiologist should be available at the time of delivery.
- Continuous electronic monitoring of all fetuses should be done if possible
- Vaginal delivery is allowed if leading twin is cephalic.
- Assess the lie and presentation of second twin by abdominal and per vaginal examination after the delivery of the first baby.
- Start oxytocin infusion if uterine contractions subsides after the delivery of first twin.
- With second twin in longitudinal lie and cephalic, do amniotomy and allow vaginal delivery.
- With second twin in breech, conduct assisted breech delivery.
- If second twin is nonlongitudinal, convert it to longitudinal by external cephalic version or internal podalic version.
- Cesarean section for second twin if second twin is larger than the first or it is in transverse lie and obstetrician is not skilled in IPV or the cervix contracts and thicken or, nonreassuring fetal heart rate develops.
- Start oxytocin infusion after delivery of all fetuses to reduce the risk of postpartum hemorrhage.
- Elective cesarean section for non-cephalic leading twin, monoamniotic twins, triplets and higher order births.
- Postpartum support to mother for taking care of two or more babies.
- Adequate maternal nutrition and supplementation of iron and calcium for 3 months.

REFERENCES

1. Martin JA, Hamilton BE, Ventura SJ. Births: Final data for 2001.Centres for disease control and prevention-Natl Vital Stat Rep Vol 51, No 2. Hyattsville, MD: National centre for health statistics, Dec 18, 2002.
2. Cunninham FG, Leveno KJ, Bloom SL, Hauth JC, Gilstrap L, Wenstrom KD. Mutiple gestation. In: Cunninham FG, Leveno KJ, Bloom SL, Hauth JC, Gilstrap L, Wenstrom KD (Eds): Williams Obstetrics, 22nd edn, Mc Graw Hill: New York 2006;911-43,
3. Hoekstra C, Zhao ZZ, Lambalk CB, et al. Dizygotic twinning. Hum Reprod Update 2008;14(1):27-47.

4. Liesbeth L, Jan Deprest. Fetal problems in multifetal pregnancy. In James DK, Steer PJ, Weiner CP, Gonk B (Eds): High risk pregnancy, Management options, 3rd edn, Elsevier (Saunders): Philadelphia 2006;524-60.
5. Platt MJ, Marshall A, Pharoah PO. The effects of assisted reproduction on the trends and zygosity of multiple births in England and Wales 1974-99. Twin Res 2001;4(60):417-21.
6. Caroline Anne Crowther, Jodie Michele Dodd. Multiple pregnancy. In James DK,Steer PJ,Weiner CP,Gonik B (Eds): High risk pregnancy, Management options, 3rd edn. Elsevier (Saunders): Philadelphia 2006;1276-92.
7. Alikani M, Ceckleniak NA, Walters E, Cohen J. Monozygotic twining following assisted conception: An analysis of 81 consecutive cases. Hum Reprod 2003;18(9):1937-43.
8. Meulemans WJ, Lewis CM, Boomsma DL. Genetic modelling of dizygotic twinning in pedigrees of spontaneous dizygotic twins. Am J Med Genetics 1996;61:258.
9. Wimalasundera RC, Trew G, Fisk NM. Reducing the incidence of twin and triplets. Best Pract Res Clin Obstet Gynaecol 2003;17(2):309-29.
10. Mackay AP,Berg J, King JC, et al. Pregnancy related mortality among women with multifetal pregnancies. Obstet Gynecol 2006;107(3):563-68.
11. Kametas SJ, McAuliffe F, Krampl E. Maternal cardiac function in twin pregnancy. Obstet Gynecol 2003;102:806.
12. Campbell DM.Maternal adaptation in twin pregnancy. Semin Perinatol 1986;10:14.
13. Krafft A, Breymann C, Streich J. Haemoglobin concentration in multiple versus singleton pregnancies. Retrospective evidence for physiology not pathology. Eur J Obstet Reprod Biol 2001;99:184-7.
14. Bdolah Y, Lam C, Raja Kumar A, et al. Twin pregnancy and risk of preeclampsia: Bigger placenta or relative ischaemia. Am J Obstet Gynecol 2008;198(4):428-36.
15. Campbel D,MacGillivray L. Preeclampsia in twin pregnancies: Incidence and outcome. Hypertens Pregnancy 1999;18:197-207.
16. Mastrobattista JM, Skupski DW, Monga M. The rate of severe Preeclampsia is increased in triplet as compared to twin pregnancy. Am J Pernatol 1997;14:263.
17. Ananth C, Demissie K, Smulian J, Vintzileos A. Placenta previa in singleton and twin births in united states, 1989 through 1998. A comparison of risk factor profiles and associated conditions. Am J Obstet Gynecol 2003;188:275-81.
18. Hruby E, Sass L, Gorbe E, et al. The maternal and fetal outcome of 122 triplet pregnancies. Ovu Hetil 2007;148(49):2315-28.
19. Strauss A, Peak B, Genzl–Boroviezeny, et al. Multifetal gestations—Maternal and perinatal outcome of 112 pregnancies. Fetal Diagn Ther 2002;17(4):209-17.
20. Shunj S, Fumi K, Nozomi O, et al. Risk of postpartum haemorrhage after vaginal delivery of twins. J Nippon Med Sch 2007;74:414-17.
21. Monde Agudelo A, BAelizan J, Linmark G. Maternal morbidity and mortality associated with multiple gestations. Obatet Gynecol 2000;95:899-904.
22. Sebire N, Thorton S, Hughes K. The prevalence and consequence of missed abortion in twin pregnanciesat 10-14 weeks of gestation. BJOG 1997;104:847-48.
23. Tummers P, De Sutter P, Dhont M. Risk of spontaneous abortion in singleton and twin pregnancies after IVF/ICSI. Hum Reprod 2003;18(8):1720-23.
24. Stein Kampf MP, Whitten SJ, Hammond KR. Effect of spontaneous pregnancy reduction on obstetric outcome . J Reprod Med 2005; 50 (8):603-6.
25. Ananth CV, Vintzieos AM, Shen-Schwarz S, et al. Standards of birth weight in twin gestations stratified by placental chorionicity. Obstet Gynecol1998;91:917-24
26. Cleary-Goldman J, D'Alton ME. Growth abnormalities and multiple gestations. Semin Perinatol 2008;32(3):2006-12.
27. Caroll SGM, Soothill PW, Abdel-Fattah SA, et al. Prediction of chorionicity in twin pregnancies at 10-14weks of gestaions. BJOG 2002;109:182-86.
28. Lynch A, McDuffie RC, Murphy J. The contribution of assisted conception,chorionicity and other risk factors to very low birth weight in twin cohort. BJOG 2003;110:405-0.
29. Fountain SA, Morrison JJ, Smith SK, Winston RM. Ultrasonography growth measurements in triplet pregnancies. J Perinat Med 1995;23:257-63.
30. Senoo M, Okamuro K, Murotsuki J, et al. Growth pattern of different chorionicity evaluated by sonography biometry. Obstet Gynecil 2000;95:656-61.
31. Victoria A, Mora G, Arias F. Perinatal outcome, placental pathology and severity of discodance in monochorionic and dichorionic twins. Obstet Gynecol 2001;97(2):310-15.

9

32. Gliniianaia SV, RanKin J, Wright C. Congenital anomalies in twins: A register based study. Hum Reprod 2008;23(6):1306-11.
33. Hall JG. Twinning. Lancet 2003;362:735.
34. Bajoria R. Abundant vascular anastomses in monoamniotic versus diamiotic placentas. Am J Obstet Gynecol 1998;179:788-93.
35. Allen VM, Windrim R, Barret J. Managment of monoamniotic twin pregnancies: Acase series and systemic review of literature. BJOG 2001;108:931.
36. Lam YH, Sin SY, Lam C, et al. Prenatal sonographic diagnosis of conjoined twins in the first trimester: Two case reports. Ultrasound Obstet Gynecol 1998;11(4):289-91.
37. Spitz L, Kiely FM. Experience and management of conjoined twins. Br J Surg 2002;89:1188-92.
38. Nik Lah Naz, Che YaaKob CA, Othman MS, Nik Mahmood NMZ. TRAP sequence. Singapore Med J 2007;48(12):335-37.
39. Quintero RA, Chmait RH, Murakoshi T, et al. Surgical management of twin reversed arterial perfusion. Tsao. Am J Obstet Gynecol 2006;194:982-91.
40. Hecher K, Lewi L, Gratacos E, et al. Twin reversed arterial perfused fetoscopic laser coagulation of placental anastomosis or the umbilical cord. Ultrasound Obstet Gynecol 2006;28:688-91.
41. Hirose M, Murata A, Kita N, et al. Successful intrauterine treatment with radiofrequency ablation in a case of acardiac twin pregnancy complicated with hydropic pump twin. Ultrasound Obstet Gynecol 2004;23:509-12.
42. Tan TY, Sepal Veda N. Acardiac twin: A systemic review of minimally invasive treatment modalities. Ultrasound Obstet Gynecol 2003;22:409-19.
43. Sullivan AE, Varner MW, Ball RG. The management of acardiac twins: A conservative approach. Am J Obstet Gynecol 2003;189:1310.
44. Larroche JC, Droulle P, Delezoide AL. Brain damage in monozygous twins. Biol Neonate 1990;57:261.
45. Bruner JP, Rosemond RL. Twin-Twin transfusion syndrome. A subset of twin oligohydoamnios–polyhydroamnios sequence. Am J O bstet Gynecol 1993;169:925.
46. Wee LY, Muslim I. Perinatal complications of monochorionic placentation. Current opinion Obstet Gynecol 2007;19(6):554-60.
47. Challis D, Gratcos E, Deprest JA. Cord occlusion techniques for selective termination in monochorionic twins. J Perinat Med 1999;27:327.
48. Donner C, Shahabi S, Thomas D. Selective feticide by embolisation in twin-twin transfusion syndrome: A report of two cases. J Reprod Med 1997;42:747.
49. Roberts D, Gates S, Kilby M, Neilson JP. Interventions for twin-twin transfusion syndrome: A Cochrane review. Ultrasound Obstet Gynecol 2008;31(6):701-11.
50. Rouse DJ, Skopee GS, Zlanik FJ. Fundal height as predictor of preterm twin delivery. Obstet Gynecol 1993;81:211,
51. Sepulveda W, Sebire N, Hughes K. The Lambda sign at 10-14 weeks of pregnancy as a predictor of chorionicity in twin pregnancies. Ultrasound Obstet Gynecol 1996;7:421-3.
52. Sepulveda W. Chorionicity determination in twin pregnancy; double trouble? Ultrasound Obstet Gynecol 1997;10:79-81.
53. LeFevre ML, Bain RP, Ewigman BG. A randomized trial of prenatal ultrasonographic screening: Impact on maternal management and outcome. RADIUS study group. Am J Obstet Gynecol 1993;169:483.
54. Roem K. Nutritional management of multiple pregnancies. Twin Res 2003;6(6):514-19.
55. Souka AP, Heath V, Flint S. Cervical length at 23 weeks in twins in predicting spontaneous preterm delivery. Obstet Gynecol 1999;94:450.
56. Wennerholm U, Holm BN, Mattsby-Baltzer I, et al. Fetal fibronectin, endotoxin, bacterial vaginosis and cervical length as predictors of pretem birth and neonatal morbidity in twin pregnancies. BJOG 1997;104:1398-1404.
57. McMahon KS, Neerhof MG, Haney EL, et al. Prematurity in multiple gestations: Identification of patients who are at low risk. Am J Obstet Gynecol 2002;186:1137.
58. Crowther C.Hospitalization for bed rest in multiple pregnancy (Cochrane Review). In Cochrane library,Issue 4, 2003, John Wiley and Sons: Chichester, UK.
59. Crowther C, Verkuyl D, Ashworth, et al. The effects of bed rest on duration of gestatation, fetal growth and neonatal morbidity in triplet pregnancy. Acta Genet Med Gemellol 1991;40:63-68.

60. Elimian A, Figueroa R, Nigam S, et al. Perinatal outcome of triplet gestation: Does prophylactic encerclage make a difference? J Matern Fetal Med 1999;8:119.
61. Newman RB, Krombach S, Myers MC, et al. Effect of cerclage on obstetrical outcome in twin gestations with shortened cervical length. Am J Obstet Gynecol 2002;186:634.
62. EsKander M, Shafiq H, Almushail MA, et al. Cervical cerclage for prevention of preterm birth in women with twin pregnancy. Int J Gynecol Obstet 2007;99(2):110-12.
63. Crowley P. Antenatal corticosteroids prior to preterm birth (Cochrane Review). In Cochrane Library; Issue 4; 2003. John Willyand Sons: Chichester, UK.
64. Stein W, Misselwitz B, Schmidt S. Twin to twin delivery time interval: Influencing factor and effect on short term outcome of the second twin. Acta Obstet Gynecol Scan 2008;87(3):346-53.
65. Leung T, Tam W. Effects of twin-to-twin delivery interval on umbilical cord blood gas in the second twin. BJOG 2002;109:1424-25.
66. Koffel B. Abnormal presentation and multiple gestation. In Chestnut DH (Ed): Obstetrical Anesthesia, 2nd edn. St Louis, Mosby, 1999;694.
67. Hutton E, Hannah M, Barret J. Use of external cephalic version for breech pregnancy and mode of delivery for breech and twin pregnancy: A survey of Canadian practitioners. J Obstet Gynecol Can 2002;24:804-10.
68. Saito K, Ohtsu Y, Amano K. Perinatal outcome and management of single fetal death in twin pregnancy: A case series and review. J Perinat Med 1999;27:473.
69. Sebire NJ, Thornton S, Hughes K, et al. The prevalence and consequences of missed abortion in twin pregnancies at 10 to 14 weeks of gestation. BJOG 1997;104:847-48.
70. Pharoah POD, Adi Y. Consequences of in utero death in a twin pregnancy. Lancet 2000;355: 1597.
71. Santema JG, Swaak AM, Wallenburg HCS. Expectant management of twin pregnancy with single fetal death. BGOG 1995;102:26.
72. Lee YM,Wylie BJ, Simpson LC,D'Alton MC.Twin chorionicity and risk of still birth.Obstet Gynecol 2008;111(2pt1):301-8.
73. Pennings G. Avoiding multiple pregnancies in ART. Multiple pregnancies: A test case of moral quality of medically assisted reproduction. Hum Reprod 2000;15(12):2466-69.
74. Evans MI, Berkowitz RL, Wapner RJ, et al. Improvement in outcome of multifetal pregnancy reduction with increased experience. Am J Obstet Gynecol 2001;184:97.
75. Dodd J, Crowther C. Reduction of the number of fetuses for women with triplet and higher order multiple pregnancies (Cochrane review). In Cochrane library, Issue 4, 2003,John Wiley and Sons: Chichester UK.

Multifetal Pregnancy

Intrauterine Growth Restriction (IUGR)

10

Abha Singh

INTRODUCTION

Intrauterine growth restriction (IUGR) is a condition in which the fetus fails to achieve its inherent growth potential. Earlier, it was known as intrauterine growth retardation which was confused with mental growth retardation of fetus, so the term has been replaced by "fetal growth restriction." It is the second most common cause of perinatal morbidity and mortality, following prematurity.[1,2]

The incidence quoted in literature varies between 3 and 10%, depending upon the population under study and the standard growth curves used as references.[3] The high risk of perinatal mortality and morbidity associated with a growth restricted fetus is due to inadequate nutrition and prematurity. Due to limited availability of treatment options for IUGR, the obstetrician has to mostly deliver the fetus prematurely. Early detection of IUGR is crucial because proper evaluation and timely management can result in a favorable outcome.

DEFINITION

Intrauterine growth restriction is used to describe a fetus whose birth weight is below the 10th percentile or < 2 SD below the mean weight for that gestational age[4] and or abdominal circumference is less than 10th percentile.

The current WHO criteria for low birth weight is a weight less than 2,500 g (5 lb, 8 oz) or weight below the 10th percentile for the gestational age.[5] Neonates below the third percentile are very small for gestational age and those between 10th and 90th percentile are appropriate for gestational age (AGA).[6,7]

Approximately 70% of fetuses with a birth weight below 10th percentile for gestational age are constitutionally small, in the remaining 30%, IUGR is pathologic.[8]

Lubchenco et al[4] plotted birth weight against gestational age at delivery and reported a high perinatal mortality and morbidity when infants were below 10th percentile for gestational age. Moreover, 25-60% of infants diagnosed as small for gestational age (SGA) are appropriately grown for gestational age when determinants of birth weight like maternal ethnic group, parity, weight and height are considered.

CLASSIFICATION OF IUGR

IUGR can begin at anytime in pregnancy. Intrauterine growth restriction (IUGR) can be broadly classified into early onset or late onset. Fetal growth has been divided into three phases.[10] The first phase is from conception to early second trimester and involves cellular hyperplasia, in which there is an increase in number of cells of all organs. Second phase involves continued hyperplasia and hypertrophy, where there is both cellular multiplication and organ growth. The third phase, i.e. beyond 32 weeks is characterized by cellular hypertrophy. The cells rapidly increase in size, there is deposition of fat and fetal weight may increase by 200 gm per week.

Early Onset or Symmetrical IUGR

The growth of the fetus is affected before 16 weeks of pregnancy. This is the time when cellular hyperplasia is arrested resulting in symmetrically growth restricted fetus, i.e. entire body of the fetus is proportionally small.

It is often due to exposure to chemicals, chromosomal or structural abnormalities, aneuploidy, maternal disease, malnutrition, intrauterine infections (TORCH) [9,10] or severe problems with the placenta.

Late Onset or Asymmetrical Growth Restriction

In asymmetrical IUGR occurring after 32 weeks of gestation, cellular hypertrophy is affected (fat and hepatic glycogen) but head is spared (brain sparing effect).[10] Here, there is preferential shunting of oxygen and nutrients to the brain, so growth of the vital organs, e.g. brain and heart is at the expense of the body e.g. liver, muscle and fat. The fetus with asymmetrical growth restriction has normal head dimension but a small abdominal circumference (decreased liver size), scrawny limbs (decreased muscle mass) and thin skin. This type of IUGR may be due to placental insufficiency which is usually related to maternal diseases such as hypertension, anemia, heart disease and APH. These neonates catch up with growth after birth. In IUGR, the growth of the baby's body and organs is limited. When blood flowing through the placenta is insufficient, there is hypoxemia and acidemia in the fetus resulting in abnormal fetal heart rate and greater risk to the baby.

Intrauterine Growth Restriction (IUGR)

Newborn babies with IUGR appear thin, pale and have loose, dry skin. The umbilical cord is usually thin and dull-looking rather than shiny and thick. Babies with IUGR may have a wide-eyed look. Some babies do not have this malnourished appearance but are overall small. These neonates are small in all parameters and after birth they catch up growth poorly.

ETIOLOGY

Fetal growth is dependent on genetic, placental and maternal factors. The maternal- placental–fetal unit acts in harmony to provide for the needs of fetus and mother. Intrauterine growth restriction results when a problem or abnormality prevents cells and tissues from growing or causes cells to decrease in size. These abnormalities could be either maternal, uterine, placental or fetal. These may occur when the fetus is deprived of the essential nutrients and oxygen needed for growth and development of organs and tissues, or due to infections. Abnormality of nutrient and oxygen transfer across the placenta, fetal uptake or regulation of growth process results in growth restriction characterized usually by reduction in cell size, but when early in onset or severe, the cell number is also affected. Some babies may be small genetically but mostly IUGR is due to other causes.

PATHOPHYSIOLOGY OF PLACENTAL INSUFFICIENCY

The number of spiral arteries supplying the placental bed is fixed relatively early in pregnancy. In order to accommodate necessary blood flow the spiral arteries undergo certain changes mediated by trophoblastic invasion. In the 1st trimester the decidual segments of the arteries undergo degeneration of internal elastic lamina, denudation of smooth muscle and elastin in the inner and outer media, which are replaced by hyaline and fibrin. In the second phase at 16-18 weeks there is extension of trophoblastic invasion into the myometrial segment of spiral arteries. In woman with placental insufficiency the trophoblastic invasion is confined to the decidual portion of the myometrium and the spiral and radial arteries do not transform into low resistance vessels. The histopathological changes seen are listed in Table 10.1.

The various factors that cause IUGR are shown in Table 10.2.[9]

Table 10.1: Histopathological changes in placenta

- Reduction in villi and stem capillaries
- Decrease in parenchyma and increase in stroma
- Clumps of syncitial villi forming knots in the intervillous space
- Trophoblastic invasion restricted to decidual segments
- Myometrial segments remain intact and responsive to vasoconstrictors
- Acute atherosis of stem villi—lipid necrosis of myometrium and smooth muscle cells
- Hyperplastic proliferation of the remaining smooth muscle cells resulting in narrowing of the lumen.

Maternal factors	Placental factors	Uterine factors	Fetal factors
• Hypertension–both chronic and acute as pre-eclampsia • Chronic renal disease • Immunological disorders SLE APLS • Advanced diabetes • Cardiovascular disease • Respiratory disease causing maternal hypoxia • Malnutrition • Chronic anemia and maternal hemo-globinopathies, e.g. Sickle cell disease. • Infection • Periodontal disease[12] • Crohn's disease, ulcerative colitis • Bacterial vaginosis • Maternal hypoxia –pulmonary disease, cyanotic cardiac diseases, high altitude • Substance abuse- alcohol, caffeine and tobacco/cigarette smoking (3.5 fold increase in IUGR) • Drugs – anticonvulsants (e.g. trimethadione, phenytoin),-folic acid antagonists (methotrexate) and anticoagulants (warfarin)	• Placental mosaicism (25%) and chorioangioma (rare) • Small placenta, single umbilical artery • Uteroplacental insufficiency resulting in decreased blood flow in the uterus and placenta • Partial placental abruption, hematoma and infarction of placenta • Placental vasculitis, edema • Placenta previa, placenta accreta • Abnormal insertion of cord, e.g. Circumvallate	• Decreased uteroplacental blood flow • Atheromatosis • Atherosclerosis of decidual spiral arterioles • Connective tissue disorders • Chronic hypertension • Preeclampsia • Fibromyoma • Morphological abnormalities	• Multiple gestation • Birth defects • Infections—Viral— rubella, CMV and HSV **Protozoal**— Toxoplasmosis gondii, Trypanosoma cruzi (Chagas disease) and malaria, **Bacterial**—Listeria, tuberculosis and syphilis • Chromosomal abnormality, Trisomy 13, 18 and 21, Triploidy, Turner's syndrome

FETAL AND NEONATAL COMPLICATIONS

Problems in Babies with IUGR at Birth

1. Fetal death—15 fold increased risk of IUD in IUGR fetus as compared to AGA fetus.[13] At 38 weeks, the neonatal mortality is 1% compared to 0.2% for appropriately grown infants.
2. Hypoxia due to decreased oxygen levels.
3. Low 5 min Apgar scores. Cesarean section for fetal distress is increased with low 5 min Apgar score, severe acidemia at delivery and neonatal resuscitation requiring intubation and admission in NICU.[14]
4. Meconium aspiration leading to respiratory distress.
5. In preterm SGA infants—Respiratory distress requiring ventilation and grade 3 and 4 intraventricular hemorrhage are increased as compared to AGA infants of the same gestational period.
6. Hypoglycemia and hypocalcemia.
7. Hypothermia and difficulty maintaining normal body temperature.

8. Polycythemia and hyperviscosity.
9. Hyponatremia and hyperbilirubinemia.
10. Sepsis, necrotizing enterocolitis. In term SGA infants, seizures in the first 24 hours of life and chances of neonatal sepsis are increased.[14]
11. Pulmonary hemorrhage.

The long-term consequences include neuromotor dysfunction, cerebral palsy, low IQ, poor concentration, hyperactivity and clumsiness especially in very low birth weight children.[15,16]

Complications in Adult Life

Recently, it has been suggested that there is a relation between IUGR and adult diseases.[15] Barker's hypothesis – Barker proposed that low birth weight IUGR infants might be at a greater risk of developing coronary artery disease, hypertension and stroke.[16] Other problems in adult life include obesity, noninsulin dependent diabetes and cardiovascular disease.[17] The proposed mechanism is congenital pancreatic deficiency manifesting as insulin resistance later in life and alteration in sympathetic nervous activity or adrenocortical function.

Postnatal growth and development of the IUGR fetus depends upon the cause of growth restriction, nutrition in infancy and the social environment. Infants with IUGR due to congenital, viral, chromosomal or maternal constitutional factors remain small throughout life, but those due to placental insufficiency will catch up growth after birth according to their inherent growth potential under optimal environment.

DIAGNOSIS OF IUGR

The identification of IUGR fetus remains a challenge and sometimes the diagnosis may not be made until delivery.

Recognition of high-risk factors is important which are:
- A previous history of IUGR—The risk of IUGR in current pregnancy is one in four with history of previous one IUGR baby, while the risk increases four-fold with previous two IUGR pregnancies.
- History of maternal malnutrition, poor socioeconomic status.
- Chronic illness like hypertension or connective tissue disorder.
- Drug abuse like amphetamines.
- History of bleeding per vaginum.

History

Accurate dating of early pregnancy is essential. The woman should have known date of last menstrual period and should have regular cycles. An early ultrasound between 8-13 weeks is most accurate for estimating the gestational age. An ultrasound done at 20 weeks has a margin of error of 7-10 days but at term there is an error of three weeks so the due date of the women should not be changed based on third trimester ultrasound.

Maternal Weight Gain

A low prepregnancy weight and low maternal weight gain during pregnancy has been associated with IUGR. Weight gained in pregnancy should be plotted on a graph. It is often a late manifestation of IUGR and is not a good screening test. Maternal weight gain in pregnancy can also indicate a baby's size. Small maternal weight gain in pregnancy may correspond with a small baby.

Clinical Evaluation

During pregnancy, fetal size can be estimated in different ways.

Uterine Fundal Height

Measurement of fundal height in pregnancy by palpation is a simple, non-invasive method that can be used to screen small for gestational age fetuses. After 20 weeks the uterus grows 1 cm per week.[15] A lag of four weeks suggests that fetus is small. This is unreliable if the mother is obese, there is excessive liquor or fetus is lying transversely.

Measurement of Symphysiofundal Height (SFH)

Serial measurement of fundal height throughout pregnancy is a safe, simple, inexpensive, quite accurate, noninvasive method that can be used to screen small for gestational age fetuses. The height is measured by a measuring tape from the upper border of symphysis pubis to the top of fundus of uterus. Between 20 and 30 weeks, this measurement in centimeters usually corresponds to the number of weeks of pregnancy. If the SFH is four cm less than the number of weeks, the baby is suspected to be having IUGR.[18] Symphysio-fundal height measurement can identify only 40% of such infants. However, if the measurement is more than 2-3 cm from the expected height inappropriate fetal growth may be expected after ruling out full bladder.

A single measurement at 32-34 weeks of gestation has a sensitivity of 70-85% and a specificity of 96% for detecting IUGR pregnancies.[19]

Abdominal girth is measured in inches, at the level of umbilicus also corresponds to the period of gestation after 28 weeks, but it may not correspond if the women is obese, having multiple pregnancy or hydramnios. Estimation of fetal size and weight by abdominal examination should alert the obstetrician regarding inappropriate growth of the fetus.

Other diagnostic procedures may include the following:

Ultrasonography

A diagnostic imaging technique using high frequency sound waves to create images of tissues and organs as they function and also assess blood flow through various vessels. Ultrasound done in early pregnancy (8-10 weeks) is most reliable and invaluable for accurate dating of pregnancy which is the first step in diagnosing IUGR. For routine screening ultrasound examination should be done at 16-20 weeks to establish gestational age and rule out congenital abnormalities. A repeat scan should be done at 32-34 weeks to evaluate fetal growth. A third trimester ultrasound, with single measurement of abdominal circumference detects 80% of IUGR fetuses.[20]

Serial ultrasounds are done to monitor fetal growth by measuring biparietal diameter (BPD), femur length (FL), head circumference (HC), abdominal circumference (AC), estimated fetal weight (EFW) and amniotic fluid volume.

If ultrasound reveals that HC, FL and AC are all reduced for the period of gestation then it is likely to be a case of symmetrical IUGR. On the other hand, in a case of asymmetrical IUGR, the FL and HC are spared, but abdominal circumference is decreased.

Individual Parameters

Biparietal diameter: Although easy to measure it is not a good tool for diagnosis of IUGR. This is because the delay in growth of the cranium is a relatively late development in IUGR. Also, the shape of the cranium is readily altered by external forces (e.g. oligohydramnios, breech presentation, etc.).

Head circumference: This parameter is better than BPD as it is not subject to intrinsic variability as is BPD.

Abdominal circumference: It is the single best parameter for detection of IUGR because it is related to liver size, which is a reflection of fetal glycogen storage.[21] It has the highest sensitivity (> 95%) for detecting small for gestational age at birth.[22] A growth rate less than one cm in two weeks identifies most IUGR babies. If it is within the normal range IUGR can be excluded. It has a false-negative rate of less than 10%.

The most accurate abdominal circumference is the smallest value obtained at the level of the hepatic vein between fetal respirations.

Measurement Ratios

1. Measurements of the fetal head and abdominal circumference are taken, HC /AC ratio is >1 before 32 weeks, between 32-36 weeks it is 1 and after 36 weeks it is < 1.
2. Femur length to AC ratio (FL/AC) is 22 $\pm$ 2 irrespective of period of gestation. If FL/AC is >24 IUGR should be suspected. FL/AC ratio is not helpful in detecting symmetrical IUGR. The ratios are compared with the growth chart to estimate fetal weight. Serial measurement of biometric growth patterns can be used to diagnose IUGR.
   HC/AC ratio and FL/AC ratio are poorer than AC or EFW alone in predicting SGA fetuses.

Estimated Fetal Weight

It can be calculated by using abdominal circumference alone (Campbell) or after addition of biparietal diameter (Shepherd) and/or femur length (AOKI / Hadlock). It has the highest odds ratio for detection of SGA fetuses.

Ponderal Index

It is calculated by the formula, birth weight (gm)/crown- heel length^3) × 100. It is most accurate for identification of IUGR.[23,24] In a study, it was shown that 40% of neonates with birth weight below the 10th percentile did not have growth restriction based on ponderal index.[24] So ponderal index correlates more closely with perinatal morbidity and mortality than birth weight percentiles, but tends to miss small and lean neonates with growth restriction.[25,26]

Serial measurements of AC and EFW (growth velocities) are superior to single estimations in prediction of FGR and predicting poor perinatal outcome.

Customized growth charts can be used, which take into account the maternal height, weight, parity, ethnic origin and fetal sex. An individual growth chart is given to each patient, thus reducing the number of false positive cases and can distinguisting between constitutionally small and growth restricted fetuses.[27]

Amniotic Fluid Volume

Amniotic fluid volume is an important diagnostic and prognostic parameter for fetuses with IUGR. Amniotic fluid volume can be measured by taking the vertical depth of largest cord-free amniotic fluid pocket.

Decreased liquor volume particularly pool depth < 2 cm is found to have abnormal outcome and mortality.[28] Changes in liquor volume usually occur late during fetal adaptation due to poor growth. Amniotic fluid volume has good negative predictive value for poor outcome (98%) in the small for gestation age fetus and so is reassuring when normal.

If increased liquor volume is found with a small fetus, fetal abnormality should be suspected, particularly syndromal associations. Sickler [29] reported that 90% of fetuses with estimated fetal weight < 10 th centile and hydramnios had major malformations at birth and antenatal detection was not possible in a quarter of cases, while one-third had chromosomal anomalies.

AFI (amniotic fluid index) is calculated by dividing the maternal abdomen into four quadrants and adding the measurement of the largest cord-free liquor pocket in all four uterine quadrants. The AFI reflects measured amniotic fluid volume better than maximum pool depth. Liquor volume should be related to gestational age and various reference ranges are available from different studies. Magann [30] has published tables and charts recently to this effect.

If AFI is less than 5, it suggests oligohydramnios. The volume of amniotic fluid denotes the amount of fetal urine production which reflects renal blood flow. A low AFI suggests less renal blood supply and hence severe degree of IUGR. It is associated with 77-83% cases of IUGR pregnancies[31-33] and is suggestive of growth failure and increased risk for fetal death. The smaller the vertical dimension of amniotic fluid pocket, the greater the perinatal mortality because of hypoxia.

Localization of Placenta

Visualization of placenta and its details is important. If placental maturity is grade III, it should alert the obstetrician that there may be placental insufficiency.

Congenital Anomalies

Fetal anomalies should be searched for like esophageal atresia, renal abnormalities especially agenesis and if detected it helps in deciding the management of the case. If abnormality detected is incompatible with life then cesarean section should not be done for termination of pregnancy.

Biochemical Studies

Measurement of maternal serum estriol, hPL, hCG and α fetoprotein levels should be done in early second trimester. Abnormal levels are associated with development of IUGR later in pregnancy. A single unexplained high value of α fetoprotein is associated with 5-10 fold increased risk of IUGR. Amniotic fluid levels of C-peptide, a fragment of proinsulin and glucose are also reduced in IUGR. A flat response to glucose tolerance test also suggests IUGR which may be due to decreased subcutaneous fat. Umbilical blood leptin concentration is significantly lower than normal fetus (leptin is stored in fetal adipose tissue which is reduced in IUGR fetuses). IUGR neonates with placental insufficiency show high levels of tumor necrosis factor (TNF) than normal neonates.

Biological Markers

Biological markers like erythropoietin (Ruth etal 1988), amino acid concentration and increased glycerol in cord blood could be risk factors in fetus for long-term morbidity and mortality.

Screening should also be done for congenital infections if fetus is growth restricted.

Doppler Blood Flow Velocimetry

Deteriorating placental function triggers a sequence of fetal protective mechanisms resulting in altered fetal cardiac function. These cardiac vascular alterations are mirrored by fetal arterial and venous Doppler studies. Doppler velocimetry is the best fetal surveillance technique for detecting hypoxemia/acidemia.

Evaluation of blood flow in uterine, umbilical and fetal middle cerebral vessels by Doppler velocimetry is used to interpret and diagnose IUGR during pregnancy.

The indices used are as follows:

Arterial Flow

1. *S/D ratio*: Systolic peak velocity/diastolic peak velocity.
2. *Resistance index (Pourcelot index)*: Systolic – End diastolic peak velocity/Systolic peak velocity.
3. *Pulsatility index*: Systolic – End diastolic peak velocity/Time averaged maximum velocity.

Venous Flow

1. *Percentage reverse flow*: Systolic time averaged velocity/Diastolic time averaged velocity × 100.
2. *Preload index*: PLI = PVA (Peak velocity in atrial contraction)/PVS (Peak velocity in ventricular systole) Normal: 0 to 0.37.
3. *Cerebroplacental Ratio*: Cerebral flow/placental or umbilical flow Normal: >1.
   i. Doppler blood flow in uterine arteries is recorded at 11-14 weeks. An early diastolic notch in the uterine arteries suggests delayed trophoblastic invasion whereas persistence of notching beyond 24 weeks is confirmatory. Thus, increased resistance in the uterine artery helps in identifying high-risk pregnancies. Notching of uterine arteries in Doppler waveform is predictive of PIH and preeclampsia,[34] suggesting increased perinatal risk after 28 weeks.
   ii. Blood flow in umbilical arteries–Systematic review and meta-analysis of randomized control trials which included 7000 patients[35] showed that use of umbilical artery Doppler causes statistically significant reduction in perinatal mortality (OR 0.62; 95% CI 0.45- 0.85).[36] Resistance in umbilical artery decreases with increasing period of gestation. A resistive index of > 0.72 is abnormal after 26 weeks of gestation.

   A study comparing resistance index with pulsatility index, S/D ratio and diastolic- average ratio has shown resistance index to be the most discriminatory for predicting poor outcome.[37]

   In conditions with increased placental vascular resistance, the low pressure flow during fetal cardiac diastole is further reduced leading to increased ratio of systolic to diastolic blood flow. The elevated umbilical

Intrauterine Growth Restriction (IUGR)

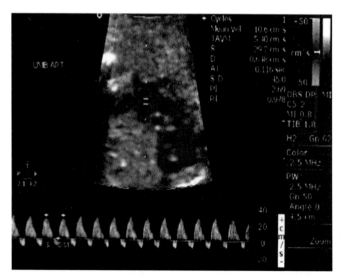

Figure 10.1: Umbilical artery Doppler blood flow showing reversed end diastolic flow

artery S/D ratio (more than 3) at term is significantly related to fetal growth restriction and adverse perinatal outcome (Fig. 10.1).

Reversed or absent end diastolic blood flow in umbilical artery has a poor positive predictive value and is associated with poor perinatal outcome and high perinatal mortality. It suggests a severely compromised fetus which should be delivered immediately to prevent intrauterine or neonatal death. In contrast, a normal S/D ratio in IUGR fetus has excellent negative predictive value and can be used as a rationale to delay delivery with some reassurance.[38-40]

In GRIT Trial,[41] suggestions from 49 European obstetricians were taken regarding the time of delivery in IUGR baby at different gestational age with a range of Doppler waveforms and CTG variability. There was uncertainy and disagreement about the time of delivery. Half of them recommended delivery in presence of reversed EDF > 29 weeks gestation or, absent EDF beyond 32 weeks and severely reduced blood flow after 35 weeks.

iii. Blood flow in the fetal brain (middle cerebral artery) can be measured with Doppler flow studies. The fetus responds to hypoxia by increasing the blood flow to the cerebral hemispheres, resulting in decrease in resistance in middle cerebral artery (MCA) –a sign of compromised fetus (called the "Brain sparing effect" or Centralization/Cephalization). Continued insult causes decrease in blood flow or reversal of brain sparing effect in fetus which is indicative of grave fetal prognosis.

Antenatal fetal blood sampling has shown a relationship between cerebral indices and hypoxemia and acidosis. These fetuses are at increased risk of fetal distress in labor and admission to neonatal intensive care.[42,43]

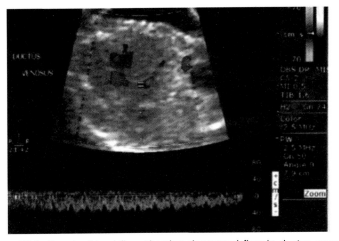

Figure 10.2: Doppler blood flow showing decreased flow in ductus venosus

iv. Blood flow in ductus venosus/inferior vena cava may be reduced in a hypoxemic fetus (Fig. 10.2).

v. Umbilical venous blood flow—There may be pulsatile wave form in umbilical vein indicating fetal acidemia and a high risk of intellectual impairment and other postnatal complications.[9]

Doppler velocimetry may be normal in IUGR fetuses with chromosomal or structural abnormalities. It has been shown to reduce both interventions and improve fetal outcome by early delivery in pregnancies at risk for IUGR.

In fetus when no anomaly is detected on ultrasound and umbilical artery Doppler is normal then the small fetus is likely to be a "normal small fetus" and not SGA. Such patients can safely be managed on an outpatient basis. Fetal monitoring can be done every fortnight.

Karyotyping

It is an invasive procedure. Nearly 19% of growth restricted babies have chromosomal abnormalities. Fetuses with structural abnormalities seen on ultrasonography should undergo karyotyping. Other indications are extremely small fetus or presence of increased liquor or growth restriction of early onset with no predisposing factors. High rates of chromosomal and structural abnormalities have been reported with abnormal umbilical artery Doppler.

MANAGEMENT OF IUGR

Management depends upon the diagnosis whether the fetus is constitutionally small or having IUGR, the severity of growth restriction, and how early the problem began in the pregnancy. Earlier the IUGR develops and more the severity of growth restriction, greater is the risk to the fetus. The challenges faced by the clinician are:

To determine whether the fetus has reached its optimum growth potential or is growth restricted.

To identify underlying cause if any.

To monitor both the fetus and mother.

To deliver at optimum time so as to minimize the damage to the baby both from adverse intrauterine factors and from prematurity.

The general principles of management of IUGR are:

1. Early detection of high-risk factors and their removal such as stress and smoking. Mother is advised to stop smoking or drinking alcohol which has a positive effect on birth weight.[44]
2. To detect the etiology of IUGR by examining fetal chromosomes or structural anomalies or intrauterine infection and other causes of impaired fetal growth. 19% of fetuses with AC and EFW less than 5th centile may have chromosomal defects[11] which can be detected on karyotyping.
3. Specific treatment of any associated bowel disease which results in malnutrition.
4. Treatment of medical disorders such as anemia and heart disease if present.
5. Accurate surveillance of fetal growth requires correct dating. The women should be sure about the date of her last menstrual period.

   First trimester USG has an accuracy of 5-7 days, while second trimester of 10-14 days and third trimester of 18-21 days for dating of pregnancy.

Antepartum Fetal Surveillance

Some of the methods to monitor the fetus for potential problems in IUGR fetuses include the following:

DFMR

Counting fetal movements by the mother is important and a reliable parameter of fetal well-being. The pregnant mother is asked to keep a record of fetal kicks and movements. The woman is explained to count the number of fetal movements over one hour after each major meal, these are added and multiplied by 4 to give the count over 12 hours. There should be at least 3 movements over one hour and a minimum of 10 movements over a period of 12 hours. A change in the number or frequency may mean the fetus is under stress.

Nonstress Test (NST)

NST is most widely used test for assessment of fetal well-being. Cardiotocographic recording of fetal heart rate is done in relation to fetal movements to assess the fetal condition. Normally, with fetal movements, there is acceleration of the fetal heart. NST is said to be reactive if the CTG shows 2 or more accelerations in fetal heart rate of 15 beats/minute and is sustained for 15 sec within a period of 20 minutes. If there are no movements perceived by the patient in 20 minutes an extended testing can be done over 40 minutes as fetus may have sleep cycle. A reactive NST predicts fetal well-being while nonreactive NST does not predict fetal compromise.

Absence of accelerations during a period of 80 minutes, absence of baseline beat-to-beat variability and presence of late decelerations following spontaneous uterine contractions are indicative of uteroplacental insufficiency. However, if NST is reactive and oligohydramnios is not severe then no intervention is required and pregnancy can be monitored by NST done twice a week.

Contraction Stress Test or Oxytocin Challenge Test (OCT)

Contraction stress test or oxytocin challenge test is based on the principle that during uterine contractions there is an increase in myometrial and amniotic pressure causing closure of myometrial vessels. If uteroplacental pathology is present oxygen exchange will be impaired during uterine contractions resulting in late fetal heart rate decelerations. In OCT a conti-nuous infusion of intravenous oxytocin is started at a rate of 0.5 mU/min and doubled every 20 minutes until satisfactory contractions are obtained and fetal heart rate tracings are taken.

OCT can be interpreted as:

Negative—No late or significant deceleration.

Positive—Presence of late deceleration in 50% of contractions.

Equivocal—Presence of late and variable deceleration.

Unsatisfactory—Less than three contractions in a period of 10 min or uninterpretable tracing.

Biophysical Profile (Manning's Score BPS)

Manning suggested a scoring system for evaluation of fetal well-being. The biophysical profile is a combination of five biophysical variables, which are evaluated over a period of 30 minutes and each parameter is given a score of 0- 2, (a score of 2 if normal and 0 if abnormal) the total score being 10 (Table 10.3).

Interpretation: A biophysical score of 0 is associated with significant fetal acidemia while scores of 8 or 10 are associated with a normal pH.

BPS does not improve the perinatal outcome. However, when done in high-risk women it has a good negative predictive value (fetal death is rare, i.e. 1/1000, if BPS is normal).[45]

A decreasing score indicates higher risk to the fetus. If the score is 8 with NST being nonreactive, it is repeated again after meals.

Modified Biophysical Profile–This test combines two parameters, the non-stress test with amniotic fluid index, which is as reliable as Manning's score. AFI is the sum of measurement of the largest cord-free vertical pockets in the

10

Intrauterine Growth Restriction (IUGR)

Table 10.3: Biophysical Profile—Its components and score		
Component	Score 2	Score 0
Nonstress test	>2 accelerations of > 15 beats/min sustained for 15 seconds in 20- 40 min.	0-1 acceleration in 20-40 min
Fetal breathing	At least 1 episode of rhythmic breathing lasting for >30 seconds within 30 minutes	< 30 seconds of breathing within 30 minutes
Fetal movement	>3 discrete body or limb movements within 30 min	< 3 discrete movements
Fetal tone	> 1 episode of extension of a fetal extremity or spine and return to flexion, or opening and closing of hand within 30 min.	No movements or no extension/flexion
Amniotic fluid volume	At least one vertical pocket measuring 2 cm	Largest single vertical pocket < 2 cm

four quadrants of uterus on ultrasound. An AFI < 5 is considered abnormal and is associated with an increased risk of Apgar score of < 7 at 5 minutes and increased perinatal mortality.

Interpretation of BPS

Score 10—Normal fetus, no need for intervention. Repeat test weekly (except in diabetes and postdated pregnancy).

Score 8 with normal liquor—No fetal indication for termination.

Score 8 with oligohydramnios-chronic fetal asphyxia is suspected, deliver the fetus if 37 weeks gestation or more.

Score 6—Suspected fetal asphyxia. If > 37 weeks gestation, deliver the fetus. Optimal mode of delivery to be decided according to amount of liquor. If liqour is normal, Bishop's scoring should be done. If cervix is favorable induce labor and deliver the fetus.

Score 4—Probable fetal asphyxia. If > 36 weeks then deliver same day.

Score 0-2—Fetal asphyxia is present. Deliver the fetus.

Umbilical Artery Doppler Flow Study

In comparison to other biophysical methods like NST or BPS, umbilical artery Doppler studies has better ability to predict poor perinatal outcome in IUGR fetuses. An increased S/D ratio in the umbilical artery is indicative of increasing fetal compromise. A patient with raised S/D ratio can be monitored with serial Doppler studies till:
1. 37 weeks maturity
2. Absent or reversed diastolic flow
3. Reversal of Doppler velocities in ductus venosus during atrial contraction

Flow chart 10.1: Management of IUGR

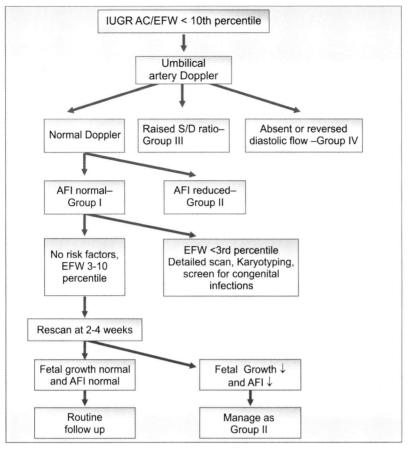

Flow chart 10.2: Management of Group II

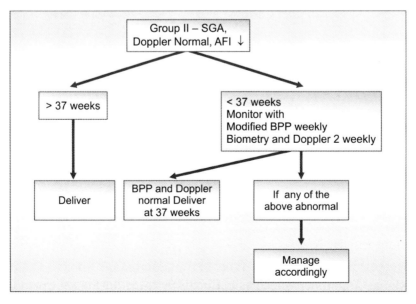

Flow chart 10.3: Management of Group III

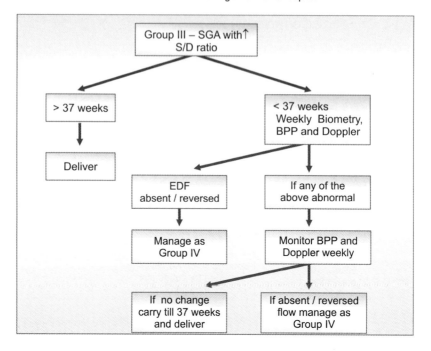

Flow chart 10.4: Management of Group IV

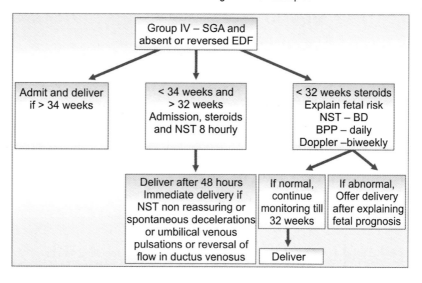

4. Umbilical venous pulsations
5. Abnormal NST or BPP.

Management of IUGR is summarized in Flow charts 10.1 to 10.4.

Treatment for IUGR

It is not possible to reverse IUGR. The management involves balancing the risks and benefits of prematurity with those of hostile intrauterine environment. The effect of a number of conservative interventions on IUGR have been studied.[46] These include bedrest, improvement in nutrition, increased intake of proteins, essential amino acids, maternal hyperoxygenation, low dose aspirin therapy and administration of insulin like growth factor.[47-50] However, except antenatal administration of corticosteroids for improving the outcome of babies born prematurely following induction of labor there is no evidence to support the use of any other conservative intervention. The premature fetus faces the risk of RDS, intraventricular hemorrhage and necrotizing enterocolitis. To improve the outcome in preterm fetus who are less than 34 weeks of period of gestation, inj. betamethasone 12 mg given, two doses 24 hours apart which helps to enhance the lung maturity. The belief that the stress of intrauterine condition enhances the maturity and protects against prematurity has not been supported by studies in neonates with IUGR.[3,38] Improving the nutrition of a pregnant woman who is poorly nourished appears to be logical. The definitive management of IUGR is to deliver the baby at an optimum time.

Timing and Mode of Delivery

There is progressive metabolic deterioration in IUGR endangering the life of the fetus and with limited intrauterine treatment options available, the timing of intervention is important. An early delivery may be necessary but the consequences of prematurity should be weighed against risk of IUD.

The long- and short-term quality of life may be affected in IUGR fetuses. Many fetuses with IUGR are hypoxemic before the onset of labor. Intrauterine chronic acidemia may be associated with impaired intellectual development in postnatal life.[51]

The perinatal survival depends upon the gestational age at decompensation. Between 24 and 32 weeks gestation, each day gained intrauterine by the fetus, increases the neonatal survival by 1-2%.

Hence, the goal is to delay delivery as long as possible to achieve fetal maturity and ensuring viability while avoiding the sequelae of fetal acidemia.[41]

1. Reduced end diastolic blood flow (raised S/D ratio):
   • Close fetal monitoring with daily NST and biweekly modified BPP and weekly Doppler studies. If above tests are normal carry pregnancy till 37 weeks.
2. Absent or reversal of end diastolic flow:
   • Admission and termination if ≥ 34 weeks period of gestation.
   • If < 34 weeks, period of gestation, admission, antenatal steroids and close fetal monitoring with NST done every 8 hours. Terminate if NST nonreactive, spontaneous decelerations on CTG, BPP < 6/10 or reversal of ductal venosus flow during atrial contraction or presence of umbilical venous pulsations.

Mode of Delivery

The mode of delivery is likely to be a cesarean section. However, every case needs to be individualized and decision taken after consulting the pediatrician.

If the women is allowed trial of labor then continuous fetal heart monitoring should be done during labor. If late or variable decelerations are present then immediate delivery should be done.

During labor, patient should be kept in left lateral position, oxygen inhalation is given, I/V fluids with oxytocin are started, and labor should be monitored closely, if required by continuous CTG. If continuous CTG monitoring is not available the fetal heart should be auscultated just after a uterine contraction, every 15 minutes in the first stage and every 5 minutes in the second stage. Cesarean should be done at the earliest indication or if ominous signs on CTG are present.

A pediatrician should be present at the time of delivery, if meconium is present there is risk of meconium aspiration so laryngeal aspiration should be done. After delivery, the condition of the neonate at birth and the degree of prematurity affect perinatal morbidity and mortality rates in fetus.

PREVENTION OF INTRAUTERINE GROWTH RESTRICTION

Some factors may increase the risks of IUGR, such as cigarette smoking, intake of liquor and poor maternal nutrition. Avoiding harmful lifestyles, eating a healthy diet and getting prenatal care may help decrease the risks for IUGR. Regular antenatal checkup for early detection of IUGR may also help in treatment and good outcome.[46]

KEY POINTS

- Intrauterine growth restriction is used to describe a fetus whose birth weight is below the 10th percentile or < 2 SD below the mean weight for that gestational age and/or abdominal circumference is less than 10th percentile.
- Diverse factors, including intrinsic fetal conditions as well as maternal and environmental factors, can lead to intrauterine growth restriction (IUGR).
- Small for gestational age fetus is at increased risk for perinatal morbidity and mortality. In formulating a comprehensive approach to the management and follow-up of the growth-restricted fetus and infant, physicians should take into consideration the etiology, timing and severity of IUGR. In addition, they should be cognizant of the immediate perinatal response of the growth-restricted infant as well as the childhood and long-term associated morbidities.
- All the pregnancies should be screened for IUGR by using serial fundal height measurements. Ultrasonography in the third trimester to monitor

growth velocity of fetus and measurement of abdominal circumference can detect 80% of IUGR fetuses.

- If on ultrasonography fetal abnormality is detected, a detailed scan to detect other fetal structural defects should be done. If IUGR is detected in early gestation or it is severe then fetal karyotyping should also be done.
- After diagnosis of IUGR is confirmed, fetal monitoring should be done with DFMR and biweekly NST. Other tests of fetal well-being include standard or modified biophysical profile, Doppler blood flow velocimetry in umbilical and middle cerebral arteries and contraction stress test.
- Management includes bedrest in lateral position, removal of risk factors like smoking and intake of alcohol and treatment of infections and medical disorders.
- Other interventions which can be tried are nutrient supplementation— like increasing protein, essential amino acids, zinc and calcium intake, addition of low dose aspirin, plasma volume expanders, maternal oxygen therapy and heparin.
- If umbilical artery Doppler velocimetry in SGA fetus shows normal blood flow and liquor is adequate, with regular monitoring pregnancy can be taken to term.
- If liquor is reduced and POG is >37 weeks, pregnancy can be terminated.
- In patients diagnosed with IUGR delivery is indicated if:
  a. Absent or reversal of end diastolic blood flow at POG > 34 weeks
  b. Abnormal BPP or NST at POG > 34 weeks
  c. Reversal of Doppler velocities in ductal venosus during atrial contraction at POG > 32 weeks
  d. Umbilical venous pulsations at POG > 32 weeks.

The timing of intervention and mode of delivery is very important and should be individualized, as there is progressive metabolic deterioration in IUGR endangering the life of the fetus. With limited options availabe for intrauterine treatment, an early delivery may be necessary but the consequences of prematurity should be weighed against risk of IUD. Delaying delivery may result in a hypoxic, acidotic infant with long-term neurological sequelae.[52]

REFERENCES

1. Bernstein I, Gabbe SG. Intrauterine growth restriction.In: Gabbe SG, Niebyl JR, Simpson JL, Annas GJ, et al (Eds). Obstetrics: Normal and Problem Pregnancies. New York: Churchill Livingstone 1996;3:863-86.
2. Wolfe HM, Gross TL. Increased risk to the growth retarded fetus. In: Gross TL, Sokol RJ, (Eds). Intrauterine Growth Retardation: A Practical Approach. Chicago: Year Book Medical Publishers 1989;111-24.
3. Creasy RK, Resnik R. Intrauterine growth restriction In: Creasy RK, Resnik R (Eds). Maternal Fetal Medicine: Principles and Practice. Philadelphia: Saunders 1994; 3:558-74.
4. Battaglia FC, Lubchenco LO. A practical classification of newborn infants by weight and gestational age. J Pediatr 1967;71:159-63.

10

Intrauterine Growth Restriction (IUGR)

5. Dunn PM. The search for perinatal definitions and standards. Acta Paediatr Scand Suppl 1985;319:7-16.

6. Ott WJ. The diagnosis of altered fetal growth. Obstet Gynecol Clin North Am 1988;15: 237-63.

7. Hoffman HJ, Stark CR, Lundin FE, Ashbrook JD. Analysis of birth weight, gestational age, and fetal viability, US. Births, 1968. Obstet Gynecol Surv 1874;29:651.

8. Subramanian KNS, Barton Aimee M, Montazami S. Extremely low birth weight infant. e medicine Pediatrics, 18 June, 2009; MD "(http://www.Emedicine.com/ped/topic 2784.htm)".

9. Weiner CP, Baschat AA. Fetal growth restriction : Evaluation and management. In: James DK, Steer PJ, Weiner CP, Gonik B (Eds). High Risk Pregnancy: Management Options. London: WB Saunders 2007.

10. Divon MY, Ferbert A. Fetal growth restriction: Etiology. Uptodate, 2005. Available at www.Uptodate.com.

11. Robert C, Vandenbosche MD, Jeffery T, Kirchner DO. Intrauterine Growth Retardation; American Academy of Family Physicians Oct 15, 1998 http://www. Aafp. Org/afp/AFP printer/981015ap/vandenbo.html.

12. Lopez NJ, Smith PC, Gutierrez J. Periodontal therapy may reduce the risk of preterm low birth weight babies in women with periodontal disease: A randomized controlled trial. J Periodontal 2002;73:911.

13. Cnattingius S, Haglund B, Kramer MS. Differences in late fetal death rates in association with different determinants of small for gestational age fetuses: Population based cohort study. BMJ 1998;316:1483-87.

14. Mc Intyre DD, Bloom SL, Casey BM, Leveno KJ. Birth weight in relation to morbidity and mortality among newborn infants. N Engl J Med 1999; 340 :1234-12.

15. Greggory R, Devore MD. IUGR: Diagnosed www.Fetal.com/IUGR/diagnosed.html

16. Barker DJ, Osmond C, Golding J, Kuh D, Wadsworth ME. Growth *in utero*, blood pressure in childhood and adult life, and mortality from cardiovascular diseases. BMJ 1989;298: 564-67(level II-3).

17. Morley R, Dwyer T. Fetal origin of adult disease? Clin Exp Pharmacol Physiol 2001;28: 962-66.

18. Belizan JM, Villar J, Nardin JC, et al. Diagnosis of intrauterine growth retardation by a simple clinical method: Measurement of uterine height. Am J Obstet Gynecol 1978;131: 643.

19. Leeson S, Aziz N. Customised fetal growth assessment. Br J Obstet Gynecol 1997;104: 648-51 (level III).

20. Pearce JM, Compbell S. A comparison of symphysis –fundal height and ultrasound as screening tests for light- for gestational age infants. Br J Obstet Gynecol 1987;94:100-04 (level II-3).

21. Snijders RJ, Sherrod C, Gosden CM, Nicolaides KH. Fetal growth retardation: Associated malformations and chromosomal abnormalities. Am J Obstet Gynecol 1993;168:547-55.

22. Chang TC, Robson Sc, Boys RJ, Spencer JA. Prediction of the small for gestational age infant: Which ultrasonic measurement is the best? Obstet Gynecol 1992;80:1030-38.

23. Miller HC. Fetal growth and neonatal mortality. Pediatrics 1972;49:392.

24. Weiner CP, Robinson D. The sonographic diagnosis of intrauterine growth retardation using postnatal ponderal index and the crown heel length as standards of diagnosis. Am J Perinatol 1989;6:380-83.

25. Walther FJ, Ramaekers LHJ. The ponderal index as a measurement of the nutritional status at birth and its relation to some aspects of neonatal morbidity. J Perinat Med 1982;108: 42-47.

26. Ballard JL, Rosenn B, Khoury JC, Miodovn KM. Diabetic fetal macrosomia: Significance of disproportionate growth. Pediatrics 1993;122:115-19.

27. Mongelli M, Gardosi J. Reduction of false positive diagnosis of fetal growth restriction by application of customized fetal growth standards. Obstet Gynecol 1996;88:844-48.

28. Baschat AA, Gembruch U, Harman CR. The sequence of changes in Doppler and biophysical parameters as severe fetal growth restriction woesens. Ultrasound Obstet Gynecol 2001;18:571-77.

29. Sickler GK, Nyberg DA, Sohaey R, Luthy DA. Polyhydramnios and fetal intrauterine growth restriction; ominous combination. J Ultrasound Med 1997;16:609-14.

30. Magann EF, Sanderson M, Martin JN, Chauhan S. The amniotic fluid index, single deepest pocket, and two – diameter pocket in normal human pregnancy. Am J Obstet Gynecol 2000;182:1581-88.

31. Chamberlain PF, Manning FA, Morrison I, Harman CR, Lange IR. Ultrasound evaluation of amniotic fluid volume.I. The relationship of marginal and decreased amniotic fluid volumes to perinatal outcome. Am J Obstet Gynecol 1984;150:245-49.

32. Varma TR, Bateman S, Patel RH, Chamberlain GV, Pillai U. Ultrasound evaluation of amniotic fluid: Outcome of pregnancies with severe oligohydramnios. Int J Gynecol Obstet 1988;27:185-92.

33. Philipson EH, Sokol RJ, Williams T. Oligohydramnios clinical associations and predictive value for intrauterine growth retardation. Am J Obstet Gynecol 1983;146:271-78.

34. Chien PFW, Arnott N, Gordon A, Owen P, Khan KS. How useful is uterine artery Doppler flow velocimetry in prediction of pre-eclampsia, intrauterine growth retardation and perinatal death? An overview. Br J Obstet Gynecol 2000;107:196-208.

35. Alfirevic Z, Neilson JP. Doppler ultrasonography in high risk pregnancies: Systematic review with meta-analysis. Am J Obst Gynecol 1995;172:1379-87.

36. Neilson JP, Alfirevic Z. Doppler ultrasound for fetal assessment of high risk pregnancies (Cochrane Review). Oxford: The Cochrane Library. Issue 2, 2002.

37. Maulik D, Yarlagadda P, Youngblood JP, Ciston P. Comparative efficacy of umbilical arterial Doppler indices for predicting adverse perinatal outcome. Am J Obstet Gynecol 1991;164:1434-38.

38. Kingdom JC, Burrell SJ, Kaufmann P. Pathology and clinical implications of abnormal umbilical artery Doppler waveforms. Ultrasound Obstet Gynecol 1997;9:271-86 (level III).

39. Karsdorp VH, Van vugi JM , Van Geijn HP, Kostense PJ, et al. Clinical significance of absent or reversed end diastolic velocity waveforms in umbilical artery. Lancet 1994; 344:1664-68.

40. Pardi G, Cetin I, Marconi AM, Lanfranchi A, Bozzetti P, et al. Diagnostic value of blood sampling in fetuses with growth retardation. N Engl J Med 1993;328:692-96.

41. The GRIT Study Group. When do obstetricians recommend delivery for a high risk preterm fetus? Eur J Obstet Gynecol Reprod Biol 1996;67:121-26.

42. Mari G, Deter RL. Middle cerebral artery flow velocity waveforms in normal and small for gestational age fetuses Am Jobstet Gynecol 1992;166:1262-70.

43. Gugmundsson S, Tulzer G, Huhta JC, Marsal K. Venous Doppler in the fetus with absent end diastolic flow in the umbilical artery. Ultrasound Obstet Gynecol 1996;7:262-67.

44. Mac Arthur C, Knox EG. Smoking in pregnancy: Effects of stopping at different stages. Br J Obstet Gynecol 1988;95:551-55.

45. Dayal AK, Manning FA, Berck DJ Mussalli, et al. Fetal death after normal biophysical profile score: An eighteen years experience. Am J Obstet Gynecol 1999;181:12316.

46. Peleg D, Kennedy Colleen M, Hunter Stephen K. Intrauterine growth restriction: Identification and management. American Family Physician. http://www.aafp.Org.

47. Laurin J, Persson PH. The effect of bed rest in hospital on fetal outcome in pregnancies complicated by intrauterine growth retardation. Acta Obstet Gynecol Scand 1987;66: 407-11.

48. Gulmezoglu AM, Hofmeyr GJ. Maternal nutrient supplementation for suspected impaired fetal growth (Cochrane Review). In: The Cochrane Library, Issue 2, 1999. Oxford: update software.

49. Gulmezoglu AM, Hofmeyr GJ. Maternal oxygen administration for suspected impaired fetal growth (Cochrane Review). In: The Cochrane Library, Issue 2, 1999. Oxford: update software.

50. CLASP. A randomized trial of low dose aspirin for the prevention and treatment of pre-eclampsia among 9364 pregnant women. CLASP (Collaborative Low- dose Aspirin Studt in pregnancy) Collaborative Group. Lancet 1994;343:619-29.
51. Robertson CM, Etches PC, Kyle JM. Eight-year school performance and growth of preterm, small for gestational age infants: A comparative study with subjects matched for birth weight or for gestational age. J Pediatr 1990;116:19-26.
52. Stephen A, Walkinshaw Lindsay Cochrane. Investigation and management of the small fetus: Recent Advances in Obstetrics and Gynaecology Vol. 22 edited by John Bonnar and William Dunlop 2003;22:41-55.

Malpresentations

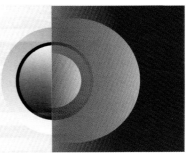

11

Usha Gupta

INTRODUCTION

The fetus at term or at onset of labor normally assumes a position of longitudinal lie with vertex presentation in a flexed attitude. In 3-5%[1,2] of cases the lie, position or attitude of the fetus is other than the normal and this is known as malpresentation. The commonest malpresentation is the breech presentation when the lie is longitudinal and the podalic pole of fetus occupies the lower uterine segment. The other malpresentations are either due to a deviation from the normal longitudinal lie like transverse and oblique lie or due to a deviation from the normal flexed attitude of head in cephalic presentation resulting in the face and brow presentations (Fig. 11.1). Sometimes more than one fetal part presents at the podalic pole resulting in compound presentation.

PREVALENCE

The prevalence varies with the type of malpresentation. Breech presentation is seen in 3-4% of cases,[2,3] transverse lie in 0.3-0.5% and face in 0.2-0.5%. Compound and brow presentations are the least common, present in less than 0.2% of cases.

ETIOLOGY

Malpresentations are due to several factors:
- Diminished space in the uterus like in low lying placenta or fundal insertion of placenta, uterine myomata and intrauterine synechiae.

- Laxity of abdominal wall as in multigravida altering the vertical axis of uterus and consequently the vertical axis of fetus.
- Contracted pelvic inlet or large fetus with resultant cephalopelvic disproportion.
- Müllerian duct abnormalities of the uterus like septate, subseptate uterus or uterus didelphys.
- Increased mobility of fetus as occurs in prematurity and hydramnios.
- Decreased mobility of fetus as in oligoamnios.
- Congenital malformation of the fetus like hydrocephalus is associated with breech presentation. Anencephaly and tumors of fetal neck can cause face presentation.
- Multiple pregnancies.
- Idiopathic.

CLINICAL PRESENTATION AND DIAGNOSIS

In the antenatal period the patient usually has no complaints. The malpresentation may be detected on routine palpation of abdomen. The earlier in pregnancy a patient is examined the higher are the chances of diagnosing malpresentations. However, when any malpresentation is observed one must look for predisposing factors like uterine malformations, placenta previa, space occupying lesions like fibroid uterus, ovarian tumor, diminished or increased liquor volume, multiple pregnancy, fetal malformations like anencephaly or hydrocephaly. In 50-75% of the cases, no predisposing or associated factor may be found.

It is important to diagnose malpresentation as it is likely to adversely impact labor. Eliciting a good history is important as it may give a clue to the possible cause of malpresentation. The patient may complain of bleeding pervaginum in case of placenta previa, pressure symptoms like dyspnea or difficulty in walking in case of excessive liquor or multiple pregnancy, discomfort in the hypochondrium or epigastric region if the patient has breech presentation at term.

A previous obstetric history of difficult labor, operative delivery, intrapartum stillbirth, asphyxiated baby, neonatal death may be elicited in case of contracted pelvis. In case of congenital malformations of uterus, it may have been diagnosed prior to conception, there may be previous history of repeated malpresentations or bad obstetric history. In case of tumors of uterus, patient may have had menstrual disturbances or bladder pressure symptoms prior to getting pregnant or documentation of uterine or ovarian mass on previous ultrasound.

She may give history of premature rupture of membranes with or without cord prolapse in her previous pregnancy or a history suggestive of prolonged labor and rupture of uterus if obstruction was not relieved. In the current pregnancy patient may be a multigravida or grandmultigravida.

The management of patient varies with the nature of the malpresentation.

The first step in the management is the correct diagnosis of the malpresentation and this can be made by careful palpation of the abdomen.

BREECH PRESENTATION

Types of Breech

Complete Breech or the Flexed Breech (Fig. 11.1)

In this the lower limbs of the fetus are flexed at both the hip and knee joint. This is the least common variety being present in 4-12% of cases. Here the presenting part comprises of the buttocks, feet and the external genitalia. As the presenting part does not fit the pelvic brim well, the risk of cord prolapse is 4-6%.

Frank Breech or the Extended Breech (Fig. 11.2)

In this the lower limbs of the fetus are flexed at the hip joint but extended at the knee joint. This is the commonest type, being present in 48–73%.[4] In this the buttocks fit the pelvic brim well and hence the chance of cord prolapse is only 0.5%.

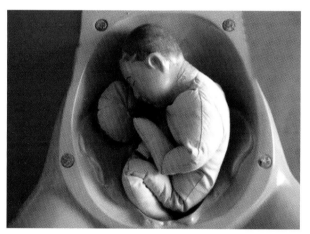

Figure 11.1: Breech presentation – Flexed breech

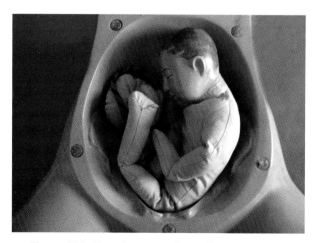

Figure 11.2: Breech presentation – Extended breech

Malpresentations

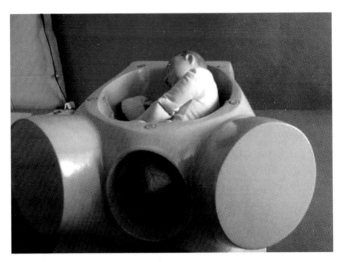

Figure 11.3: Breech presentation – Footling breech

Incomplete Breech or the Footling Breech (Fig. 11.3)

In this the lower limb is extended at the hip joint and the foot or the knee is the presenting part. This is seen in 12-38% of the cases. Here the presenting part fits poorly in the pelvis and so the risk of cord prolapse is highest being 15-18%.

Clinical Examination

Palpation of Abdomen

The height of uterus corresponds to the period of gestation unless the fetus has associated intrauterine growth restriction, congenital anomalies, hydramnios or multiple pregnancy.

The fetal lie is longitudinal. Leopold's maneuvers show hard globular, smooth, rounded and ballotable head of the fetus in the fundal grip. The lateral grip is suggestive of back on one side and limbs on the other side. On superficial pelvic grip, broad, soft, irregular podalic pole of fetus which is not ballotable is appreciated. Deep pelvic grip shows the relationship of the fetal pole to the pelvic brim. When breech is extended the head may not be well-appreciated as the limbs are alongside the head. The fetal heart is heard at the level of the umbilicus or slightly above it.

Pervaginum Findings

The broad, soft, irregular breech is felt in extended breech, whereas the limbs and external genitalia are felt along with the breech in complete breech or footling presentation. The extended breech has to be distinguished from the face. The anal opening may be mistaken for the mouth. In face presentation the mouth is surrounded by the hard alveolar ridges and forms the apex of a triangle with the malar prominences forming the base of the triangle. The examining finger may appreciate the sucking motion of the mouth if the membranes are ruptured. On the other hand, finger in the anus feels the muscular resistance and it is in line with the two ischial tuberosities. The spinous processes of the fetal sacrum can be palpated easily and are diagnostic of breech presentation and its position. The examining finger in the anus may be stained with meconium.

The breech must be differentiated from the shoulder presentation and this can be done by feeling for the ribs which have a grid iron feel. One must also look for cord presentation if membranes are intact or for cord prolapse and cord pulsations if membranes are ruptured. The average risk of prolapse of cord in breech is 3-5% as compared to only 0.3% in cephalic presentation. The risk is highest in footling presentation and least in frank breech.

Imaging Techniques

Ultrasound examination is justified even if the diagnosis is made clinically in order to get additional information on issues which will influence the management. One must find out if there are any congenital anomalies in the fetus which are two to three fold higher in breech as compared to cephalic presentation. The type of breech, estimated weight of fetus, hyperextension of fetal head, multiple pregnancy and placental localization all can be better appreciated on ultrasound.

Mechanism of Labor

The denominator is the sacrum and as in vertex presentation there are eight positions, the right and left sacroanterior, sacroposterior, sacrolateral positions, direct sacroanterior and direct sacroposterior positions. The commonest position is the right sacroanterior.

During labor the bitrochanteric diameter of the fetus engages in the right oblique diameter of the maternal pelvis. With increasing uterine contractions there is descent of the buttocks till the anterior buttock touches the pelvic floor at the level of ischial spines when it undergoes an internal rotation of 45 degrees so that the bitrochanteric diameter comes to lie in the antero-posterior diameter of outlet of maternal pelvis. Now the anterior buttock hinges below the symphysis pubis and the posterior buttock is born by lateral flexion and the anterior buttock slips out from beneath the symphysis pubis.

Delivery of the shoulders take place next. The bisacromial diameter is 12 cm and engages in the same oblique diameter, undergoes descent and internal rotation as the bitrochanteric diameter. The anterior shoulder hinges below the symphysis pubis and the posterior shoulder and the arm sweep over the perineum and are born.

The head now prepares to deliver. One of the two diameters, i.e. the sub-occipitofrontal diameter which is 10 cm or the suboccipito bregmatic which is 9.5 cm engages in the left oblique diameter of the maternal pelvis, followed by descent and flexion. When the occiput touches the pelvic floor, it rotates by 45 degrees so that the sagittal suture lies in the anteroposterior diameter of maternal pelvis with the occiput anterior. Now the subocciput hinges below the pubic symphysis and the head is born by flexion.

Antenatal Management

Patients with breech presentation need close follow-up in antenatal period as there is increased risk of premature rupture of membranes and preterm labor.

External Cephalic Version (ECV)

The risk of perinatal mortality is higher with breech vaginal delivery compared to delivery as vertex therefore if it persists at 35-36 weeks, correction of breech by ECV should be attempted. ECV is one of the most effective procedures in modern obstetrics.

Before attempting version, the contraindications to it should be excluded.

Contraindications are:
- History of antepartum hemorrhage.
- High blood pressure or PIH.
- Scarred uterus as in cesarean section, previous myomectomy or uteroplasty.
- Multiple pregnancy.
- Previous bad obstetric history.
- Uterine malformations.
- Oligohydramnios or polyhydramnios.
- Severe pelvic contraction or pelvic deformity.
- Nonreassuring fetal status.
- Intrauterine death.
- Intrauterine growth restriction.

Timing of ECV

It can be done anytime from 32-41 weeks of gestation, however the best time is 37-38 weeks.

From 32-34 weeks, risk of reversion after version is high and repeated attempts at it may be required and should any complication which requires termination of pregnancy occur, the fetus will be preterm with attendant risks of prematurity.

At 37-38 weeks, the fetus is term and pregnancy can be terminated without any risk of prematurity and the risk of reversion to breech is significantly reduced however the chances of failure of the procedure are higher as liquor is reduced. To improve the success rate of, ECV at term, use of tocolytics is advocated.

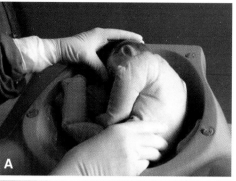
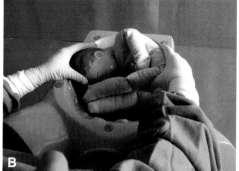
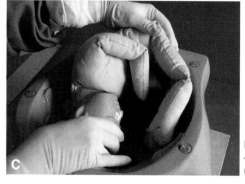

Figures 11.4A to C: (A) External cephalic version – step I, (B) External cephalic version – step II, (C) External cephalic version – step III

Procedure (Figs 11.4 A to C)

ECV should be carried out at a place where facilities for emergency cesarean section are available. The patient should be counseled and consents taken. The procedure is explained to allay anxiety. The bladder should be emptied and patient placed in dorsal supine position with legs flexed to 45 degrees at the hip joint. Abdomen is exposed and fetus palpated to ensure the exact position of the back. The fetal heart is heard or fetal cardiotocography should be carried out. If the version is done at 37 weeks or more, it is preferable to use ultrasound to monitor the fetal heart and the fetal movements. It is preferable to rotate the fetus in the direction of its face called "the forward roll," to maintain an attitude of flexion. The head is held by one hand and the other hand supports the buttocks, and the head is turned down and the podalic pole is turned upwards till the fetal head comes to occupy the pelvis and the podalic pole occupies the fundus of the uterus. The fetal heart is observed as soon as the version is completed. There should be no or minimal discomfort to the mother.

Complications of ECV
- Abruptio placentae: Patient will complain of severe pain in the abdomen. One should look for any bleeding pervaginum, fetal heart sounds and any area of tenderness and rigidity on the abdomen.
- Fetal distress: It may result from cord entanglement around the neck or other body parts of the fetus. If fetal distress is present, watch the fetal

heart for 30 sec, if it does not settle and cord entanglement is suspected revert the fetus to its original position in an attempt to undo the cord entanglement.

• Premature labor pains or premature rupture of membranes.

If there are no complications the patient may be sent home with the advice to come back after one week to check the presentation of the fetus. Patient is also advised to report if there is any complaint like decreased fetal movements, leaking pervaginum, or bleeding pervaginum.

In case the version is not successful due to increased tendency of the uterus to contract, ECV may be done under cover of tocolytic agents. The commonly used tocolytic agents are terbutaline and ritodine. Terbutaline can be given as subcutaneous injection of 250 micrograms prior to version.

A placebo controlled randomized trial showed that terbutaline given before an attempted version in women at term with noncephalic presentations significantly increased the initial success rate of version and decreased the rate of cesarean delivery in labor.[5]

Success of version is reported to be 60-80%. It may fail due to a deeply engaged breech which may be difficult to disimpact, undiagnosed multiple pregnancy, oligoamnios with big baby, congenital malformations of uterus like septate uterus, obesity, posterior position of the fetal back, extended legs and anterior placenta.

Fetomaternal hemorrhage occurs in about 6% of women hence anti-D should be given to Rh-negative patients in a dose of 300 micrograms. Wherever possible, Kleihauer-Betke test should be done to determine the degree of hemorrhage as approximately 1% of patients require additional dose of anti-D.

Management of Breech at Term

Elective Cesarean Section

It is first line of management in:
• Footling breech presentation: In this the progress of labor is slow as the presenting part acts as a poor cervical dilator, chances of premature rupture of membranes and cord prolapse are high and delivery of fetal parts before full dilatation of cervix and entrapment of fetal head are high therefore LSCS is justified.
• Breech with hyperextended head: In this the risk of fetal spinal injury is very high (21%) therefore CS is done.
• Low birth weight breech: CS for breech weighting 1000-1500 gm have less risk of trauma than for vaginal delivery. At some places less than 2000 gm is taken as the cut off for CS.
• Large fetus usually more than 3.5 kg.
• Any degree of contracted pelvis or unfavorable shape of the pelvis; CS is indicated for even minor degrees of contracted pelvis and there is no place for trial of labor.

- Associated medical conditions like PIH, BOH are indications for CS.
- Prolonged pregnancy.
- Nonreassuring fetal heart rate.

Planned Vaginal Delivery

Term Breech Trial Collaborative Group[6] did a randomised multicenter trial to compare planned cesarean section and planned vaginal birth for breech presentation at term. The group reported a significantly lower perinatal mortality, neonatal mortality or serious neonatal morbidity for planned cesarean section group as compared to planned vaginal birth group but found no differences in terms of maternal mortality or serious maternal morbidity between the groups. They therefore concluded that planned cesarean section is better than planned vaginal birth for a term fetus in breech presentation. After this study, a number of countries included these recommendations in their hospital protocol for managing term breech deliveries with resultant increase in rate of LSCS from 20-80%.

American College of Obstetricians and Gynecologists recommend that cesarean delivery is the preferred mode of delivery in breech presentation by most physicians because of the diminishing expertise in breech vaginal delivery. Planned vaginal delivery of a term singleton breech fetus may be reasonable where the health care provider is an expert at it and hospital protocol and guidelines for both eligibility and labor management are fulfilled. Prior to undertaking a vaginal breech delivery the women should be informed about the risk of perinatal or neonatal mortality and that the short-term serious neonatal morbidity may be higher than that of planned cesarean delivery and obtain her consent.

Management of Breech in Labor

If a patient has any indication of CS as mentioned above the patient is taken up for emergency CS. Vaginal delivery is considered in a set up where facilities for emergency CS exist provided:
- Estimated weight of fetus is between 2.0-3.5 kg.
- Frank breech.
- Fetal head is flexed.
- Pelvis is adequate.
- Absence of any associated obstetric complications like PIH.

It is desirable to score the patient by Zatuchni-Andros score. If score is 4 or more patient can be left for vaginal delivery. Bird and Mclein conducted a prospective study over six years employing the Zatuchni-Andros Breech Scoring Index and observed that when patients with a score of 4 or more were allowed to go in labor under meticulous supervision, a high rate of successful vaginal deliveries resulted and fetal mortality and morbidity rates were markedly reduced.[7,8]

11

Malpresentations

On the other hand, when the score was 3 or less chances of successful delivery were poor so the authors recommended that patients whose breech score was 3 or less should have immediate cesarean section. Further the authors were of the opinion that this breech assessment method was a valid method for selecting cases for vaginal delivery. They also observed intravenous oxytocin could be safely used when necessary if the breech score was 4 or more.

The Zatuchni-Andros score is calculated in Table 11.1.

It is important to ensure that expertise is available for conducting breech vaginal delivery.

The following should be kept ready for vaginal delivery:
- An IV line with 16-18 G needle should be placed.
- Crossmatched blood.
- Facilities for continuous electronic fetal monitoring or enough help for frequent auscultation of fetal heart.
- Anesthetist should be readily available. There is no contraindication to use of epidural analgesia once true labor is well-established.
- Pediatrician should be alerted.
- Facilities for neonatal resuscitation should be available.
- Instrument trolley should have all the instruments for any normal vaginal delivery with an additional extra towel and a pair of long forceps preferably Piper's forceps.

Monitoring Progress of Labor

It is preferable to maintain a partogram once labor starts. A careful watch is kept on the following:
- Vitals of mother.
- Nutrition of mother which should consist of small quantities of liquid diet that is rich in calories and electrolytes.
- The uterine contractions should be recorded. Their intensity and duration should progressively increase and interval decrease till about 3 contractions per 10 minutes are attained by late first stage of labor. If uterine contractions are inadequate and suggest hypotonia, augmentation with oxytocin drip can be done.

Table 11.1: Zatuchni-Andros score			
Parameter	Score		
	0	1	2
Parity	Nullipara	Multipara	
Gestational age	39 wks or more	38 wks	37 weeks
Previous history of Breech	none	one	two
Estimated fetal weight	8 lbs	7-8 lbs	7lbs
Cervical dilatation at admission	2 cm	3 cm	4 cm or >
Station of breech	minus 3 or >	minus 2	minus 1 or less

- The fetal heart sounds should be auscultated frequently or continuous fetal electronic monitoring is done. If labor is progressing normally the site of maximum intensity of fetal heart shifts to progressively lower level in the abdomen.
- Patient should be encouraged to labor in the left lateral position. When membranes rupture a pervaginum examination is done to exclude cord prolapse and at the same time the cervical dilatation, effacement and station of breech are noted.
- If labor is progressing normally, no interference is done till patient enters second stage of labor.
- The patient is shifted to delivery table once the anterior buttock starts climbing the perineum.

Conduct of Breech Delivery

Cardinal rules of breech delivery:
- Watchful expectancy, with no unnecessary interference.
- Teams comprising of anesthetist, pediatrician and an obstetrician well-versed with the art of breech vaginal delivery are present at delivery.
- Never pull the breech from below.
- Always encourage patient to push.
- Ask the assistant to apply fundal or suprapubic pressure whenever required.

When Breech Starts Climbing the Perineum

- Give liberal episiotomy after infiltration of the perineum with local anesthetic agent, pudendal block may be used.
- Allow the breech to deliver spontaneously till the umbilicus (Fig. 11.5 A).

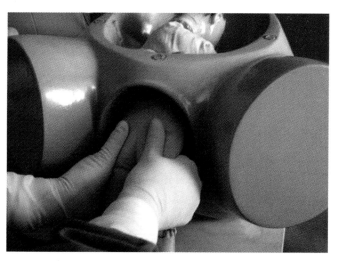

Figure 11.5 A: Assisted breech delivery—Fetopelvic grip

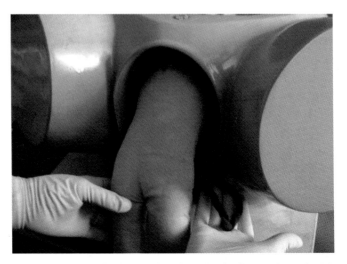

Figure 11.5B: Umbilical cord—length and pulsations to be looked for

- Now pull out a loop of cord to check for cord pulsations and length of cord and start timing the delivery from here (Fig. 11.5B). From now on the delivery of the fetus should be completed within 3-5 minutes. Too rapid delivery runs the risk of tearing of tentorium cerebelli and hence intracranial hemorrhage.
- Cover the baby with a towel so that it is easy to hold the baby and it reduces the external stimulus for it to start premature attempts to breathe.
- The uterine contractions are monitored closely. If inadequate, oxytocin drip can be started or if already on flow the rate is increased to obtain good contractions. During contractions, encourage the patient to bear down and give fundal pressure. This is called Kristellar's maneuver.
- As trunk starts emerging from below the symphysis pubis look for the inferior angle of scapula. If it is parallel to the spine it means the arms are flexed. If there is winging of the inferior angle of scapula, it means the arms are extended.
- As soon as the axilla is visible look for the arms across the chest of the fetus and gently deliver them out. Now the trunk and shoulders are disengaged.
- Suprapubic pressure is given in backward and downward direction so that attitude of flexion of fetal head is maintained. Fetal head is now delivered using the Burns and Marshall technique.
- Delivery of placenta, inspection of placenta and perineum and stitching of episiotomy is completed.
- Oxytocic agents are given.
- Patient is watched for postpartum hemorrhage (PPH).

Overcoming Difficulties in Breech Delivery

Difficulty in Delivery of Buttocks

Breech impacted low in the pelvis or the outlet. In this case a liberal episiotomy may relieve the impaction. In some cases, groin traction (single or double) may be required. Index fingers of one or both the hands of operator are placed in groins of the baby and steady gentle traction is applied on the pelvis and not the femur of the baby as this can result in fracture of this bone (Fig. 11.6A).

Difficulty in Delivery of Legs

This is likely when the legs are in extended position. The legs get splinted alongside of the abdomen and chest. In this case the two fingers of right hand of the birth attendant should be passed up the thighs and the middle and index finger press popliteal fossa to flex the knee joint and sweeping the knee in a backwards and outwards direction across the trunk of the fetus. This brings down the leg which can then be delivered easily. The second leg may deliver on its own or may require same treatment as first leg. This is called Pinard's maneuver (Fig. 11.6B).

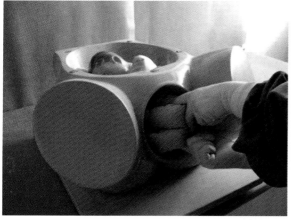

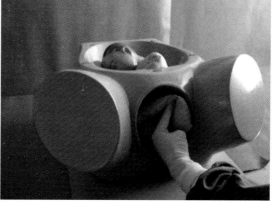

Figure 11.6A: Groin traction for extended legs impacted at outlet – note the pressure of the indexfingers of the operator are towards pelvis to prevent injury to thighs

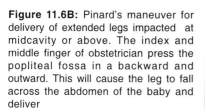

Figure 11.6B: Pinard's maneuver for delivery of extended legs impacted at midcavity or above. The index and middle finger of obstetrician press the popliteal fossa in a backward and outward. This will cause the leg to fall across the abdomen of the baby and deliver

Extended Arms

One or both arms may be extended. This usually happens when traction is applied at the baby too early or when the cervix is not fully dilated.

Methods of Delivery

There are two methods of delivery. The obstetrician must know which method to select.

Classical Method

This method is done under general anesthesia. In this the legs of the fetus are grasped by one hand of the obstetrician and body of the fetus is carried slightly upwards and medially towards the abdomen of mother. This depresses the posterior shoulder. It is important not to pull the trunk too low down in the pelvis as it will jam the shoulders along with the head making delivery of arms very difficult. The other hand is passed in the sacral hollow and the index and middle finger are passed along the dorsal aspect of the shoulder of the posterior arm of the fetus till it reaches beyond the elbow joint (Fig. 11.7). Then the forearm is pressed so that the elbow joint flexes and the forearm drops across the face and chest of the fetus and is delivered. It is important not to catch the fingers or the humerus to pull on them for bringing down the arm as this will cause fracture of the arm. The anterior arm may now be delivered from beneath the symphysis pubis. The arm is rotated in oblique diameter of maternal pelvis, child is depressed and two fingers passed

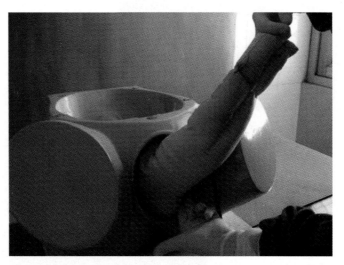

Figure 11.7: Classical method of delivery of extended arms. The baby is gently lifted by its feet and its ventral aspect carried towards the abdomen of mother. This increases the space in sacral hollow. The index and middle fingers of left hand of obstetrician are carried up the posterior arm of baby and passed above the elbow. The forearm is swept across the face of baby and delivered

212

Management of High-Risk Pregnancy—A Practical Approach

over anterior shoulder and is disengaged in the same manner as the posterior arm. If not possible the fetus is rotated by 180° so that anterior arm becomes posterior and is delivered in the same way. For rotation of the child it is important to push up the trunk slightly so that the chin does not enter the pelvic brim at the same time. The child should be held by the trunk with both hands, the thumbs are placed over the back and the fingers grasp the pelvis by the pelvifemoral grip and rotated and the arm delivered as described for posterior arm.

Lovset's Maneuver (Figs 11.8A to C)

This is an extrapelvic maneuver. This works on the principle that the posterior arm is at lower level in the pelvis so when the fetus is rotated through 180° the

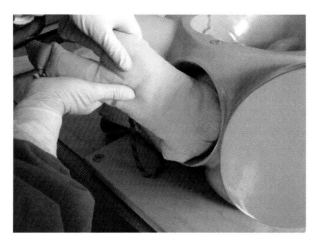

Figure 11.8A: Lovset's maneuver for delivery of extended arms. (A) The baby is gently lifted up so that the posterior arm descends down in the sacral hollow

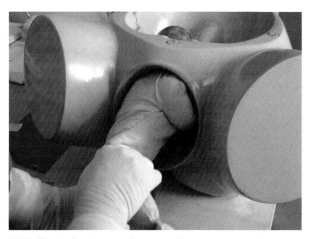

Figure 11.8B: The baby is rotated so that the posterior arm becomes anterior

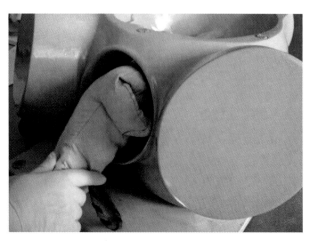

Figure 11.8C: As the rotation is nearing completion gently depress the baby so that posterior arm which now becomes anterior descends below the symphysis pubis and delivers

posterior arm will fall below the symphysis pubis and deliver as the anterior pelvis is deficient.

The fetus is grasped by the fetopelvic grip and drawn down till the inferior angle of the anterior scapula is visible below the symphysis pubis, and is lifted and rotated by applying further traction to the trunk and carrying it away from the shoulder in question. Rotation should be in such a way that the back remains anterior and as it nears completion through 180° the fetus is suddenly depressed so that the elbow, shoulder and arm deliver in succession below the symphysis pubis. The other arm is hooked out from the sacral hollow. If any difficulty is encountered fetus is again rotated in similar fashion as with each rotation of 180° the shoulders descend and one can repeat it 3-4 times.

Nuchal Displacement of the Arm

Here the arm is displaced behind the occiput. Rotation of the fetus is done in the direction of fingers, this causes the occiput to slip past the arm and the arm is brought in easy reach for delivery as in extended arms.

Delivery of the Head

Burns and Marshall technique: This method works well for an average-sized baby. The patient is brought to the edge of the table and baby allowed to hang by its weight (Fig. 11.9A). An assistant gives suprapubic pressure in backwards and downwards direction so that head enters the pelvic brim in well-flexed position. When the nape of the neck is seen then the feet of the baby are grasped between the index and ring finger with the middle finger between the two feet, a steady outwards traction is maintained and the body of the baby carried in an arc-shaped manner over the mother's abdomen (Fig. 11.9B). It is important to ensure that the fulcrum is the nape of the neck and it rotates over the symphysis

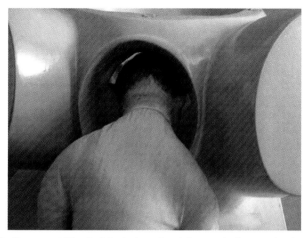

Figure 11.9A: Burns and Marshall technique for delivery of after coming head of breech. (A) Patient is on edge of delivery table and baby is allowed to hang till nape of neck is seen

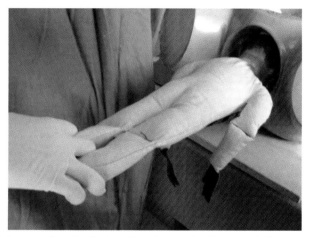

Figure 11.9B: Baby is held by the feet and traction applied in outward direction and subocciput hinges below the symphysis pubis

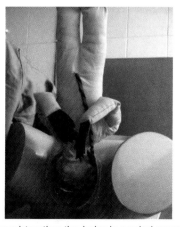

Figure 11.9C: Maintaining outward traction the baby is carried across the abdomen of the mother in a wide arc with the fulcrum of rotation at subocciput. Note the fulcrum should be subocciput and not the cervical vertebrae to prevent injury to the cervical spine and spinal cord

Malpresentations

pubis. If traction is not maintained over the body once the nape of the neck is seen it slips beneath the symphysis pubis and the rotation of the baby may occur over cervical vertebrae causing fracture of the neck and difficulty in delivery of the head (Fig. 11.9C). If the baby is large or the nape of neck not seen even when the baby is suspended by its own weight for 1-2 min, delivery of the head should be done by an alternative method.

Delivery of the aftercoming head of breech by forceps: This method is superior to all other methods of delivery of the head as the pull is made directly to the head and flexion of the head is maintained with forceps. On the other hand, with all other methods the traction is through the spinal column which is much more dangerous for the child.

For applying the forceps it is very important that the head is in the pelvic cavity. The trunk and abdomen are wrapped in a towel and the assistant holds it upwards so that it does not interfere with the application of the forceps (Fig. 11.10A). The blades of the forceps are applied from ventral aspect of the fetus (Fig. 11.10B). In this the blades lie in the mentovertical plane. The pull

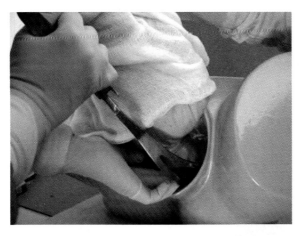

Figure 11.10A: Forceps application for delivery of after coming head of breech. (A) The baby is wrapped in a sheet and gently lifted up to prevent it from interferring in the forcep application. The right blade of long midcavity or Piper forceps is introduced from the posterolateral aspect of maternal pelvis

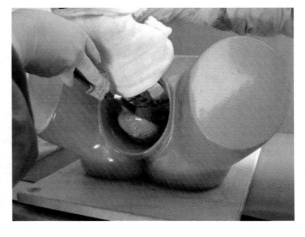

Figure 11.10 B: Cephalic application of both blades of forceps locked in position. Traction is first applied in downward and backward till chin appear and then in upward and outward towards direction

is applied downwards and backwards till the chin appears then the child is carried upwards towards the mother's abdomen.

Mauriceau-Smellie-Veit Maneuver: In this the assistant gives gentle suprapubic pressure. Then the obstetrician places the body of the child astride the left arm with one leg on either side of the forearm and places the index and middle fingers on the malar prominences of the baby and applies pressure on them, thus maintaining an attitude of flexion (Fig. 11.11A). The middle finger of the right hand is placed on the cervical spine and the occiput whereas the ring and index finger are placed on the shoulders on either side. This splints the spine and provides protection to it. Traction is now exerted in a backward and downward direction till the nape of the neck is seen below the symphysis pubis. Now the baby is carried in upwards direction towards the mother's abdomen (Fig. 11.11B). As the traction to the baby is through its spine, hence the chances of cervical injury are more than with the application of forceps.

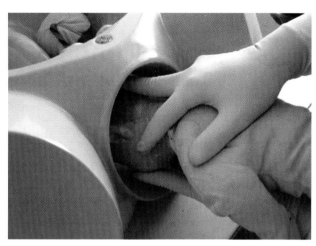

Figure 11.11A: Mauriceau Smellie Veit technique for delivery of after coming head of breech. (A) The obstetrician places the body of the baby astride the left arm with one leg on either side of the forearm and puts the index and middle fingers on the malar prominences to flex the head. The right hand is placed on the head with middle finger on the occiput and neck to splint it. The index and ring finger rest astride the shoulders

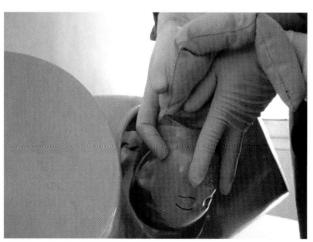

Figure 11.11B: The left hand flexes the head and right hand is used for traction to deliver the head

Delivery of head with occiput posterior: On rare occasions during delivery of the trunk the back rotates posteriorly an event which can be prevented by facilitating anterior rotation of back once trunk is delivered till the umbilicus.

The infants shoulders are grasped between the fingers and thumb of one hand and the feet grasped with other hand. Supra-pubic pressure is given and traction is applied in upwards and forwards direction and baby carried 360° across the abdomen of mother and baby delivered.

Breech Extraction

This procedure is done when delivery of the baby is done by the obstetrician without waiting for spontaneous delivery. This is seldom done nowadays as it is associated with a high perinatal mortality (20%).

Indications

- Cord prolapse in second stage of labor and when delivery occurs in clinic/health center with no facilities for cesarean section.
- Second twin in breech presentation with fetal distress.

Technique (Figs 11.13B and C)

This requires complete relaxation of the uterus hence it is done under general anesthesia using halothane or amyl nitrate or nitroglycerin. One hand is inserted into the uterine cavity and the anterior leg is followed to the foot. The heel of the foot is then grasped between the fingers and the thumb and traction is applied to it while the external hand steadies the uterus and applies counterpressure. It is important not to bring down the posterior leg as the anterior buttock will get caught at the symphysis pubis and hinder in extraction of the baby and the cord should be kept out of the way by pushing it against the wall of the uterus if it is palpated during breech extraction. Steady gentle pressure is applied backwards in line of Curve of Carus and then forwards and upwards till the knee is visible at the introitus, now the thigh is grasped with the fingers on one side and thumb on the other side and traction is continued till the groin is visible. The leg is now hooked out by groin traction. This brings down the other leg and when the posterior buttock distends the perineum, the anterior leg is pulled upwards so that enough room is there to deliver the posterior leg. No attempt should be made to bring the leg down, rather the pelvis is delivered and then if the leg is extended it is delivered by Pinard's maneuver. Sometimes traction on one leg may not allow other leg to come down if it is impacted or being held up by any fetal part. In this case traction may have to be applied to the other heel and both legs brought down together.

Once both legs are born the baby is covered with towel and held with fetopelvic grip and delivery completed as for assisted breech delivery, delivering trunk, arms and head by maneuver described above.

Following delivery of baby, placenta is delivered and inspected, perineum explored for lacerations and episiotomy stitched as in normal delivery and usual precautions taken for preventing PPH.

Cesarean Section for Breech

It is done in routine manner. The difficulty may be encountered in extraction of a preterm breech baby when the lower segment is not well-formed. An adequate uterine incision is required to deliver the head otherwise the same injuries as vaginal breech delivery will occur and benefit of CS lost. A C-shaped incision is given after carefully reflecting the lower uterine segment peritoneum. A low vertical incision has been suggested as an alternative when lower uterine incision is not well-formed but in these cases there is a danger of extension into upper segment.The breech should be delivered with care as injuries and difficulty can occur even when LSCS is done.

Perinatal Outcome in Breech Delivery

Vaginal birth is associated with three times higher perinatal mortality as compared to cephalic presentation. The perinatal mortality is 40.9 per 1000 breech deliveries and 25% of all stillbirths are due to breech delivery. The lowest perinatal mortality is in frank breech, intermediate in flexed breech and is highest in footling breech.

Causes of perinatal morbidity and mortality:
- *Birth asphyxia*: This can be due to arrest of the aftercoming head or entrapment of the head due to incompletely dilated cervix, the latter being more common with preterm breech when the relatively small fetal body delivers before cervix is fully dilated. The other causes of birth asphyxia are cord compression, cord prolapse or prolonged labor.
- *Head injury*: Intracranial hemorrhage due to fracture of skull bones or due to sudden decompression leading to tentorial tears of the unmoulded head.
- *Congenital malformations*: Lethal malformations like hydrocephalus, anencephaly and meningomyelocele are more common with breech presentation.
- Fracture of bones like fracture of femur, humerus, pelvis, clavicle, skull, spine or any other bones and their effects.
- Spinal cord injuries like lacerations or transections.
- Intraventricular hemorrhage or hemorrhage into the adrenals.
- Injury to viscera like liver, spleen, muscles and genitalia.
- Injuries to nerve plexus leading to cervical or brachial nerve paralysis.
- Nonlethal malformations affecting the fetus.

TRANSVERSE LIE

When long axis of fetus is perpendicular to the long axis of uterus, it is called transverse lie (Fig. 11.12). In this the cephalic pole occupies the lumbar region

Malpresentations

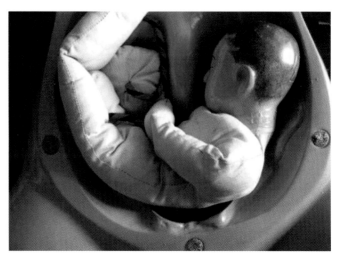

Figure 11.12: Transverse lie—Dorsoinferior position

or iliac fossa and podalic pole occupies the opposite pole. The denominator is the acromian. The position of fetus is determined by its back being dorso-anterior when back is anterior, dorsoposterior when back is posterior, dorsosuperior when back is superior and dorsoinferior when back is inferior.

Incidence

It is 1 in 300 pregnancies at term.

Etiology is same as for breech presentation.

Diagnosis

On inspection of the abdomen the uterine ovoid appears wide and the height of uterus appears relatively shortened. On palpation the height of uterus appears less than period of gestation. On Leopold maneuvers the head is in one flank and breech in other. The back is readily palpable in dorso-anterior and dorsosuperior positions while it is less clearly palpable in dorsoposterior and dorsoinferior positions. Fetal heart is heard through the shoulder and hence in dorsosuperior position it is along fundus of the uterus and in dorsoinferior it is low down in the pelvis. The position of fetal heart may first raise the suspicion of the presence of transverse lie. This is especially important if liquor is drained and fetal parts are not clearly defined.

On pervaginum examination, the bag of membranes may be conical in shape and the membranes often rupture prematurely. Cervix is not well-applied to the presenting part and the soft parts are felt high up. The ribs of the thorax have a grid iron feel and this is a diagnostic feature of shoulder presentation. At other times vertebra of the spine are felt and in neglected cases the arm may be prolapsed.

Diagnosis can be confirmed on ultrasound.

Management

Antenatal Period

An attempt should be made to correct the transverse lie by external version, if there is no contraindication to it from 34 weeks of gestation onwards. If ECV fails or is contraindicated, elective LSCS is done at 38-39 weeks of gestation.

Intrapartum Period

If patient comes in early labor and membranes are intact, ECV can be tried if there are no contraindications for vaginal delivery.

If however, patient comes in late first stage of labor or in second stage or with rupture of membranes and liquor is drained with fetal heart still present, it is safer to do cesarean section.

If the patient presents with a prolapsed arm and neglected shoulder presentation, the patient is carefully examined for any features of obstructed labor.

On general examination, patient usually appears dehydrated, has tachycardia, fever and acidotic breathing. The urine is high-colored and may show presence of acetone. Abdominal examination may show Bandl's ring due to stretching of lower uterine segment. Abdominal palpation reveals the fetus to be in transverse lie. Often the liquor is completely drained hence it may be difficult to feel fetal parts. There may be tenderness in lower uterine segment if it is stretched. Occasionally, if uterus is ruptured, uterine contour may not be made out properly, fetal parts may be felt superficially and retracted uterus may be felt separately. On auscultation, there may be fetal distress or the fetal heart may be absent. The arm of the fetus prolapses out of the introitus and may get swollen and discolored. Pervaginal examination reveals the presence of fetal thorax or spine at brim or impacted in the pelvis.

Management will depend on features of obstruction and on the presence or absence of fetal heart sounds.

If there are features of obstructed labor like presence of Bandl's ring, LSCS is indicated even if FHS is absent as the risk of rupture uterus is very high with IPV and breech extraction. If rupture of uterus has already occurred laparotomy with removal of fetus and placenta is done followed by repair of uterus or hysterectomy depending on the circumstances.

If fetal heart is absent but there are no features of obstructed labor, management will depend on the duration of rupture of membranes and the amount of liquor that has drained from the uterine cavity. If liquor is adequate and shoulder is not impacted in pelvis the prolapsed arm is replaced and internal podalic version is done under general anesthesia and relaxation of the uterus (Figs 11.13A to C).

If however liquor is drained, decapitation of the fetus can be tried if the fetal neck is within easy reach. For this the prolapsed arm is pulled downwards

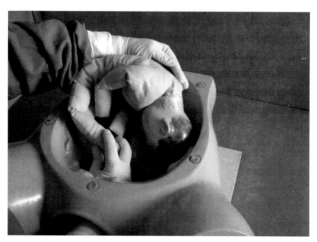

Figure 11.13A: Internal podalic version. (A) The anterior leg of the baby is grasped by its feet. Note that posterior leg should not be brought down first as the anterior buttock will hinge against the symphysis pubis and prevent delivery of the baby

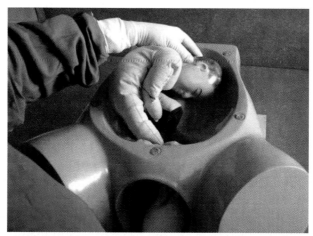

Figure 11.13B: The fundus of the uterus is steadied and leg brought down

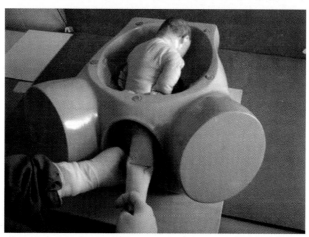

Figure 11.13C: Maintain traction on the anterior leg till posterior leg comes within reach for delivery

and away from the neck by the assistant and the decapitation knife either Jardin's hook or the Gigley's saw is negotiated above the neck under cover of the left hand which is placed in the anterior vaginal wall to protect it from damage. The hook is then rotated through 90° and the left hand is shifted to the posterior vaginal wall. The neck is then severed off from the body by rotatory movements. Embryotomy scissors can also be used for cutting the neck. The body is then extracted by pulling on the prolapsed hand. The head is removed by putting finger in the mouth or crochet can be used for it.

After removal of the placenta the uterine cavity and genital tract should be explored in all the cases to detect any genital tract injury. In all these cases, prophylactic oxytocic agents are used to prevent postpartum hemorrhage.

FACE PRESENTATION

Face presentation occurs when the lie of fetus is longitudinal and attitude of head is in complete extension, mentum is the denominator and the engaging diameter is submentobregmatic (Fig. 11.14).

The incidence of face presentation varies from 1 in 150 to 1 in 900 live births.

Etiology: Exact cause is not known, some predisposing factors are:
- Contracted pelvis.
- Multiparity with lax abdominal wall.
- Congenital malformations of the fetus like anencephaly, congenital bronchocele, hydrocephaly and meningocele.
- Congenital tumors of the neck like goiter or multiple loops of cord or tight loop of cord round neck.
- Shape of the fetal head—like dolichocephaly.
- Prematurity.

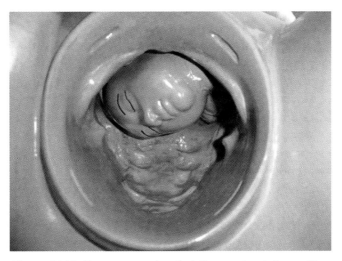

Figure 11.14: Face presentation depicting mentoanterior position

Management

It is very important to diagnose this condition especially at onset of labor. There are six positions in face presentation:

Right and left mentoanterior – commonest accounts for 60-80% of the cases.
Right and left mentoposterior – 20-25% are mentoposterior.
Right or left mentolateral – 10-12% are mentotransverse.

Clinical Diagnosis

General physical examination of the patient will be normal except if she comes late in labor with unfavorable face position like mentoposterior position or with contracted pelvis, when there may be evidence of obstructed labor.

Abdominal Findings

It is often difficult to diagnose the condition as the extended head distends the lower uterine segment causing slight tenderness on palpation hence the muscles of lower abdomen may not relax to permit proper examination.

In face presentation, the occipital eminence is prominent and felt on a higher level than the sinciput. In the vertex presentation, the occiput and back form one continuous curve with a slight depression at the neck whereas in face presentation, the continuity of the back is broken by a deep grove between the back and the occiput. This deep prominence can be mistaken for sinciput of a well-flexed head but a careful examination will reveal limbs of the baby to be on the opposite side of the prominence in face presentation whereas in vertex presentation the limbs will be on the same side as the sincipital prominence.

In mentoanterior positions, the chest will appear as prominent on side opposite to back and fetal heart may be palpated through it. In mentoposterior position chest is difficult to define and fetal heart is not well-heard. In mentolateral positions, fetal heart is heard best on the side of limbs rather than through the back as in vertex positions.

On pervaginum examination: If the membranes are intact, the bag of membranes will appear conical instead of saucer-shaped as the presenting part does not fit well in the pelvis. There is usually premature rupture of membranes or the membranes rupture early in the course of labor. The smooth rounded head is not palpated. Irregular parts are felt which are difficult to make out if the cervix is not dilated or only slightly dilated. When the cervix dilates and the presenting part lies within easier reach, one can palpate the opening of the mouth which is surrounded by the hard alveolar ridges unlike the anal opening which has no such hard bony landmarks. The anal opening lies in line with the ischial tuberosities and forms the base of the triangle, the apex of which is formed by the tip of sacrum. The mouth on the other hand forms the apex of a triangle, the base of which is formed by the orbital ridges. The sucking movements may be appreciated by the finger in the mouth whereas the finger in the anus may be stained with the meconium on withdrawing it. The ridge of nose and chin may also be palpable and distinguishable if there is no edema of the face.

Diagnosis can be confirmed by ultrasound or by radiography. The latter shows hyperextended head with facial bones at pelvic inlet. Early diagnosis improves perinatal outcome.

Mechanism of Labor

The commonest position in face presentation is left mentoanterior. The lie is longitudinal, denominator is mentum and the engaging diameter is submentobregmatic and it engages in right oblique diameter of maternal pelvis. With increasing uterine contractions, the face descends to the level of ischeal spines and then undergoes internal rotation through one eighth of a circle and crowning takes place. The submentum comes to lie under the surface of symphysis pubis and the face is delivered by flexion. Rest of the delivery occurs as in the vertex presentation.

Management in Labor

If any degree of contracted pelvis is associated with face presentation, LSCS should be considered as facial bones cannot undergo moulding in labor, to overcome the mild pelvic contraction.

If the face is in mentoposterior position, the likelihood of forward rotation to convert to anterior position sometimes late in labor is only 25% therefore, if baby is large and pelvis is borderline CS is justified.

In favorable face position and normal pelvis, vaginal delivery is permitted. The patient is allowed to go into spontaneous labor and is watched very carefully. Labor is often prolonged so a careful partogram is kept to watch for progress of labor and for evidence of fetal distress. If possible, continuous electronic fetal heart rate monitoring should be done. No internal maneuvers should be done to convert face into vertex presentation. If progress of labor is arrested an evaluation of its cause should be done and fetal heart auscultated. If progress is arrested with good uterine contractions, LSCS should be done as the face cannot undergo moulding and hence is less likely to deliver without risk to the fetus. If non-progress of labor is due to hypotonic uterine contractions, careful augmentation with oxytocin is done.

The perinatal mortality for viable pregnancies varies from 0.6-5%.

BROW PRESENTATION

When the part of fetal head between the orbital ridges and the anterior fontanel and the coronal sutures presents, it is brow presentation (Fig. 11.15). It is the rarest presentation. The engaging diameter on fetal skull is the mentovertical which is 14 cm and is the longest diameter, therefore engagement cannot

Malpresentations

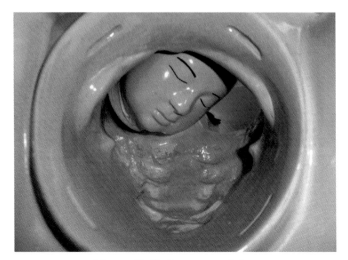

Figure 11.15: Brow presentation

take place and fetus cannot deliver. It can deliver by converting to vertex presentation. Etiology is same as for face presentation.

Diagnosis

Abdominal Palpation

The chin and occiput can be palpated easily and are at same level.

Vaginal Examination

The orbital ridges and root of the nose are easily palpated on one side and the anterior fontanel and coronal suture is palpated on the other side. The mouth and chin cannot be reached.

Management

Cesarean section is indicated in persistent brow presentation.

COMPOUND PRESENTATION

When a limb of fetus is present along with the major presenting part it is termed as compound presentation. The most common combination is an upper limb with the vertex.

Diagnosis

It may be detected during routine pervaginal examination at the beginning of labor or more commonly it is suspected if there is arrest of progress of labor in the active phase or if there is failure of presenting part to engage in spite of good uterine contractions.

Diagnosis is made by vaginal examination when limb is palpated along with the larger presenting part.

Compound presentation is most frequently associated with prematurity. It can also occur with external cephalic version of breech presentation.

Management

- Primary cesarean section is indicated if there is associated prolapse of cord or nonreassuring fetal heart is present.
- In early labor if no complications are present, one can wait and watch closely for the limb to retract on its own above the presenting part. During this stage however as the risk of cord compression or prolapse is high, continuous fetal monitoring is essential.
- In late first stage, the limb can be gently pushed up and reposited above the presenting part.
- If limb cannot be pushed up and/or signs of obstruction appear or if complications like cord prolapse or fetal distress occur, cesarean section is the delivery of choice.

    Perinatal loss is increased as a result of cord prolapse, preterm delivery and obstetric manipulation which may cause traumatic delivery.

KEY POINTS

- When fetus assumes a position other than the normal longitudinal lie with vertex presentation in a flexed attitude in labor, it is called malpresentation and occurs in 3-5% of cases.
- The commonest malpresentation is breech presentation.
- Other malpresentations are the transverse and oblique lie, the face and brow presentations and the compound presentation. Brow and compound presentations are the least common.
- Predisposing factors for malpresentations are uterine abnormalities or space occupying lesions, site of placental insertion, multigravida with lax abdominal wall, contracted pelvic inlet, congenital malformations of the fetus and amniotic fluid abnormalities and multiple pregnancies.
- The first step in the management of malpresentation is its correct diagnosis as it is likely to impact labor adversely.
- A good history, clinical examination of the abdomen and pelvis and imaging techniques like ultrasound help in correct diagnosis of the type of malpresentation.
- Breech presentation in the antenatal period or early labor should be corrected by ECV.
- Contraindications for ECV are antepartum hemorrhage, PIH, scarred uterus, multiple pregnancy, BOH, uterine malformations, pelvic contraction, prolonged leaking and nonreassuring fetal status.

- ECV should be carried out where facilities for emergency CS are available.
- Complications of ECV are abruptio placentae, fetal distress and premature labor pains or premature rupture of membranes.
- Rh-negative patients should be given anti-D after ECV.
- Elective cesarean section for breech presentation is indicated for footling breech presentation, hyperextended head, low birth weight breech, large fetus more than 3.5 Kg, any degree of contracted pelvis or unfavorable shape of the pelvis, associated medical conditions, post-dated pregnancy and non-reassuring fetal heart rate.
- As per ACOG guidelines, planned vaginal delivery of a term singleton breech fetus may be reasonable where the health care provider is an expert at it and hospital protocol and guidelines for both eligibility and labor management are in place.
- Prior to undertaking a vaginal breech delivery the women should be informed about the risk of perinatal or neonatal mortality or that the short-term serious neonatal morbidity may be higher than that of planned cesarean delivery and her informed consent should be documented.
- Perinatal mortality is three times higher for vaginal breech delivery as compared to vertex delivery. The causes of perinatal morbidity and mortality are birth asphyxia, head, spinal cord, visceral and nerve injuries, fracture of long bones and other bones and congenital malformations.
- Transverse lie in antenatal period should be corrected by external version, if there is no contraindication to it from 34 weeks of gestation onwards.
- If ECV fails or is contraindicated, elective LSCS should be done at term.
- If patient comes with transverse lie in early labor and membranes are intact, ECV should be tried if there are no contraindications to it.
- If patient comes late in labor with rupture of membranes and liquor drained out with fetal heart present, LSCS is the treatment of choice.
- If patient comes very late in labor or with neglected shoulder presentation and with features of obstruction LSCS is justified even if FHS is absent due to risk of rupture of uterus.
- Face presentation should be differentiated from breech presentation by careful abdominal and vaginal examination.
- If any degree of contracted pelvis is associated with face presentation, LSCS should be done as facial bones cannot undergo moulding in labor, to overcome the mild pelvic contraction.
- If the face is in mentoposterior, the likelihood of forward rotation to convert to anterior position sometimes late in labor is only 25% therefore, if baby is large and pelvis is borderline CS is justified.
- Cesarean section is indicated in persistent brow presentation.
- Primary cesarean section is indicated in compound presentation if there is associated prolapse of cord or nonreassuring fetal heart is present.

- In early labor if no complications are present in compound presentation, wait and watch for the limb to retract on its own above the presenting part. During this stage however, as the risk of cord compression or prolapse is high continuous fetal monitoring is essential.

REFERENCES

1. Breech Presentation in Oxoford hand book of Obstetrics and Gynaecology. Arulkumaran S, Symonds I, Fowlie (Eds). A publishers Oxford University Press, 2007;221-25.
2. Lanni SM, Seeds JW. Malpresentations in Obstetrics Normal and Problem pregnancies. Steven G Gabbe, Jennifer K Niebyl, Joe Leigh Simpson (Eds): illustrated by Mikke Senkariak and Micheal Cooley 4th edn. Churchill Livingstone, 2002.
3. James D, Steer P, Weiner C, Gonik B (Eds). Breech Presentation in High-Risk Pregnancy. 3rd edn. 2006;1334-56.
4. Shah PK, Sardeshpande NS. Breech presentation in Textbook of Obstetrics. Salhan S (Ed), 1st edn, Jaypee Brothers Medical Publishers (P) Ltd, 2007;575-94.
5. Fernandez CO, Bloom SL, Smulian JC et al. A randamised placebo controlled evaluation of terbutaline for external cephalic version.Obstet and Gynecol 1997,90:775-79.
6. Hannah ME, Hannah WJ, Hewson SA, Hodnett ED, Saigal S, Willan AR. Planned caesarean section versus planned vaginal birth for breech presentation at term: a randomised multicentre trial. Term Breech Trial Collaborative Group. Lancet 2000;356(9239):1375-83.
7. Bird CC, McElin TW. A six-year prospective study of term breech deliveries utilizing the Zatuchni-Andros Prognostic Scoring Index. Am J Obstet Gynecol 1975;121(4):551-58.
8. Bird CC, McElin TW. 500 consecutive term breech deliveries. Use of the Zatuchni-Andros prognostic scoring index. Obstet Gynecol 1970;35(3):451-57.

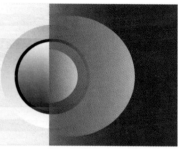

Pregnancy with Previous Cesarean Section

12

Ritu Rana

INTRODUCTION

Pregnancy with previous cesarean section remains a topic of widespread public and professional concern. Globally the increase in rates of cesarean section over the last couple of decades have led to an increase in proportion of women having pregnancies with previous cesarean and thus increasing the pool of high-risk obstetric population. The cesarean section rates have increased by 25-30% in USA in the last decade, doubled to 22% in UK and reached upto 35% in Brazil and 25% in India. This increase is attributed to an increasing use of elective cesarean sections for indications like previous cesarean section.[1] Previous cesarean section (CS) contributes to 29% in India, 40% in USA and 29% in UK to overall cesarean section rates. Nearly 60% of all elective cesarean sections have previous cesarean section as an indication and up to 14% of emergency cesareans are in women with a previous cesarean. Vaginal birth-after-cesarean section (VBAC) has been advocated as a means of reducing the CS rate.[2] Multiple cesarean sections are a known cause of increased maternal and neonatal morbidity and mortality and there is a systematic shift towards reducing cesarean section rates not only based on evidence, but also to reduce costs. We as obstetricians are faced with the important and difficult challenge of making choices, to be able to facilitate healthy outcome for the mother and child. The current chapter explores the pool of evidence and current guidelines on management of pregnancy with previous cesarean section.

EFFECT OF FUTURE FERTILITY

One of the key concerns for all women and to the obstetricians is the likely effect of any medical or surgical intervention including cesarean sections on conception and future pregnancies. Women who deliver by cesarean sections have been noted to be less likely to have a subsequent pregnancy and this has led to the debate whether such observations are a result of individual choices due to previous obstetric experience or pathological. There is very scanty evidence to suggest the relationship of previous cesarean delivery and future pregnancy rate and most of the studies are limited by several confounding factors including the indications for the cesarean section and the choice of the women.[1,3-6] It is also been observed that infertile women have a higher rate of operative deliveries as compared to fertile women. A retrospective Cohort study in Scotland with a mean follow-up duration of 13 years, absence of conception was voluntary in 69% (CI 66-73%) of the cases.[6] A systematic review of Cohort studies has shown that women with previous cesarean section have got a 46% higher chance of not having or having fewer children after five years of first cesarean delivery (RR:1.46; 95%CI: 1.07-1.99). The sterilization rates were also higher in these women.[3] It is also postulated that women who had their first child by cesarean section may take longer to conceive because of pelvic adhesions, infections or placental bed disruption which in turn may be influenced by the indication for cesarean section.[7] As most of the evidences suggesting decrease in fertility are at the most of level II[a], it may be assumed that association between cesarean section and subfertility is more likely to be caused by confounding rather than being causal.

ANTENATAL COMPLICATIONS

As an obstetrician, it is essential that we are well aware of all the potential complications one can come across in post CS pregnancies, not only to be able to look for and be prepared for all eventualities but also to inform the parents and counsel them. Some of these complications are elaborated in the following sections.

As stated above, previous operative interventions can lead to postoperative infections which can lead to changes in the tubal lining and also, healing can cause fibrosis and adhesions leading to inflammation of pelvic organs and formation of scars and adhesions and these are likely to affect implantation during early pregnancy and subsequent development of the placenta.

Ectopic Pregnancy

Cesarean section is a risk factor for subsequent ectopic pregnancies. Post-operative inflammation and infection seems to be the most likely cause. Although the risk is small, but due to the serious consequences of ectopic pregnancy it is a clinically important factor.[8-10]

---

[a]Levels of Evidence

Cesarean Scar Pregnancy

With increasing cesarean section rate, this is getting more common than before. The pregnancy implants at the site of cesarean scar and usually presents as early as 5 weeks to as late as 16 weeks with symptoms of painless vaginal bleeding and abdominal pain. It can cause massive uncontrolled bleeding if uterine curettage is undertaken in the absence of diagnosis which can occur in many cases.[10-12]

The cesarean section scar has been reported to cause pathological changes like lymphocyte infiltration, capillary dilatation, infiltration of the endometrial tissue and polyp formation.[13] These in turn cause suboptimal implantation of the placenta, impaired decidualization, increased vascular malformations which are known risk factors for placenta previa, placental abruption and placenta accreta.[14] Placenta location should be noted in patients with a history of prior uterine surgery. Placenta accreta should be ruled out in patients having placenta previa.

Placenta Previa

The incidence of placenta previa is 0.4-0.8% for women with a previous cesarean section as compared to 0.2-0.5% for women with a previous vaginal birth.[15-17] There is an exponential increase in risk of placenta previa with number of cesarean sections and women with the combination of high parity and multiple repeat cesarean deliveries have the greatest likelihood of placenta previa (Table 12.1). Shorter interdelivery time also increases the risk of placenta previa among such women.[15,18,19]

Placental Abruption

Placental abruption complicates 1 in 100 pregnancies and is known to recur in subsequent pregnancies.[20-22] Abruption rates in pregnancy with a previous cesarean section have been reported to be significantly higher than one with previous vaginal birth (0.95% *vs* 0.74%). Getahun et al reported that the risk of abruption in third pregnancy increases by 30% after two consecutive cesarean deliveries (RR 1.3, 95% CI 1.0–1.8) and abruption rates increase if interdelivery period is less than a year (Table 12.2). This increase is by 52% if previous delivery was vaginal and by 111% if previous delivery was by cesarean section [RR 1.5, 95% CI 1.1–2.3].[23]

Placenta Accreta

Overall incidence of placenta accreta is 1 in 2500 pregnancies. Placenta accreta is usually associated with placenta previa and causes significant morbidity and mortality due to severe postpartum hemorrhage that can lead to hysterectomy.[24] There are very few case series reports on the incidence of placenta accreta in women with previous CS.[25,26] The risk of placenta accreta has been reported to increase from 4.1% in women with no previous CS to 60% in patients with three or more cesarean sections (Fig. 12.1).[24]

Table 12.1: The association between the number of prior cesarean deliveries and placenta previa based on the three indicator variables for number of prior cesarean deliveries[18]

Number of previous cesarean deliveries	1 (n = 1171)	2 (n = 675)	Parity 3(n = 265)	4 + (n = 171)
0	1.0	1.0	1.0	1.0
1	1.28 (0.82-1.99)	1.10 (0.47-2.55)	1.60 (1.15-2.22)	1.72 (1.12-2.64)
2		2.02 (1.16-3.53)	2.56 (1.33-4.93)	2.96 (1.26-6.97)
3			4.09 (1.53-10.96)	5.09 (1.41-18.39)
4 +				8.76 (1.58-48.53)

(Adjusted odds ratio and 95% confidence intervals stratified by parity)
Age ≥ 35 vs other, smoker vs nonsmoker, and any prior induced abortion are included in the adjusted model

Table 12.2: Association between cesarean delivery and placental abruption in subsequent pregnancies

First birth	Second birth	Median inter-pregnancy interval (y)	Total births (N)	Placental abruption	Risk of placental abruption in subsequent pregnancy Unadjusted RR (95% CI)	Adjusted RR (95% CI)
First 2 pregnancies	(n = 156,475)					
Vaginal	-	2.2	116,003	0.74	1.0 (Reference)	1.0 (Reference)
Cesarean	-	2.4	40,472	0.95	1.3 (1.1-1.4)	1.3 (1.2-1.5)
First 3 pregnancies	(n = 31,102)					
Vaginal	Vaginal	2.0	22,332	0.91	1.0 (Reference)	1.0 (Reference)
Vaginal	Cesarean	2.1	1,826	1.31	1.5 (1.0-2.2)	1.5 (0.9-2.2)
Cesarean	Vaginal	2.2	2,341	0.73	0.8 (0.5-1.3)	0.9 (0.5-1.4)
Cesarean	Cesarean	2.2	4,603	1.06	1.2 (0.9-1.6)	1.3 (1.0-1.8)

RR—Relative risk; CI—Confidence interval.
Relative risks are adjusted for maternal age, race, education, prenatal care, marital status, interpregnancy interval, and smoking and drinking during pregnancy.

Stillbirth

Stillbirth rate in women who had no previous cesarean section was 2 per 1000 compared to 4 per 1000 among women who had a previous cesarean section. This risk depends on gestational age and increases especially after 34 weeks of gestation (hazard ratio 2.23, 95% CI 1.48 to 3.36).[27] It is important to remember that the absolute excess risk is still less than 1/1000. One of the recent studies by Salihu et al however did not find any increase in stillbirth in women with previous cesarean section.[28]

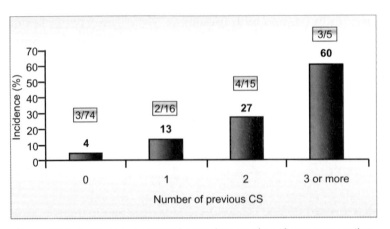

Figure 12.1: Incidence of accreta by previous number of cesarean section

MODE OF DELIVERY AFTER PREVIOUS CESAREAN SECTION—VBAC OR ERCS

In 1916, Cargin quoted 'once a cesarean, always a cesarean'. However, this was due to the fact that almost all cesarean sections were performed by classical uterine incision. The turning point came in 1978 when Merrill and Gibbs safely attempted vaginal delivery in 83% of their patients with previous cesarean section.[29] In 1980 the National Institute of Health convened a conference called the National Consensus Development Conference on Cesarean Birth which released a report, recognizing VBAC as the safe mode of delivery.[30,31] The cesarean section rate however continued to rise in spite of NIH report and ACOG consensus on VBAC. By 1996, the cesarean delivery rate in the United States was 20.7%, reached 29.1% in 2004 and is still increasing. The reason most likely is inability to make VBAC a norm in well-selected patients. This in turn is due to the lack of clear and robust evidence which prevents establishment of a uniform protocol for VBAC and each case needs to be individualized. Physicians therefore find it difficult to give a confident explanation and women are afraid to take chances with this uncertainty about the grave outcomes of uterine rupture or failed VBAC. Medicolegal implications do not help either. It therefore becomes extremely important to have a full and evidence-based knowledge of factors that decide the safety and success of VBAC in order to enhance our counseling and decision making.

There are many studies pertaining to VBAC. However, the two landmark clinical studies which form most of the evidences for VBAC are from the research undertaken by Landon et al and Macones et al.[32,33] In 2005, Macones did a large multicenter retrospective cohort study in North-East United States of over 25,000 patients with a history of at least one prior cesarean delivery and studied the maternal complications as well as factors determining success of VBAC.[32] The second study done by Landon et al was a prospective cohort study of almost 46,000 women with a history of a prior cesarean delivery within the Maternal-Fetal-Medicine Units Network in US which looked not only at the maternal outcomes but also the neonatal outcomes and factors determining success rates of VBAC.[33] The latter is quoted as a stronger study as it was prospective and in addition to maternal outcomes it also assessed the neonatal outcomes.

Factors Predicting Success Rates

The success rates of VBAC after one cesarean section is approximately 72-76%. This has been shown by systematic reviews.[34-37] The knowledge of factors predicting success rates would enable us to apply them to an individual woman. A good idea of the success rate of VBAC can be done at the first antenatal visit. The best available evidence still remains to be Level 2 and 3 as discussed below.

Antenatal Factors

Previous vaginal birth, particularly previous VBAC, is the single best predictor for successful VBAC and is associated with an approximately 87-90% planned VBAC success rate.[38-40] The success rate ranges from 63.3% with women having no previous VBAC to 91.6% for women with 4 or more prior VBAC. It is important to note that though the success rate increases, so do the rate of uterine scar dehiscence and rupture. As the number of prior VBAC increases, there is a greater probability of VBAC success as well as a lower risk of uterine rupture and perinatal complications in the current pregnancy (Fig. 12.2).[41,42] However, this decrease in risk is mainly after first VBAC. The risk of scar rupture being 0.87% with no history of VBAC and 0.45%, 0.38%, 0.54% and 0.52% after one, two, three and four or more successful VBAC respectively.

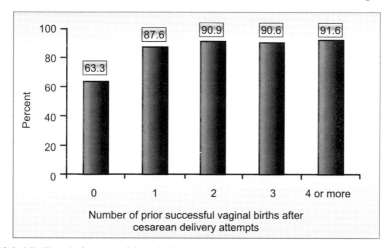

Figure 12.2: Likelihood of successful vaginal birth after cesarean delivery (VBAC) according to the number of prior successful VBAC attempts[41]

Favorable modified Bishop's score is related to increase chance in VBAC being successful. First pelvic examination in labor can give some idea whether VBAC is likely to be successful or not. Bujold et al in his study showed the success rates being 57.8%, 64.5%. 82.5%, and 97% for modified Bishop's score being 0-2, 3-5, 6-8 and 9-11 respectively.[43] The success rate of VBAC is 81% *vs* 67% in women with spontaneous labor and induced labor respectively. Further augmented labor with oxytocin has been shown to have a better success rate than induced labor but is less than that of spontaneous labor (Table 12.3).[39]

Table 12.3: Factors related to VBAC success rates[39]		
Characteristic	*n (VBAC Success %)*	*Odds ratio (95% CI)*
Previous cesarean delivery		
Dystocia	2940 (63.5)	0.34 (0.30-0.37)
Nonreassuring fetal wellbeing		
(NRFWB)	2231 (72.6)	0.51 (0.45-0.58)
Other	1718 (77.5)	0.67 (0.58-0.76)
Malpresentation	2856 (83.8)	1.0
Prior scar		
Transverse	8688 (72.5)	0.71 (0.64-0.79)
Unknown*	2002 (78.7)	1.0
Previous cesarean delivery		
≤ 2 years	2338 (67.8)	0.70 (0.64-0.76)
> 2 years*	7831 (75.2)	1.0
Previous vaginal delivery		
Yes*	6121 (86.6)	1.0
No	4499 (60.9)	0.24 (0.22-0.23)
Previous VBAC		
Yes*	4166 (89.6)	1.0
No	5924 (64.4)	0.21 (0.19-0.23)
Maternal disease[1]		
Yes	1652 (70.1)	0.81 (0.74-0.90)
No*	9038 (74.3)	1.0
Labor type		
Induction	2569 (67.4)	0.50 (0.45-0.55)
Augmented	3854 (73.9)	0.68 (0.62-0.75)
Spontaneous*	4266 (80.6)	1.0
Admit cervical dilation (cm)		
<4	5384 (66.8)	0.39 (0.36-0.48)
≥ 4*	4980 (83.8)	1.0
Epidural anesthesia		
Yes*	7850 (73.4)	1.0
No	1007 (50.4)	0.37 (0.33-0.41)
Birth weight (g)		
< 2500	267 (77.2)	1.14 (0.89-1.47)
2500 – 3999*	9486 (74.9)	1.0
≥ 4000	935 (62.0)	0.55 (0.49-0.61)
Gestational age (wk/d)		
37 0/7 – 40 6/7*	9340 (75.0)	1.0
≥ 41	1350 (64.8)	0.61 (0.55-0.68)

* Reference group
[1] Maternal diseases was defined as diabetes, asthma, thyroid disease, seizure disorder, pregestational chronic hypertension treated with medication, renal disease, connective tissue disease

Factors Related to Unsuccessful VBAC

Antenatal

Many predictive nomograms have been suggested in the literature which are simple and can calculate the VBAC success rate as soon as the first antenatal visit on the basis of simple variables. These models however have their own limitations and therefore have not yet gained popularity.[40,44-47] They are applicable only to women at term with a previous uncomplicated cesarean section. No previous vaginal birth as described earlier has got the VBAC success rate of only 63%.[41] Body mass index greater than 29 has been shown to decrease the success rate. These patients are almost 50% less likely to have VBAC success than their underweight counterparts [odds ratio 0.53, 95% confidence interval 0.29-0.98, P = 0.043].[48]

Previous cesarean section for dystocia decreases the success rates of VBAC.[39] Cervical dilatation achieved at the primary cesarean section has also been found to play a role and there has been controversy about the amount of cervical dilatation in previous pregnancy before cesarean section to the success rate of VBAC in current pregnancy. As a more generalization, the success rate of VBAC in women with previous cesarean section for cervical dystocia in first and second stage is 75% and 65% respectively compared to 82% success rates when cesarean section was done for other indication apart from cervical dystocia.[49] No correlation of the amount of cervical dilatation at previous cesarean section and successful VBAC was found.[50] Previous preterm cesarean birth has comparable success rates but is associated with higher scar rupture rates.[51,52] Interdelivery period of less than 24 months from previous cesarean birth is associated with lower VBAC success rate of 67%. Fetal weight of more than 4000 gm is also associated with decreased VBAC rates to as low as 62%.[39,53] Advanced maternal age, nonwhite ethnicity, short stature and fetus of male sex have all shown to reduce success rates.[54]

Intrapartum

Apart from antenatal factors, certain indicators during intrapartum period can affect the success rate of VBAC. Induction of labor decreases the rate of successful VBAC to 67% (OR 0.50, 95% CI 0.44-0.55) as compared to 80% in spontaneous labor. On the other hand, augmented labor has got a VBAC success rate of 73.9% (OR 0.68, 95% CI 0.62-0.75). The MFMU Cesarean Registry also showed the following intrapartum factors related to decreased success of VBAC. In post-mature gestation, i.e. 41 weeks or more of gestation, the VBAC success rates decrease to 65% as compared to that of 75% between 37 weeks to 40 weeks and 6 days (OR 0.61,95% CI0.55-0.68). Landon in his study also showed that epidural anesthesia increases the success of VBAC to 73% as compared to 50% in women with no epidural anesthesia (OR 0.37, 95% CI 0.33-0.41). When women present in labor with cervical dilatation of ≥ 4 cm, the chances of favorable outcome is increased. When all these unfavorable factors are present, successful VBAC is achieved in as few as only 30% of women (Table 12.3).[39]

Risks and Benefits of VBAC

The main evidence of VBAC on neonatal and pregnancy outcomes came from study by Landon as shown in the Figure 12.2.[33]

Maternal Risks

Maternal morbidity and mortality: This is usually associated with failure to achieve successful VBAC as morbidity otherwise is very low in cases of successful vaginal birth. The morbidity is mainly due to uterine rupture, emergency cesarean section, blood transfusion and endometritis (Table 12.4). According to the best available evidence the rate of significant maternal complications for women undergoing VBAC are 5.5% compared with only 3.6% in women who had elective repeat cesarean section (ERCS) (Table 12.5). Maternal mortality does not increase significantly in women undergoing VBAC to those having planned ERCS.[33]

Risk of uterine rupture: Uterine rupture is the most dreaded complication of trial of scar. This results in severe maternal and neonatal morbidity. Risk of uterine rupture is 0.2-0.7% in planned VBAC after one previous cesarean section and zero in women undergoing ERCS.[35,42,55-59] This is much higher

Outcomes	Number of prior VBACs			P value*
	0 (n = 9,012)	1 (n = 2,900)	2 or more (n = 1,620)	
VBAC success	63.3	87.6	90.9	< 0.001
Uterine rupture	0.87	0.45	0.43	0.01
Uterine rupture if induced	1.37	0.37	0.68	0.03
Uterine dehiscence	0.94	0.24	0.25	< 0.001
Hysterectomy	0.23	0.17	0.06	0.15
Surgical complications[1]	0.45	0.17	0.12	0.008
Thromboembolism[2]	0.09	0	0	0.07
Transfusion	1.89	1.24	0.99	0.002
Endometritis	3.68	1.17	1.30	< 0.001
Maternal death	0.02	0	0	0.71
5 minute Apgar score ≤ 5	2.50	2.11	1.86	0.07
Cord arterial pH ≤ 7.00[3]	2.34	1.63	1.62	0.17
Neonatal intensive care unit admission	15.1	12.9	14.6	0.08
Hypoxic ischemic encephalopathy	0.17	0.07	0	0.05
Infant death	0.64	0.59	0.44	0.35

Table 12.4: Pregnancy and neonatal outcomes according to number of prior successful vaginal birth after cesarean delivery attempts[33]

* P value from Mantel-Haenszel test for trend
[1] Broad ligament hematoma, cystotomy, or bowel or ureteral injury
[2] Deep vein thrombosis or pulmonary embolus
[3] N=3249857 and 432 for umbilical cord arterial pH.

Table 12.5: Maternal complications in women undergoing VBAC[39]

Complications	Trial of labor (n = 17,898) n (%)	Elective repeat cesarean delivery (n = 15,801)	Odds Ratio (95% CI)	P value
Uterine rupture	124 (0.7)	0	-	< 0.001
Uterine dehiscence[1]	119 (0.7)	76 (0.5)	1.38 (1.04-1.85)	0.03
Hysterectomy	41 (0.2)	47 (0.3)	0.77 (0.51-1.17)	0.22
Thromboembolism[2]	7 (0.04)	10 (0.1)	0.62 (0.24-1.62)	0.32
Transfusion	304 (1.7)	158 (1.0)	1.71 (1.41-2.08)	< 0.001
Endometritis	517 (2.9)	285 (1.8)	1.62 (1.40-1.87)	<0.001
Maternal death	3 (0.02)	7 (0.04)	0.38 (0.10-1.46)	0.21
Other maternal adverse events[3]	64 (0.4)	52 (0.3)	1.09 (0.75-1.57)	0.66
One or more of the above	978 (5.5)	563 (3.6)	1.56 (1.41-1.74)	<0.001

[1] Not all women underwent examination of their scars after vaginal delivery
[2] Includes deep vein thrombosis or pulmonary embolus
[3] Includes broad ligament hematoma, cystotomy, or bowel or ureteral injury

Table 12. 6: Maternal complications according to the outcome of trial of labor[39]

Complications	Failed vaginal delivery (n = 4759) n (%)	Successful vaginal delivery (n = 13,139)	Odds ratio (95% CI)	P value
Uterine rupture	110 (2.3)	14 (0.1)	22.18 (12.70-38.72)	< 0.001
Uterine dehiscence	100 (2.1)	19 (0.1)	14.82 (9.06-24.23)	< 0.001
Hysterectomy	22 (0.5)	19 (0.1)	3.21 (1.73-5.93)	< 0.001
Thromboembolism	4 (0.1)	3 (0.02)	3.69 (0.83-16.51)	0.09
Transfusion	152 (3.2)	152 (1.2)	2.82 (2.25-3.54)	< 0.001
Endometritis	365 (7.7)	152 (1.2)	7.10 (5.86-8.60)	< 0.001
Maternal death	2 (0.04)	1 (0.01)	5.52 (0.50-60.92)	0.17
Other maternal adverse events	63 (1.3)	1 (0.01)	176.24 (24.44-1271.05)	< 0.001
One or more of the above	669 (14.1)	309 (2.4)	6.81 (5.93-7.83)	< 0.001

than risk of rupture 1/10,000 to 1/20,000 in unscarred uterus. However, the more recent study by Macones et al found the rate of uterine rupture in women attempting VBAC with one single prior cesarean as 0.98%.[32] Maternal complications are shown in Table 12.5.

Risk associated with failed VBAC: The most important detrimental effect on morbidity in cases of trial of VBAC is because of failed VBAC. Women who had successful VBAC had an overall morbidity of 2.4% whereas women who had failed attempted VBAC had a 14.1% incidence of morbidity (Table 12.6).[39]

Long-term complications of VBAC: Vaginal birth may cause adverse effects on pelvic floor and bladder functions. However, this in context to VBAC and ERCS still needs to be studied further.

Fetal Risks

Antepartum stillbirth: As explained earlier in the chapter, the risk of stillbirth (excluding malformations) is 2/1000 in VBAC and 0.8/1000 in ERCS (RR with VBAC 2.45;95% CI 1.25-4.78; p = 0.007).[21,33] The risk is primarily due to increased chances of stillbirth after 34 weeks.

Delivery-related perinatal death: Though the risk of delivery related perinatal death is increased by 12 fold in VBAC group than ERCS, however, the absolute risk is 1.3/1000. Only 30% of these are due to uterine rupture. There is a further chance of 10% babies having severe asphyxia among the cases with uterine rupture which would lead to hypoxic ischemic encephalopathy or death.[27,59,60]

Maternal and Fetal Benefits

The benefits are primarily shorter hospital stay and prevention of operative morbidity. The respiratory morbidity in the newborn due to transient tachypnea of newborn is decreased in cases of successful VBAC.

Risks and Benefits of ERCS

Maternal Risks

Women having ERCS have complication rate of 3.6% which is higher than women having successful VBAC.[33,55] This is attributed to routine complications of surgery like bleeding, thromboembolism, febrile morbidity, long-term bladder dysfunction and prolonged recovery. In addition, there is an increased risk of future placental problems, subfertility and ectopic pregnancies, as highlighted in the previous sections. Anesthetic complications are very rare, irrespective of planned VBAC or ERCS.

Maternal Benefits

Elective repeat cesarean section avoids the risks of failed VBAC and consequently all the complications associated with emergency cesarean section. It also avoids pelvic floor and perineal trauma. Moreover, it is done under controlled circumstances with a full knowledge of time of delivery and woman can, therefore, plan relatively well.

Fetal Risks

Respiratory problems: This is the main cause of morbidity in babies delivered by ERCS. ERCS is associated with 5 fold increase in TTN (transient tachypnea of the newborn) or respiratory distress syndrome (RDS).[61] Absolute risk of morbidity in ERCS group is 3.5–3.7% compared with 0.5–1.4% for VBAC.[60-62] Risk is more if cesarean is performed before labor and in the earlier weeks of gestation after term. It is seen that the risk of asthma in neonates admitted with TTN is doubled as compared to those who are not.[62-64] The respiratory morbidity is 11.4%, 6.2% and 1.5% at 37, 38 and 39 weeks of gestation, respectively.

Hypoxic ischemic encephalopathy: The incidence of intrapartum HIE at term is significantly greater in planned VBAC (7.8/10,000) compared with ERCS (zero rate).[55]

Fetal Benefits

They are from avoidance of any morbidity from scar rupture.

Planned VBAC in Special Circumstances

In cases where previous cesarean section was done by an uncomplicated low transverse incision with an otherwise present uncomplicated pregnancy, the success and complication rates have been studied by many published series.

Preterm Birth

Preterm (24–36 weeks of gestation) planned VBAC has higher success rates when compared with women at term undergoing planned VBAC (82% *vs* 74%). The risk of uterine rupture is also decreased though non-significantly.[65] Perinatal outcomes were similar with preterm VBAC and preterm ERCS. The Bishop's score of cervix should be taken into account as these women can have unfavorable cervix resistant to induction. Also the risks of scar rupture associated with induction should be discussed well with the patient. However, women with preterm gestation who are in labor have got a higher chance of successful VBAC and lesser rate of uterine rupture.

Twin Gestation

It was initially thought that women with previous cesarean delivery and currently having twin pregnancy should be delivered by cesarean section, however the evidence does not show any benefit of doing so. Also the success rate of VBAC in twins has been controversial. However, two recent studies by Cahil et al and Varner et al show no increased maternal risk associated with twins and comparable success rates of 75.7% in twins *vs* 75.4% in singletons.[66-68]

Macrosomia

The concern for women with previous cesarean section and macrosomic baby (> 4000 gram) is primarily the decreased success rate of VBAC and secondly increased rate of rupture. In the study done by Landon et al, the success rate of trial of VBAC is 55-67% for pregnancies with infants weighing 4000 g or more compared to 75-83% with smaller infants.[33] However, we do not have enough data to support the concern regarding increased rupture rates. It should, however, be acknowledged that antenatal estimation of fetal weight by ultrasound is not very accurate. It is important to be cautious in cases where the progress of labor is suboptimal as cephalopelvic disproportion could be one of the causes. There is however no significant difference in the maternal and perinatal morbidity.

Short Interdelivery Interval

Pregnancies in quick succession after previous cesarean delivery can cause suboptimal healing of the scar and increased chances of scar dehiscence and scar rupture. Studies have shown a two- to three-fold increased risk of uterine scar rupture for women with a short interdelivery interval (below 12-24 months) from their previous cesarean.[69]

Contraindications to VBAC

There is limited evidence on safety of VBAC in more than one previous cesarean sections or type of previous uterine scar and therefore absolute risks are not known.[33,34,39,55,67,70] According to best possible evidence available, planned VBAC is contraindicated in:
1. Previous uterine rupture increases the risk of recurrent uterine rupture although the absolute rate is not known.
2. Previous high vertical classical cesarean section (200–900/10,000 risk of uterine rupture).
3. Two or more previous cesarean deliveries (reliable estimate of risks of rupture unknown).
4. In certain extreme circumstances (such as miscarriage, intrauterine fetal death) for some women in the above groups, the vaginal route (although risky) may not necessarily be contraindicated.
5. Previous inverted T or J incision (190/10,000 risk of uterine rupture).
6. Prior low vertical incision (200/10,000 risk of uterine rupture).

The current practice in most units is to do an elective cesarean section in women where uterine cavity was opened during myomectomy. However the evidence is insufficient and conflicting information on whether the risk of uterine rupture is increased in women with previous myomectomy or prior complex uterine surgery.[71]

VBAC in Previous Two Cesarean Sections

There have been many published studies advocating vaginal delivery after multiple previous cesarean deliveries. These show an insignificant increased risk of scar rupture with VBAC after two previous cesarean sections as compared to VBAC after one cesarean section (92/10,000 vs 68/10,000) and also slightly decreased success rates of VBAC (66% in previous two cesareans vs 74% in previous one cesarean).[39] A study by Macones et al, also showed an insignificant increase in scar rupture between previous 2 LSCS and 1 cesarean section, i.e. 1.8% vs 0.9%.[72] VBAC is therefore not a contraindication and can be offered to women in certain cases but this decision has to be done by the consultant after proper evaluation of the risks and benefits. Still very few obstetricians permit trial of VBAC after two previous cesarean sections. Cesarean section with three or more cesarean deliveries is not advocated.

Uterine Rupture and Previous Cesarean Section

Uterine rupture is defined as separation of the entire thickness of the uterine wall with extrusion of any portion of the fetal-placental unit, intraperitoneal or vaginal hemorrhage, need for a hysterectomy, or bladder injury. As mentioned earlier the uterine rupture rate in women undergoing trial of VBAC varies from 0.2-0.7%. It is an obstetric catastrophe that is associated with serious complications like blood transfusions, hysterectomy, and damage to the genitourinary tract, severe neonatal morbidity and even maternal and perinatal mortality. Chauhan et al reviewed literature from 1989 to 2001 to find the morbidity related to uterine rupture and found that per thousand trial of VBAC the morbidity related to uterine rupture was 1.8 for packed red blood cell transfusion, 1.5 for pathologic fetal acidosis (cord pH < 7.00), 0.9 for hysterectomy, 0.8 for genitourinary injury, 0.4 for perinatal death, and 0.02 for maternal death.[35] Moreover, prompt delivery is needed to avoid permanent neonatal damage or death. It is by far the most common reason for women refusing trial of VBAC. There is lack of robust evidence in absence of randomized controlled trials, inadequately powered studies and most data in form of meta-analysis of retrospective studies.

There are certain predisposing factors which can increase this risk and we need to know them to counsel women accordingly and safely. All the factors which contraindicate VBAC increase the chance of uterine rupture if VBAC is still attempted. The type of previous uterine scar is an important factor determining the scar rupture rates. In study done by Landon et al, the rates of rupture were 0.7% for women with one prior low transverse incision, 2% for those with a prior low vertical incision, 1.9% with a prior classical, inverted T, or J incision who either presented in advanced labor or refused a repeated cesarean delivery, and 0.5% for those with an unknown type of prior incision. In women with previous classical cesarean section, it would be advisable to do an ERCS earlier than 39 weeks as there is a chance of silent scar rupture and also to minimize the risk of them going into labor before elective cesarean section. A previous preterm cesarean delivery significantly increases the risk of subsequent uterine rupture as compared to women with previous cesarean section at term (0.58% compared with 0.28%, P < 0.001).[52] The reason primarily is due to suboptimal healing of a poorly formed lower segment in these women, as the risk of rupture was higher in women who had not gone into labor prior to cesarean section. This together with a shorter inter delivery period compounds the risk. Previous single layer closure has been found to increase the risk of uterine rupture by up to 6 times.[73] The risk of uterine rupture is also inversely related to inter delivery interval.[69] As discussed later in the chapter, induction of labor with prostaglandins increases scar rupture rates. A woman having successful vaginal birth, in any order, has got a protective factor from scar rupture and her chance of having it is five times less. Maternal age greater than 30 years is also associated with increased scar rupture. The risk is 3 times higher than for women younger than 30 years old undergoing trial of VBAC.[74] Maternal fever after previous cesarean section seems to be associated with increased risk of scar rupture but needs further studies.

MANAGEMENT

Antenatal Counseling

The antenatal counseling is based on the evidence given earlier in the chapter regarding success rates, complications, risks and, benefits and suitability of the patient for trial of VBAC or ERCS. It is vital to apply this evidence to the individual woman, according to her circumstances. Women with previous one uncomplicated lower-segment transverse cesarean section with an otherwise uncomplicated pregnancy, with no other contraindication for vaginal delivery can be given an option of planned VBAC or elective repeat cesarean section (ERCS) at term. An estimate of the likelihood of a successful trial of labor should be discussed. This is important because the increased risk for morbidity in women attempting VBAC is primarily found in those who fail to achieve successful vaginal birth. The discussion should be well-documented in the notes.

Previous operation notes should be seen to find the details of previous cesarean section surgery. Any divergence from the routine low transverse incision should be noted.

Discussion should also be done regarding continuous intrapartum monitoring.[50] Future reproductive choices should be discussed as this can be important in decision making. In women planning future pregnancies, multiple cesarean sections increase the risks of severe maternal morbidity and mortality, e.g. placenta previa, placenta accreta or percreta. Proper documentation is vital from medicolegal aspects. The decision should be made before term at least few weeks before term.

Monitoring in Antenatal Period

Role of USG

In women with placenta previa, possibility of placenta accreta should be ruled out by ultrasound or MRI. A consultant should be present during the cesarean section with placenta previa/accreta with previous scar. Blood should be cross matched, senior anesthetist should be present and interventional radiologist should be kept available if possible.

Scar Thickness

There have been few observational studies showing the possible benefit of measuring scar thickness before trial of VBAC.[75-77] Even an arbitrary cut-off of 3.5mm scar thickness has been used by some authors for selecting patients for trial of VBAC and showed good negative predictive value for scar rupture. However, the evidence is not robust enough for routine clinical practice, but some units do use it.

Timing of Elective Repeat Cesarean Section or Planned VBAC

As up to 10% of women scheduled for ERCS go into labor before the 39th week, it is good practice to have a plan for the event of labor starting prior to the scheduled date. For the same reason, 39 weeks seems to be a reasonable gestation to perform elective cesarean section. The risk of respiratory morbidity in the neonate appears to be very low. However, in cases of planned VBAC pregnancy should go till term and plan for induction of labor should be undertaken weighing the risks and benefits of postdated pregnancy with risks and benefits of induction of labor. Apart from these factors routine monitoring according to hospital protocol should be done.

Management of Labor

Intrapartum Support and Intervention during Planned VBAC

VBAC should be conducted in a well-staffed and equipped delivery suite with a good consultant support. Knowing that there is a risk of 0.5–1.0% of scar rupture and consequent risk of fetal demise, there should be adequate facilities for immediate cesarean section and neonatal and maternal resuscitation. Intravenous access with grouping and cross matching of blood should be done in all these cases. Continuous cardiotocography is recommended as abnormality in the cardiotocograph is the most consistent finding in uterine rupture. CTG abnormalities are present in 55–87% of such cases.[42] Although abnormal cardiotocograph is usually the earliest warning sign, presence of any of the following should raise the suspicion of uterine scar rupture.
1. Abnormal CTG
2. Severe abdominal pain, especially if persisting between contractions
3. Chest pain or shoulder tip pain
4. Sudden onset of shortness of breath
5. Scar tenderness
6. Abnormal vaginal bleeding or hematuria
7. Cessation of previously efficient uterine activity

8. Maternal tachycardia, hypotension or shock
9. Loss of station of the presenting part.

Epidural anesthesia is not contraindicated in planned VBAC. There is no evidence to show that masking of symptoms of uterine rupture due to epidural anesthesia increases the risk of maternal or perinatal morbidity. The routine use of intrauterine pressure catheters in the early detection of uterine scar rupture is not recommended.

Induction and Augmentation

Induction of labor (regardless of the method of induction) and augmentation of labor with oxytocin are associated with a significantly greater risk of uterine rupture than with spontaneous labor without oxytocin augmentation (P<0.001 for both).[21,33] Induction should be done after analyzing the risks and benefits of induction of labor. Women should be informed that there is a two- to three-fold increase in risk of uterine rupture and 1.5-fold increase in emergency cesarean section due to induction and/or augmentation of labor compared with spontaneous labor[78] (Table 12.8). However, some studies in literature do not suggest a significant increase in uterine rupture rate between women undergoing induction of labor with or without previous cesarean section.[79] As the evidence is not strong enough, hence caution should be taken before induction of labor. The decision should be consultant led and induction should happen preferably in the labor ward.

Prostaglandin Induction

The risk of uterine rupture is 0.4% in women with spontaneous labor. There has been controversial evidence with some authors suggesting no significant increase in uterine rupture in women with previous cesarean section when induction using prostaglandins is done under strict protocol. However the best available evidence suggests a higher rupture rate in these cases. Prostaglandin induction with or without oxytocin augmentation compared with non-prostaglandin induction has a higher risk of uterine rupture of 1.4% *vs* 0.9% respectively. In another study, the uterine rupture rate was found to be 0.87% *vs* 0.29%. Prostaglandin induction is also associated with a higher risk of perinatal death from uterine rupture. Prostaglandin E2 (dinoprostone) is associated with an increased risk of uterine rupture and should not be used except in rare circumstances.[59] Prostaglandin E1 (misoprostol) is found to have a high risk of uterine rupture and should not be used for induction of labor after cesarean section.[80] The results of NICHD on prostaglandin induction are shown in the Table 12.7. Hence looking at the overall evidence, prostaglandin E2 can be used with great caution using the safe dose, usually single dose, for induction in women with previous scar. Misoprostol should not be used in these women for induction of labor at term.

Table 12.7: National institute of child health and human development (NICHD) study[21,33]			
Outcome	Spontaneous labor	Augmented labor	Induced labor
Uterine rupture rate	0.4%	0.9%	1.0%
Cesarean section rate	19%	26%	33%

Nonprostaglandin Induction

Induction of labor with oxytocin may be associated with an increased risk of uterine rupture. However, the exact rate of increase is not known.[69] Foley's catheter may be safely used to ripen the cervix in a woman planning a VBAC.

Table 12.8: Rates of uterine rupture according to labor status				
Type of labor	No. of patients	Uterine rupture no. (%)	Odds ratio (95% CI)	P value
Spontaneous	6685	24 (0.4)	1.00	-
Augmented	6009	52 (0.9)	2.42(1.49-3.93)	< 0.001
Induced	4708	43 (1.0)	2.86 (1.75-4.67)	< 0.001
With any prostaglandin, with or without oxytocin	926	13 (1.4)	3.95 (2.01-7.79)	< 0.001
With no prostaglandins*	1691	15 (0.9)	2.48 (1.30-4.75)	< 0.001
With oxytocin alone	1864	20 (1.1)	3.01 (1.66-5.46)	< 0.001
Not classified	496	0	-	-

*Induction with no prostaglandins includes mechanical dilation with or without oxytocin

Augmentation of Labor

Oxytocin augmentation is not contraindicated in women undergoing a VBAC according to SOGC guidelines but it should be a consultant led decision. Oxytocin rate should be titrated such that it should not exceed the maximum rate of four contractions in 10 minutes. Early recognition and intervention for labor dystocia can prevent a proportion of uterine ruptures among women attempting VBAC and therefore progress of labor should be carefully assessed. Misoprostol (PGE1) should not be used for augmentation of labor as it increases the risk of uterine rupture.[80]

Management of Third Stage of Labor

Due to the presence of scar and its inability to contract, the possibility of post- partum hemorrhage is increased and therefore active management of third stage is recommended. Following interventions should be considered:
- Oxytocics at delivery of the shoulders.
- Delivery of placenta immediately after appearance of the separation signs of placenta.
- Consider routine use of 10 units oxytocin in 500 ml of normal saline at the rate of 125 ml/hr for 4 hours after delivery in absence of any contraindication.

It is important not to attempt delivery of the placenta if there are no signs of placental separation. Scan reports should be reviewed to see the site of placenta and possibility of placenta accreta should be kept in mind especially if the placenta is anterior. In case of such suspicion following should be done:

- 4 units of blood should be cross matched.
- Explain to the patient about placenta accreta and the possible interventions that can be done and obtain consent from the patient.
- Consultant should be informed.
- Operation theater should be arranged for exploration and consent should be taken for manual removal of placenta and possible interventions in case of placenta accreta should be clearly explained.

Manual removal should only be done if a clear plane of cleavage is found between the uterus and placenta. If no such plane is found then it is extremely important not to attempt any separation, as this might lead to massive bleeding.

In cases of placenta accreta the management options are discussed below.

- *Hysterectomy*: Evidence supports an aggressive surgical approach by means of hysterectomy in such cases unless preserving fertility is an issue. However if the patient is not bleeding or fertility is an issue expectant management can be one.
- *Expectant*: There have been many case reports and case series published where expectant management of placenta accreta has been used especially where conserving fertility is an issue.[81] This would involve leaving the whole placenta in and cutting the cord as close to the placenta as possible. However close monitoring is required by means of weekly scans and monitoring for infection. The expectant management can be continued until placenta gets resorbed which could take up to 6-10 months or until patient develops any signs or symptoms of infection or heavy bleeding. Role of methotrexate to help resorption is not known although some authors' have advocated its use in form of weekly injections. Beta hCG although has been used by some authors to see the resorption of placenta however it does not have any effect on the complications like heavy bleeding.
- *Blunt dissection and curettage*: This can be done in cases of late identification of placenta accreta where removal of placenta has already been proceeded with. The placenta is removed manually as much as could be. Oxytocics should be given in these cases to contract the uterus and intrauterine pressure balloon can be inserted for 24 hours. Antibiotic cover should be given and once the bleeding stops blunt curettage should be considered. Complications like uterine rupture while curettage and infection can occur therefore it should be done with great care.
- *Conservative surgery*: Uterine artery embolization, internal artery ligation or embolization and subendometrial vasopressin are other methods which have been reported in the literature. In many cases after conservative surgery, a relaparotomy followed by hysterectomy is done under a more controlled situation and with less bleeding and morbidity.

Manual Exploration of Scar after Cesarean Section

Although a lot of controversy exists on this issue our current practice is not to routinely examine the lower uterine segment in a woman after a successful VBAC. The reasons are primarily no knowledge about the sensitivity and specificity of a manual assessment of the lower uterine segment for an occult rupture, secondly vigorous manual examination can damage or perforate the lower uterine segment. There would be a question of repairing it if the patient remains well.[67] There is also no evidence as to what would be the impact of this finding on future vaginal birth.

POSTNATAL VISIT

All women undergoing emergency cesarean sections for failed VBAC should be briefed about the events surrounding delivery and should be counseled about safe interdelivery time.

COST OF VBAC COMPARED WITH REPEAT CS

Although vaginal birth after cesarean section are known to be cost effective as compared to ERCS however it is important to understand that VBAC is associated with high maternal and perinatal morbidity if there are not adequate facilities for close intrapartum monitoring and continuous cardiotocography monitoring in these women. This would in turn increase the costs incurred in further management of the mother and baby. It is therefore important for individual units to work out their own cost effectiveness.

AUDIT AND RESEARCH

It is important to audit the practice around VBAC and ERCS. Further research needs to be done in form of randomized controlled trials to find more hard evidence.

Pending Relevant Trials[78]

Evidence for VBAC can hopefully be more robust after results of following trials:

- *BAC (Birth after cesarean):* Planned vaginal birth or planned cesarean section for women at term with a single previous cesarean birth. Professor C Crowther, University of Adelaide, Australia. ISRCTN53974531.
- *The twin birth study:* A multicenter randomized controlled trial comparing planned cesarean section with planned vaginal birth for twins at 32–38 weeks of gestation. Dr J Barrett, Toronto, Canada. DIAMOND (Decision Aids for Mode of Next Delivery). ISRCTN 84367722, Dr A Montgomery, Bristol, UK. ISRCTN 74420086.

12

Pregnancy with Previous Cesarean Section

- *CAESAR (Cesarean section surgical techniques):* Dr P Brocklehurst, National Perinatal Epidemiology Unit, Oxford, UK. ISRCTN 11849611.

KEY POINTS

- There is a 46% higher chance of not having or having fewer children after five years of first cesarean section delivery.
- The adjusted RR of placenta previa in subsequent pregnancy is 1.28 after 1 LSCS in primiparous, 2.0 after 2 previous cesarean section only and 4.0 after 3 previous cesarean sections only. The risk increases with parity irrespective of nature of delivery, though the risk is highest with cesarean deliveries in all previous pregnancies.
- Abruption rates in pregnancy with a previous cesarean section are 0.95%, significantly higher than 0.74% with previous one vaginal birth. The risk of abruption in third pregnancy increases by 30% after two consecutive cesarean deliveries. If interdelivery interval is less than an year there is an increase in abruption rates by 52% if previous delivery was vaginal and by 111% if previous delivery was by cesarean section.
- The risk of placenta accreta is 4% after vaginal delivery, 13% after one cesarean section, 27% after two cesarean section and 60% after 3 cesarean sections.
- The success rates of VBAC after one cesarean section is approximately 72-76%.
- Amongst many factors previous vaginal birth, particularly previous VBAC, is the single best predictor for successful VBAC and is associated with an approximately 87–90% planned VBAC success rate.
- Successful VBAC had an overall morbidity of 2.4% whereas women who had failed attempted VBAC had a 14.1% incidence of morbidity.
- Maternal risk of ERCS is primarily related to future reproductive problems. Fetal risks are primarily respiratory morbidity associated with 5 fold increase in TTN (transient tachypnea of the newborn) or RDS.
- Risk of delivery related perinatal death is increased by 12 fold in VBAC group than ERCS however the absolute risk is still small.
- VBAC between 26-37 weeks is associated with decreased scar rupture rates.
- Any previous uterine incision apart from lower segment transverse incision is a contraindication of planned VBAC.
- There is no clear evidence on safety of VBAC after myomectomy.
- ERCS section should be planned at around 39 weeks in usual circumstances.
- Trial of VBAC should be done in well-staffed unit with consultant support and adequate available resources for immediate cesarean section and advanced neonatal and maternal resuscitation.
- There is a two- to three-fold increased risk of uterine rupture and around 1.5-fold increased risk of cesarean section in induced and/or augmented labor compared with spontaneous labor.

- As far as the method of induction is concerned prostaglandins carry a higher rate of rupture than ARM or oxytocin induction.
- Continuous monitoring by cardiotocograph should be done in women with trial of VBAC as FHR abnormality is the most consistent finding in uterine rupture and is present in 55-87% of these events.

End notes

Planned VBAC: Planned VBAC (vaginal birth after cesarean) refers to any woman who has experienced a prior cesarean birth who plans to deliver vaginally rather than by ERCS (elective repeat cesarean section).

Successful and unsuccessful planned VBAC: A vaginal birth (spontaneous or assisted) in a woman undergoing planned VBAC indicates a successful VBAC. Delivery by emergency cesarean section during labor indicates an unsuccessful VBAC.

Elective repeat cesarean section: Planned cesarean section usually at around 39 weeks and prior to onset of labor.

Uterine rupture: Disruption of the uterine muscle extending to and involving the uterine serosa or disruption of the uterine muscle with extension to the bladder or broad ligament.

Uterine dehiscence: Disruption of the uterine muscle with intact uterine serosa.

Other outcomes: Hysterectomy, thromboembolism, hemorrhage, transfusion requirement, viscus injury (bowel, bladder, ureter), endometritis, maternal death.

Term is defined as, at or beyond 37 completed weeks of gestation.

Term delivery-related perinatal death is defined as the combined number of intrapartum stillbirths and neonatal deaths per 10,000 live births and stillbirths, at or beyond 37 completed weeks of gestation.

Birth-related perinatal mortality rates exclude antepartum stillbirths and deaths due to fetal malformation unless otherwise stated.

Neonatal respiratory morbidity is defined as the combined rate of transient tachypnea of the newborn (TTN) and respiratory distress syndrome (RDS).

REFERENCES

1. Oral E, Elter K. The impact of cesarean birth on subsequent fertility. Curr Opin Obstet Gynecol 2007;19:238-43.
2. Dodd J, Crowther C. Vaginal birth after Caesarean versus elective repeat Caesarean for women with a single prior Caesarean birth: A systematic review of the literature. Aust N Z J Obstet Gynaecol 2004;44:387-91.
3. Jolly J, Walker J, Bhabra K. Subsequent obstetric performance related to primary mode of delivery. Br J Obstet Gynaecol 1999;106:227-32.

12

Pregnancy with Previous Cesarean Section

4. Hemminki E. Impact of caesarean section on future pregnancy—A review of cohort studies. Paediatr Perinat Epidemiol 1996;10:366-79.
5. Collin SM, Marshall T, Filippi V. Caesarean section and subsequent fertility in sub-Saharan Africa. BJOG 2006;113:276-83.
6. Bhattacharya S, Porter M, Harrild K, et al. Absence of conception after caesarean section: Voluntary or involuntary? BJOG 2006;113:268-75.
7. Murphy DJ, Stirrat GM, Heron J. The relationship between Caesarean section and subfertility in a population-based sample of 14,541 pregnancies. Hum Reprod 2002;17:1914-17.
8. Hemminki E, Merilainen J. Long-term effects of cesarean sections: Ectopic pregnancies and placental problems. Am J Obstet Gynecol 1996;174:1569-74.
9. Kendrick JS, Tierney EF, Lawson HW, et al. Previous cesarean delivery and the risk of ectopic pregnancy. Obstet Gynecol 1996;87:297-301.
10. Maymon R, Halperin R, Mendlovic S, et al. Ectopic pregnancies in a Caesarean scar: Review of the medical approach to an iatrogenic complication. Hum Reprod Update 2004;10:515-23.
11. Halperin R, Schneider D, Mendlovic S, et al. Uterine-preserving emergency surgery for cesarean scar pregnancies: Another medical solution to an iatrogenic problem. Fertil Steril 2008.
12. Ash A, Smith A, Maxwell D. Caesarean scar pregnancy. BJOG 2007;114:253-63.
13. Morris H. Surgical pathology of the lower uterine segment caesarean section scar: Is the scar a source of clinical symptoms? Int J Gynecol Pathol 1995;14:16-20.
14. Nicola Jackson. SP-B. Physical sequelae of caesarean section. Best Practice and reserach Clinical Obstet and Gynaecology 2001;15:49-61.
15. Rasmussen S, Albrechtsen S, Dalaker K. Obstetric history and the risk of placenta previa. Acta Obstet Gynecol Scand 2000;79:502-07.
16. Rageth JC, Juzi C, Grossenbacher H. Delivery after previous cesarean: A risk evaluation. Swiss Working Group of Obstetric and Gynecologic Institutions. Obstet Gynecol 1999;93: 332-37.
17. Lydon-Rochelle M, Holt VL, Easterling TR, et al. First-birth cesarean and placental abruption or previa at second birth(1). Obstet Gynecol 2001;97:765-69.
18. Gilliam M, Rosenberg D, Davis F. The Likelihood of Placenta Previa With Greater Number of Cesarean Deliveries and Higher Parity. Acogjnl 2002;99:976-80.
19. Ananth CV, Smulian JC, Vintzileos AM. The association of placenta previa with history of cesarean delivery and abortion: A metaanalysis. Am J Obstet Gynecol 1997;177:1071-78.
20. Ananth CV, Savitz DA, Williams MA. Placental abruption and its association with hypertension and prolonged rupture of membranes: A methodologic review and meta-analysis. Obstet Gynecol 1996;88:309-18.
21. Ananth CV, Berkowitz GS, Savitz DA, et al. Placental abruption and adverse perinatal outcomes. JAMA 1999;282:1646-51.
22. Rasmussen S, Irgens LM, Dalaker K. The effect on the likelihood of further pregnancy of placental abruption and the rate of its recurrence. Br J Obstet Gynaecol 1997;104:1292-95.
23. Getahun D, Oyelese Y, Salihu HM, et al. Previous cesarean delivery and risks of placenta previa and placental abruption. Obstet Gynecol 2006;107:771-78.
24. Zaki ZM, Bahar AM, Ali ME, et al. Risk factors and morbidity in patients with placenta previa accreta compared to placenta previa non-accreta. Acta Obstet Gynecol Scand 1998;77:391-94.
25. Clark SL, Koonings PP, Phelan JP. Placenta previa/accreta and prior cesarean section. Obstet Gynecol 1985;66:89-92.
26. Miller DA, Chollet JA, Goodwin TM. Clinical risk factors for placenta previa-placenta accreta. Am J Obstet Gynecol 1997;177:210-14.
27. Smith GC, Pell JP, Dobbie R. Caesarean section and risk of unexplained stillbirth in subsequent pregnancy. Lancet 2003;362:1779-84.
28. Salihu HM, Sharma PP, Kristensen S, et al. Risk of stillbirth following a cesarean delivery: Black-white disparity. Obstet Gynecol 2006;107:383-90.
29. Merrill BS, Gibbs CE. Planned vaginal delivery following cesarean section. Obstet Gynecol 1978;52:50-52.
30. The National Institutes of Health Consensus Development statement on cesarean childbirth. A summary. J Reprod Med 1981;26:103-12.
31. NIH consensus development statement on cesarean childbirth. The Cesarean Birth Task Force. Obstet Gynecol 1981;57:537-45.

32. Macones GA, Peipert J, Nelson DB, et al. Maternal complications with vaginal birth after cesarean delivery: A multicenter study. Am J Obstet Gynecol 2005;193:1656-62.

33. Landon MB, Hauth JC, Leveno KJ, et al. Maternal and perinatal outcomes associated with a trial of labor after prior cesarean delivery. N Engl J Med 2004;351:2581-89.

34. Guise JM, Hashima J, Osterweil P. Evidence-based vaginal birth after Caesarean section. Best Pract Res Clin Obstet Gynaecol 2005;19:117-30.

35. Chauhan SP, Martin JN, Jr., Henrichs CE, et al. Maternal and perinatal complications with uterine rupture in 142,075 patients who attempted vaginal birth after cesarean delivery: A review of the literature. Am J Obstet Gynecol 2003;189:408-17.

36. Mozurkewich EL, Hutton EK. Elective repeat cesarean delivery versus trial of labor: A meta-analysis of the literature from 1989 to 1999. Am J Obstet Gynecol 2000;183:1187-97.

37. Guise JM, Berlin M, McDonagh M, et al. Safety of vaginal birth after cesarean: A systematic review. Obstet Gynecol 2004;103:420-29.

38. Gyamfi C, Juhasz G, Gyamfi P, et al. Increased success of trial of labor after previous vaginal birth after cesarean. Obstet Gynecol 2004;104:715-19.

39. Landon MB, Leindecker S, Spong CY, et al. The MFMU Cesarean Registry: Factors affecting the success of trial of labor after previous cesarean delivery. Am J Obstet Gynecol 2005;193:1016-23.

40. Smith GC, White IR, Pell JP, et al. Predicting cesarean section and uterine rupture among women attempting vaginal birth after prior cesarean section. PLoS Med 2005;2:e252.

41. Mercer BM, Gilbert S, Landon MB, et al. Labor outcomes with increasing number of prior vaginal births after cesarean delivery. Obstet Gynecol 2008;111:285-91.

42. Guise JM, McDonagh MS, Osterweil P, et al. Systematic review of the incidence and consequences of uterine rupture in women with previous caesarean section. BMJ 2004;329:19-25.

43. Bujold E, Blackwell SC, Hendler I, et al. Modified Bishop's score and induction of labor in patients with a previous cesarean delivery. Am J Obstet Gynecol 2004;191:1644-48.

44. Durnwald C, Mercer B. Vaginal birth after Cesarean delivery: Predicting success, risks of failure. J Matern Fetal Neonatal Med 2004;15:388-93.

45. Hashima JN, Eden KB, Osterweil P, et al. Predicting vaginal birth after cesarean delivery: A review of prognostic factors and screening tools. Am J Obstet Gynecol 2004;190:547-55.

46. Dinsmoor MJ, Brock EL. Predicting failed trial of labor after primary cesarean delivery. Obstet Gynecol 2004;103:282-86.

47. Macones GA, Cahill AG, Stamilio DM, et al. Can uterine rupture in patients attempting vaginal birth after cesarean delivery be predicted? Am J Obstet Gynecol 2006;195:1148-52.

48. Juhasz G, Gyamfi C, Gyamfi P, et al. Effect of body mass index and excessive weight gain on success of vaginal birth after cesarean delivery. Obstet Gynecol 2005;106:741-46.

49. Bujold E, Gauthier RJ. Should we allow a trial of labor after a previous cesarean for dystocia in the second stage of labor? Obstet Gynecol 2001;98:652-55.

50. Sachs BP, Kobelin C, Castro MA, et al. The risks of lowering the cesarean-delivery rate. N Engl J Med 1999;340:54-57.

51. Kwee A, Smink M, Van Der Laar R, et al. Outcome of subsequent delivery after a previous early preterm cesarean section. J Matern Fetal Neonatal Med 2007;20:33-57.

52. Sciscione AC, Landon MB, Leveno KJ, et al. Previous preterm cesarean delivery and risk of subsequent uterine rupture. Obstet Gynecol 2008;111:648-53.

53. Zelop CM, Shipp TD, Repke JT, et al. Outcomes of trial of labor following previous cesarean delivery among women with fetuses weighing >4000 g. Am J Obstet Gynecol 2001;185:903-05.

54. Srinivas SK, Stamilio DM, Sammel MD, et al. Vaginal birth after caesarean delivery: Does maternal age affect safety and success? Paediatr Perinat Epidemiol 2007;21:114-20.

55. McMahon MJ, Luther ER, Bowes WA, Jr., et al. Comparison of a trial of labor with an elective second cesarean section. N Engl J Med 1996;335:689-95.

56. Wen SW, Rusen ID, Walker M, et al. Comparison of maternal mortality and morbidity between trial of labor and elective cesarean section among women with previous cesarean delivery. Am J Obstet Gynecol 2004;191:1263-69.

57. Turner MJ, Agnew G, Langan H. Uterine rupture and labour after a previous low transverse caesarean section. BJOG 2006;113:729-32.

58. Gardeil F, Daly S, Turner MJ. Uterine rupture in pregnancy reviewed. Eur J Obstet Gynecol Reprod Biol 1994;56:107-10.
59. Smith GC, Pell JP, Pasupathy D, et al. Factors predisposing to perinatal death related to uterine rupture during attempted vaginal birth after caesarean section: Retrospective cohort study. BMJ 2004;329:375.
60. Smith GC, Pell JP, Cameron AD, et al. Risk of perinatal death associated with labor after previous cesarean delivery in uncomplicated term pregnancies. JAMA 2002;287:2684-90.
61. Smith GC, Wood AM, White IR, et al. Neonatal respiratory morbidity at term and the risk of childhood asthma. Arch Dis Child 2004;89:956-60.
62. Morley GM. Mode of delivery and risk of respiratory diseases in newborns. Obstet Gynecol 2001;97:1025-26.
63. Levine EM, Ghai V, Barton JJ, et al. Mode of delivery and risk of respiratory diseases in newborns. Obstet Gynecol 2001;97:439-42.
64. Richardson BS, Czikk MJ, daSilva O, et al. The impact of labor at term on measures of neonatal outcome. Am J Obstet Gynecol 2005;192:219-26.
65. Quinones JN, Stamilio DM, Pare E, et al. The effect of prematurity on vaginal birth after cesarean delivery: Success and maternal morbidity. Obstet Gynecol 2005;105:519-24.
66. Varner MW, Leindecker S, Spong CY, et al. The Maternal-Fetal Medicine Unit cesarean registry: Trial of labor with a twin gestation. Am J Obstet Gynecol 2005;193:135-40.
67. Cahill AG, Macones GA. Vaginal birth after cesarean delivery: Evidence-based practice. Clin Obstet Gynecol 2007;50:518-25.
68. Cahill A, Stamilio DM, Pare E, et al. Vaginal birth after cesarean (VBAC) attempt in twin pregnancies: Is it safe? Am J Obstet Gynecol 2005;193:1050-55.
69. Bujold E, Mehta SH, Bujold C, et al. Interdelivery interval and uterine rupture. Am J Obstet Gynecol 2002;187:1199-1202.
70. Spaans WA, van der Vliet LM, Roell-Schorer EA, et al. Trial of labour after two or three previous caesarean sections. Eur J Obstet Gynecol Reprod Biol 2003;110:16-19.
71. Seracchioli R, Manuzzi L, Vianello F, et al. Obstetric and delivery outcome of pregnancies achieved after laparoscopic myomectomy. Fertil Steril 2006;86:159-65.
72. Macones GA, Cahill A, Pare E, et al. Obstetric outcomes in women with two prior cesarean deliveries: Is vaginal birth after cesarean delivery a viable option? Am J Obstet Gynecol 2005;192:1223-28; discussion 8-9.
73. Gyamfi C, Juhasz G, Gyamfi P, et al. Single- versus double-layer uterine incision closure and uterine rupture. J Matern Fetal Neonatal Med 2006;19:639-43.
74. Zelop CM, Shipp TD, Repke JT, et al. Effect of previous vaginal delivery on the risk of uterine rupture during a subsequent trial of labor. Am J Obstet Gynecol 2000;183:1184-86.
75. Rozenberg P, Goffinet F, Phillippe HJ, et al. Ultrasonographic measurement of lower uterine segment to assess risk of defects of scarred uterus. Lancet 1996;347:281-84.
76. Rozenberg P, Goffinet F, Philippe HJ, et al. Echographic measurement of the inferior uterine segment for assessing the risk of uterine rupture. J Gynecol Obstet Biol Reprod (Paris) 1997;26:513-19.
77. Rozenberg P, Goffinet F, Philippe HJ, et al. Thickness of the lower uterine segment: Its influence in the management of patients with previous cesarean sections. Eur J Obstet Gynecol Reprod Biol 1999;87:39-45.
78. Royal College of Obstetricians and Gynaecologists. Birth after previous caesarean birth. Green-top Guideline No 45, Feb 2007.
79. Locatelli A, Regalia AL, Ghidini A, et al. Risks of induction of labour in women with a uterine scar from previous low transverse caesarean section. BJOG 2004;111:1394-99.
80. SOGC clinical practice guidelines. Guidelines for vaginal birth after previous caesarean birth. Number 155 (Replaces guideline Number 147), February 2005. Int J Gynaecol Obstet 2005;89:319-31.
81. Kayem G, Davy C, Goffinet F, et al. Conservative versus extirpative management in cases of placenta accreta. Obstet Gynecol 2004;104:531-36.

Rh Negative Pregnancy

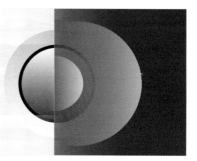

13

Aruna Nigam

INTRODUCTION

Rh isoimmunization occurs when a Rh negative woman's immune system is sensitized to Rh factor present on the surface of the fetal erythrocytes, stimulating the production of immunoglobulin G (IgG) antibodies. The most common routes of maternal sensitization are via blood transfusion or fetomaternal hemorrhage associated with delivery, trauma, spontaneous or induced abortion, ectopic pregnancy or invasive obstetric procedures. These antibodies can cross the placenta during subsequent pregnancies in alloimmunized women and if the fetus is positive for the erythrocyte surface antigens, result in hemolysis of fetal erythrocytes and anemia. This IgG antibody mediated hemolysis of fetal erythrocytes, known as hemolytic disease of the fetus and newborn (HDFN), can have a varied degree of manifestations which are the result of anemia and hyperbilirubinemia. In severe cases, hemolysis may lead to extramedullary hematopoiesis leading to hepatosplenomegaly, decreased liver function and ensuing hypoproteinemia, ascites and anasarca in the fetus. When associated with high output cardiac failure and pericardial effusion, this condition is known as hydrops fetalis. Intensive neonatal care, including emergency exchange transfusion is required many times, without which this condition is often fatal.

Cases of hemolysis in the newborn that do not result in fetal hydrops can still lead to kernicterus in which there occurs deposition of unconjugated bilirubin in the brain because of absence of placental clearance and immature fetal bilirubin-conjugating ability. The manifestations include poor feeding, inactivity, loss of the Moro reflex, a bulging fontanelle and seizures of the infants who survive 10% may develop spastic choreoathetosis, deafness and mental retardation.

PREVALENCE

Though antibodies to D antigen remains most common, smaller families[1] and the widespread use of immunoprophylaxis has decreased the incidence and enhanced other antigen groups causing isoimmunization.

The incidence of alloimmunization varies greatly among the populations. Rates of Rh negativity among ethnic and racial groups are as follows:

- White—15-16%
- African American—8%
- African—4%
- Basque (region of Spain/France)—30-35%
- Asian—Less than 1%
- Asian American—1%
- American Indian—1-2%
- Eurasian—2-4%
- Indians—3-5.7%.[2]

In India, the incidence of Rh sensitization during pregnancy is 1.9% and the perinatal loss has been reported to be between 1 and 2.5%.[3] The main causes of Rh sensitization in India in present era are: lack of awareness and omission of routine testing of pregnant females for ABO and Rh group especially in rural setups, scarcity of facilities for laboratory testing for isoimmunization, ignorance about use of anti-D for the prevention of isoimmunization in various situations.

PATHOPHYSIOLOGY

There are several classes of antigens which can cause fetal or neonatal hemolytic disease as delineated in Table 13.1. Of the existing Rh antigens, D antigen is the most immunogenic. Three pairs of Rh antigens are known, with varying gene frequencies and possible combinations. Interestingly, with respect to the c and e alleles of the Rh locus, both c and C as well as e and E antigens exist. With

Table 13.1: Antigens causing fetal or neonatal hemolytic disease[4]
Common
• Rhesus family: D, C, E, c, e (d antigen is nonexistent)   • Kell: K.k, Ko,
Uncommon
• JK[a](Kidd)   • Fy[a](Duffy)   • Kp[a or b]   • k   • S
Rare
• Do[a] Di[a or b], Fy[b], Hutch, Jk[b] Lu[a] M, N,S. s, U, yt

respect to the *D* allele, *d* actually refers to the absence of the *D* allele, as no *d* antigen is known to exist. When referring to the different alleles, the capital and small letters are used. For example, a patient with the *cDE* complex would be considered to have little c, capital D, and capital E antigens.

The primary immune response to the D antigen is weak and occurs over 6 weeks to 12 months. The initial antibodies are of IgM type that does not cross the placenta, as a result first pregnancy is not typically at great risk. IgG become detectable within 6 month time. A second antigen challenge generates amnestic response that is both rapid and almost exclusive IgG which can cross the placenta, thus posing the greater risk of severe fetal disease.

There are three phases of fetal hematopoiesis: Mesoblastic, hepatic and myeloid related to three major organs. Erythropoiesis commence in the yolk sac at day 21 (mesoblastic phase), then moves to the liver (hepatic phase) and finally to the bone marrow at the 16 weeks of gestation (myeloid phase). The decreasing contribution of the liver is characterized by the exponential decrease in the number of erythroblasts. The Rh antigens are well-developed by day 30 of gestation, in contrast to ABO antigens which are poorly expressed on the fetal RBC. Anti-D antibody triggered hemolysis is not complement mediated, rather anti-D coated RBC are destroyed extravascularly by a reticuloendothelial system at a rate faster than normal. The response of the affected fetus is quite variable depending on the quantity and subclass of IgG antibody (amount of fetomaternal hemorrhage), the efficiency of placental passage, the avidity with which the antibody binds to the antigen site, the maternal HLA make up, coexistence of ABO incompatibility, the maturity and efficiency of reticuloendothelial system, prophylaxis given in previous pregnancies and perhaps even the fetal sex.[4]

Hemolytic anemia may occur whenever the erythrocyte lifespan declines below 70 to 90 days and hematopoietic system can no longer meet the demands. Erythropoiesis may occur anywhere in the fetoplacental unit. Both the liver and the spleen are enlarged secondary to extramedullary erythropoiesis and congestion. Erythroblasts are released into peripheral circulation, hence the term erythroblastosis fetalis. The greater the number of erythroblasts in the circulation, the greater the likelihood that an antenatal transfusion therapy may be necessary. All fetal sequelae of hemolytic disease relate to development of anemia. In general, fetus tolerates mild to moderate anemia well. However, other metabolic alterations develop as the anemia worsens. As the fetal RBCs are principal fetal buffer, metabolic acidemia with hyperlactatemia develops in fetus with extreme anemia. Most important causative factor in the development of fetal hydrops is cardiac dysfunction, probably secondary to insufficient oxygen carrying capacity. This dysfunction is detectable immediately prior to development of hydrops and resolves rapidly after transfusion with increase in the fetal oxygen carrying capacity.

Hyperbilirubinemia secondary to hemolysis is an important part of alloimmune hemolytic disease. Heme pigment is first converted to biliverdin by heme oxygenase and then to water-insoluble and lipid-soluble bilirubin (the indirect fraction) by biliverdin reductase. Both the fetus and the neonates have reduced levels of glucuronyl transferase, the enzyme necessary for the production of water-soluble diglucuronide. Indirect bilirubin unbound to albumin penetrates the lipid neuronal membrane and produce cell death. Thus the neonates with severe hyperbilirubinemia are at risk of developing encephalopathy (kernicterus). Kernicterus and jaundice are not the component of erythroblastosis fetalis during intrauterine life, since accumulation of the pigment is prevented by its removal through the placental circulation and metabolism in the maternal liver. However after birth the newborn, liver cannot effectively handle the large amount of pigment released during the brisk hemolytic process and this leads to rapid increase in serum bilirubin and eventual tissue deposition. The concentration of bilirubin necessary to cause kernicterus rises with the gestational age. Thus, whereas term neonate can tolerate a total bilirubin of 25 mg/dl, the extremely preterm neonate are at risk of developing kernicterus at 12 mg/dl. Affected neonates are initially lethargic and then become hypertonic, lying with their neck hyperextended, their back arched and their knees, elbows and wrist flexed. They suck poorly and ultimately develop apneic episodes. Neural tissue in the auditory center is particularly sensitive to indirect bilirubin. Survivors often have profound neurosensory deafness and choreoathetoid spastic cerebral palsy.

Causes of maternal alloimmunization include the following:
- Blood transfusion
- Fetomaternal hemorrhage
  - Antepartum
  - Intrapartum
- Abortion
  - Therapeutic—in 4-5% of cases
  - Spontaneous—in 2% of cases
  - Threatened—There is some risk but less understood, administration of Anti-D is recommended.
- Ectopic pregnancy
- Multiple pregnancy
- Abdominal trauma
- Intrauterine death
- Obstetric procedures
  - Amniocentesis
  - Chorionic villus sampling (CVS)
  - Percutaneous umbilical blood sampling
  - External cephalic version-risk is 2-6%
  - Manual removal of the placenta
  - During cesarean section.

The blood type and Rh group should be done in all the pregnant women at their first prenatal visit at least twice which are in agreement and an antibody screening is also recommended. Detection of the antibodies to D antigen can be done by several methods which are as following:

Agglutination Test

Saline

Rh positive red blood cells suspended in saline agglutinate when serum containing IgM is added to it.

Colloid

Rh positive red cells suspended in colloid medium such as bovine albumin agglutinate if serum containing either IgM or IgG is added as the pretreatment of the serum with dithiothreitol disrupts the sulfhydryl bonds of IgM (but not of IgG) and prevents its binding to the red blood cells.

Antiglobulin or Coombs' Test

Indirect

Maternal plasma is incubated with Rh positive red blood cells and with serum rich in antiglobulin antibodies (Coombs' serum) and the red cells will agglutinate if the Rh antibodies are present in the maternal plasma. The IgG antibodies have relatively small molecular weight and are not capable of bridging the intercellular distance of 250 Å that exists between the red cells in solution to cause agglutination. The distance results from red cells repelling each other because of their negative surface charge or zeta potential. The addition of Coombs' serum to the maternal plasma decreases the intercellular distance and facilitates the agglutination of the cells when anti-Rh antibodies are present.

Direct

Antihuman antiglobulin is added directly to the red cells from the patient. Agglutination indicates antibody is bound to the red cells.

The concentration of antibodies is determined by a titration procedure in which progressively double dilutions of maternal serum incubated with group O Rh+ ve erythrocytes and the agglutination of erythrocytes is used as the endpoint of the reaction. Titer values correspond to the greatest dilution with positive agglutination. There are variations of antibody titers among different laboratories and the obstetrician managing an immunized pregnancy should use the same laboratory for all of the antibody titer determinations of a given patient. For maximum accuracy, serum samples should be stored and the

13

Rh Negative Pregnancy

procedure repeated in the original sample each time that a titer is determined in a subsequent sample.

PRINCIPLES OF TREATMENT

Rh negative women presenting for obstetrical care can be categorized in two different groups:

1. Rh negative nonimmunized women.
2. Rh negative immunized women.

There could be another group of Rh positive women immunized against non-D Rh antigens or against other blood group systems.

Management of Rh Negative Nonimmunized Women (Flow chart 13.1)

The first step is to determine the Rh phenotype status of husband where the paternity is certain. If the husband is Rh negative, the baby will be Rh negative and pregnancy should be managed like any other normal pregnancy without any further testing. If the baby's father is Rh positive, irrespective of the zygosity, the fetus will inherit one copy of the RhD gene and therefore Rh alloimmunization may occur during pregnancy. Thus, it is not necessary to determine the Rh genotype of the father because in the best of the circumstances (father heterozygous for the D antigen), the probability that the fetus will be Rh positive is substantial and the plan of management will be same. Thus it is important to detect occurrence of Rh alloimmunization during the first 28 weeks of pregnancy and prevent it during last 12 weeks and at the time of delivery when fetomaternal bleeding is more common by taking prophylactic measures as mentioned below.

Flow chart 13.1: Management of Rh negative nonimmunized women

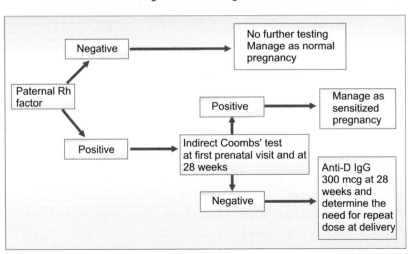

Prophylaxis following Sensitizing Events before Delivery

Anti-D immunoglobulin should be given to all nonsensitized RhD negative women after the following potentially sensitizing events during pregnancy:
- Invasive prenatal diagnosis (amniocentesis, chorion villus sampling, fetal blood sampling)
- Other intrauterine procedures (e.g. insertion of fetal shunts, embryo reduction)
- Antepartum hemorrhage
- External cephalic version of the fetus
- Closed abdominal injury
- Intrauterine death.

A dose of 50 mcg is recommended for prophylaxis following sensitizing events up to 12 weeks of pregnancy. For all events after 12 weeks, 300 mcg of anti-D immunoglobulin should be given followed by a test to identify fetomaternal hemorrhage (FMH) greater than 4 ml red cells and additional anti-D IgG should be given as required.[5]

Anti-D immunoglobulin is best given intramuscularly into the deltoid muscle as injections into the gluteal region often only reach the subcutaneous tissues and absorption may be delayed. For successful immunoprophylaxis, anti-D immunoglobulin should be given as soon as possible after the sensitizing event but always within 72 hours. If it is not given before 72 hours, every effort should still be made to administer the anti-D immunoglobulin, as a dose given within 28 days may provide some protection.

Detection of Rh Alloimmunization

Possibility of Rh sensitization during antenatal period is very small, thus antibody screening is performed at 28 weeks before the administration of anti-D immunoglobulin. Current guidelines for the management of Rh negative women is that if antibody screen is negative at first prenatal visit, the screen is repeated at 28 weeks and 300 mcg anti-D administered if it remains negative.

Prevention of Rh Alloimmunization

After the antepartum administration of anti-D immunoglobulin, the antibody screening will detect anti-D antibodies in the patient's serum, but the titer should not be greater than 1:4 at term. An antibody titer greater than 1:4 at term most probably results from alloimmunization rather than anti-D immunoglobulin administration.

The Rh negative gravida who remains unsensitized during pregnancy and receive anti-D immunoglobulin antenatally should be administered anti-D immunoglobulin in the postpartum period only when the following conditions are fulfilled:[6]
1. Infant is Rh positive
2. Direct Coombs' test on umbilical cord blood is negative.

13

Rh Negative Pregnancy

The usual dosage of 300 mcg anti-D immunoglobulin is capable of neutralizing the antigenic potential of up to 30 ml of fetal blood (15 ml of fetal red cells) and prevents Rh alloimmunization in 90% of cases. In less than 1% of cases in which the volume of fetomaternal hemorrhage exceeds 30 ml, Kleihauer-Betke test is used to quantitate the volume of FMH and the appropriate amount of anti-D IgG (i.e. 10 mcg/ml fetal blood) is administered accordingly. The basic principle behind this test is that acid denatures the adult hemoglobin present in RBC as compared to fetal hemoglobin which is resistant to it. The maternal blood is examined on a counting chamber after fixation with 80% of ethanol and hematoxylin staining. The amount of fetal blood cell in the maternal circulation can be approximated from the number of red cells per grid using formula:

$$\text{Fetal cells/no of maternal cells} = \frac{\text{Estimated blood loss}}{\text{Estimated maternal blood volume in milliliters (85 ml/kg)}}$$

Flow cytometry offers an alternative technique for quantifying the size of FMH.[7] It has a number of advantages in that the results are more accurate and more reproducible than those from the Kleihauer test and that it detects RhD positive cells, making it particularly helpful in patients with high HbF levels. Not all hospitals will have ready access to a flow cytometer. Flow cytometry is most effectively employed in those cases where a Kleihauer screening test indicates a large FMH which requires accurate quantitation and follow-up. The rosetting technique is a relatively simple serological method which offers another alternative for quantifying FMH of RhD positive red cells greater than 4 ml.

Anti-D immunoglobulin administration in postpartum period may be withheld if the last administration was given less than 21 days previously and passively acquired antibodies are still demonstrable on the antibody screen.[4] The rosette test may also be performed in maternal blood to assess the need for further administration of anti-D immunoglobulin.

Management of Rh Negative Immunized Pregnant Women (Flow chart 13.2)

Management in this category first requires the determination of the paternal and fetal Rh phenotype and genotype followed by observing that whether it is a first affected pregnancy or woman already had a previously affected pregnancy.

Paternal Rh Phenotype and Genotype

If the Rh typing of the father is negative there is no need of further evaluation. If the father is Rh positive one might go for the determination of zygosity for the RhD gene. If the couple had an Rh negative infant with previous pregnancy, it can be concluded that the father is heterozygous.

Flow chart 13.2: Management of the Rh negative immunized women

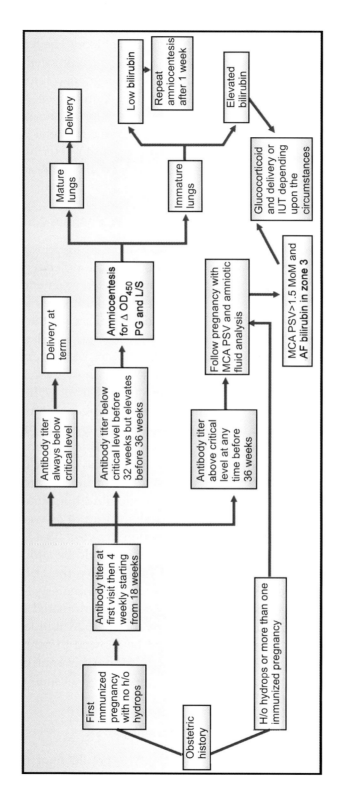

The fetal phenotype can be determined by using blood. The fetal Rh genotype can be determined using cells collected by CVS or amniocentesis. Although CVS has the advantage of being done early in pregnancy, it increases the risk of alloimmuinzation if the fetus is Rh positive. Amniocentesis is a method of choice to obtain fetal cells for Rh factor determination because of its simplicity and safety. PCR test can also be used to determine the fetal genotype in the amniocytes. In the near future it may be possible to determine the fetal Rh genotype from the free fetal DNA that is present in the maternal plasma using PCR technology.[8,9]

First Affected Pregnancy Determined by the Positive Antibody Titers

Only in these cases, Rh antibody titers can be used to determine the risk of fetal anemia. The rationale being that the association between the antibody titers and fetal affection that exists in the first affected pregnancy is lost during subsequent gestations. Also, in majority of first immunized pregnancies the anti-Rh antibody concentration is low and rarely exceeds the critical level of most laboratories. The critical level is that level below which no death due to fetal hemolytic disease has occurred within 1 week of delivery:

- Serum antibody titers are done in these women every 4 weeks until the titers are found to be at or above the critical level (1:16) on the initial evaluation, exceeds this level anytime during pregnancy or there is significant rise in titer between 2 consequent samples (two tube dilution), even if the upper dilution does not reach the critical level.
- If any of the above conditions occur, there is no further use of antibody titer and the pregnancy is further monitored by middle cerebral artey peak systolic velocity (MCA-PSV) and amniotic fluid bilirubin concentration.
- If antibody titers remains below critical level up to 36 weeks, the patient should be delivered by elective induction between 38-40 weeks and the birth of unaffected or mildly affected fetus should be anticipated.
- If there is sudden rise of antibody titers above the critical level after 34 weeks but before 37 weeks of gestation, amniocentesis is done to assess the fetal lung maturity. Pregnancy should be terminated if the lungs are mature, but if the lungs are immature and the bilirubin level is low (less than 0.5 mg/dl), the pregnancy should be allowed to continue as long as weekly amniocentesis shows fetal pulmonary immaturity and a low bilirubin concentration. Delivery is contemplated as soon as these fetuses achieve lung maturity.

Women with Previous Affected Pregnancy

After the first affected pregnancy, the ability to predict fetal anemia from the maternal anti-D antibody titers is lost and now these pregnancies should be monitored by MCA-PSV and amniotic fluid bilirubin concentration. In these cases, past obstetric history is the predominant indicator of the outcome. Patients with normal past obstetrical history and titers remaining at or below 64 have a 4% incidence of intrauterine death whereas with similar titers but with histories of affected deliveries the incidence increases to 32% before 37 weeks. Patients with normal obstetric history and titer above 64, have a 17.2% incidence of stillbirth, whereas those women with affected obstetric history have a 67.8% stillbirth rate.

Middle Cerebral Artery Peak Systolic Velocity

It is a noninvasive tool for the diagnosis of fetal anemia. The principle behind this test is that there is increased velocity of blood flow in the anemic fetuses due to increased cardiac output in an attempt to enhance the oxygenation. In their studies[10,11] of the middle cerebral artery (MCA), Mari et al demonstrated that increases in peak velocity of systolic blood flow in the MCA can be used to detect moderate and severe anemia in nonhydropic fetuses. The MCA is utilized because it can be evaluated using a minimal angle of insonation.

Technique

The ultrasound probe is used to obtain a view adequate for the measurement of biparietal diameter and the vascular structures are identified with color Doppler. The MCA of the cerebral hemisphere closer to the ultrasound transducer is interrogated few millimeters after its origin from the internal carotid artery but without including any part of this artery and taking care of that angle of insonation is as close as possible to zero. The fetus should be resting, since activity will cause falsely elevated PSV values.[12] It is better to examine proximal one-third part of MCA far from the ultrasound probe.[13] Typical waveforms are obtained and the PSV of at least three of them measured and averaged.

The threshold for the diagnosis of fetal anemia is a value equal to or greater than 1.5 multiples of median (MoM) for the gestational age. Abnormally elevated MCA-PSV has a sensitivity of 100% and a false-positive rate of 12% for the diagnosis of fetal anemia. Some investigators recommend cordocentesis and intrauterine transfusion (IUT) as the next step following an abnormal MCA-PSV. Application of the invasive tools can be minimized to 30% if MCA Doppler studies are routinely involved.

Reliable MCA-PSV values can be obtained as early as 18 weeks gestation. False positive rate of MCA-PSV increases after 35 weeks gestation, and consideration should be given to converting to amniocentesis. MCA Doppler studies can be done every 1-2 weeks depending on the trend.

Invasive Evaluation

- Indirect—amniotic fluid spectrophotometry
- Direct—cordocentesis.

Each method has its advantages and disadvantages, proponents and opponents. The method selected should reflect the facilities available and the physician's experience.

Amniotic Fluid Spectrophotometry (AFS)

It detects the presence and severity of fetal hemolysis and anemia. By the middle of the second trimester, amniotic fluid consists predominantly of fetal urine and tracheopulmonary effluent, thus the amniotic fluid bilirubin is also elevated if the fetal hemolysis is there. Amniotic fluid containing high levels of bilirubin, such as that found in fetuses with severe hemolytic disease, is yellowish-brown. This observation by Liley in 1961 led to the development of a method to predict the severity of fetal hemolysis using spectrophotometric measurements of bilirubin in amniotic fluid (Fig. 13.1). Because the wavelength at which bilirubin absorbs light is 420-460 nm, the amount of shift in optical density from linearity at 450 nm (ΔOD_{450}) in amniotic fluid samples can be used to estimate the degree of fetal hemolysis. The Queenan curve is a modification of the Liley curve to adjust for the relative inaccuracy of ΔOD_{450} readings in the early to middle second trimester (Fig. 13.2).

The interface between the different zones has a negative slope; this is secondary to the increased ability of the fetus to metabolize the breakdown products of hemoglobin. Thus, the same value of ΔOD_{450} is more worrisome for hemolysis at a later gestation.

The principal advantage of amniocentesis is that most of the obstetricians are familiar with the technique. Amniotic fluid is obtained by ultrasound guided amniocentesis, transported to the laboratory in a light resistant container to prevent degradation of bilirubin, centrifuged and filtered.

The determination of the fetal hemolytic disease by AFS has several disadvantages which are as following:

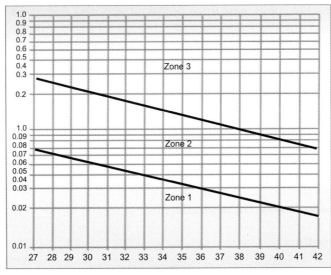

Figure 13.1: Liley's graph to estimate severity of fetal anemia

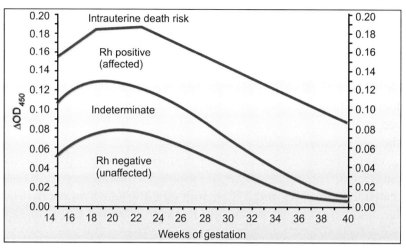

Figure 13.2: Queenan curve
Curve for ΔOD 450 values from 14-40 weeks of gestation

1. It is an indirect test for fetal anemia.
2. Its application requires serial invasive procedures over the space of several weeks. Each procedure carries a risk of enhanced maternal sensitization as well as loss from either amnionitis or rupture of membranes, fetal bleeding, fetal bradycardia requiring emergency cesarean delivery, preterm labor, spontaneous abortion.
3. This is modelled on anti-D alloimmunization. Fetuses with Kell alloimmunization have lower serum bilirubin concentrations and lower reticulocyte count for their level of anemia compared to D alloimmunized fetuses.
4. It is subjected to a variety of intrinsic errors that can interfere with laboratory measurements, e.g. maternal hyperbilirubinemia and specimen contaminated with blood or meconium.

During normal pregnancy ΔOD_{450} values changes with gestational age and it is necessary to use adequate norms to correlate the laboratory values with fetal situation. In his original description, Liley recorded the ΔOD_{450} of 101 immunized patients on a semilogarithmic paper (gestational age in weeks on X-axis and ΔOD_{450} values on the Y-axis) and divided the graph in 3 zones. Mild or no hemolytic disease occurs in zone 1; intermediate disease in zone 2 (transitional between mild and severe hemolysis); and severe disease, including the development of hydrops within a week, in zone 3.

If the amniotic fluid values shows a ΔOD_{450} in zone 1 there is no immediate danger to the fetus and the procedure should be repeated in 4 weeks. If the ΔOD_{450} remain in zone 1 in repeated amniocentesis carried out every 4 weeks, the patient should be delivered at term gestation and the birth of unaffected or a mildly affected baby should be anticipated. If at any time the amniotic fluid shows a ΔOD_{450} in zone 2, the procedure should be repeated in 1 week, since values in this zone may correspond to moderately or severely affected infants. If the following amniocentesis shows ΔOD_{450} in zone 1, there is no need to repeat the amniocentesis before 4 weeks. If the following amniocentesis shows a decreasing trend but still remain in zone 2, amniocentesis should be repeated in 2 weeks. If the following amniocentesis shows same value as previous one and remain in zone 2 (horizontal trend), procedure should be repeated in another week and if the horizontal trend continues, cordocentesis and fetal hematocrit evaluation is indicated with exception of those patients who have achieved fetal lung maturity and better managed by immediate delivery.

If the initial amniotic fluid examination shows a ΔOD_{450} in zone 3 or if any ΔOD_{450} value previously in zone 1 or 2 moved to zone 3 (rising trend), the infant may be in immediate danger of intrauterine death. Fetal blood sampling is indicated in these cases and IUT performed if the fetal hematocrit is less than 30%. Termination of the pregnancy is the treatment of choice where lung maturity has been achieved.

The main limitation of the Liley's curve is that it starts at 26 weeks of gestation and extrapolation of the lines to earlier gestational ages is inaccurate. Queenan have developed a curve for fetal assessment from 14 to 40 weeks, divided into 4 zones. The lower, first zone correspond to nonaffected Rh negative fetuses. Values in the second zone are indeterminate and do not permit a determination whether the fetus is affected or not. The third zone corresponds to affected Rh +ve fetus. The upper zone corresponds to the fetuses at risk of intrauterine death. In general, ΔOD_{450} greater than 0.15 indicates severe immunization and the need for cordocentesis and early transfusion. Values below 0.09 indicates mild disease or no disease. Values between 0.09 and 0.15 will require repeat amniocentesis in 1 week. After 26 week the need for intervention can be determined by Liley's graph.

Amniotic fluid bilirubin and MCA-PSV can be used together in the diagnosis of fetal anemia. MCA-PSV should be the initial test because it is noninvasive and better predictive value than the amniotic fluid bilirubin concentration. When MCA-PSV is above normal limits, amniocentesis should be performed before cordocentesis to avoid invasive procedure in nonanemic fetuses.

Ultrasonography

Ultrasonography can be utilized in the management of Rh negative pregnancies to assess gestational age, fetal wellbeing, diagnose hydrops and guide amniocentesis, fetal blood sampling, and intrauterine transfusions. In this capacity, ultrasonography has improved both the safety and success rate of noninvasive procedures and has helped to minimize invasive procedures. The sonographic findings consistent with hydrops include ascites, pleural and pericardial effusions and edema. Several other sonographic findings have been proposed as possible indicators of the future development of hydrops. These include polyhydramnios, increased placental thickness (>4 cm), dilation of the cardiac chambers, dilation of the umbilical vein, chronic enlargement of the spleen and liver and visualization of both sides of the fetal bowel wall. Serial ultrasound can be used to document the progression of the disease.

Fetal Blood Sampling (FBS)

The only definitive means of diagnosing fetal anemia and acidosis is via FBS, also known as cordocentesis or percutaneous umbilical blood sampling, which was first performed in the early 1980s. FBS is especially useful in cases of anti-Kell alloimmunization and before 26-28 weeks gestational age when ΔOD_{450} values of amniotic fluid are not as reliable. The other advantage of FBS is that the same procedure can be used to transfuse blood to the fetus. This procedure is not used routinely because of concerns regarding fetal and maternal complications which include fetomaternal hemorrhage, fetal loss (0.5-2% per procedure), placental abruption, acute refractory fetal distress and amnionitis with maternal adult respiratory distress syndrome.

Intrauterine Transfusion (IUT)

Fetal transfusion therapy is done whenever the fetus is hydropic with significant anemia, i.e. hematocrit < 30% because it is below the 2.5 percentile for all gestational ages greater than 20 weeks.

There are two types of IUT: Intraperitoneal and intravascular. In both methods, the procedure is carried out under visual control with real time ultrasound. In intraperitoneal transfusion the blood is injected in the peritoneal cavity and transported by lymphatic system into the fetal bloodstream. In intravascular transfusion, the blood is injected directly in the umbilical circulation. They complement each other and either one or both of them may be used depending on the circumstances. Although the direct intravascular transfusion is the procedure of choice, it is not without problems and it is preferable to perform and intraperitoneal transfusion if the approach to umbilical cord is difficult (posterior placenta, maternal obesity) or if a sample of blood cannot be obtained after several attempts. In the severly hydropic fetus, the intravascular approach offers the best possibility for successful fetal therapy. If access into the umbilical cord is difficult, it is possible to transfuse through intrahepatic portion of umbilical vein. When everything fails, access is done through the right ventricle of heart.

The blood to be transfused should be fresh when available and compatible with both mother and the fetus. The blood is prepared on the day of transfusion, rendered leukocyte poor and washed several times in the saline to remove the particles associated with viral transmission. The amount of blood to be transfused can be calculated once the hematocrit or hemoglobin results are obtained. In general, 30-60 ml/kg of nonhydropic fetal weight is transfused because volumes higher than this may be difficult for the fetus to tolerate in intravascular transfusion. Intraperitoneal transfusions require a greater volume of blood, roughly calculated as the following:

(Number of weeks' gestation – 20) × 10 ml

After the transfusion fetus should be monitored with continuous fetal monitoring for the ensuing 4 hours because decelerations of the fetal heart rate are common and must be managed cautiously.

The goal of the procedure is to maintain the fetal hemoglobin value at greater than 9 g/dl. Serial IUTs are usually performed until 34 weeks gestation, beyond which time the risk of the procedure likely outweighs the benefits. This leads to delivery of the fetus at 34-37 weeks gestation and occasionally, even earlier if fetal lung maturity is documented.

Early Delivery and Glucocorticoids

Use of corticosteroid is recommended if the delivery is anticipated before 34-35 weeks of gestation. But corticosteroids causes decrease in ΔOD_{450} values and give false sense of security, thus fetal lung maturity should be assessed generously after 34 weeks by amniocentesis.

Other Treatment Modalities

Where there are high initial titers of antibody and history of fetal hydrops, plasmapheresis and promethazine and IgG have been tried. The best evidence of benefit is for Ig G administration. Voto et al[14] treated 69 women with extremely severe Rh alloimmunization. Thirty received IgG before 20 weeks, 400mg/kg/day for 5 consecutive days every 2-3 weeks, followed by IUTs after 20 weeks and 39 received IUT only. They found significantly lower incidence of number of fetal deaths in women treated with the combination of IUT and IgG.

ABO Incompatibility and Minor Blood Group Antigens

ABO incompatibility rarely causes fetal disease because the antibodies are often IgM which are not strongly expressed on the fetal erythrocyte. Lewis antibodies are most common of all the minor blood group antigens but they are almost always IgM and do not pose a risk for fetal disease as the antigen is poorly expressed on erythrocytes. Therefore risk for hemolysis is low.

Kidd, Kell and Duffy are the most common minor antigens that cause perinatal hemolytic disease. Kell alloimmunization is of particular interest because of its different pathophysiology and particularly unpredictable clinical course as the anti-Kell antibodies damage or inhibit erythrocyte progenitors. Severe anemia and hydrops in this condition develops with low antibody titers and ΔOD_{450} values. Management is similar to Rh isoimmunization with monitoring and intervention tailored to the individual circumstances.

KEY POINTS

- Maternal alloimmunization, also known as isoimmunization, occurs when a woman's immune system is sensitized to foreign erythrocyte surface antigens, stimulating the production of immunoglobulin G (IgG) antibodies.
- The most common routes of maternal sensitization are via blood transfusion or fetomaternal hemorrhage (FMH).
- Only IgG class antibodies cross the placenta and bind to the fetal red blood cells. Anti-D alloimmunization remains the most important cause of fetal hemolytic disease.
- All sequelae of the disease (hydrops fetalis, reflecting cardiac and hematologic events) are secondary to hemolysis or severe anemia.
- All complications of fetal hemolytic anemia are potentially preventable, i.e cardiac dysfunction which occurs before development of hydrops, resolves after fetal transfusion.
- The blood type and Rh group should be done in all the pregnant females at their first prenatal visit and an antibody screening is also recommended using a combination of indirect and direct methods.
- Anti-D immunoglobulin effectively prevents maternal alloimmunization. It should be given after amniocentesis, at 28 weeks of gestation, episodes of vaginal bleeding and after delivery of Rh positive child.
- The dose for the prevention of Rh alloimmunization in first trimester is 50 mcg and thereafter 300 mcg after 20 weeks of gestation or more according to amount of fetomaternal hemorrhage.
- The management of the pregnant alloimmunized woman utilizes both invasive and noninvasive methods of maternal/fetal evaluation.
- The first affected pregnancy is the only pregnancy in which Rh antibody titers can be used to determine the risk of fetal anemia. In these pregnancies indirect Coombs tests are performed at monthly intervals after 18 weeks of gestation until the critical titer for laboratory is exceeded.
- MCA-PSV is performed weekly once the critical titer is exceeded.
- Amniotic fluid bilirubin and MCA-PSV can be used together in the diagnosis of fetal anemia.
- MCA-PSV should be the initial test because it is noninvasive and has better predictive value than the amniotic fluid bilirubin concentration. When MCA PSV is above normal limits, amniocentesis should be performed before cordocentesis to avoid an invasive procedure in nonanemic fetuses.
- An MCA PSV > 1.5 MoM or bilirubin concentration in zone 3 of the Liley's curve strongly suggests the presence of fetal anemia and should be followed by cordocentesis.
- The treatment of the significant fetal anemia (hematocrit <30%) prior to 34 weeks of gestation is intrauterine transfusion.
- Successful transfusion eliminates the antenatal and largely the postnatal complications of fetal anemia.

13

Rh Negative Pregnancy

- Intravascular transfusion is the procedure of choice.
- Delivery may be safely delayed until 37-38 weeks of gestation if intravascular transfusion is done.
- By maintaining the hematocrit at high end, fetal erythropoiesis is minimized, reducing the risk of postnatal hyperbilirubinemia.

REFERENCES

1. Joseph KS, Kramer MS. The decline in Rh hemolytic disease: Should Rh prophylaxis get all the credit? Am J Public Health 1998;88:209-15.
2. Salvi V. The clinician's approach to rhesus isoimmunization. In: Shah D, Salvi V, (Eds). The Rh factor. Mumbai: Perinatology Committee FOGSI 1998;99.
3. Shah D, Shroff S. New approaches in the management of rhesus alloimmunization. In Saraiya UB, Rao KA, Chatterjee A (Eds). Principles and Practice of Obstetrics and gynaecology for Postgraduates. FOGSI Publication. New Delhi: Jaypee Brothers, Medical Publishers (P) Ltd. 2004;137.
4. Weiner CP. Fetal hemolytic disease.High Risk Pregnancy, 3rd edn, 2006; 291-311.
5. RCOG Green Top Guidelines. Use of Anti D immunoglobulin for Rh prophylaxis (22) Revised May 2002.
6. Arias F, Daftary SN, Bhinde AG. Rh alloimmunization. Practical Guide to High Risk Pregnancy and Delivery 3rd edn, 2008;358-72.
7. Johnson PR, Tait RC, Austen EB, Shwe KH, Lee, D. Flow cytometry in diagnosis and management of large feto-maternal haemorrhage. J Clin Path 1995; 48:1005-08.
8. Lo YM, Hjelm NM, Fidler C, et al. Prenatal diagnosis of fetal RhD status by molecular analysis of maternal plasma. N Eng J Med 1998;339:1734-38.
9. Finning KM, Martin PG, Soothill PW, et al. Prediction of fetal D status from maternal plasma: Introduction of new non-invasive fetal RHD genotype service. Transfusion 2002;42:1079-85.
10. Mari G and the Collaborative Group for diagnosis of fetal anemia with Doppler ultrasonography. Noninvasive diagnosis byDoppler ultrasonography of fetal anemia due maternal red-cell alloimmunization. N Eng J Med 2000; 342:9-14.
11. Mari G, Detti L, Oz U, et al. Accurate prediction of fetal hemoglobin by Doppler ultrasonography. Obstet Gynecol 2002;99:589-93.
12. Sallout BI, Fung KFK, Wen SW, et al. The effect of fetal behavioural status on middle cerebral artery peak systolic velocity.Am J Obstet Gynecol 2004;191: 1283-87.
13. Abel DE, Grambow SC, Brancazio LR, et al. Ultrasound assessment of fetal middle cerebral artery peak systolic velocity: A comparison of the near field versus far field. Am J Obstet Gynecol 2003; 189:986-89.
14. Voto LS, Mathet ER, Zapaterio JL, et al. High dose gammaglobulin (IVIG) followed by intrauterine transfusions (IUTs). A new alternative for the treatment of severe haemolytic disease. J Perinat Med 1997;25:85-88.

Anemia in Pregnancy

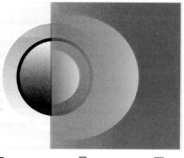

14

Manju Puri, Nidhi Malhotra

INTRODUCTION

Anemia is the commonest medical disorder in pregnancy. In developing countries it contributes to 40-60% of all maternal deaths directly or indirectly.[1,2] In India 16% of maternal deaths are directly due to anemia.[3] Anemia is associated with an increase in incidence of preterm birth, IUGR and low Apgar at birth with resultant increase in perinatal morbidity and mortality. Anemic mothers give birth to anemic infants who are more likely to suffer from cognitive and affective dysfunction and possibly long-term morbidities in the form of diabetes and cardiovascular disease.[4,5] Although in 1997, United Nations declared anemia as a major public health problem needing total elimination, a decade later it still remains an important factor contributing significantly to adverse maternal and perinatal outcome.

PREVALENCE OF ANEMIA

Anemia is more common in developing countries as compared to developed countries. It is estimated that all over the world about 500 million women in reproductive age group are anemic.[6] WHO estimates 56% of all women in developing countries as anemic.[7] In India, National Family Health Survey (NFHS-3) in 2005-2006 has shown that 55% of Indian women are anemic.[8] This is as compared to only 2-4% women in USA.[9]

As pregnancy is associated with augmented erythropoiesis it imposes an increased demand on erythropoietic factors. Thus the prevalence of anemia is further increased in pregnancy. It ranges between 50-90% in developing countries compared to 18-20% in developed countries. According to NFHS-3

59% of pregnant women are anemic.[8] In India, a Steering Committee report has shown that 13% of pregnant women have a hemoglobin level of less than 5 gm% and 34% have values less than 8 gm%.[10]

DEFINITION

Anemia is defined as a condition when the circulating levels of hemoglobin are qualitatively or quantitatively lower than normal. The criteria for defining anemia are as shown in Table 14.1.

Table 14.1: Criteria for defining anemia	
Nonpregnant women	Hb < 12 gm%
Pregnant women (WHO)[11]	Hb < 11 gm%; hematocrit < 33%
Pregnant women (CDC 1999)[12]	Hb < 11 gm% (first and third trimester)
	Hb < 10.5 gm% (second trimester)

The severity of anemia has been graded by Indian Council of Medical Research (ICMR) as shown in Table 14.2.

Table 14.2 : Classification of anemia according to severity (ICMR)[13]	
Severity	Hemoglobin levels (g/dl)
Mild	10.0 – 10.9
Moderate	7 – 9.9
Severe	< 7
Very severe	< 4

ETIOPATHOGENESIS OF ANEMIA IN PREGNANCY

Pregnancy is associated with a marked increase in blood volume, 40-45% above the prepregnant level. It is due to an increase in both plasma and red cell mass. As the increase in plasma is more marked compared to red cell mass despite an increase in total hemoglobin content, there is a resultant dilutional decrease in hemoglobin levels. The increase in red cell mass is consequent to augmented erythropoiesis with associated increase in demand of various erythropoietic factors like iron, proteins, vitamins like folic acid, vitamin B_{12}, vitamin C, vitamin A, pyridoxine and trace elements like copper, zinc, cobalt. Inadequate dietary intake of these can result in nutritional deficiency anemia in pregnancy. It is the commonest type of anemia in pregnancy. Iron deficiency is most prevalent followed by folic acid and vitamin B_{12} deficiency. Most often there is a combined deficiency manifesting as dimorphic anemia.

During pregnancy in addition to the routine daily iron requirement an additional about 1000 mg of iron is required. Of this, approximately 300 mg is actively transported to the fetus and placenta, 500-600 mg is used for increase in red cell mass and 100-250 mg is lost during delivery. About 150-300 mg of iron is conserved as a result of amenorrhea during pregnancy. Thus an additional requirement of 4-6 mg/day of iron is there during pregnancy. This is lower in early pregnancy 2-3 mg/day compared to 6-7 mg/day in late pregnancy. A normal diet contains about 14 mg of iron. The average absorption of iron from normal diet is about 5-10% (1-2 mg) and is only 3-4% if the diet is purely vegetarian. Iron absorption is increased in iron deficient states but normal diet is inadequate in providing additional iron requirement during pregnancy and a daily supplement of 40-60 mg of elemental iron is needed by women during pregnancy.

The requirement of folic acid is also increased during pregnancy (400-800 µg/day). In developing countries the diet is poor in folic acid due to low consumption of green leafy vegetables, fruits, nonvegetarian foods like liver, kidney, etc. There is further reduction in dietary folic acid due to prolonged cooking. Pregnancy induced nausea and vomiting, malabsorption, worm infestation, use of goat's milk, and use of drugs like antiepileptics also contribute to decreased levels of folic acid during pregnancy.

During pregnancy vitamin B_{12} is actively transported from the placenta to the fetus. Vitamin B_{12} is found in foods of animal origin like meat, fish, eggs and milk and is not destroyed by heating. The daily requirement of vitamin B_{12} (3 µg/day) is easily met by diet in nonvegetarians. However in strict vegetarians vitamin B_{12} deficiency may be there.

Other causes of anemia in pregnancy include chronic and acute blood loss. Chronic blood loss can result from parasitic infections like hookworm, trichuriasis, vesical and intestinal schistosomiasis, etc. Acute blood loss is usually related to previous abortions or conditions like antepartum hemorrhage (APH) or postpartum hemorrage (PPH) in previous pregnancies. Infections cause anemia by impairing erythropoiesis. Chronic or recurrent infections like urinary tract infection and malaria are a common cause of anemia.

Genetic factors like thalassemia, sickle cell trait and glucose 6 phosphate dehydrogenase deficiency can also cause anemia in pregnancy. These may be coexistent with nutritional deficiency anemia. Certain pregnancy related conditions like pregnancy induced hypertension may be associated with hemolytic anemia. Aplastic anemia is rarely seen in pregnancy. The classification of anemia based on the etiology is shown in Table 14.3.

Table 14.3: Classification of anemia in pregnancy according to etiology	
Acquired	*Inherited*
Nutritional deficiency anemia • Iron deficiency • Folic acid deficiency • Vitamin B_{12} deficiency • Combined	Hemoglobinopathies • Thalassemia • Sickle cell disease • Others
Hemorrhagic • Acute or chronic blood loss	Membrane defects • Spherocytosis • Elliptocytosis
Hemolytic • PIH	Enzyme defects • G6PD deficiency • Pyruvate kinase deficiency
Others • Infection	

CLINICAL FEATURES OF ANEMIA IN PREGNANCY

The spectrum of clinical presentation of anemia during pregnancy ranges from a completely asymptomatic woman with mild anemia to a very sick decompensated woman with severe anemia. It essentially depends upon the severity of anemia. Although all pregnant women are at risk of developing anemia, those at higher risk are as shown in Table 14.4.

Table 14.4: Pregnant women at high risk of anemia
• Young adolescent mothers • Multiparous women • Women with multiple pregnancy • Women from poor socioeconomic status

Women with mild to moderate anemia are usually asymptomatic. Those with severe anemia may complain of increasing pallor, weakness, easy fatiguability, breathlessness, palpitation, swelling feet or swelling all over the body. There may be no signs in mild anemia. However, in moderate to severe anemia there may be pallor, facial puffiness, raised JVP, tachycardia, tachypnea, crepts in lung bases, hepatosplenomegaly, pitting edema of abdominal wall and legs. Signs of various nutritional deficiencies like glossitis, stomatitis, chelosis, etc. may be present.

WORKUP OF PREGNANT WOMEN WITH ANEMIA

History and Examination

A detailed history and thorough examination is important to assess the severity of problem and the probable cause of anemia. The onset of symptoms whether acute or insidious and the duration of symptoms should be inquired. The important points to be elicited in the history to arrive at a probable cause of anemia are as listed in Table 14.5.

Table 14.5: Important points to be elicited in history	
Probable cause	*Points elicited in history*
Presence of infections (Malaria, UTI, TB)	Recurrent fever with chills and rigors, urinary complaints, prolonged cough
Chronic loss of blood	Bleeding gums, piles or worm infestation.
Malabsorption	Bulky stools, chronic diarrhea
Bleeding or coagulation disorder	Petechiae, bruises, ecchymosis
Hemoglobinopathies	Repeated blood or blood component transfusion in self or family
Hemolysis	High-colored urine, discoloration of sclera, drug intake
Dietary deficiency	Detailed dietary history, cooking habits, etc.
Menstrual history	Cycle length, duration, amount of bleeding, clots, etc.
Obstetric history	Abortions, repeated child birth, any complications like APH, PPH, blood transfusion, etc. in previous or current pregnancies
Contraceptive history	Use of IUCD with menorrhagia

A thorough head to toe general physical examination should be followed by a systemic examination. The various signs to be looked for are listed in Table 14.6.

Table 14.6: Clinical examination in a pregnant woman with anemia	
General physical examination	*Systemic examination*
Pulse rate, BP and respiratory rate	Chest examination
Skin and mucosa	–Sternal tenderness
–Pallor	–Any crepts fine basal or coarse apical
–Color of palmar creases	CVS examination
–Petechiae, ecchymosis	–Murmurs
Eyes	
–Pallor	Per abdomen
–Icterus	–Edema of abdominal wall
Oral cavity for	–Hepatosplenomegaly
–Glossitis	–Presence of free fluid
–Stomatitis	Obstetrical examination
–Cheilosis	–Height of uterus
Nails	
–Pallor	–Tone of uterus
–Platynychia or koilonychia	–No. of fetuses
–Clubbing	–Presentation
Neck	
–Lymphadenopathy,	–Amount of liquor
–JVP	–FHS
–Thyroid enlargement	
Legs	
–Edema	
–Ulcers	
–Peripheral neuropathy	

Investigations

The primary investigations in all pregnant women with anemia aim at assessing the:
- Severity of anemia
- Type of anemia
- Bone marrow activity
- Cause of anemia.

Severity of Anemia

Hemoglobin levels and hematocrit estimation are two simple investigations done to confirm the presence of anemia and assess the severity of anemia. During antenatal period hemoglobin estimation should be done thrice, at first visit, at 28-30 weeks and at 36 weeks.

Type of Anemia

A complete blood count including blood indices and a peripheral smear help in the diagnosis of type of anemia. According to the peripheral smear report, anemia can be classified into microcytic, macrocytic, dimorphic, normocytic or hemolytic. The differential diagnosis according to the type of anemia is as shown in Table 14.7.

Table 14.7: Differential diagnosis according to the type of anemia	
Type of anemia	*Cause of anemia*
Microcytic	Fe deficiency, thalassemia, chronic infections
Macrocytic	Megaloblastic: Folic acid deficiency, vitamin B_{12} deficiency
	Non-megaloblastic: Liver disease, hypothyroidism, myelodysplasia
Normocytic	Post-hemorrhagic, renal or hepatic disease, impaired marrow response, e.g. early iron deficiency, marrow hypoplasia, infiltrative disorder, myelodysplasia
Dimorphic	Combined iron and folic acid deficiency
Hemolytic	Inherited: Thalassemia, sickle cell disease, spherocytosis, G6PD deficiency, pyruvate kinase deficiency
	Acquired: Microangiopathic as in PIH, cardiac hemolytic, auto immune, pregnancy induced, infections, drugs
Pancytopenia	Megaloblastic: Folic acid and vitamin B_{12} deficiency
	Aplastic: Drugs, viral infections, exposure to toxic substances, etc.

Bone Marrow Activity

It is assessed by the reticulocyte count. The normal reticulocyte count is 0.2-2%. An increased reticulocyte count indicates increased bone marrow activity as is seen in cases of hemolytic anemia, following acute blood loss and in women with iron deficiency anemia on treatment.

Cause of Anemia

The cause of anemia should be systematically found out and treated.The various investigations required for finding out the cause of anemia are listed in Table 14.8.

Table 14.8: Investigations required for finding out the cause of anemia	
Investigation	*Cause of anemia*
Peripheral smear	Malarial parasite, sickle cells, spherocytes, evidence of hemolysis
Liver function tests	Liver disease, hemolysis
Renal function tests	Renal disease
Serum proteins	Hypoproteinemia
Electrophoresis/high performance liquid chromatography	Abnormal hemoglobins
Urine examination	Urinary tract infection (UTI), occult hematuria, schistosomiasis
Stool examination (3 consecutive days)	Ova and cyst, occult blood
Bone marrow aspiration	Abnormal cells, iron, stores
X-ray chest (after shielding abdomen)	Pulmonary tuberculosis

Further investigations are done depending on the type of anemia and the differential diagnosis thereof. The algorithm of an approach to anemia in pregnancy is summarized in the Flow chart 14.1.

MATERNAL AND FETAL COMPLICATIONS

Anemia is an important cause of an increase in maternal and perinatal morbidity and mortality. It is associated with an increase in incidence of

Flow chart 14.1: Algorithm of approach to anemia in pregnancy

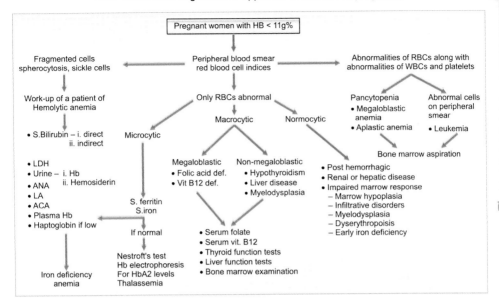

obstetric complications like preeclampsia, abruptio placentae and preterm labor in antepartum period.[13] As these women are immunosuppressed they are predisposed to infections such as UTI and puerperal sepsis.[13,14] There is an increase in risk of PPH, subinvolution of uterus, puerperal sepsis, thromboembolism, lactation failure and maternal mortality.[15]

The critical periods for women with severe anemia to decompensate are: 3rd trimester at 28-30 weeks, in labor, immediately after delivery or in early puerperium. The congestive cardiac failure is due to inability of the hypoxic cardiac muscles to cope with the increase in pregnancy induced cardiac load. The various causes of maternal mortality in anemic women during pregnancy and labor are congestive cardiac failure, cerebral anoxia, sepsis and thromboembolism.

As regards the fetus, most of the nutrients are actively transported to the fetus across the placenta. There is placental hypertrophy associated with maternal anemia which provides for an increase in oxygen transport to the fetus to compensate for decrease in circulating hemoglobin. An increased incidence of spontaneous abortions, prematurity, intrauterine growth restriction and intrauterine death have been reported with anemia. These children are more predisposed to have anemia and more susceptible to infections.[16] Infants born to anemic mothers are more likely to suffer from cognitive and affective dysfunction and possibly long-term morbidities in the form of diabetes and cardiovascular disease.[4,5]

IRON DEFICIENCY ANEMIA

This is the most common type of anemia in pregnancy. Pregnancy is associated with an increase in iron demand consequent to augmented erythropoiesis and growing fetus and placenta. Women with normal hemoglobin levels but poor iron stores manifest as overt iron deficiency anemia during pregnancy.

Etiopathogenesis

Iron deficiency can be consequent to factors like dietary deficiency, malabsorption, increased iron demand, infections and blood loss. Dietary deficiency can result from poor dietary content of iron due to factors like poverty, lack of knowledge of iron rich food and intake of vegetarian diet rich in inhibitors of iron absorption. This is further aggravated by factors like malabsorption syndromes, infections like hookworm infestation, amoebiasis, tuberculosis, malaria, etc. and poor iron stores due to excessive blood loss during menstruation and bleeding complications in previous pregnancies. More than 50% of women from developing countries have a negative iron balance in nonpregnant state.[8] With each pregnancy the women's iron reserves are further depleted. Thus, too many and too soon pregnancies result in a high prevalence of iron deficiency anemia in developing countries.

Diagnosis

The diagnosis of iron deficiency anemia is largely based on the reports of complete blood count, red blood cell indices and peripheral smear (Table 14.9). Serum iron studies are indicated in women not responding to iron therapy. Bone marrow aspiration is the most rapid and reliable method for assessing iron stores but it is an invasive procedure and is rarely indicated in women with refractory anemia. Serum ferritin estimation is an excellent non invasive tool for assessing the iron stores. It is the first investigation to be affected in iron deficiency anemia, even before hemoglobin levels fall. It has the advantage of not being affected by recent iron intake. Certain other investigations like free erythrocyte protoporphyrin estimation and serum transferrin receptor assay are also used for diagnosing iron deficiency.

Table 14.9: Laboratory profile of iron deficiency anemia [17,18]		
Investigation	*Normal value*	*Iron deficiency anemia*
RBC count	4.0-5.2×10^{12}/cumm	$< 4.0 \times 10^{12}$/cumm
MCV	80-102 fl	< 80 fl
MCH	27-34 pg	< 27 pg
MCHC	31-37 g/dl	< 33 g/dl
RDW	11.5-14.5%	>14.5%
Peripheral smear	Normocytc normochromic RBC	Microcytic hypochromic RBC with anisocytosis, target cells
Serum iron studies:		
Serum iron	50-150 µg/dl	< 30 µg/dl
Serum ferritin	50-200 µg/l	< 15 µg/l
TIBC	300-360 µg/dl	> 400 µg/dl
Transferrin saturation (%)	30-50%	< 10%
Serum transferrin receptor (%)	5-9 µg/l	↑ed
Bone marrow iron	Present	Absent

Treatment

Prevention of Iron Deficiency Anemia

The various strategies to prevent iron deficiency anemia should aim at improving the diet, increasing the bioavailability of dietary iron, prevention and treatment of infections like hookworm infestation and malaria and iron and folic acid supplementation in young girls and pregnant women. Food fortification with iron and genetic modification of food is also being evaluated.

All adolescent girls should be screened for the presence of anemia and those with a hemoglobin level of < 12 g% should be treated. They should be counseled regarding dietary modifications and general hygiene. The diet should be balanced and contain all nutrients like folic acid, iron, ascorbic acid, vitamin A, etc. Iron in diet is present in two forms heme and nonheme iron. Heme iron is present in animal food and is better absorbed. The absorption of nonheme iron from vegetarian diet is influenced by iron absorption enhancers and inhibitors. Bioavailability of iron from vegetarian diet can be increased by taking iron rich diet with iron absorption enhancers like citrus fruit rich in vitamin C and avoiding iron absorption inhibitors like phytates, phosphates, oxalates and calcium present in tea, coffee, eggs, cereals, etc.

Diet rich in iron includes jaggery, green leafy vegetables like spinach, mustard leaves, methi, cereals, sprouts and pulses. Moreover cooking in iron utensils also seem to increase the iron content of the diet.[19]

Iron Prophylaxis or Iron Supplementation

It is an effective intervention for reducing the prevalence of iron deficiency anemia in both pregnant and nonpregnant women. Government of India in 1970 initiated the National Nutritional Anemia Prophylaxis Program (NNAPP). Under this program all pregnant women, lactating women, contraceptive acceptors and children (1-11 year) are provided iron and folic acid supplements.[13]

Routine iron supplementation during pregnancy has shown to improve maternal and perinatal outcome. WHO recommends universal oral iron supplementation of 60 mg of elemental iron and 400 µg of folic acid once daily for 6 months during pregnancy and for additional 3 months postpartum in all developing countries with prevalence of anemia of > 40%.[20] Currently the Ministry of Health and Family Welfare, Government of India has recommended routine iron prophylaxis to all pregnant women with 100 mg elemental iron and 500 µg of folic acid for at least 100 days in second half of pregnancy.

Once or twice a week oral iron supplementation has also been found to be an effective intervention with better compliance compared to daily supplementation.[21] Iron supplementation with 30 doses administered at weekly interval over 7 months have been found to be as effective as 90 doses given over 3 months.[22]

Drug Treatment

The therapeutic dose of elemental iron for treatment of anemia is 180-200 mg per day. Iron can be administered by either oral or parenteral route. The route of administration depends on period of gestation, patient's ability to tolerate oral iron, patient's compliance, any associated malabsorption syndromes and cost. However, the preferred route is oral.

Oral Iron Therapy

Various oral iron preparations are available in the market. The daily dose of each preparation should be decided according to the elemental iron content of each tablet. There is no significant difference between various preparations. Table 14.10 show the percentage of elemental iron present in different salts.

Table 14.10: Iron content of different salts		
Salt	Dose of salt in mg	Elemental iron in mg
Ferrous fumarate	100	30
Ferrous gluconate	100	10
Ferrous glycine sulfate	100	15
Ferrous succinate	100	35
Ferrous sulfate	100	30
Ferrous ascorbate	100	12

Oral iron intake is associated with side effects like nausea, vomiting, gastritis, diarrhea and sometimes constipation. The newer preparations like carbonyl iron are better tolerated. This is because penta carbonyl iron is reduced to fine microspheres of < 5 microns in diameter by heating. These are better absorbed and associated with lesser gastrointestinal symptoms. Iron ascorbate has an edge over other preparations due to its ascorbate content which enhances iron absorption and possibly protects the gastrointestinal mucosa due to its antioxidant property. It has been shown to have higher bioavailability of iron.[23,24]

Sustained release preparation reduce the overall absorption of iron by releasing iron beyond the most actively absorbing regions of the intestines that is the first part of duodenum. Ferrous sulfate, ferrous fumarate and ferrous ascorbate are preferred preparations.

For maximizing the iron absorption, women should be advised to take iron tablet either empty stomach or in between two meals with a glass of orange juice or lemon water. To minimize the side effects and improving the compliance, the treatment may be started with a lower dose or prescribing the tablet with meals or given less frequently. Sometimes changing the preparation also helps in reducing side effects.

Parenteral Iron Therapy

The preferred route of administration of iron is oral but in certain conditions parenteral therapy is indicated (Table 14.11). The main advantage of parenteral iron therapy is the certainty of its administration and possibly early restoration of body stores.

Table 14.11: Indication of parenteral therapy
Poor tolerance to oral iron therapy
Poor absorption: Malabsorption syndromes
Noncompliance
Women with moderate to severe anemia near term
Women on recombinant erythropoietin

It is available in the market as iron dextran complex, iron sorbitol complex, iron sucrose complex and iron gluconate. Iron dextran and iron sorbitol have been largely replaced by iron sucrose due to decreased side effects and negligible risk of anaphylactic reactions with it. Cost is the only limiting factor. Iron dextran by intramuscular route is associated with pain at injection site, risk of abscess formation, staining of skin, arthralgia, fever, painful lymphadenopathy etc. Intravenous administration can result in severe anaphylactic reaction. Iron dextran should be administered after a test dose of 0.5 mg im 24 hours before the first dose followed by 100 mg OD deep im by Z technique. Test dose for total dose intravenous infusion is given by slow intravenous infusion and observing the patient for any adverse reactions like chills, rigors, breathlessness, hypotension, hemolysis etc. Iron sucrose is administered as intravenous infusion 2-3 times a week in the dose of 200-300 mg per dose to a maximum of 600 mg per week. It does not require any test dose.

The total dose of parenteral iron needs to be calculated carefully to avoid the potential risk of iron overload and side effects. The elemental iron requirement in milligram can be calculated by any of the formulae given below:

- Weight of patient in kg × (normal hemoglobin – patient's hemoglobin in g/dl) × 2.21 + 1000 mg for stores
- Weight of patient in pounds × hemoglobin deficit in percentage × 0.3. Add 50% more of the calculated dose, for the stores
- 200 mg of elemental iron is required for raising the hemoglobin level by 1g%. Total dose is calculated according to hemoglobin deficit and additional 500 mg is added for stores.

The route of administration of parenteral iron can be intramuscular or intravenous depending upon the preparation used. The elemental iron content and route of administration of different preparation of parenteral iron are given in Table 14.12.

Anemia in Pregnancy

Table 14.12: Elemental iron content, route of administration and absorption of different preparations of parenteral iron		
Preparation	Strength	Route of administration
Iron dextran complex	2 ml ampoule 50 mg/ml 10 ml multidose vial	im or iv
Iron sorbitol citric acid complex	1.5 ml ampoule 50 mg/ml	im
Iron sucrose	5 ml ampoule 20 mg/ml	iv
Iron gluconate	5 ml ampoule 12.5 mg/ml	iv

Assessment of Response to Therapy

The response to therapy can be assessed clinically or by hematological indices. Clinically the woman looks better, feels better and her appetite improves. The reticulocyte count increases within 5-10 days and hemoglobin rises at the rate of 1g/dl per week. It takes about 4-10 weeks for the hemoglobin levels to be restored to normal.

Reasons of Failure to Respond

If the woman fails to respond the possible causes can be:
- Non iron deficiency anemia
- Noncompliance
- Faulty absorption
- Persistent blood loss, e.g. worm infestation, NSAIDs
- Coexisting infection
- Concomitant folate or vitamin B_{12} deficiency
- Pyridoxine deficiency.

Recent studies comparing oral iron therapy with parenteral therapy using newer preparations show that parenteral iron therapy with iron sucrose is costly, has no serious side effects, better tolerated, restores iron stores faster and more effectively than oral iron.[25] Recent Cochrane database (2007) concluded that it is not possible to draw well-informed balance of benefits and harms of oral *vs* parenteral therapy.[26]

MEGALOBLASTIC ANEMIA

The incidence of megaloblastic anemia in pregnant anemic women in developing countries is about 25% compared to only 3-4% in developed world. Megaloblastic anemia is due to folic acid and or vitamin B_{12} deficiency.

Etiopathogenesis of Megaloblastic Anemia

Folic acid and vitamin B_{12} are coenzymes required for the synthesis of thymidine, one of the four bases found in DNA. Deficiency or impaired metabolism of folic acid and vitamin B_{12} can affect DNA synthesis resulting in impaired nuclear maturation. As the cytoplasmic maturation is normal there is resultant nuclear cytoplasmic asynchrony with formation of megaloblasts in the bone marrow. These are released in the blood as macrocytes. As a large number of megaloblasts fail to mature they are destroyed in the bone marrow resulting in ineffective erythropoiesis and megaloblastic anemia.

Folic acid deficiency can result from inadequate dietary intake, increased demand, poor absorption or impaired metabolism. In women from poor socioeconomic status, the dietary folic acid is inadequate to meet the enhanced metabolic demand during pregnancy. This is further aggravated by prolonged cooking, less intake of raw vegetables, pregnancy induced nausea and vomiting, malabsorption syndromes and vitamin C deficiency. Certain drugs like antiepileptics, pyrimethamine and trimethoprim can also cause folic acid deficiency. Multiple pregnancy, repeated child birth, hemoglobinopathies, hemolytic anemia, worm infestation, bleeding piles, all increase the demand of folic acid. Its requirement is also increased in women with iron deficiency anemia on iron therapy.

The minimum daily requirement of folic acid is 50 µg-100 µg and is increased several fold during pregnancy (300 µg/day) and lactation (150 µg/day). The growing fetus and placenta extract folate from maternal body stores very effectively. Even when mother is severely anemic the fetus is not anemic. Green leafy vegetables, sprouts, beans, liver, kidney, fruits, cereals, nuts, etc. are rich sources of folic acid. It is absorbed from duodenum and upper jejunum.

Vitamin B_{12} is a complex organometallic compound known as cobalamin. The absorption of vitamin B_{12} requires intrinsic factor which is secreted by parietal cells of the mucosa of the fundus of the stomach. Human beings are totally dependent on dietary animal products for their vitamin B_{12} requirements. Plants and vegetables contain little cobalamin except that contributed by microbial contamination. Hence, strict vegetarian or macrobiotic diets do not contain adequate amount of this essential nutrient.

The daily requirement of vitamin B_{12} is 2 to 3 µg. Inadequate intake in the diet as in strict vegans, impaired absorption as in intrinsic factor deficiency, pernicious anemia, gastrectomy, malabsorption, ileal resection, fish tapeworm parasitic infestation, bacterial overgrowth in blind loops and diverticule of bowel and increased requirement as in pregnancy, hypothyroidism, disseminated cancer and chronic infections cause vitamin B_{12} deficiency.

Diagnosis of Megaloblastic Anemia

The diagnosis is made on the basis of peripheral smear report and red cell indices. The Hb levels are usually < 10 g% and peripheral smear may show pancytopenia, macrocytosis, anisocytosis, hypersegmented neutrophils (> 5 lobes), giant cell polymorphs, neutropenia and thrombocytopenia. RBCs may show basophilic stippling, Howell Jolly bodies and Cabbot rings.

Serum homocystiene and LDH levels are raised in both folic acid and vitamin B_{12} deficiency. The red cell indices show increased MCV> 100 fl, increased MCH and normal MCHC 31-37 g/dl. The reticulocyte count is low.

The differentiation between folic acid and vitamin B_{12} deficiency can be done clinically by presence of neurological symptoms in case of vitamin B_{12} deficiency secondary to the degeneration of the posterior and lateral columns of spinal cord and are irreversible if prompt therapy is not instituted. These features are absent in folic acid deficiency. Low serum folate levels (< 2.5 µg/L) and low RBC folate levels < 160 µg/L) are diagnostic of folic acid deficiency. Whereas serum levels of vitamin B_{12} of < 200 ng/L indicate vitamin B_{12} deficiency. In the absence of availability of these tests serum methylmalonic acid levels can also differentiate between the two, as its levels are raised in vitamin B_{12} deficiency. Examination of bone marrow reveals megaloblastic erythropoiesis. The Schilling test done to assess the cause of malabsorption of vitamin B_{12} is done in the post partum period.

Treatment

Preventive

Women should be counseled to take diet rich in folic acid like green leafy vegetables, beans, etc. WHO recommends a daily intake of 400 µg of folic acid per day for all pregnant women in antenatal period and for 3 months in postnatal period[20.] Ministry of Health and Family Welfare, Government of India recommends a daily supplementation of 500 µg of folic acid and 100 mg of elemental iron in antenatal period.[13] Periconceptional folic acid supplementation of 400 µg daily in low-risk women and 5 mg daily in high-risk women is an effective intervention for preventing neural tube defects. Routine supplementation of vitamin B_{12} is not recommended but vegetarian women should be encouraged to increase intake of dairy products during pregnancy and lactation.

Curative

In megaloblastic anemia due to folic acid deficiency a daily intake of 5 mg of folic acid is sufficient. It is important to supplement vitamin B_{12} 1000 µg per week by parenteral route to prevent worsening of peripheral neuropathy in case deficiency of vitamin B_{12} is coexisting. There is no consensus on the dose of vitamin B_{12} for the women with megaloblastic anemia however a dose of 1000 µg per week intravenously or intramuscular for 8 weeks followed by 1000 µg every month for 8 doses is sufficient. Oral preparations are also available and are prescribed in the dose of 1000-2000 µg per day. In the presence of neuropathy initial dose of 1000 µg daily or every alternative day for 5-7 doses may be given. Blood transfusion is indicated in women with severe anemia near term.

Response to Therapy

The response to therapy with folic acid and vitamin B_{12} is evident by a fall in LDH levels and an increase in reticulocyte count within 3-5 days. The associated thrombocytopenia also improves within 5-7 days.

THALASSEMIA

Thalassemia is a heterogeneous group of genetic disorders of hemoglobin synthesis characterized by absent or decreased synthesis of one or more globin chains. Thalassemia can be classified as α or β depending on the globin chain affected.

In India, β thalassemia comprises 80-90% of all cases of thalassemia. The frequency of occurrence of β thalassemia in general population is 3.5–15%[27] and that of α thalassemia is 0.05-0.98%. The communities commonly affected are Gujaratis, Maharashtrians, Sindhis, Goaneses, Bengalis and people from northern states like Haryana, Punjab, UP and Rajasthan.

Etiopathogenesis

Hemoglobin is a tetrameric protein compound comprising of 2 pairs of globin chain, each attached to a heme complex. There are various types of globin chains α, β, γ, δ, etc. In adults 95% of circulating hemoglobin is HbA ($\alpha_2 \beta_2$), 2-3% is HbA_2 ($\alpha_2 \delta_2$) and < 2 % is HbF ($\alpha_2 \gamma_2$).[28] The genes controlling the synthesis of these chains are located on chromosome 11 and 16. There are 4 genes located on chromosome 16 that control the synthesis of α globin chains. Of these two are derived from each parent. Synthesis of β globin chains is controlled by 2 genes located on chromosome 11, one gene derived from each parent. β thalassemia is a mutation disorder whereas α thalassemia is a deletion disorder resulting in absent or reduced synthesis of globin chains.

The clinical presentation in α thalassemia depends upon the number of genes deleted. The severity of disease increase with an increase in the number of genes deleted. When all the 4 genes are deleted, α globin chains are absent. None of the hemoglobins HbA, HbA_2, HbF can be synthesized; instead tetramers of γ chains known as Hb Bart (γ_4) are synthesized. This condition is incompatible with life. In β thalassemia presence of mutant genes result in reduced or absent β globin chains and excess of α globin chains. There is decreased production of HbA ($\alpha_2 \beta_2$) and increased production of HbA_2 ($\alpha_2 \delta_2$) and HbF ($\alpha_2 \gamma_2$). The pathophysiology of β thalassemia is depicted in the Flow chart 14.2.

Clinical Presentation

α Thalassemia

α Thalassemia trait: There are normally 4 functioning α globin genes. If one or two of these genes are missing the result is α thalassemia trait. These traits can not be detected on hemoglobin electrophoresis as no abnormal

Flow chart 14.2: Pathophysiology of β thalassemia

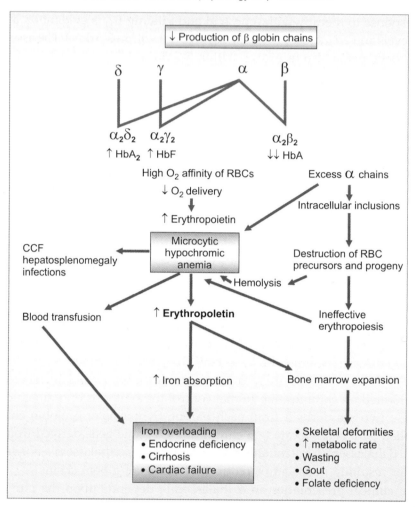

hemoglobin is synthesised. In addition, there is neither excess nor lack of any normal hemoglobin.

HbH disease: Deletion of three α globin genes result in HbH disease, manifesting as chronic hemolytic anemia with normal life expectancy. This can be detected on Hb electrophoresis. Cholelithiasis is commonly associated with HbH disease. The pregnant women are predisposed to hemolytic crisis in conditions like fever, infection, drug intake, etc.

Hb Bart's disease: Deletion of all 4 α globin genes result in Hb Bart's disease. Tetramers of γ chain known as Hb Bart (γ_4) are produced. In this condition no α chain is synthesized, so Hb F, Hb A and Hb A_2 are not synthesized. This disease is incompatible with life and results in intrauterine hydrops. Serious obstetric complications like preeclampsia, polyhydramnios, placentomegaly and difficult delivery due to large fetus and placenta can occur.

β Thalassemia minor: In β thalassemia minor, only one mutant gene is present. It is a heterozygous state. The obstetric outcome or complications are the same as that in the general population but it causes microcytic hypochromic anemia. There is increase in the incidence of anemia and doubtful increase in neural tube defects consequent to relative folate deficiency.[29]

β Thalassemia major: Women with β thalassemia major have high morbidity and mortality. Although these women are usually subfertile, pregnancies have been reported.[30] Increased incidence of early pregnancy losses, IUGR and prematurity due to maternal anemia and associated chronic placental hypoxia have been reported.[31] Women are predisposed to heart failure, hypersplenic crisis and venous thrombosis (in splenectomized women due to thrombocytosis). These women are small in stature and have small pelvic bones which may be responsible for increased rate of cesarean delivery in these women. Use of iron chelating agents can lead to retardation of bone ossification, vertebral aplasia and bifurcation or fusion of ribs in the fetus.[32]

14

Diagnosis

Thalassemia should be suspected in pregnant women with following findings:
- History of transfusion dependent anemia in self or family
- Women with mild to moderate microcytic anemia not responding to oral iron
- α thalassemia should be suspected in pregnant women with mild anemia with low MCV, not responding to oral iron and with normal Hb electrophoresis.

The diagnosis of β thalassemia is confirmed by Hb electrophoresis or automated high performance liquid chromatography (HPLC), which show raised HbA_2 levels > 3.5% of total hemoglobin.

α thalassemia trait cannot be diagnosed by Hb electrophoresis or HPLC and requires molecular genetic testing for detecting α globin gene deletion. The iron studies usually show normal serum iron and serum ferritin levels. There may be evidence of hemolysis in thalassemia major.

Recommendations for Screening for Thalassemia in Pregnancy

The following recommendations are based on good and consistent scientific evidence (Level A):[33]
- Routine screening should be carried out in populations with increased risk for being carriers of hemoglobinopathies like in populations with high prevalence of thalassemia in India, e.g. Gujaratis, Sindhis, Bengalis, North Indians, etc.

Anemia in Pregnancy

- A complete blood count and hemoglobin electrophoresis are appropriate laboratory tests for screening for hemoglobinopathies. Red cell indices such as MCH < 27 pg and MCV < 80 fl are good measures to select women for HPLC.
- Couples at risk for having a child with thalassemia should be offered genetic counseling to review prenatal testing and reproductive options. Prenatal diagnosis of hemoglobinopathies is best accomplished by DNA analysis of cultured amniocytes or chorionic villi.[33]

Delhi government has implemented thalassemia screening program which includes subjecting all pregnant women to NESTROFT (naked eye single tube rapid osmotic fragility test) with 0.36% buffer solution. Those testing positive are followed by hemoglobin electrophoresis and husband's blood for NESTROFT.

Management of Pregnancy with Thalassemia

α Thalassemia Trait

Pregnancy is well-tolerated. Folate supplementation is recommended for all women during pregnancy however iron supplementation should be advised only if iron deficiency is documented. Parenteral iron is contraindicated. Genetic screening of partner should be done. If both parents are carriers of heterozygous α^0 thalassemia trait(--/αα) there is a 25% chance of the fetus being affected by Hb Bart's disease. Prenatal diagnosis should be offered and MTP is advised if fetus is affected by Hb Bart's disease. In case both parents are homozygous α+ thalassemia trait (-α/-α), there is no risk of HbH and Bart's disease and fetal testing is not required.

HbH Disease

Women with HbH disease are likely to have acute exacerbation of chronic anemia during pregnancy. Periconception high dose folate supplementation (5 mg/day) is recommended. Iron supplementation is advised only in presence of iron deficiency. Blood transfusion is indicated in the presence of severe anemia. The partner should be subjected to genetic screening for a carrier state. If the partner tests positive for carrier state, prenatal diagnosis should be offered to the women for early diagnosis of fetus with HbH or Hb Bart's disease and medical termination of pregnancy is offered accordingly.

β Thalassemia Minor

In pregnant women with β thalassemia minor, screening of partner should be adviced. If the partner is a carrier, prenatal diagnosis (CVS, amniocentesis, cordocentesis) should be offered. In couples who are heterozygous carriers of β thalassemia have a 25% chance of having a baby with thalassemia major and 50% chance of having a baby with thalassemia minor. Folate supplementation is recommended for all pregnant women and iron supplementation in women with documented iron deficiency. Blood transfusion is indicated if the Hb level is < 8 gm% near term.

β *Thalassemia Major*

In women with thalassemia major, the partner is screened. Prenatal diagnosis is offered if partner is a carrier. These women should undergo a baseline evaluation before conceiving including cardiac, endocrine and liver functions. These are again repeated at the initial visit after conception and then in the second and third trimesters. Chelation with desferrioxamine should be stopped as soon as pregnancy is confirmed or in the midcycle when ovulation induction is being done due to its teratogenic effects. However, in women with myocardial dysfunction the risk of stopping chelation therapy outweighs the risk of teratogenecity on continuing the drug. The women are subjected to complete blood count every two weeks and transfusion therapy is continued to maintain Hb levels at 10 gm%. Prompt recognition and management of factors that precipitate hemolytic crisis like fever, infection and ingestion of oxidative compounds should be avoided.

SICKLE CELL ANEMIA

Sickle cell anemia is an inherited chronic hemolytic anemia due to presence of an abnormal hemoglobin HbS. The clinical manifestations are as a result of polymerization of hemoglobin S and deformation of RBCs into a characteristic sickle shape. It has highest prevalence in tropical Africa. In India it is prevalent in the tribal population of central India. The sickle cell trait provides survival benefit in areas endemic for falciparum malaria. The sickle hemoglobin containing red cells inhibit proliferation of plasmodium falciparum and the infected cells are more likely to become deformed and removed from circulation.

Etiopathogenesis

Sickle cell disease is caused due to homozygosity of hemoglobin S. It is caused by a point mutation of the β globin gene on chromosome 11 that produces an amino acid change at position 6, changing glutamic acid to valine acid and results in production of HbS. In sickle cell disease polymerization of hemoglobin S in the deoxygenated state is increased and leads to sickling and increased rigidity of red blood cells. Sickle cells exhibit abnormal adherence to vascular endothelium and lead to vasoocclusion, sickling induced membrane fragmentation and complement mediated lysis causing intravascular hemolysis. Poorly deformable sickle cells get entrapped extravascularly and phagocytosed by macrophages and monocytes and results in extravascular hemolysis.

Investigations

The dignosis is made on the basis of peripheral smear report which shows sickle cells, target cells, cigar-shaped cells and ovalocytes. The reticulocyte count is raised due to increased bone marrow activity consequent to hemolysis. Mean reticulocyte count is 10% with average ranging between 4-24%.

Management

At the first antenatal visit, a detailed history particularly with respect to prior sickle cell crisis, their nature, frequency and management is noted. Baseline complete blood count, reticulocyte count, serum iron levels, renal and liver function tests are obtained. Woman is screened for HIV and hepatitis.

The woman's partner should be screened for presence of sickle cell trait. If partner is positive for sickle cell trait, prenatal diagnosis is offered in the form of CVS or amniocentesis. Folic acid supplementation 1 mg/d is given to all women. Routine iron supplementation is given in the absence of any iron overload.

Patients are counseled regarding the importance of maintaining good hydration and prevention of infections, as dehydration and infections precipitate sickle cell crisis. Early diagnosis and prompt treatment of infections should be done. Pregnancy is carefully supervised for early detection of complications like preeclampsia, abruption, IUGR, preterm labor or any sickle cell disease activity.

During labor, intravenous fluids and oxygen supplementation help in preventing dehydration and maintaining an adequate circulation. Vaginal delivery is preferred. General anesthesia is avoided due to the risk of hypoxia associated with it, regional block is preferred.

In the postpartum period early mobilization is encouraged. Analgesics are given for pain relief and breastfeeding is encouraged.

MANAGEMENT OF LABOR IN ANEMIA

The general principles of management of labor in women with mild or moderate anemia are essentially the same as that of nonanemic women. Extra precautions need to be taken to prevent infection and minimize the blood loss in third stage of labor. Strict aseptic precautions are observed and per vaginum examinations should be kept to a minimum. Blood is kept cross matched and the third stage of labor is managed actively.

The management of labor in a pregnant woman with severe anemia is challenging. The relatives are counseled about the high risk to the mother and fetus and an informed high risk consent is taken. Adequate blood, preferably packed blood cells is arranged. The woman is nursed in a propped up position and administered intermittent oxygen by mask. Intravenous access is established but intravenous fluids are avoided. Prophylactic antibiotics may be given. In women who are decompensated, diuretics like frusemide 40 mg is given intravenously and packed cells may be started under diuretic cover. The flow rate should not exceed 15-30 drops per minute. Maternal and fetal condition and progress of labor is carefully monitored. The labor is usually easy and short in anemic women. The woman is observed for any signs of cardiac decompensation due to increased cardiac load during labor. Cardiac decompensation is suspected if pulse rate is > 100/ min, respiratory rate > 24 /min, JVP is raised and there are fine basal crepts in lungs.

The second stage may be cut short by application of ventouse or outlet forceps to avoid cardiorespiratory embarrassment. The third stage is managed actively. Oxytocics are kept ready. Injection methergin is contraindicated in women with congestive cardiac failure and per rectal misoprostol is preferred. If required concentrated infusion of oxytocin 20 units in 500 ml of RL is administered at the rate of no more than 125 ml per hour, i.e. 30 drops per min.

Women with severe anemia tolerate the blood loss poorly and even the normal blood loss in third stage can amount to postpartum hemorrhage in these women. The blood loss should be promptly replaced by packed blood cells transfusion.

These women are likely to go into failure immediately after delivery due to increased cardiac load consequent to release of pressure of the gravid uterus from the inferior vena cava and blood from the placental bed. These women should be kept propped up and observed carefully for any signs of decompensation immediately after delivery. Diuretics, frusemide 40 mg intravenously may be administered immediately after delivery of placenta to reduce the cardiac load.

Postnatal Care and Contraception in Anemic Women

Women with severe anemia are predisposed to infections and other complications. They need to be carefully observed for complications like sub-involution of uterus, puerperal sepsis, congestive cardiac failure, thromboembolism and lactation failure. Early ambulation is encouraged. Breastfeeding is not contraindicated.

Blood transfusion is avoided even with severe anemia if the woman is compensated except if there is any associated sepsis. Oral hematinic therapy is continued in therapeutic dose till the hemoglobin level is more than ≥ 12 gm%. It is continued for another 3 months after this for replenishing the body stores. The woman and her relatives are counseled regarding the importance and need for continuing hematinics.

Anemic women are counseled to avoid pregnancy for at least 2 years. A combination of lactational amenorrhea method (LAM) and barrier contraception is a good option for the first six months along with continued hematinic therapy. Once her hemoglobin levels are restored to normal any contraceptive can be advised. Progestin only pills can also be started after 3 weeks of delivery and continued for first 6 months and then switched over to combined oral contraceptive pills. Copper IUCD is avoided till the anemia

14

is corrected for the risk of associated menorrhagia however progesterone containing IUCD can be given. If she has completed her family, sterilization may be done provided her hemoglobin is 8 gm% or more as per eligibility criteria laid down by government of India.

KEY POINTS

- Anemia is the commonest medical disorder in pregnancy.
- Prevalence of anemia in pregnancy ranges from 20% in developed countries to 50-90% in developing countries.
- Nutritional iron deficiency anemia is the commonest type of anemia in pregnancy.
  Anemia is associated with an increase in maternal and perinatal morbidity and mortality.
- The clinical presentation of anemia may vary from a completely asymptomatic woman with mild anemia to a severely decompensated woman with severe anemia.
- Overall improvement in diet is an important intervention to tackle nutritional anemia.
- Routine iron and folic acid supplementation is recommended for all pregnant women in antenatal and postnatal period in countries with a high prevalence of anemia.
- The cause of anemia should be systematically identified and treated.
- Labor should be carefully supervised, observing strict asepsis and third stage is managed actively to minimize blood loss.
- Patient is counseled to continue hematinic therapy in the postpartum period and avoid next pregnancy for at least 2 years.

REFERENCES

1. Bhatt R. Maternal mortality in India- FOGSI-WHO Study. J Obstet Gynaecol Ind 1997, 47:207-14.
2. Viteri FE. The consequences of iron deficiency and anaemia in pregnancy. Adv Exp Med Biol 1994; 352: 127-39.
3. Abou Zahr C , Royston E. Maternal mortality. A global factbook. Geneva: World Health Organization,1991.
4. Prema K, Neela KS,Ramalaxmi BA. Anaemia and adverse obstetric outcome . Nutr Rep Int 1981; 23: 637-43.
5. Lozoff B, Jiminez E, Wolf AW. Long term developmental outcome of infants with iron deficiency. N Engl J Med 1992; 325:687-94.
6. UN Standing Committee on Nutrition 5th annual report on the world nutrition situation: Nutrition for improved developmental outcomes. March 2004.
7. World Health Organization. The prevalence of anemia in women: A Tabulation of Available Information; 2nd edn. Geneva: WHO, 1992. (WHO/MCH/MSM/92.2).
8. National Family Health Survey (NFHS) 3, India .website http://www.nfhsindia.org/ NFHS-3%20Data/NFHS-3%20NKF/Report.pdf
9. Kennedy E. Dietary reference intakes: Development and uses for assessment of micronutrient status of women—a global perspective. Am J Clin Nutr 2005; 81 (suppl):1194S-7S.
10. Report of steering committee on nutrition for tenth five year plan (2002-2007). Government of India, Planning commission. Micronutrient deficiencies. Sept 2002: 75-107.

11. WHO, Iron deficiency anaemia: Assessment, prevention and control. WHO/NHD/01.3, Geneva.2001.
12. Centres for Disease Control. Criteria for anemia in children and childbearing aged women MMWR 1989;38:400-04.
13. Indian Council of Medical Research. Evaluation of the National Nutrition Anemia Prophylaxis programme. Task force study. New Delhi. ICMR, 1989.
14. Patra S, Pasrija S, Trivedi S S, Puri M. Maternal and perinatal outcome in patients with severe anemia in pregnancy. Int J Gynaecol Obstet 2005;91 (2):164-65.
15. Joanne F, Ian A G. Thromboembolism in pregnancy: Problems prevention and treatment In: John Studd Progress in Obstet and Gynaecol (Ed) Churchill Livingstone 2003;15: 57-74.
16. Lops V R, Hunter L P, Dixon L R. Anemia in pregnancy. Am Fam Physician 1995; 51: 1189-97.
17. L Kasper DL,, Braunwald E, Fauci AS, et al. Harrison's Principles of Internal Medicine, 16th edn. 2005;586-592,601-06.
18. Hilman RS, Adult KA, Rinder HM, Iron deficiency anemia. Haematology in Clinical Practice, 4th edn. 2005; 53-64.
19. Sharma JB. Medical complications in pregnancy. In Sharma JB. (Ed) The obstetric Protocol, 1st edn. Jaypee Brothers Medical Publishers (P) Ltd. 1998; 78-98
20. Stoltzfus R, Dreyfuss ML. Guidelines for use of iron supplement to prevent and treat iron deficiency anaemia. Geneva: INACG, WHO, UNICEF,1998.
21. Ridwan E, Schultink W, Dillon D, Gross R. Effects of weekly iron supplementation on pregnant Indonesian women are similar to those of daily supplementation. Am J Clin Nutr1996; 63: 884-90.
22. Sloan NL, Jordan EA, Winikoff B. Does iron supplementation make a difference? Mother care project, 15 Arlington, VA, USA.1992.
23. Hallberg L, Hulthen L. Prediction of dietary iron absorption: An algorithm for calculating absorption and bioavailability of dietary iron. Am J Clin Nutri. 2000; 71 : 1147-60.
24. Olivares M, Pizarro F, Pineda O, Name JJ. Hertramph E, Walter T. Milk inhibits and ascorbic acid favors ferrous bioglycine chelate bioavailability in humans. J Nutr. 1997; 127(7) : 1407-11.
25. Ragip A. Al, Eylem Unlubilgin, Omer Kandemir, Serdar Yalvac, Leyla Cakir, and Ali Haberal, Intravenous versus oral Iron for treatment of anemia in pregnancy. Obs. and Gynecology 2005;106:1335-40.
26. Reveiz L, Gyte GML, Cuervo LG. Treatments for iron-deficiency anaemia in pregnancy. Cochrane Database of Systematic Reviews 2007, Issue 2. Art. No. CD003094. DOI: 10.1002/14651858.CD003094.pub2.
27. Ambedkar SS, Phadke MA, Mokashi GD, et al. Pattern of haemoglobinopathies in Western Maharashtra. Indian Paediatrics.2001;38(5):530-34.
28. Steiberg MH, Benz EJ. Pathobiology of the human erythrocyte and its hemoglobins. Hoffman J (Ed) Haematology: Basic principles and practice, 3rd edn. 2000; 356-66.
29. Ibba RM, Zoppi MA, floris M, et al. Neural tube defects in the offspring of thalassemia carriers. Fetal Diagn Ther 2003; 18:5-7.
30. Rappaport VJ, Velazquez M, Williams K. Hemoglobinopathies in pregnancy in Obstetric Gynecol. Clin N America. 2004;31:287-317.
31. Warwood M, Hoffbrand AV. Iron metabolism, iron deficiency and disorders of hemosynthesis. Postgraduate hematology 5th edn. 2005:26-43.
32. Leung, Tse N a; Lau, Tze K b; Chung, Tony KH â Thalassaemia screening in pregnancy. Current Opinion in Obstetrics & Gynecology.2005, 17(2):129-34.
33. Hemoglobinopathies in pregnancy. ACOG Practice Bulletin No. 78. American College of Obstetricians and Gynecologists. Obstet Gynecol 2007;109:229–37.

14

Anemia in Pregnancy

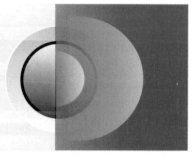

Hypertensive Disorders of Pregnancy 15

SS Trivedi, Monika B Nagpal

INTRODUCTION

Hypertension is a common medical disorder that affects 10% of all pregnancies and covers a spectrum of conditions namely gestational hypertension, preeclampsia, eclampsia, chronic hypertension and preeclampsia superimposed on chronic hypertension. They form one of the deadly triad along with hemorrhage and infection, which contribute greatly to both perinatal and maternal morbidity and mortality worldwide. Approximately 30% of hypertensive disorders in pregnancy are due to chronic hypertension and 70% are due to gestational hypertension-preeclampsia[1]. The spectrum of gestational hypertension-preeclampsia ranges from mildly elevated blood pressures with minimal clinical significance to severe hypertension and multiorgan dysfunction. There is no single, reliable, cost-effective screening test for gestational hypertension-preeclampsia and there are no well-established measures for primary prevention. Delivery remains the ultimate treatment but expectant management may be chosen depending on gestational age, fetal status and severity of maternal condition at the time of evaluation. Access to prenatal care, early detection of the disorder, careful monitoring and appropriate management are crucial elements in the prevention of hypertension related morbidity and mortality. This chapter presents the most widely accepted and current understanding on maternal and fetal risks and the management of hypertension in pregnancy.

DEFINITION

Hypertension

Hypertension is defined as a diastolic blood pressure of at least 90 mm Hg or a systolic BP of at least 140 mm Hg. Severe hypertension is defined as systolic blood pressure of ≥160 or diastolic blood pressure ≥110 mm Hg. Diastolic blood pressure is the pressure at which the sound disappears (Kortotkoff Phase 5). It is important to take certain precautions for an accurate reading of the blood pressure as enumerated below.

Measurement of Blood Pressure

- A range of sphygmomanometer cuff sizes should be available. Too small a size will overestimate blood pressure; too large will underestimate it (ideally bladder length should encompass 80% of arm circumference and width should be 40% of the arm circumference).
- Measurements should be taken in the sitting position after a period of rest with the arm supported at the heart level. Measurements are not significantly different if the woman is lying with lateral tilt and the arm is at the heart level.
- While inflating the cuff, the radial pulse should be palpated to get an approximate of the systolic blood pressure.
- During auscultation the cuff should be inflated to a pressure 20 mm Hg more than the estimated systolic pressure by palpation.
- The first appearance of repetitive sounds is taken as the systolic blood pressure (K1; rounded upwards to the nearest 2 mm Hg).
- The disappearance of these sounds is taken as the diastolic pressure (K5; rounded to the nearest 2 mm Hg).
- If K4 and K5 are markedly different, confusion can be avoided by recording both.

Proteinuria

Abnormal proteinuria in pregnancy is defined as excretion of 300 mg or more protein in 24 hours. The protein excretion may vary through the day. The most accurate measurement of proteinuria is obtained with a 24 hour collection and it is the preferred method. When semiquantitative dipstick measurement is used, which is less accurate, a value of 1+ or greater correlates with 30 mg/dl. Proteinuria with dipstick is defined as 1+ or more on at least two different occasions 6 hours apart but no more than 1 week apart. Care should be taken to collect a clean sample because blood, vaginal secretions and bacteria can increase the amount of protein in the urine. Others causes of a false-positive test by dipstick include contamination of the urine by chlorhexidine preparations, very alkaline urine or very concentrated urine (specific gravity >1.030). On the other hand a very dilute urine (specific gravity < 1.010) may produce false-negative results. Another way of assessing proteinuria is to measure the urinary protein: creatinine ratio. A value of >30 mg protein/mmol creatinine reflects a quantitative proteinuria of >0.3 gm/24 hours.

Edema

Though edema has been eliminated as a diagnostic criterion by the modified classification systems because it occurs too commonly during pregnancy in the dependent parts, but nondependent edema on face and arms is mostly pathologic.

CLASSIFICATION

The classification system of hypertension in pregnancy was proposed originally by the ACOG committee on Terminology in 1972. Further modifications by NHBPEP (National High Blood Pressure Education Program) working group in 2000 arrived at the classification scheme we use today.[2] It is based on 4 important features—hypertension, proteinuria, onset of hypertension, persistence of hypertension beyond 12 weeks postpartum. It is presented in the Table 15.1.

Table 15.1: Classification of hypertension in pregnancy

Gestational Hypertension

Hypertension detected for the first time after 20 weeks of gestation.

Distinguished from preeclampsia by the absence of proteinuria.

Working diagnosis only during pregnancy.

Gestational hypertension resolves by 12 weeks postpartum.

Preeclampsia

Hypertension that occurs after 20 weeks of gestation in a woman with previously normal blood pressure. Systolic blood pressure ≥ 140 mm Hg or diastolic blood pressure ≥ 90 mm Hg on two occasions at least 6 hours apart

Proteinuria, defined as excretion of ≥ 0.3 g protein in a 24 hour urine sample. This finding usually correlates with a finding of 1+ or greater on dipstick

Can be classified as mild and severe

Eclampsia

New onset grand mal seizures in a woman with preeclampsia which cannot be attributed to other causes.

Superimposed preeclampsia-eclampsia

Preeclampsia or eclampsia that occurs in a woman with a preexisting chronic hypertension.

Chronic hypertension

Hypertension with onset before pregnancy or before 20 weeks of gestation.

Persistence of hypertension beyond 12 weeks postpartum.

Preeclampsia is further classified into mild and severe which is presented in Table 15.2.

Table 15.2: Classification of preeclampsia	
Mild preeclampsia	*Severe preeclampsia*
Blood pressure ≥ 140/90 mm Hg but ≤ 160/110 mm Hg on two occasions at least 6 hours apart	Blood pressure ≥ 160 mm Hg systolic or ≥ 110 mm Hg diastolic
Proteinuria ≥ 300 mg/24 hours but < 5 g/24 hours	Proteinuria of 5 g or higher in the 24 hour urine specimen or 3 + or greater with dipstick
Asymptomatic	Oliguria (< 500 ml in 24 hours)
	Cerebral or visual disturbances
	Pulmonary edema or cyanosis
	Epigastric or right upper quadrant pain
	Impaired liver function
	Thrombocytopenia
	HELLP syndrome
	Fetal growth restriction

ETIOPATHOGENESIS

The etiologic agent responsible for the development of preeclampsia is unknown. Several theories have been proposed which include:
- Abnormal cytotrophoblast invasion
- Abnormal or increased immune response
- Endothelial cell injury
- Genetic predisposition
- Abnormal coagulation or thrombophilias
- Alterations in prostaglandin activity
- Alterations in nitric oxide levels
- Increased oxygen-free radicals
- Abnormal calcium metabolism
- Dietary deficiencies.

The syndrome is characterized by vasospasm, hemoconcentration and ischemic changes in the placenta, kidney, liver and brain. Recent studies have suggested that excess secretion of naturally occurring antiangiogenic molecules of placental origin referred to as soluble fms-like tyrosine kinase-1 may contribute to the pathogenesis of preeclampsia.[3] This leads to angiogenesis imbalance further leading to failure of trophoblast invasion and physiological remodelling of uterine spiral arteries hampering their normal physiological vasodilatation and this in turn leads to placental hypoxia which leads to further increase in fms-like tyrosine kinase-1 and maternal endothelial dysfunction. The vascular endothelium is known to supply all organ systems and this explains the widespread aspects of the syndrome. The sequence of events is summarized in Flow chart 15.1

The pathologic changes seen in various organ systems due to widespread endothelial damage and vasoconstriction are as follows[4]:

Hypertensive Disorders of Pregnancy

Flow chart 15.1: Pathogenesis of preeclampsia[3]

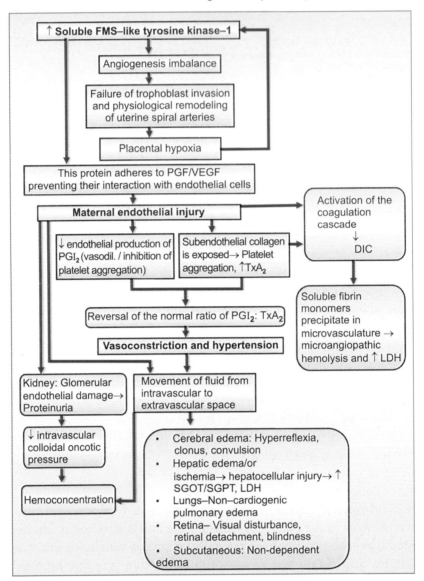

- *Brain*: Fibrinoid necrosis, thrombosis, microinfarcts, petechial hemorrhage, cerebral edema, subarachnoid hemorrhage and interventricular hemorrhage.
- *Liver*: Sinusoidal fibrin deposition in periportal areas with surrounding hemorrhage and portal capillary thrombi, centrilobular necrosis and subcapsular hematoma.
- *Kidney*: Glomeruloendotheliosis, i.e. swelling and enlargement of glomerular capillary endothelial cells.
- *Eyes*: Retinal vasospasm, retinal edema, retinal detachment

- *Heart*: Absence of normal intravascular volume expansion, hemo-concentration and loss of normal refractoriness to endogenous vasopressors including angiotensin II.
- *Uteroplacental circulation*: Acute atherosis, endothelial cell damage, basement membrane disruption, mural thrombi, increase in smooth muscle cells with vasospasm that leads to a decreased vessel lumen.

PREDICTION

Many clinical, biophysical, hematological and biochemical tests have been used for prediction of preeclampsia. An ideal predictive test should be simple, noninvasive, rapid, inexpensive, easy to perform early in pregnancy and reproducible with high sensitivity and predictive value. Currently there is no single screening test for preeclampsia that is reliable, valid and cost effective.[5] Thus an accurate and thorough maternal history with identification of risk factors (shown below) is the most cost-effective screening method. This should be done at first contact and women's level of risk for preeclampsia should be evaluated so that the plan for her subsequent schedule for antenatal appointments can be formulated.[4]

Risk Factors for Preeclampsia

- Age < 20 years or > 35 years
- Nulliparity
- History of preeclampsia in previous pregnancies
- Multiple gestations
- Family history of preeclampsia
- Chronic hypertension
- Trophoblastic disease
- Diabetes mellitus
- Obesity
- Renal disease
- Thyroid disease
- Collagen vascular disease
- Antiphospholipid syndrome
- Thrombophilias.
  The various tests which have been used for prediction are as follows:

Biophysical Tests

- Roll over test
- Angiotensin II infusion test
- Isometric exercise
- Uterine artery Doppler
- Mid-pregnancy mean arterial pressure (MAP)

Hematological and Biochemical

- Increased maternal serum uric acid
- Elevated second trimester MSAFP/β-HCG
- Decreased urinary calcium excretion
- Higher fasting insulin levels.

Perhaps the best test available is the use of Doppler ultrasound of the uterine arteries. The presence of a persistent notching pattern at 18-22 weeks gestation is thought to reflect failure of the second wave of trophoblast invasion and increased peripheral vascular resistance. It has sensitivity of 75%, specificity of 96%, although the positive predictive value is only 28%. It can be useful for screening pregnant women who are at high risk for pre-eclampsia.

PREVENTION

The observed alteration in the ratio of vasoconstrictive and vasodilatory prostaglandins in preeclampsia led the investigators to study different approaches for the prevention of preeclampsia including use of low-dose aspirin, calcium and magnesium supplements, a low-salt diet and antioxidants. Calcium is essential in the synthesis of nitric oxide, a potent vasodilator believed to contribute to the maintenance of reduced vascular tone in pregnancy. Calcium supplementation may offer protection for calcium-deficient women, but there is no benefit in patients with adequate daily calcium intake.[6] Similarly, low-dose aspirin which reverses the imbalance between vasoconstrictor thromboxane A_2 and the vasodilator prostacyclin have been tried but there has been conflicting evidence regarding its use. A recent systematic review concluded that there is a small to moderate benefit of low aspirin in preventing preeclampsia in women at high risk such as those with a history of chronic hypertension and preeclampsia in a previous pregnancy.[7] Initial promising data related to a potential benefit of antioxidants (vitamins C and E) is not supported by a recent Cochrane review.[8]

MANAGEMENT

The only definitive therapy for gestational hypertension/preeclampsia is delivery. In case of preterm pregnancies, the main objective of expectant management is to improve neonatal outcome if the risks for the mother and child remain acceptable. The decision between delivery and expectant management depends on fetal gestational age, fetal status and severity of maternal condition at the time of evaluation. Management plan for mild and severe preeclampsia has been illustrated in flow charts 15.2 and 15.3 respectively.

Goals of Management

- Prevention of convulsions.
- Prevention of complications like cerebrovascular hemorrhage, pulmonary edema, renal failure, abruption, intrauterine death of fetus.
- Deliver a surviving baby with minimal maternal trauma.

Flow chart 15.2: Summary of management protocols of mild gestational hypertension/preeclampsia

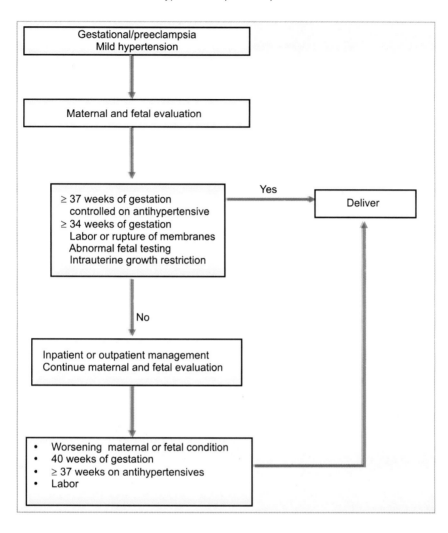

Assessment

Women with overt hypertension ≥140/90 with or without proteinuria should be admitted to the hospital for two-three days to evaluate the severity of new onset hypertension. After serial assessment, the setting for continued management can be determined. Those with mild gestational hypertension/ preeclampsia who are remote from term, outpatient management may be an option. Among those with severe disease, some women will have a stabilization of the disease and would be eligible for expectant management. Conversely, some others will have rapid deterioration of the maternal/fetal condition that will necessitate expeditious delivery regardless of the gestational age.

After admission, the first step is to evaluate the maternal and fetal status.

Flow chart 15.3: Summary of management protocols of severe gestational hypertension/preeclampsia

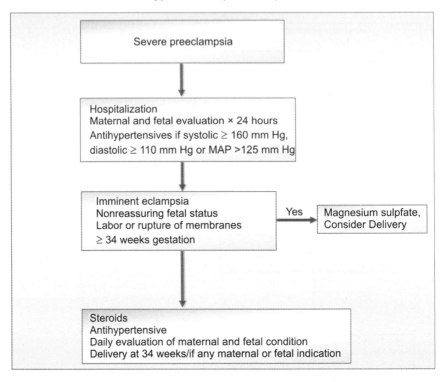

Maternal evaluation

Includes taking a complete history including evaluation of end organ damage if any, physical evaluation including obstetric examination, laboratory evaluation including hematocrit, platelet count, liver function tests, serum creatinine, uric acid, coagulation studies, 24 hour urinary protein and fundus examination.

Fetal evaluation

History of decreased fetal movements, on obstetric examination—evaluation of symphysiofundal height, abdominal girth, amount of liquor, estimated fetal weight, fetal heart sounds, non stress test/biophysical profile (after 28 to 30 weeks of gestation), USG for fetal weight and amount of liquor, umbilical artery Doppler waveform in suspected intrauterine growth restriction.

Expectant Management

In patients diagnosed with mild gestational hypertension/preeclampsia at term (≥ 37 weeks), the general consensus is to deliver the woman. For the patient who is preterm (< 37 weeks), controversy arises regarding management with respect to the level of activity, hospitalization, antihypertensive and anticonvulsants. Usually these patients do not require immediate delivery and expectant management is advocated.

Patients with severe preeclampsia at 23-34 weeks gestation receive individualized treatment based on their initial assessment.

Outpatient Management/Hospitalization

Prolonged hospitalization for the duration of pregnancy allows rapid intervention in case of fulminant progression to hypertensive crisis, eclampsia or abruption placentae. These complications are rare in women who have mild disease. Outpatient management at home or at a day care unit has been evaluated as an option for monitoring women with mild gestational hypertension or preeclampsia remote from term. A number of studies suggest a place for ambulatory management in carefully selected women.[9] Thus women with mild disease who are:

- Compliant
- Asymptomatic
- Have normal laboratory results
- Have readily available round the clock transportation

can be managed in an ambulatory setting. Such management should include frequent maternal and fetal evaluation and access to health care providers. At the time of initial and subsequent visits, the women should be educated and instructed to immediately report to the hospital in case they develop any of the warning symptoms like nausea, vomiting, persistent severe headache, right upper quadrant pain, epigastric pain, scotoma or blurred vision, decreased fetal movements, bleeding per vaginum, leaking per vaginum or labor pains. Indicatiors of disease progression evident on BP records, laboratory tests; fetal compromise on fetal surveillance like intrauterine growth restriction or oligohydramnios are not suitable for ambulatory management.

On the other hand management of patients with severe gestational hypertension/preeclampsia is best accomplished in a tertiary care setting.

Surveillance

During expectant management close monitoring of both mother and fetus is initiated by evaluating the clinical symptoms, signs and laboratory findings and the decision to continue pregnancy must be reevaluated daily. The frequency of testing depends on the severity of disease and its progression.

Maternal surveillance: Includes monitoring for clinical symptoms like headache, blurring of vision, epigastric pain, nausea, vomiting, decrease urine output and shortness of breath. Blood pressure should be measured every four hours. Daily weight and intake output should be recorded. Serial assessment of complete blood count, liver function tests and kidney function test should be performed weekly in case of mild disease with no progression, sooner if the disease progression is questionable and every other day or daily in case of severe disease. Clotting studies are not required if platelet count is more than 100000/mm^3 and liver enzymes are normal.[10]

Fetal surveillance: The woman is instructed to keep a daily fetal movement count. Weekly symphysio-fundal height and abdominal girth is charted. Non-stress test for fetal well being is done weekly in mild disease, twice weekly for suspected growth restriction or oligohydramnios and alternate day or daily for severe disease depending upon the progression of the disease with weekly amniotic fluid index (AFI) determinations. Ultrasound examination for fetal growth is done every 3-4 weeks in mild disease and every 2-3 weeks in severe disease. Umbilical artery Doppler is done depending upon the presence and severity of intrauterine growth restriction.[11]

Steroids

In attempts to enhance fetal lung maturation glucocorticoids have been administered to women with severe hypertension who are < 34 weeks of gestation. Treatment does not worsen maternal hypertension and a reduction in the incidence of respiratory distress and intraventricular hemorrhage and improved fetal survival has been found.[12]

Bedrest

Complete or partial bedrest for the duration of pregnancy was recommended in the past for women with gestational hypertension/preeclampsia. However, various studies have shown that strict bedrest in the hospital for pregnant women with preeclampsia does not appear to lower rates of perinatal morbidity and mortality including preterm birth, endotracheal intubations, or neonatal intensive care unit (NICU) admissions.[13] On the other hand prolonged bed rest for the duration of pregnancy increases the risk of thromboembolism. Thus, women with proteinuric or nonproteinuric hypertension are instructed to restrict their activity, not complete bedrest.

Antihypertensives

Antihypertensive therapy is used to protect the mother from effects of severe hypertension such as cerebrovascular hemorrhage, cardiac failure, abruption and eclampsia. The value of antihypertensives in mild to moderate disease (diastolic BP 90 to 109 mm Hg) is unclear. Maternal death and stroke is rare and eclampsia is unusual in these women. Various researchers have used antihypertensive drugs for mild hypertension. Unfortunately drug treatment for mild preeclampsia has been disappointing as shown by the Cochrane review which concluded that treatment induced decrease in blood pressure may adversely affect fetal growth.[14] Thus though the risk benefit profile in mild to moderate disease needs to be re-examined, ACOG recommends antihypertensives when diastolic blood pressure is 105-110 mm Hg or higher[11] although many clinicians start antihypertensives at diastolic blood pressure of 100 or higher.

On the other hand there is consensus that antihypertensives should be prescribed when systolic blood pressure is ≥ 160 mm Hg or diastolic blood pressure is ≥ 110 mm Hg with the aim to keep the blood pressure below the severe range (systolic blood pressure at 130-150 mm Hg and diastolic blood pressure 80-100 mm Hg) or mean arterial pressure less than 125 mm Hg as the maternal risk decreases with anti-hypertensive therapy.[15] A step-wise approach to the use of antihypertensives is required.

- First line is either methyldopa or labetalol
- Second line is usually nifedipine
- Third line is methyldopa or adenoreceptor antagonist depending on which of these agents was used as first line therapy.

A suitable regime is labetalol 200 mg twice daily, increasing to 300mg four times daily as required. If blood pressure is not controlled then nifedipine is added. Such therapy is usually sufficient; if blood pressure is not adequately controlled on this combination, the disease is usually sufficiently advanced to warrant delivery. However, occasionally a third line agent is required and in this situation methyldopa is added at a dose of 0.25 gm two to three times daily increasing upto 500 mg four times a day. Where an adrenoceptor antagonist is contraindicated, methyldopa is used as first line therapy. ACE inhibitors must not be used antenatally especially during second and third trimester. Reported complications with ACE inhibitors include oligohydramnios, fetal growth restriction, bony malformations, limb contractures, persistent PDA, pulmonary hypoplasia, respiratory distress syndrome, prolonged neonatal hypertension and neonatal death.[16]

The following Table 15.3 summarizes the various antihypertensive drugs used for long-term nonemergency oral treatment.

Table 15.3: Antihypertensive drugs				
BP medication	Dosage	MAX dose	Benefits	Adverse effects
Methyldopa (α₂ -Adrenergic agonists- central inhibition of sympathetic drive)	250-500 mg po q6-12h	4 g/24h	Proven to be safe, and efficacious; decreased second-trimester fetal losses	Maternal fatigue, depression, orthostatic hypotension, xerostomia, elevated liver enzymes (5-10%)
Nifedipine (Calcium channel blocker-inhibits extracellular calcium influx into cells through slow calcium channels)	10-20 mg oral q4-6 hour	240 mg/24h	Effective for refractory HTN; Potent tocolysis in preterm labor; lowers BP without effects on blood flow in the umbilical artery	Maternal side effects-flushing headache palpitations; interaction with magnesium-sulfate: profound hypotension; no increase risk of congenital malformations
Labetalol (α and β) blocker-reduction in cardiac output)	100 mg po bid	2400 mg/ 24 hour	Effective BP control; lowers BP without altering cerebral autoregulation; lower risk of arrhythmia than with vasodilatory agents	Fetal bradycardia, neonatal hypoglycemia, impaired fetal response to hypoxia, decreased uteroplacental flow; avoid in patients with asthma and CHF[17]

Oral or intravenous therapy can be decided on the basis of the presentation.

Hypertensive crisis can be classified as:

Hypertensive urgency which is defined as severely elevated blood pressure in a patient with no signs or symptoms or laboratory evidence of end organ damage. Oral drugs should be used here.

Hypertensive emergency, is said to be present when elevated blood pressure is responsible for signs, symptoms or laboratory evidence of end organ damage. Rapid but controlled reduction in BP using intravenous medication is required. One should target to reduce MABP by 25% within 1 hour of presentation. If initial reduction is well-tolerated, reduction to normal levels can be achieved over ensuing 24 hours.

The objective of treating acute severe hypertension is to prevent potential cerebrovascular and cardiovascular complications such as encephalopathy, hemorrhage and congestive heart failure. Antihypertensive therapy is recommended by some for sustained systolic BP values of at least 180 mm Hg and for sustained diastolic values of at least 110 mm Hg. The definition of sustained hypertension is not clear ranging from 30 min to 2 hours. Others use mean arterial pressure to guide management. Antihypertensive therapy should be initiated urgently if mean arterial pressure is more than 140 mmHg as above this cerebral autoregulation of pressure is not reliable. Agents used for treatment of acute severe hypertension should be initiated at low doses, given that women with preeclampsia are intravascular volume depleted and are at increased risk for hypotension. A latest review has generated uncertainty about the agent of first choice among them but labetalol and nifedipine are usually preferred as compared to hydralazine which is associated with more adverse outcomes[15].

The following Table 15.4 depicts the therapeutic options in the treatment of acute severe hypertension

Table 15.4: Ttreatment of acute severe hypertension			
Medication	Onset of action	Dosage	Adverse effects
Labetalol	5 min	20 mg iv bolus then 40 mg after 10 min, then 80 mg every 10 min upto a maximum total dose of 220 mg, a continuous infusion of 1-2 mg/min may also be used	See Table 15.3
Nifedipine	10 min	10 mg po can be repeated in 30 min, then 10-20 mg q4-6h with a maximum dose of 240 mg/24 hours	See Table 15.3

Contd...

Contd...

Medication	Onset of action	Dosage	Adverse effects
Nitroglycerine		Initial infusion rate of 10 mg/min and titrated to the desired pressure by doubling the dose very five minutes	Methemoglobinemia may result from high dose (>7 mg/kg/min) iv infusion
Hydralazine	10-20 min	5-10 mg iv every 15-20 min until a desired response is obtained	Profound maternal hypotension and oliguria, fetal distress; Maternal pyridoxine-responsive polyneuropathy and drug-induced lupus, neonatal thrombocytopenia and lupus
Sodium nitroprusside	0.5 to 5 min	0.2-5µg/kg/min infusion; for use in refractory hypertension	Fetal cyanide and thiocyanate toxicity

The blood pressure and pulse rate should be monitored every 5 min and the goal of therapy is to decrease the diastolic BP to 90-100 mm Hg.

Anticonvulsants

Magnesium sulfate is the drug of choice to prevent convulsions in women with preeclampsia. The rate of seizures in women with mild preeclampsia not receiving magnesium sulfate is very low, about 1 in 200 and as such the benefit to risk ratio does not support the routine use of magnesium sulfate in mild preeclampsia.[18] On the other hand among women with severe preeclampsia and those with features of imminent eclampsia are the best candidates to receive magnesium sulfate prophylaxis as the number needed to be treated to prevent one case of eclampsia is 36. Most authorities now recommend prophylactic magnesium sulfate in all women with severe preeclampsia once a delivery decision has been made and in the immediate postpartum period especially if there is concern about the risk of eclampsia.[10,19] There is no agreement in the literature regarding the optimal time to initiate magnesium sulfate, the dose to use (both loading and maintenance), the route of administration (intramuscular or intravenous), as well as the duration of therapy in these women. Use for 24 hours at admission in women with severe preeclampsia is recommended by some experts. Others start it once the decision for delivery is made. The various regimens are discussed in section on eclampsia.

Delivery

Indications and Timing

Mild disease: In general, women with mild disease developing at 37 weeks gestation or later have a pregnancy outcome similar to that found in normotensive pregnancy. Thus, those who have a favorable cervix should undergo induction of labor and delivery. In addition, cervical ripening with prostaglandins and induction of labor can be used in women with an

Hypertensive Disorders of Pregnancy

unfavorable cervix at 37 weeks or more because the mother is at slightly increased risk for development of abruptio placentae and progression to severe disease. If the cervix is unfavorable, disease is stable and the woman is compliant, expectant management may be continued upto 40 weeks (but not beyond 40 weeks) with close monitoring of maternal and fetal condition.

Thus the indications for delivery in gestational hypertension/mild preeclampsia are as follows:[20]

- 37 weeks gestation controlled on antihypertensives
- Abnormal results of fetal testing
- Worsening preeclampsia or hypertension
- Labor or rupture of membranes

Severe disease: The presence of severe disease mandates immediate hospitalization. The maternal and fetal condition is assessed and a decision is made regarding the need for delivery. Patients with gestational age below 23 weeks should be counselled and offered termination of pregnancy in view of poor prognosis. Patients at 33-34 weeks are given corticosteroids and then delivered after 48 hours. Patients with gestational ages of 23-32 weeks should receive individualized treatment based on their clinical response during 24 hour observation period. If BP is adequately controlled and fetal tests are reassuring, the patients are observed closely in the antepartum high-risk ward until 34 weeks gestation or till development of a maternal or fetal indication for delivery as enumerated in Table 15.5[21]

Table 15.5: Indications for delivery in severe preeclampsia
Maternal indications
Uncontrolled severe hypertension
Eclampsia
HELLP syndrome
Persistent oliguria
Abruptio placentae
Platelet count < 1,00,000/mm^3
Elevated liver enzymes with epigastric pain or right upper quadrant tenderness
Pulmonary edema
Persistent severe headache or visual changes
Fetal death
Spontaneous labor
Rupture of membranes
Gestational age $\geq$ 34 weeks
Fetal indications
Repetitive late deceleration
Severe variable deceleration
Biophysical score $\leq$ 4 on two occasions 4 hours apart
Estimated fetal weight $\leq$ 5th percentile
Reversed end diastolic flow
Severe oligohydramnios

Mode of Delivery

In women with gestational hypertension/preeclampsia without contraindications to labor, vaginal delivery is the preferred approach. Cervical ripening agents and oxytocin are used as needed. Blood pressure stabilization prior to induction should be done. The decision to perform cesarean delivery should be individualized and based on gestational age, maternal and fetal condition, presence of labor and Bishop score. Cesarean section is reserved for cases in which the maternal and fetal conditions are adverse and deteriorating and for patients with preterm gestation and an unripe cervix. Regional anaesthesia is preferred in the absence of coagulopathy. General anesthesia increases the risk of aspiration and failed intubation due to airway edema and is associated with marked increase in systemic and cerebral pressures during intubation and extubation. If general anesthesia is given then antihypertensive therapy should be used before intubation to prevent further increase in blood pressure during intubation.[10]

Intrapartum Management

The goals of treatment of women with gestational hypertension/ preeclampsia are early detection of fetal heart rate abnormalities, early detection of progression from mild to severe disease and prevention of maternal complications. Therefore, all these women should receive continuous fetal heart rate monitoring with special attention to hyperstimulation and development of vaginal bleeding during labor. Blood pressure should be recorded every hour and women should be questioned about the new onset of symptoms suggesting severe disease. Maternal pain relief during labor and delivery can be provided by systemic opioids or epidural analgesia. A strict intake output record should be maintained and to avoid pulmonary edema rate of intravenous fluids should not exceed 100 ml/hour. Invasive hemodynamic monitoring (pulmonary artery catheterization) may be used in women with preeclampsia who have severe cardiac/renal disease, pulmonary edema, refractory hypertension or oliguria not responding to fluid challenge. The control of acute severe hypertension has been discussed above. The use of magnesium sulfate during labor and 24 hours postpartum in all women with severe preeclampsia has been discussed above.

CARE FOLLOWING DELIVERY

During the immediate postpartum period, women with preeclampsia should receive close monitoring of blood pressure and those with symptoms consistent with severe disease and imminent eclampsia, accurate measurements of fluid intake and urine output is indicated as there is mobilization of extracellular fluid leading to increased intravascular volume for the first 24-48 hours. As a result, these women especially those with abnormal renal function and capillary leaks are at increase risk for pulmonary edema and exacerbation of severe hypertension. In general most women with gestational hypertension become normotensive during the first week following delivery whereas those with preeclampsia take a longer time to resolve. The antihypertensive regime used antenatally can be continued and dose adjusted and a second line agent is introduced as required to control the blood pressure. As the blood pressure settles, the drugs are gradually tapered and then withdrawn under supervision usually as an outpatient. Calcium channel blockers are most commonly used as methyldopa has unwanted side effects like postpartum depression. Blood pressure is monitored one to two times per week. If hypertension persists beyond 12 weeks postpartum, the patient is classified as having chronic hypertension and referred to a specialist for investigation to rule out any underlying medical condition such as renal disease and followed up accordingly.[20] The women have to be explained about the risk of recurrence. The earlier preeclampsia is diagnosed during index pregnancy the greater the likelihood of recurrence. The risk in nullipara where diagnosis is made before 30 weeks is upto 40%. In HELLP syndrome it is 5-27%.[22]

LONG-TERM COMPLICATIONS

The long-term cardiovascular prognosis depends on whether preeclampsia has occurred in nulliparous or multiparous women, as the risk of chronic hypertension and death related to hypertension has been found to be increased in multiparous women. Those with recurrent pregnancy induced hypertension are at increased risk for chronic hypertension whereas those who remained normotensive during subsequent pregnancy are at decreased risk.[22]

SUMMARY OF MANAGEMENT PROTOCOLS

Summary of management protocols of mild and severe gestational hypertension/preeclampsia is presented in Flow charts 15.2 and 15.3.[23]

ECLAMPSIA

Eclampsia is defined as the development of convulsions and/or unexplained coma during pregnancy or postpartum in patients with signs and symptoms of preeclampsia. The estimated incidence of eclampsia is 1 to 3 per 1,000 preeclamptic patients. It continues to be a major cause of maternal and perinatal morbidity and mortality worldwide. The maternal mortality rate is 4.2%. The perinatal mortality rate is higher ranging from 13 to 30%. It occurs more commonly as term approaches. Eclampsia can occur antepartum (50%), intrapartum (25%) or postpartum(25%) but when the first convulsion occurs more than 48 hours postpartum, other causes should be excluded.

Clinical Course

The usual clinical presentation is development of classical prodrome of headache, epigastric pain, visual disturbance followed by convulsions on a background of variable signs and symptoms of preeclampsia. However, the signs and symptoms of preeclampsia are not necessary for the development of convulsions. Complications include placental abruption, neurological deficits, aspiration pneumonia, pulmonary edema, cardiopulmonary arrest, acute renal failure and maternal death.

Differential Diagnosis

Other causes of convulsions which are enumerated below must be considered in the differential diagnoses depending upon the clinical presentation:

- Epilepsy
- Intracranial hemorrhage
- Meningitis
- Encephalitis
- Thrombosis
- Rupture of cerebral aneurysm
- Hyperventilation syndrome
- Cerebral tumor

Management

Definitive treatment of eclampsia includes the following:
- Avoidance of injury
  - Padded bedside rails
  - Physical restraints
  - Padded tongue blade
- Maintenance of oxygenation to mother and fetus
  - Oxygen at 8-10 l/min by face mask.
  - Monitor oxygenation by transcutaneous pulse oximetry and metabolic status with arterial blood gas measurement.
- Minimize aspiration
  - Lateral decubitus position.
  - Suctioning of vomitus and oral secretion.
- Initiate magnesium sulfate treatment to prevent recurrent seizures.
- Control severe hypertension.
- Stabilize maternal condition
- Initiate the delivery process.
  Vaginal delivery is the preferred route after an eclamptic seizure. Cesarean delivery should be performed for obstetric indications only. Induction of labor should be performed with oxytocin or prostaglandins. Magnesium sulfate is the drug of choice and has been shown to be superior to both phenytoin and

diazepam for the prevention of eclamptic seizures.[24] The exact mechanism of action is unclear but it appears to have a peripheral action at the neuromuscular junction.

Magnesium sulfate dosing schedules which are used for severe preeclampsia and eclampsia include:

Continuous Intravenous Infusion

1. Give 4 to 6 g loading dose of magnesium sulfate diluted in 100 ml of iv fluid administered over 15-20 minutes.
2. Begin 1-2 gm/hour in 100 ml of iv maintenance infusion.
3. Measure serum magnesium level at 4-6 hour and adjust infusion to maintain levels between 4-7 mEq/l (4.8 – 8.4 mg/dl).
4. Magnesium sulfate is discontinued 24 hour after delivery.

Intermittent Intramuscular Injections

1. Give 4 gm of magnesium sulfate ($MgSO_4.7H_2O$ USP) as a 20% solution intravenously at a rate not to exceed 1 gm/min.
2. Follow promptly with 10 gm of 50% magnesium sulfate solution, one half (5 gm) injected deeply in the upper outer quadrant of both buttocks through a 3 inch long, 20 gauge needle (addition of 1.0 ml of 2% lignocaine minimizes discomfort). If convulsions persist after 15 minutes, give 2 gm more intravenously as a 20% solution at a rate not to exceed 1gm/min. If the woman is large, upto 4 gm may be given slowly.
3. Every 4 hour thereafter give 5 gm of a 50% solution of magnesium sulfate injected deeply in the upper outer quadrant of alternate buttocks, but only after ensuring that:
   1. patellar reflex is present
   2. respiration is not depressed
   3. urine output in the last 4 hour exceeded 100 ml.
4. Magnesium sulfate is discontinued 24 hours after delivery.

Patients receiving magnesium sulfate are at increased risk of postpartum hemorrhage due to uterine atony. This should be anticipated and blood should be cross-matched. Patients should be monitored for signs of magnesium toxicity throughout the course of administration. The serum magnesium levels and associated clinical findings are as given below:

- 8-12 mg/dl: Loss of patellar reflex
- 9-12 mg/dl: Feeling of warmth, flushing
- 10-12 mg/dl: Double vision, somnolence
- 10-12 mg/dl: Slurred speech
- 15-17 mg/dl: Muscular paralysis
- 15-17 mg/dl: Respiratory difficulty
- 30-35 mg/dl: Cardiac arrest.

If a patient develops signs of magnesium toxicity the following steps should be initiated:
- Stop magnesium sulfate.
- Begin supplemental oxygen administration.
- 1 g calcium gluconate (10 cc of 10% calcium gluconate) by slow intravenous push.
- Check serum magnesium level.
- Repeat calcium gluconate administration if necessary.
- If respiratory arrest occurs begin cardiopulmonary resuscitation.

HELLP SYNDROME

HELLP syndrome is used to describe preeclampsia in association with hemolysis, elevated liver enzymes and low platelet count. The incidence is 10% among pregnancies complicated by preeclampsia. It is a severe form of preeclampsia and may develop in patients with only mild to moderate blood pressure elevations and occasionally in the absence of proteinuria. HELLP syndrome develops antepartum in 70% of patients and postpartum in the rest. The hallmark of HELLP syndrome is liver involvement that may lead to liver failure and in most severe cases, liver rupture, which is associated with high maternal and fetal mortality rates.

Criteria for Diagnosis of HELLP syndrome[25]

- Hemolysis
  - Abnormal peripheral smear
  - Lactate dehydrogenase > 600 U/L
  - Serum bilirubin ≥ 1.2 mg/dl.
- Elevated liver enzyme levels
  - Serum aspartate aminotransferase >70 U/L
  - Lactate dehydrogenase > 600U/L
- Low platelets
  - Platelet count < 100,000/mm.[3]

Clinical Features

The clinical picture is highly variable, the signs and symptoms include the following:[26,27]
- Right upper quadrant pain or epigastric pain (86-90%)
- Nausea or vomiting (45-84%)
- Headache (50%)
- Right upper quadrant tenderness on palpation (86%)
- Diastolic blood pressure greater than 110 mm Hg (67%)
- Proteinuria greater than 2+ on dipstick (85-96%)
- Edema (55-67%)

Hypertension may be absent in as many as 20% of patients. HELLP syndrome is associated with an increased risk of many adverse outcomes including complications like abruption, pulmonary edema, adult respiratory distress syndrome, ruptured liver hematoma, acute renal failure, DIC, eclampsia, intracerebral hemorrhage and maternal death. It needs to be differentiated from other conditions which might have overlapping features as given below.

Differential Diagnosis of HELLP Syndrome[25]

- Acute fatty liver of pregnancy
- Appendicitis
- Cerebral hemorrhage
- Diabetes insipidus
- Gallbladder disease
- Gastroenteritis
- Glomerulonephritis
- Hemolytic uremic syndrome
- Hyperemesis gravidarum
- Idiopathic thrombocytopenia
- Pancreatitis
- Pyelonephritis
- Systemic lupus erythematosus
- Thrombophilias
- Thrombotic thrombocytopenic purpura
- Viral hepatitis including herpes.

Management

The clinical course of women with HELLP syndrome is usually characterized by progressive and sometimes sudden deterioration in maternal and fetal condition. Therefore, patients with suspected diagnosis of HELLP syndrome should be hospitalized immediately.

Management includes the same principles of treatment as for severe preeclampsia.

- The first priority is to assess and stabilize the maternal condition particularly coagulation abnormalities.
- Fetal assessment
- Control of hypertension
- Initiation of magnesium sulfate
- Plan the delivery process.

Patients ≥ 34 weeks gestation should be delivered immediately. In patients less than 34 weeks and without proven lung maturity, glucocorticoids should be given for fetal benefits and delivery planned within 48 hours provided no worsening of maternal or fetal status occurs. In patients with a favorable cervix, regardless of the length of gestation should undergo induction of labor with either oxytocin or prostaglandins. Elective cesarean section should be considered in patients with very early gestation who have an unfavorable cervix. In addition the following precautions should be taken for a patient with HELLP syndrome requiring cesarean section.[4]

- General anesthesia is preferred if platelet count < 75,000/mm.[3]
- Platelets 5-10 units should be transfused before surgery if platelet count < 50,000/mm.[3]
- Vesicouterine peritoneum (bladder flap) should be left open.
- Subfascial drain should be put.
- Secondary closure of skin incision or subcutaneous drain.
- Postoperative transfusions should be given as needed.
- Close monitoring for at least 48 hours postpartum.

  For pain management during labor, intravenous narcotics can be given to achieve analgesia. Local infiltration can be used during vaginal deliveries and vaginal repairs. Pudendal block should be avoided due to potential for unrecognised bleeding into this area. Regional anesthesia should be used with caution in patients with low platelet count. In the postpartum period, these patients require close hemodynamic monitoring for 48 hours and serial laboratory evaluation for worsening of abnormalities.

Subcapsular Liver Hematoma

The clinical features include referred pain from phrenic nerve, hepatomegaly and features of peritoneal irritation. Pain to the pericardium, peritoneum, pleura, shoulder, gallbladder and esophagus are consistent with referred pain from the phrenic nerve.[4] Diagnosis is confirmed by the use of ultrasound, CT scan or MRI. A hemodynamically stable patient (unruptured hematoma) requires close hemodynamic monitoring, serial evaluation of coagulation profile and serial evaluation of the size of hematoma and can be kept on conservative management. Whereas on the other hand, a patient with suspected rupture or a hemodynamically unstable patient requires immediate intervention in the form of an emergency laparotomy with a multidisciplinary approach involving the general surgeon and the vascular surgeon. These patients require correction of coagulopathy, massive blood transfusions, packaging and drainage. Despite immediate intervention maternal and fetal mortality is > 50%.

CHRONIC HYPERTENSION

Chronic hypertension complicates as many as 5% of pregnancies. It is characterized by a history of high blood pressure before pregnancy, elevation of blood pressure during first 20 weeks of pregnancy or high blood pressure that lasts longer than 12 weeks after delivery. It is classified as: [28]

Mild: Systolic blood pressure ≥ 140 mm Hg
                     Diastolic blood pressure ≥ 90 mm Hg

Severe: Systolic blood pressure ≥ 180 mm Hg
                Diastolic blood pressure ≥ 110 mm Hg

In women with chronic hypertension an attempt should be made to look for any underlying disorder by appropriate history, physical examination and laboratory tests. The Table 15.6 gives the causes of chronic hypertension.[29]

Table 15.6: Etiology of chronic hypertension
Idiopathic
Essential hypertension
Vascular disorders
Renovascular hypertension
Aortic coarctation
Endocrine disorders
Diabetes mellitus
Hyperthyroidism
Pheochromocytoma
Primary hyperaldosteronism
Hyperparathyroidism
Cushing's syndrome
Renal disorders
Diabetic nephropathy
Chronic renal failure
Acute renal failure
Tubular necrosis
Cortical necrosis
Chronic pyelonephritis
Chronic glomerulonephritis
Nephrotic syndrome
Polycystic kidney
Connective tissue disorders
Systemic lupus erythematosus

End Organ Damage

Next step is to evaluate the end organ damage to *eyes, kidneys, and heart.*
Abnormal Renal Function
Proteinuria (>300 mg/24 hour, > 1+ dip stick, > 30 mg/dl)
Creatinine Clearance < 110 ml/min, serum creatinine > 0.8 mg/dl.

Cardiac Involvement

Left ventricular hypertrophy.

Eye Involvement

Retinopathy

Maternal and Fetal Risks

Pregnancy complicated with chronic hypertension may be associated with several adverse outcomes including premature birth, intrauterine growth restriction, fetal demise, placental abruption, superimposed preeclampsia, worsening or malignant hypertension, cerebral hemorrhage, cardiac decompensation, renal deterioration or failure and cesarean delivery. The incidence of these potential adverse effects is related to the degree and duration of hypertension and associated end organ damage. The outcome is usually good in patients with mild chronic hypertension and no other complication but the outlook is less favorable in women with severe hypertension early in pregnancy and in those with evidence of end-organ compromise.

To make the diagnosis of superimposed preeclampsia, the patient should have increasing or difficult to control blood pressure, HELLP syndrome, symptoms such as headache, right upper quadrant pain, or visual disturbances, new onset proteinuria, or significant increase in preexisting proteinuria.

Management

Ideally these women should be evaluated before conception so that blood pressure is optimized and lifestyle changes are initiated. Once the diagnosis is made the management is individualized. The general guidelines are:

Lifestyle Modifications

The patient is advised to adopt a healthy lifestyle and maintain an ideal body weight. She should also be advised to avoid alcohol, tobacco and restrict sodium intake to 2-3 gm/day.

Antihypertensives

Women with sustained blood pressure ≥180/110 mm Hg or those with end organ damage may be at higher risk for serious complications and are candidates for antihypertensive medication,[30] however clinicians use a lower threshold of 150/100 mm Hg for instituting therapy though the evidence so far indicates that it is not beneficial in improving perinatal outcome. Choice of antihypertensives is same as discussed in section on preeclampsia.

Antenatal Visits

Women with mild hypertension should be seen every 2-4 weeks till 34 weeks and weekly thereafter whereas women with severe disease need to be seen every 2-3 weeks till 28 weeks and weekly thereafter. At each visit the women is inquired about symptoms of preeclampsia and her blood pressure, urine protein and fetal growth is checked. Antepartum fetal surveillance is started at 32-34 weeks with weekly NST/BPP and USG for fetal growth every 4 weeks, for women with mild hypertension. For women with severe hypertension USG is generally recommended every 4 weeks after 26 weeks and weekly NST/BPP after 28 weeks. On the other hand ACOG recommends if growth restriction is not present and superimposed preeclampsia is excluded these tests are not indicated.[31] The patient needs to be hospitalized if blood pressure is uncontrolled or she develops superimposed preeclampsia.

Delivery

The timing of delivery depends on the development of confounding complications, women with uncomplicated chronic hypertension of a mild degree generally can be delivered vaginally at 39-40 weeks, whereas women with severe hypertension should be delivered at 38 weeks. On the other hand delivery should be considered in all women with superimposed severe preeclampsia at or beyond 28 weeks of gestation and in women with mild superimposed preeclampsia at or beyond 37 weeks of gestation. Women with chronic hypertension complicated by significant cardiovascular or renal disease require special attention to fluid load and urine output because they may be susceptible to fluid overload with pulmonary edema.

REFERENCES

1. Sibai BM. Chronic hypertension during pregnancy. In Sciarra J (Ed). Gynecology and Obstetrics. Philadelphia: JB Lippincott 1989; 1-8.
2. Report of the National High Blood Pressure Education Program Working Group on Pregnancy. Am J Obstet Gynecol 2000; 183:S1-S22 (Level III).
3. Bdolah Y, Karumanchi SA, Sach's BP. Recent advances in understanding of preeclampsia. Croat Med J 2005; 46: 728-36.
4. Moldenhauer JS, Sibai BM. Hypertensive disorders of pregnancy. In Gibbs RS, Karlan BY, Haney AF, Nygaard Y, Danforth's (Eds) Obstetrics and Gynecology, 10th edn. Lippincott Williams and Wilkins, 257-71.
5. Agustin Conde-Agudelo, MPH*, José Villar, MPH, Marshall Lindheimer. World Health Organization Systematic Review of Screening Tests for Preeclampsia Obstetrics and Gynecology 2004;104:1367-91.
6. Levine RJ, et al. Trial of calcium to prevent preeclampsia. N Engl J Med 1997;337:69.
7. RUANO, Rodrigo, FONTES, Rosana S and ZUGAIB, Marcelo. Prevention of preeclampsia with low-dose aspirin: A systematic review and meta-analysis of the main randomized controlled trials. Clinics [online]. 2005, vol. 60, no. 5 [cited 2008-08-30],407-14.
8. Rumbold A, Duley L, Crowther CA, Haslam RR. Antioxidants for preventing pre-eclampsia. Cochrane Database Syst Rev. 2008;(1):CD004227.
9. Barton JR, Witlin AG,Sibai BM. Management of mild preeclampsia. Clin Obstet Gynecol 1999;42:465-69.
10. Barron WM, Heckerling P, Hibbard JU, Fisher S. Reducing unnecessary coagulation testing in hypertensive disorders of pregnancy. Obstet Gynecol 1999; 94:364-70.
11. Diagnosis and Management of Preeclampsia and Eclampsia. Clinical Management Guidelines for Obstetrician Gynecologist. ACOG practice Bulletin, Number 33, January 2002; 159-64.
12. Haddad B, Sibai BM. Expectant management of severe preeclampsia: Proper candidates and pregnancy outcome. Clin Obstet Gynecol 2005;48(2):430-40.
13. Cabrera ML, Todd McDiarmid, Mackler Does bed rest for preeclampsia improve neonatal outcomes? Journal of Family Practice 2007;56:938.
14. Abalos E, Duley L, Steyn DW. Antihypertensive drug therapy for mild to moderate hypertension during pregnancy. Cochrane Database of Systematic Reviews 2001, Issue 2, Art No CD 002252.

15. von Dadelszen P, Magee LA. Antihypertensive medications in management of gestational hypertension-preeclampsia. Clin Obstet Gynecol 2005;48(2):441-59.
16. Greer IA. Pregnancy induced hypertension. In Turbull's Obstetrics, 4rd edn. Chamberlain G, Steer PJ. Churchill Livingstone, Edinburgh, 2005;333-53.
17. Wagner LK. Diagnosis and management of preeclampsia. Am Fam Physician 2004;70: 2317-24.
18. Baha MS. Magnesium sulphate prophylaxis in preeclampsis: Evidence from randomized trials. Clinical Obstetrics and Gynecology 48:478-88.
19. Tuffnell DJ, Shennan AH, Waugh JJ, Walker JJ. The management of severe preeclampsia/eclampsia. London (UK): Royal College of Obstetricians and Gynaecologists; 2006 Mar. 11 p. (Guideline; no. 10(A).
20. Walfish A, Hallak M. Hypertension. In: High Risk Pregnancy Management Options 3rd edn. James DK, Steer PJ, Weiner CP, Gonik B, Philadelphia Elsevier Inc, 772-89.
21. Shennan A. Hypertensive disorders. In dewhurst's Textbook of Gynecology and Obstetrics, 7th Ed. Edmond K. USA, Blackwell Publishing 2007;227-35.
22. Hypertensive Disorders in Pregnancy. In William's Obstetrics, 22nd edn Cunningham FG, Leveno KJ, Bloom SL, Hauth JC, Gilstrap III LC, Wenstrom KD, Mc Graw Hill, New York, 2005;761-800.
23. Sibai BM. Diagnosis and management of gestational hypertension and preeclampsia. Obstet Gynecol 2003;102:181-92.
24. Eclampsia Trial Collaborative Group. Which anticonvulsant for women with eclampsia? Evidence from the collaborative eclampsia trial. Lancet 1995;345:1455-63.
25. Sibai BM. The HELLP syndrome (Hemolysis, elevated liver enzymes and low platelets): Much ado about nothing? Am J Obstet Gynecol 1990;162:311-16.
26. Weinstein L Preeclampsia/Eclampsia with hemolysis, elevated liver enzymes, and thrombocytopenia. Obstet Gynecol 1985;66:657-60.
27. Sibai BM, Taslimi MM, El- Nazera, et al. Maternal-Perinatal outcome associated with the syndrome of hemolysis, elevated liver enzymes and low platelets in severe preeclampsia-eclampsia. Am J Obstet Gynaecol 1986;155:501-09.
28. Ferrer RL, Sibai BM, Mulrow CD, Chiquette E, Stevens KR, Cornell J. Management of mild chronic hypertension during pregnancy: A review. Obstet Gynecol 2000;96:849-60.
29. Miller DA. Hypertension in pregnancy. In Current Diagnosis and treatment: Obstetrics and Gynecology, 10th edn. Decherney AH, Nathan L, Goodwin TM, Laufer N. New York, McGraw Hill, 2007;318-27.
30. Sibai BM, Anderson GD. Pregnancy outcome of intensive therapy in severe hypertension in first trimester. Obstet Gynecol 1986;67:517-22.
31. Chronic hypertension in pregnancy. Obstet Gynaecol 2001;98:177-85.

15

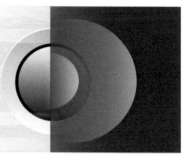

Diabetes Mellitus with Pregnancy 16

Manju Puri, Kazila Bhutia

INTRODUCTION

Diabetes mellitus is a metabolic disorder consequent to decrease in insulin secretion or increase in insulin resistance or both, resulting in abnormalities of carbohydrate, protein and lipid metabolism. Diabetes mellitus in pregnancy is associated with increased maternal and fetal morbidity and mortality.

It is classified broadly into 2 types—pregestational and gestational diabetes mellitus. Pregestational diabetes mellitus can be type 1 and type 2. Women with diabetes mellitus prior to pregnancy, i.e. pregestational diabetes mellitus may have difficulties in conceiving and pregnancy *per se* may worsen the diabetic status of the woman and precipitate certain diabetic complications. Fetuses born to diabetic mothers are at increased risk of congenital malformations, metabolic and developmental problems. There has been a significant increase in the prevalence of gestational diabetes mellitus (GDM) as well as type 2 diabetes mellitus over the past few decades.

Pregnant women with diabetes mellitus should be managed by combined efforts of a team consisting of obstetrician, endocrinologist, neonatologist and dietician. However, it is essential for all obstetricians to have adequate knowledge of this disorder to provide optimum care and treatment to pregnant women with diabetes mellitus even in lesser set ups.

PREVALENCE OF DIABETES MELLITUS

The epidemic of diabetes is now spreading to become a pandemic affecting people from both developed and developing countries. This increase in prevalence is consequent to obesity, sedentary lifestyle and increasing life expectancy. The global prevalence of diabetes mellitus in 2000 was 2.8% which is likely to increase to 4.4% in 2030.[1] The reported prevalence of diabetes mellitus in pregnancy in United States ranges from 1-14%.[2] A statistically significant increase in prevalence of diabetes mellitus during pregnancy has been reported over time in United States.[3] Of all cases of diabetes mellitus complicating pregnancy, gestational diabetes mellitus accounts for 88%.[4] In India the prevalence of GDM ranges from 0.25–5.5%.[5-9] However, in a study conducted by Seshiah et al (2004)[10], a prevalence rate of 18.9% was reported. The women who had gestational diabetes mellitus in previous pregnancy have a 33.5% likelihood of recurrence in subsequent pregnancy.[11]

CLASSIFICATION OF DIABETES MELLITUS IN PREGNANCY

Priscilla White[12] published first best known classification of diabetes in pregnancy, which was subsequently modified by her in 1965 and 1971 in order to predict effect of severity of diabetes mellitus on pregnancy outcome. However, this classification was too cumbersome for general use and is no longer considered in management decisions.

Recently diabetic pregnancies have been classified by the American Diabetes Association (ADA) and WHO based on the etiology.[13,14] The WHO classification differs from ADA by additionally recognizing impaired glucose tolerance even before pregnancy. Table 16.1 gives the ADA classification of diabetes in pregnancy.

Table 16.1: Classification of diabetes in pregnancy
I Pregestational diabetes
-   Type 1 diabetes (insulin dependent)
-   Type 2 diabetes (noninsulin dependent)
-   Secondary diabetes
II Gestational diabetes
III Impaired glucose tolerance during pregnancy.

Pregestational diabetes mellitus affects the women before pregnancy whereas gestational diabetes mellitus develops during pregnancy and resolves after delivery. Pregestational diabetes mellitus can be Type 1, i.e. insulin dependent or Type 2, i.e. noninsulin dependent. Secondary diabetes is also a form of pregestational diabetes mellitus but due to causes like pancreatitis, cystic fibrosis, hemochromatosis, pancreaotomy, neoplasm, hyperthyroidism, Cushing's syndrome, Klinefelter's syndrome, etc. Impaired glucose tolerance occurs when the glucose level reaches 140 mg/dl to 199 mg/dl at the 2 hour value during oral glucose tolerance test (OGTT).

Carbohydrate Metabolism in Pregnancy[15,16,25]

Pregnancy is a diabetogenic condition due to alteration in carbohydrate metabolism due to hormones. Several changes in glucose metabolism are observed during pregnancy. Effect of pregnancy on carbohydrate metabolism is shown in flow chart 16.1.

Development of insulin resistance is a major change. There is an approximately 50% reduction in insulin sensitivity by third trimester. This change is due to several hormones of maternal and placental origin. Maternal hormones are raised levels of estrogen, progesterone, prolactin and cortisol and placental hormones are human placental lactogen (HPL) and placental growth hormone variant. Other factors contributing to insulin resistance are increase in caloric intake and increased body weight during pregnancy. Development of insulin resistance serves to shunt nutrients preferentially to the growing fetus, while simultaneously allowing for the accumulation of caloric storage in maternal adipose tissue.

Flow chart 16.1: Effect of pregnancy on carbohydrate metabolism

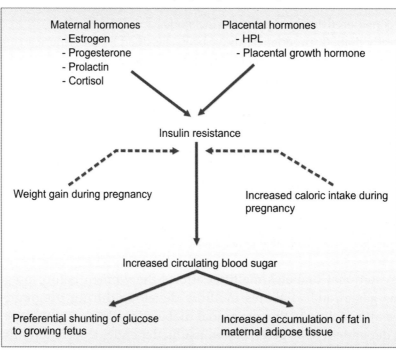

In fasting state two important additional changes in maternal carbohydrate metabolism occur, i.e. decrease in plasma glucose concentration and increase in fat catabolism. This decrease in plasma glucose further accelerates preferential shunting of nutrients to fetomaternal unit even at low circulating levels of plasma glucose. Simultaneously, fat catabolism or lipolysis is stimulated to ensure adequate nutrient supply to the mother. Hence, this ultimately ensures adequate nutrient supply to the mother and fetus but predisposes the pregnant woman to ketosis at the time of starvation.

Carbohydrate Metabolism in Diabetic Pregnancy[15,17,25]

Women who fail to sufficiently increase insulin secretion from pancreas to overcome pregnancy induced insulin resistance, develop postprandial hyperglycemia and subsequently gestational diabetes mellitus. This occurs because the insulin resistance in pregnancy imposes an additional burden on the already depleted beta cells. There is a three-fold increase in insulin requirement in women with type 1 diabetes mellitus in late pregnancy. In pregnant women with type 2 diabetes mellitus who already have pre-existing insulin resistance, there is further deterioration due to pregnancy-related insulin insensitivity and most of these women either require insulin early in pregnancy or their insulin requirement increases.

EFFECT OF PREGNANCY ON DIABETES MELLITUS[18,19,25]

There is a risk of progression of diabetic complications like established severe proliferative retinopathy and advanced nephropathy especially if coexisting with hypertension. Pregnancy is poorly tolerated by women who have severe autonomic dysfunction and those with preexisting active coronary artery disease. Early pregnancy nausea, vomiting and infections mainly urinary tract infection may precipitate diabetic ketoacidosis and result in poor perinatal outcome in women with preexisting nephropathy.

EFFECT OF DIABETES MELLITUS ON PREGNANCY

The abnormal metabolic environment created by hyperglycemia has a profound impact on both the mother and the fetus. Maternal effects include obstetric and medical complications.

Maternal Effects: Obstetric Complications[20,25]

Fertility is impaired in women with uncontrolled diabetes mellitus. However, in women who conceive, the incidence of spontaneous abortions is high especially in those with poor control of diabetes. The prevalence of preeclampsia is directly proportional to the severity of the diabetes and with the presence of proteinuria at the onset of pregnancy. Often diabetic pregnancies are complicated by hydramnios, probably due to fetal polyuria resulting from fetal hyperglycemia.

Iatrogenic and spontaneous preterm delivery is increased in pregnant women with diabetes as compared with nondiabetic pregnant women (22% vs 3%, 16% vs 11% respectively). One-third of all preterm deliveries are due to

16

Diabetes Mellitus with Pregnancy

325

hypertensive complications. This increased incidence of preterm labor may be attributed to hydramnios, poor glycemic control and infections.

Maternal Effects: Medical Complications

Various microvascular complications coexisting with pregestational diabetes may get exacerbated in pregnancy.

Retinopathy

The prevalence of retinopathy in diabetes depends upon the duration of the diabetes. The prevalence was found to be 17% in those where diabetes was diagnosed before the age of 30 years and duration of disease was 5 years. This progressively increased to 90% with increase in duration of disease to 15 years.[21] There are two well-characterized stages of retinopathy: non-proliferative or background retinopathy and proliferative retinopathy. In pregnancy the progression of retinopathy depends on factors like duration of diabetes, severity of preexisting disease, presence of hypertensive disorders, degree of metabolic control as well as rapidity in normalization of blood glucose. Hence, preconception evaluation of retinopathy is mandatory for all diabetic women who are planning a pregnancy, to initiate timely management before conception. If established retinopathy is there, rapid normalization of glucose should be avoided as it is associated with progression of retinopathy. Evaluation for presence of any high-risk factors should also be done so that intensive monitoring can be done.[22]

Nephropathy[23]

Early diabetic nephropathy and mild to moderate renal dysfunction (serum creatinine 1.4mg/dl and creatinine clearance over 90 ml/min) does not progress during pregnancy, whereas more advanced nephropathy with coexisting hypertension may deteriorate. In patients with chronic renal failure or advanced proteinuria, the glomerular filtration rate may decline rapidly during pregnancy. Overt nephropathy is defined as persistent proteinuria (more than 500 mg/24 hours of total protein or more than 300 mg/24 hours of urinary albumin excretion) observed in the first 20 weeks of pregnancy in the absence of urinary tract infection.[24] This condition adversely affects fetal and maternal outcome. Patients on ACE inhibitors should be switched over to methyldopa after confirmation of pregnancy due to the possibility of its teratogenic effects.

Neuropathy[23, 25]

Pregnancy does not worsen the neuropathy, except in women with preexisting carpel tunnel syndrome and those with advanced autonomic neuropathy and severe gastroparesis. The occurrence of gastroparesis is the most worrisome aspect of diabetic neuropathy, as it is associated with severe maternal and fetal morbidity and needs special consideration during preconception period. Preeclampsia, hypoglycemic attacks, ketoacidosis, congenital malformations, polyhydramnios, IUGR, preterm delivery, fetal loss and perinatal mortality are found to be almost double in these patients as compared to controls. Hence, pregnancy is a relative contraindication in patients with severe gastroparesis.

Cardiovascular Disease [23]

All diabetic women with proven preexisting macrovascular disease should undergo extensive cardiovascular evaluation by a cardiologist before conception. Revascularization should be considered if significant myocardial ischemia is detected which may significantly improve maternal and perinatal outcomes. Even though, recent review of a literature on pregnancy with arteriosclerotic heart disease suggests that it is not associated with a poor prognosis but pregnancy should be considered a relative contraindication in these patients considering a high mortality associated with it.

Diabetic Ketoacidosis [26]

Diabetic ketoacidosis (DKA) is one of the life-threatening complications for both the mother and the fetus in a diabetic pregnancy. The overall prevalence of DKA is difficult to evaluate. Various workers report a prevalence ranging from 1–10%. DKA is more common in type 1 and type 2 diabetes mellitus whereas it is rare in GDM, and when it presents with GDM, the possibility of unrecognized preexisting diabetes should be suspected.[27] The obstetrician must be aware of various factors that precipitate DKA, so that adequate preventive measures can be taken to prevent the onset of this disease process. The various high-risk factors include hyperemesis gravidarum, underlying infection, use of beta sympathomimetics, poor patient compliance, insulin pump failure or error in clinical judgement.

DKA has classical clinical findings; hence there is no better substitute for a detailed history and physical examination for diagnosing DKA. Patients usually present with vomiting, polyuria, hyperventilation, altered mental status, weakness and dehydration. This clinical presentation can be further confirmed with laboratory findings. There is hyperglycemia (plasma blood glucose level of ≥ 300 mg/dl sometimes at even > 200 mg/dl), acidosis (pH < 7.3), anion gap with acidosis, elevated base deficit on blood gas analysis, increased serum and urinary ketones, dyselectrolytemia and decreased serum bicarbonate levels ≤ 15 mEq/l. Due to dehydration and renal failure blood urea and serum creatinine level may be elevated.

Treatment involves aggressive fluid management, insulin administration and identification and treatment of precipitating factor. The initial fluid used for replacement is normal saline. Overall fluid deficit can be calculated as 100 ml/kg body weight.[28] Isotonic normal saline should be administered at rate of 1000 to 2000 ml/hour for first 1 to 2 hours followed by 250-500 ml/hour so that 75% of fluid deficit can be corrected over a 24 hour period. Isotonic normal saline can be used till glucose level is < 250 mg/dl, following which 5% dextrose should be started. Regular insulin with a bolus dose of 0.1U/kg followed by 0.1U/kg/hour as maintenance dosage should be started. If glucose level does not fall by 50 to 75 mg/dl over the first hour, then hourly infusion rate should be doubled. Dyselectrolytemia should be corrected. Serum potassium level should be maintained at 4 to 5 mEq/l. The need for replacement of other electrolytes like magnesium and calcium is debatable. Role of administration of bicarbonate for correction of metabolic acidosis in DKA is also debatable.

It is important that no intervention should be done for fetal indication unless the mother is stabilized so that she can withstand the process of delivery. The main aim is to first treat and stabilize the mother because most of the fetal heart rate abnormalities will be corrected with the stabilization of maternal status.

Fetal and Neonatal Effects

The congenital malformations are seen in 4 to 10% of diabetic pregnancies. The incidence is three to five times higher than in the general population and account for about 50% of all perinatal deaths in this population. Glycosylated hemoglobin (HbA1c) values of greater than 8% are associated with three to six times greater risk of congenital malformations in the fetus than when maintained at less than this cut off point.[29-31] However a value of HbA1c in the normal range (4-6%) and positively not more than 1% of the upper limit of normal range, i.e. 7% is desirable for a woman planning to conceive.[39] Malformations often involve the heart and central nervous system and are potentially lethal. Caudal regression syndrome, although very rare, is seen almost exclusively in diabetic pregnancies, and is sometimes associated with failure of femur to develop normally.[32] Neural tube defects are also more common compared to that in general population. Hence, optimizing diabetic control before conception is essential to lower the rate of congenital malformations and miscarriages to that of the background population.

Fetuses who are exposed to chronic maternal hyperglycemia are macrosomic (birth weight > 4kg).[33] Incidence of fetal macrosomia is 45% as compared to 8-9% in controls. The risk of shoulder dystocia and operative intervention is increased with fetal macrosomia and is associated with increase in perinatal asphyxia and birth trauma. On the contrary, diabetic vasculopathy and excessively tight control of diabetes mellitus in pregnancy has been linked to intrauterine growth restriction. The incidence of intrauterine fetal death and unexplained stillbirths is also higher, usually after 36 weeks and particularly in women with poor glycemic control. It is probably due to poor placental perfusion consequent to villus edema.[33]

Babies born to diabetic mothers are at increased risk of neonatal metabolic complications such as hypoglycemia, hyperbilirubinemia, hypocalcemia and hypomagnesemia. Respiratory distress syndrome (RDS) is more common in babies of diabetic mothers, compared with gestational age matched infants born before 38.5 weeks. The long-term effects include diabetes mellitus in later life, neurological deficits and childhood obesity.[34]

SCREENING AND DIAGNOSIS

Screening[11,35]

Despite decades of research, there is no consensus regarding the optimal approach to screening for gestational diabetes. The major issues include whether screening should be universal or selective, timing of screening and method of screening. Fourth International Workshop Conference on gestational diabetes mellitus (1997), recommended a selective screening strategy based on risk assessment for detecting gestational diabetes mellitus.

Risk assessment should be done at the first prenatal visit. Women with clinical features consistent with high risk of gestational diabetes mellitus like marked obesity, strong family history of diabetes, prior gestational diabetes mellitus, persistent glycosuria, macrosomia, unexplained stillbirth, hydramnios, congenitally malformed baby, etc. should undergo glucose testing as soon as feasible. If they are not found to have diabetes mellitus at initial screening, they should be retested between 24 and 28 weeks of gestation. Women of average risk (Hispanic, African, South or East Asian origins) should have testing at 24 to 28 weeks of gestation. Low-risk status requires no glucose testing, but this category is limited to women with:

- Age < 25 years.
- Normal prepregnant weight.
- Not a member of ethnic group with high prevalence of gestational diabetes mellitus (like women of Hispanic, African, Native American, South or East Asian, or Pacific Islands ancestry).
- No known history of diabetes in first degree relatives.
- No history of abnormal glucose metabolism.
- No history of poor obstetrical outcome.

Screening for gestational diabetes mellitus can be done either by one step or two step approach.

Perform diagnostic OGTT (oral glucose tolerance test) without prior GCT (Glucose Challenge Test). This approach may be cost-effective in high-risk patients or populations. The test should be done in the morning after an overnight fast of more than 8 hours after at least 3 days of unrestricted diet, consuming more than or equal to 150 gm of carbohydrate per day. Patients should not smoke before the test and should remain seated during the test. This is to avoid carbohydrate depletion, which could cause spuriously high values on the OGTT. A fasting blood glucose sample is drawn. The pregnant woman is given 100 gram of glucose in juice and the samples drawn at 1, 2 and 3 hour respectively. The recommended criteria for interpretation of oral glucose tolerance test are described in Table 16.2.

Table 16.2: Interpretation of OGTT[35]				
Status	O'Sullivan and Mahan (1964) 100gm (3hr) mg/dl	NDDG (1979) 100gm(3hr) mg/dl	C & C (1982) 100gm(3hr) mg/dl	ADA&ACOG(1997) 75gm(2hr) 100gm(3hr) mg/dl mg/dl
F	90	105	95	95 95
1hour	165	190	180	180 180
2hour	145	165	155	155 155
3hour	125	145	140	- 140

NDDG- National Diabetes Data Group, C&C- Carpenter and Coustan, ADA- American Diabetes Association.

Diagnosis of diabetes mellitus is made if two or more values are abnormal on 100 gm oral glucose tolerance test during pregnancy. All values mentioned above depict plasma blood sugar levels except O'Sullivan and Mahan which mentions venous whole blood. The blood sugar values in mg/dl can be converted to mmol/l by dividing the value by 18, e.g. 180 mg/dl=10mmol/l. Measurement of blood glucose level in capillary blood by glucometer has made screening test easy and simple as it can be done in office setting and does not require elaborate laboratory facilities. It is important to know that capillary blood glucose levels are comparable to venous blood glucose levels during fasting state but are higher after meals.[11] In the 4th International Workshop Conference on GDM in 1997, a consensus was reached on replacing NDDG criteria by C&C criteria which has lower threshold values for the diagnosis of GDM so as to diagnose more cases of GDM.[36]

Two Step Approach[11]

In this approach the first step is to subject all women to a glucose challenge test and then a selected few to OGTT.

1st step – In this test pregnant woman is administered 50 gram of glucose irrespective of the time of last meal and the blood sample is drawn after 1 hour (A cut off value of plasma blood glucose of $\geq$ 140 mg/dl identifies 80% of all women with GDM whereas a value of $\geq$ 130 mg/dl identifies 90% of all women with GDM.

2nd step – A diagnostic OGTT (oral glucose tolerance test) is performed on the subset of women with GCT value of more than the threshold value ≥ 130 mg/dl.
(It is important to note that if the GCT value is > 200 mg/dl, OGTT should not be done).

Diagnostic Criteria for Diabetes during Pregnancy

According to American Diabetes Association (2004) the criteria for diagnosis of overt diabetes during pregnancy is as follows:[37]

1. Random plasma glucose level >200mg/dl and classic symptoms like polydipsia, polyuria and unexplained weight loss.
2. Fasting blood glucose >125mg/dl.
3. Two or more abnormal values on 100 gm oral glucose tolerance test during pregnancy.

This diagnostic criteria is the same as in nonpregnant diabetic women except that in nonpregnant women a 75 gm oral GTT is done.

If a pregnant woman reports for the first time in 3rd trimester, she may be screened with GCT in the absence of high-risk factors. However in those with high-risk factors for diabetes mellitus, OGTT may be done after initial screening with fasting and postprandial blood sugar levels.

Management of Pregnancy with Diabetes Mellitus

The management of pregnancy in women with diabetes mellitus remains a challenging problem. A multidisciplinary team approach consisting of obstetrician, dietician, endocrinologist and pediatrician should be followed. The management should be initiated from the preconception period and continued till the postpartum period. The plan of management of pregnant women with diabetes mellitus is outlined in flow chart 16.2 with regard to specific considerations in addition to the routine management of a normal pregnant woman.

Preconception Counseling[23]

Goal of preconception counseling is to optimize the fetomaternal outcome of pregnancy in a diabetic mother. Preconception counseling and management should include the following:
- Emphasis on the fact that it is a high-risk pregnancy.
- Need for regular follow ups and compliance to treatment.
- Evaluation of end organ damage at the first visit.

The various investigations advised for evaluation of end organ damage are listed as below:

Diabetic nephropathy: 24 hour urinary protein, creatinine clearance, BUN and urine culture.

Diabetic retinopathy: Fundus examination.

Flow chart 16.2: Management of pregnancy with diabetes mellitus

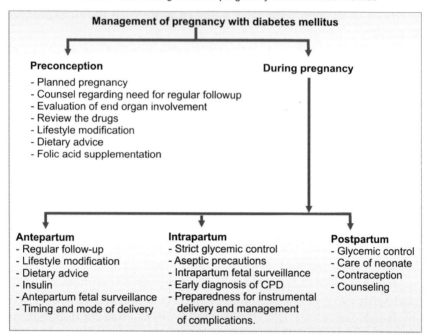

Cardiovascular system: Blood pressure is recorded. Those with pre-existing diabetes of more than 10 years, presence of hypertension or vasculopathy should be evaluated with EKG. Any suspicion of presence of coronary artery disease should be further evaluated by echocardiography, stress test, etc.

Autonomic dysfunction: Presence of symptoms like excessive nausea, vomiting, lack of awareness of hypoglycemia and orthostatic hypotension should prompt further evaluation for autonomic dysfunction.

- Explain to the couple the need to plan pregnancy with a good glycemic control so as to minimize the risk of congenital anomalies in the newborn. In women with good glycemic control HbA1c level should be in the normal range (4–6%)[38] and positively not more than 1% of the upper limit of normal range, i.e. 7%.[39] The premeal plasma blood glucose level of 80-110 mg/dl and 2 hour postprandial target of less than 155 mg/dl is optimum.[40]
- When pregnancy is planned in a patient on oral hypoglycemic agents, patient is switched over to insulin therapy. Oral hypoglycemic agents are not currently recommended during pregnancy because of lack of adequate information regarding their safety in pregnancy. However, a recent metaanalysis suggests that use of oral hypoglycemics is not associated with increased risk of congenital malformations.[41] In addition it is essential that all medications should be checked and discontinued if not essential or teratogenic.
- Lifestyle modification in the form of weight management, daily exercise, cessation of smoking and reduced alcohol intake is advised.
- Folic acid supplementation in the dose of 5 mg daily for the prevention of neural tube defects is prescribed for 3 months prior to conception.

Potential contraindications to pregnancy in diabetic women include coronary artery disease, untreated proliferative retinopathy, serious renal insufficiency or proteinuria, and severe gastroenteropathy. These women should be adviced against planning a pregnancy.

MANAGEMENT DURING PREGNANCY

Antepartum Considerations

Patient should be registered as early as possible and advised to attend antenatal clinic regularly. The frequency of follow up depends on the glycemic control and any coexisting obstetric complications. In the first visit, the patient should be thoroughly evaluated for any end organ damage particularly retinopathy and nephropathy. Preexisting retinopathy may progress rapidly in pregnancy. Therefore, medical termination of pregnancy may be offered to a pregnant woman with retinopathy requiring laser therapy.[42] Screening for nephropathy is done with an overnight or 24 hour urine sample for albuminuria or an albumin/creatinine ratio on an early morning sample of urine.[43] Patients with preexisting microalbuminuria are more likely to develop preeclampsia.[44,45] If renal function is significantly impaired (creatinine > 3.6 mg/dl), the woman is at an increased risk of requiring dialysis during pregnancy, so MTP should be offered to these women in early pregnancy. Evidence of macrovascular disease should be looked for through detailed history and examination. The woman should be subjected to detailed cardiovascular assessment if required. Significant coronary artery disease should be treated before pregnancy.[46] Thyroid function should be measured in all women with type 1 diabetes mellitus as thyroid abnormalities are common in diabetics and may adversely affect pregnancy outcome.[47] The possibility of any other coexistent autoimmune diseases (e.g. celiac disease) in women with type 1 diabetes mellitus should also be considered.[48]

Self-monitoring of blood sugar is advocated (four to six times per day). The metabolic goal during pregnancy is premeal plasma blood glucose level of 70-105 mg/dl or 60-95 mg/dl of whole blood before meals and no higher than a plasma level of 130 mg/dl or whole blood level of 120 mg/dl at 2 hours postprandial.[49, 50] The HbA1c concentration should be monitored every 4 to 6 weeks with the goal of maintaining it at a normal level (< 6%).[49, 50] Pregnant women with gestational diabetes mellitus can be controlled either on only dietary therapy or on a combined dietary and insulin therapy depending on the degree of derangement. However, eventually as the pregnancy progresses, many women on dietary therapy require insulin therapy. In pregnant women with type 1 diabetes mellitus and type 2 diabetes mellitus, insulin requirement continues to increase as the pregnancy progresses due to metabolic changes associated with pregnancy which have already been described before. All pregnant women with diabetes have more frequent antenatal check ups, the frequency of which can be decided on factors like control of blood sugar levels and any associated complications.

Dietary Therapy[51-53]

Adequate understanding of the importance of dietary therapy by the patient is important, especially the association between certain types of carbohydrates and glucose excursions. A formal consultation with a dietician should be done. The diet should consist of 30 to 35 kcal/kg/day in the form of three major meals and two to three minor meals. The diet should consist of 50–60% carbohydrates, less than 30% fat and adequate amount of dietary fiber. According to ADA, daily caloric intake by a pregnant diabetic woman can be calculated according to the proportion of the current body weight of the woman to prepregnancy ideal body weight for her height. For a woman with current body weight as 80-120% of ideal body weight, the calorie requirement is 30 kcal/kg, compared to 36-40 kcal/kg in women who are < 80% of the desirable body weight, 24 kcal/kg for those who are 120-150% and 12-18 kcal/kg for those who are more than 150% of desirable body weight.

Lifestyle Modifications

Regular physical exercise within tolerable limits should be encouraged.

Oral Hypoglycemic Agents

Till 2000, the use of oral hypoglycemic drugs during pregnancy was contraindicated. It is only recently that the use of oral hypoglycemic agents in pregnancy has been accepted at various scientific fora.[54] A recent randomized study demonstrated that the glycemic control with glyburide and insulin is comparable with a perinatal outcome similar to that in general population.[55]

Sulphonylureas[54,56]

Glyburide: This is a class B drug. It acts by enhancing insulin secretion and peripheral tissue sensitivity to insulin. The usual starting dose of glyburide is 2.5 mg orally daily, which can be increased by 2.5 mg in the following week and thereafter by 5 mg weekly up to a maximum of 20 mg per day to achieve glycemic control. The onset of action is within 2 hours, with a maximal decrease in blood sugar occurring between 3 to 4 hours. The blood glucose lowering effect lasts for 24 hours following a single morning dose in nonfasting diabetic patient. Its absorption is not affected by food intake and it does not cross the placenta. Its main side effect is hypoglycemia which is dose-related. Other side effects are like nausea, heart burn, muscle pain, joint pain, and allergic skin reactions including angioedema. Ideal patient for starting glyburide is a normal weight or an obese diabetic woman who has been hyperglycemic for less than 5 years and willing to follow strict dietary regimen.

Biguanides[54]

Metformin: It is an insulin sensitizer and a class B drug. It crosses the placenta and is also transferred in breast milk. However it has a minimal effect on the fetus. Till date no randomized study has been done to address the effect of use of metformin on organogenesis. Many workers have used this drug in pregnancy with the aim of improving the outcome of pregnancy in women with polycystic ovarian disease without any adverse effects on the baby. Nausea and dyspepsia associated with the use of this drug makes it difficult for the pregnant women to take this in first trimester of pregnancy.

Thiazolidenediones[54]

This is a class C drug and crosses the placenta. No study has been reported till date on the use of this drug in pregnancy.

Oral hypoglycemic agents make an ideal agent to treat early stages of type 2 diabetes mellitus and GDM patients. Glyburide is currently the only drug shown not to cross the placenta and studied clinically in properly designed randomized controlled trials.

Insulin Therapy

In the women with pregestational diabetes, insulin is the mainstay of therapy. The insulin used in the treatment of diabetes mellitus is mostly biosynthetic human insulin. The various types of insulins available are short-acting insulin (regular), rapid acting insulin (insulin analogs like insulin lispro, insulin aspart, insulin glulisine), long-acting insulin (i.e. NPH, Lente or Ultralente) and mixtard containing 30% short-acting insulin and 70% intermediate acting insulin). The onset and duration of each of these types is shown in Table 16.3.[57]

Types	Onset of action (hr)	Peak of action (hr)	Duration of action (hr)
Table 16.3: Types of Insulin			
Rapid-acting			
- Lispro	<0.25	0.5-1.5	3-4
- Insulin aspart	<0.25	0.5-1.5	3-4
Short-acting			
- Regular	0.5-1.0	2-3	3-6
Intermediate-acting			
- NPH (Neutral Protamine Hagedon)	2-4	6-10	10-16
- Lente	3-4	6-12	12-18
Combinations			
- 70/30: 70%NPH, 30% Regular	0.5-1	dual	10-16
- 50/50: 50%NPH, 50% Regular	0.5-1	dual	10-16

Short or rapid-acting insulin is administered before meals to reduce glucose excursions associated with the meal and allow utilization of consumed fuels,

Diabetes Mellitus with Pregnancy

whereas longer acting insulin is basal insulin, used to restrain hepatic gluconeogenesis in between meals and in the fasting state.

When to start insulin [58]

The American Diabetes Association currently recommends insulin therapy when nutritional therapy fails to maintain self-monitored glucose at the levels as shown in table 16.4:

Table 16.4: Blood glucose levels for initiating insulin therapy		
	Whole blood	*Plasma*
Fasting blood glucose	≥ 95 mg/dl	≥ 105 mg/dl
1 hour postprandial blood glucose	≥ 140 mg/dl	≥ 155 mg/dl
2 hour postprandial blood glucose	≥ 120 mg/dl	≥ 130 mg/dl

How to Initiate Insulin Therapy

Pregnant women with type 1 diabetes mellitus lack endogenous insulin secretion so administration of basal exogenous insulin is essential for regulating glycogen breakdown, gluconeogenesis, lipolysis and ketogenesis. Before conception the daily insulin requirement is approximately 0.5 to 1U/kg body weight.[57] In 1st trimester insulin requirement increases to 0.7U/kg pregnant weight of patient, by 2nd trimester it rises to 0.8U/kg which further goes upto 0.9 to 1U/kg pregnant weight per day in the 3rd trimester.[58] Various insulin regimens have been used however none has reproduced the precise insulin secretory pattern of the pancreatic islet. One commonly used regimen consists of twice daily injections of intermediate insulin mixed with short-acting insulin before the morning and evening meal. This regimen prescribes two-thirds of the daily insulin dose in the morning (two-third as intermediate acting and one-third as short-acting) and one-third before the evening meal (one half given as intermediate and one half as short-acting).[57]

In diet controlled type 2 diabetes mellitus and GDM with normal sugar profile, management should start with dietary therapy and exercise, with weekly blood sugar monitoring. Those who fail to maintain optimum blood sugar levels should be started on insulin therapy. Because endogenous insulin secretion continues and is capable of providing some coverage to the meal time calorie intake, insulin is started at a lower dose as compared to type 1 diabetes mellitus. The starting dose of insulin is decided on the degree of derangement of blood sugar profile of the pregnant woman. To compensate for postprandial hyperglycemia, short-acting or rapid-acting insulin can be used. Approximately 1 U of insulin is required for every 30mg/dl rise in blood glucose level above the normal expected level. For example, if a patient's 2 hour postprandial blood glucose level is 200 mg/dl, she needs approximately 2 units of insulin before the meal to bring her closer to the desired level of 130mg/dl.[59] It is prudent to start the woman on smaller doses and then titrate it according to the blood sugar levels. The best treatment regimen is mixtard insulin, a mixture of short-acting and intermediate- or long-acting insulin that is administered once or twice a day and premeal short-acting regular insulin or rapidly acting analogs as required.

A method for deciding initial insulin dose is based on the anticipated carbohydrate content of the meal (carbohydrate counting), the blood glucose reading before and after meal, and any anticipated activity level after the meal. In early pregnancy for every 15 gm of carbohydrate consumed in a meal 1 unit of insulin may suffice, however as pregnancy progresses, the carbohydrate: insulin ratio may decrease to 10:1 or less due to progressively increasing insulin resistance and insulin dose requirement increases accordingly.[25]

It is best for the patient to take the insulin at the same injection site each day to reduce the site specific variation in absorption of insulin. Absorption is most rapid from the abdomen (15–30 minutes) compared to the arm (30–45 minutes) and thigh (45–60 minutes). The patient can be advised to take her breakfast dose at abdomen, lunch and dinner in her arms and her bed time injection in her thigh.[59]

Insulin analogs like insulin lispro which is a rapidly acting insulin, are also available. They have considerable advantage over regular insulin. It can be injected at the start of a meal and the peak effect corresponds to the highest glucose excursion after a meal. This is as compared to regular insulin that must be taken 30 minutes before a meal and has its peak effect in 2 to 4 hours. Regular insulin also has a longer duration of action 6 to 8 hours increasing the likelihood of hypoglycemia long after its injection. So, patient's compliance with insulin lispro injections is 100% as compared to 60% with regular insulin. However, insulin analogs are more expensive than regular insulin.[59,60]

How to titrate insulin[25,61,62]

Insulin dosage should be adjusted according to glycemic trends every 2 to 3 days as assessed by blood glucose profile. Glucose profile is done every 2–3 days. It comprises of 5 or 7 samples. A 5 sample glucose profile includes a fasting sample, 3 postmeal samples and one 2 am sample. Whereas, 7 samples glucose profile includes 2 premeal samples, i.e. prelunch and predinner level as well. The dose of insulin is adjusted till an optimum control is obtained, i.e. a fasting, premeal and 2 am plasma glucose level of ≤ 105 mg/dl (whole blood 60-95 mg/dl) and 2 hour postprandial plasma values of ≤ 130 mg/dl (whole blood <120 mg/dl). If the control is unsatisfactory, potential sources of the problem such as faulty diet, concurrent medication, intercurrent illness or infections, stress, lack of exercise and faulty lifestyle need to be explored and rectified. For a single abnormal blood glucose value, dietary readjustment is advisable.

Antepartum Fetal Surveillance[63-65]

Antepartum fetal surveillance in first trimester aims at accurate dating of pregnancy and a thorough screening for fetal anomalies. Stepwise approach of screening for congenital anomalies begins in 1st trimester. Nuchal translucency, MSAFP, unconjugated estriol and inhibin A is indicated at 10–13 weeks. This is followed by an ultrasonography for fetal morphology at 18–20 week and a fetal echocardiogram at 20 to 22 weeks.

A follow up ultrasound scan at 28 to 30 weeks and 34 to 36 weeks is indicated to identify fetal macrosomia and polyhydramnios. As regards antepartum fetal surveillance there is no data from randomized trials to make specific evidence-based recommendation on type, initiation or frequency of testing. Many institutions initiate routine fetal surveillance at or near term. However, daily fetal movement count or fetal kick count is an inexpensive and easy way to evaluate fetal wellbeing in the third trimester. Perception of more than 10 movements by mother in a 10 hour period is generally considered reassuring. Some authors suggest that daily kick count should be started by 26 to 28 weeks of gestation in pregnancies complicated by diabetes mellitus and those with decreased fetal activity should be evaluated by fetal nonstress testing or biophysical profile (BPP).

Fetal nonstress test (NST) may be initiated twice a week from 34 weeks onwards. It has a positive predictive value of 50–70%. Biophysical profile does not carry as much significance in monitoring pregnant woman with diabetes mellitus as in a nondiabetic pregnant woman because of poor reliability of AFI as a predictor of fetal wellbeing. The current evidence suggests the use of Doppler flow studies in patients with diabetes mellitus who have pregnancies complicated by hypertensive disease, fetal growth restriction or vasculopathy. It is not recommended as a routine method of fetal surveillance.

Timing of Delivery[66]

The primary goal to time delivery is to prevent stillbirth. The risk of unexplained intrauterine death and stillbirth increases after 36 weeks of gestation in pregnant women with diabetes mellitus. However, elective termination of pregnancy has to be weighed against the risk of delayed lung maturity and respiratory distress syndrome.

Insulin treated diabetes

Elective delivery at 38 weeks is indicated with the primary intention of reducing the risk of stillbirth however there are some other additional advantages like reduction of infant size and associated lower rate of shoulder dystocia and cesarean section.

Amniocentesis should be done to document fetal maturity if gestational age is uncertain or elective delivery is done before 38 weeks gestation. Delivery may be carried out even without documented fetal lung maturity if maternal or fetal compromise places the life of mother or fetus at significant risk. Maternal factors like severe preeclampsia, eclampsia and other factors where maternal wellbeing is compromised by continuing the pregnancy and proven severe fetal compromise like intrauterine growth restriction with absent or reversed diastolic flow on Doppler and nonreassuring fetal heart rate pattern at a time when fetal survival after delivery is considered possible are indications for termination of pregnancy.

Mild diet treated gestational diabetes

In these women, the risk of stillbirth is not increased. The decision for elective labor induction depends on estimated fetal weight. Based on Cochrane database, there is little evidence to support elective labor induction at 38 weeks. Although elective labor induction does not increase maternal and fetal risk, however the benefits of this practice also remains unclear.[67] These women can carry their pregnancies to term, i.e. 40 weeks.

Mode of Delivery[63,64]

Vaginal delivery is preferable unless there is an obstetric or medical contraindication. Elective cesarean section should be considered for macrosomic fetuses to prevent the potential risk of shoulder dystocia and birth trauma. The ACOG considers elective cesarean delivery if estimated fetal weight is more than 4500 gm in a diabetic mother. In women with diabetes and history of shoulder dystocia, elective cesarean section should be seriously considered.In those with estimated baby weight between 4000 gm and 4500 gm, place of elective cesarean delivery remains controversial.

Intrapartum Considerations

As diabetic women are predisposed to infections, strict asepsis should be maintained during labor. The number of per vaginum examination should be restricted. It is essential to carefully watch for progress of labor and maintain a partogram. The likelihood of diabetic woman to have cephalopelvic disproportion due to fetal macrosomia is high. Cephalopelvic disproportion should be suspected if the dilatation of cervix slows down in late first stage and the cervix is not well-applied to the presenting part or there is arrest of labor in second stage. An early decision for cesarean should be taken. Obstetricians should be well-versed and well-prepared with the management of shoulder dystocia while delivering a diabetic woman.

Glycemic Control during Labor[59]

A strict glycemic control during labor is important to prevent neonatal hypoglycemia after birth. Insulin requirement during labor is less than the routine daily requirement due to fasting status of the mother and use of energy during labor. It is important to reduce or delete the dose of long-acting insulin on the day of termination of pregnancy or if the patient goes into spontaneous labor. The morning fasting blood sugar sample is sent and further management planned accordingly. The aim is to maintain a plasma blood sugar level of 70 to

100 mg/dl. The various methods of maintaining good glycemic control in diabetic women on insulin during labor are as given below.

1. An individualized dosage regime can be estimated from woman's total daily insulin requirement. Using this method, 50 % of the total daily dose is divided by 24 hours to calculate an initial hourly requirement of insulin. Dextrose infusion (D5W) at 75-125 ml/ hour should be provided to prevent catabolism.

2. One can start with intravenous fluids based on the fasting blood glucose levels. An infusion of 5% dextrose is started at the rate of 125 ml/hour if the blood sugar level is < 100 mg/dl, no insulin is required. If the fasting blood sugar level is more than 140 mg/dl patient is started on normal saline instead of 5% dextrose. If blood sugar level is between 100 to 140 mg/dl, insulin infusion is given by a calibrated pump or microdrip set at a rate of 1U/hour. Insulin infusion rate is further increased by 0.5 U for each increase of blood glucose level by 40 mg/dl. The solution is prepared by adding 25 U of regular insulin in 250 ml of normal saline which contains 1U of insulin/10 ml. Blood glucose level must be checked hourly during intravenous infusion and maintained at 70-100 mg/dl. Urine sugar and ketone should be checked 2 to 4 hourly for any evidence of ketonuria. In case of nonavailability of infusion pump it is advisable to give insulin infusion in a dilute solution (10 units in 100 ml of normal saline). Insulin may also be administered by a subcutaneous infusion pump.

Glycemic Management of Diabetes during Cesarean Section[59]

Elective cesarean section should be scheduled as the first case on the morning list. The usual dose of intermediate insulin is given on the night prior to surgery. The patient is kept fasting after midnight, her usual morning dose of insulin is withheld. Regional anesthesia is preferred because an awake patient permits earlier detection of hypoglycemia. A fasting blood glucose and serum electrolytes are sent. The blood sugar levels are maintained between 70-100 mg/dl during surgery.

Management of Preterm Labor[69-71]

The commonly used tocolytic agents like beta mimetic drugs terbutaline, ritodrine, etc. lead to maternal hyperglycemia. However, drugs like nifedipine and magnesium sulfate can be used safely. Nifedipine can be administered in a dose of 10 mg orally every 20 minutes upto 4 doses followed by a maintenance dose of 20 mg every 4 to 8 hourly to a maximum of 120 to 180 mg per 24 hours. Magnesium sulfate can be used as a loading dose of 4-6 gm intravenously and then maintained by an infusion at the rate of 2 gm/hour. Corticosteroids used for accelerating fetal lung maturity can also cause maternal hyperglycemia and increase the risk of ketoacidosis. The blood sugar level starts rising within 6-12 hour of administration of corticosteroids and may persist up to 5 days. However, corticosteroids are indicated in women with diabetes mellitus and preterm labor.

All delivered women should be hydrated adequately in postpartum period irrespective of the route of delivery. After surgery glucose levels are monitored every two hours. There is marked decrease in insulin requirement during the first 24-48 hours postpartum; hence the dose of insulin needs to be assessed carefully to prevent hypoglycemia. Patients who have type 1 diabetes mellitus will remain insulin dependent even after delivery so insulin is restarted at approximately 0.5-0.6U/kg postpartum weight. Postpartum glycemic target can be relaxed to fasting and postprandial level of 100 and 150 mg/dl respectively.

A significant fall in blood glucose level may occur during breastfeeding, therefore the mother should be encouraged to test her blood sugar before and after breastfeeding so that requirement of maintaining higher blood glucose level during breastfeeding can be ascertained. For those with type 2 diabetes mellitus, diet alone can achieve good glycemic control. Blood glucose level should be monitored to evaluate the need for medication. In a breastfeeding mother insulin is preferred however, WHO states that oral hypoglycemic agents are not contraindicated in a lactating mother. In patients on metformin, monitoring of baby for hypoglycemia is required as it is secreted in the milk.[73,74]

In women with gestational diabetes mellitus, most women have adequate glycemic control immediately following delivery. An oral GTT at 6 weeks postpartum with 75 gm glucose is recommended to determine whether glucose tolerance has returned to normal or not and then repeated at 1 year and then at a minimum of every 3 years thereafter. Patient should be counseled regarding the likelihood of recurrence of gestational diabetes mellitus in approximately 50% of subsequent pregnancies and a 50-60% lifetime risk for developing type 2 diabetes mellitus.[75]

After completing pregnancy, the woman should be encouraged to reduce weight, continue positive lifestyle modification and dietary habits. They should be encouraged to maintain normal glucose levels and should be explained that this will prevent or slow down the rate of progression of diabetic complications. Exercise programs should be initiated depending upon patient's health status, age, physical fitness and feasibility.

Contraception

It is important to discuss contraception before discharging the patient from hospital. There is no evidence that any of available contraceptive methods are contraindicated in women with diabetes. The ACOG[52] recommends use of combined low dose OCPs in those diabetic women who do not smoke, are less than 35 years old, and do not have hypertension or vasculopathy. For these women, progestin only pill is recommended which is shown to have a minimal effect on glycemic control, lipid metabolism and cardiovascular risk factors. Barrier contraceptive is also a good method of contraception.

Intrauterine contraceptive devices have no systemic side effects and metabolic effects, they offer an ideal method for diabetic women with vascular disease such as hypertension, retinopathy or hyperlipidemia. No studies have found any evidence of increase rate of pelvic infection or decreased efficacy with use of IUD's in woman with diabetes mellitus.[76]

Neonatal Management[25]

A newborn infant of a diabetic mother may develop one or more of the following complications. Thorough evaluation to look for earliest signs and symptoms need to be done.

- Hypocalcemia
- Hypomagnesemia
- Hyperbilirubinemia
- Polycythemia
- Macrosomia
- Birth trauma injury
- Respiratory distress
- Hyaline membrane disease
- Hypertrophic cardiomyopathy
- Hypoglycemia.[77]

Most of these infants display transient hyperinsulinism and are consequently at risk of hypoketonemic hypoglycemia. Screening should be undertaken for at least the first 24 hours of life and the blood glucose concentration maintained at >2.6 mmol/l (47mg/dl). Testing may be discontinued once satisfactory blood glucose concentrations are maintained without supplementary feeds or intravenous therapy. If a newborn is unwell or shows signs of hypoglycemia manifested by apnea, cyanosis, jitteriness, or convulsions (symptomatic hypoglycemia) blood glucose should be measured urgently, and if it is below 2.6 mmol/l, 10% glucose infusion should be administered as soon as possible intravenously at the rate of 2ml/kg over 2-3 minutes. Monitor the blood glucose and adjust the rate of infusion accordingly. Blood glucose level should be maintained at 70-100mg/dl. Continue normal feeding as soon as possible.

Implications for the Offspring[78,79]

Diabetes during pregnancy have health implications on a child in infancy as well as in adult life. Studies have shown that obesity, impaired glucose tolerance and type 2 diabetes mellitus are more prevalent in those who were exposed to hyperglycemic state during their fetal development. Long-term lifestyle modification may minimize the risk of diabetes later in life.

- Diabetes mellitus in pregnancy is associated with increased maternal and perinatal morbidity and mortality.
- Pregnancy is a diabetogenic condition due to alteration in carbohydrate metabolism due to hormones.
- The abnormal metabolic environment created by hyperglycemia has a profound impact on both the mother and the fetus.
- There is a risk of progression of diabetic complications like established severe proliferative retinopathy and advanced nephropathy especially if coexisting with hypertension.
- The incidence of obstetric complications like spontaneous abortions, preeclampsia, hydramnios, and preterm delivery is increased in pregnant women with diabetes as compared with nondiabetic pregnant women.
- Diabetic ketoacidosis (DKA) is one of the life-threatening complications for both the mother and the fetus in a diabetic pregnancy.
- The various factors that precipitate DKA include hyperemesis gravidarum, underlying infection, use of beta sympathomimetics, poor patient compliance, insulin pump failure and error in clinical judgement.
- In DKA on laboratory findings there is hyperglycemia (plasma blood glucose level of $\geq$ 300 mg/dl sometimes at even > 200 mg/dl), acidosis (pH < 7.3), anion gap with acidosis, elevated base deficit on blood gas analysis, increased serum and urinary ketones, dyselectrolytemia and decreased serum bicarbonate level (<15 mEq/l).
- Treatment of DKA involves aggressive fluid management, insulin administration and identification and treatment of precipitating factor.
- The fetal and neonatal effects of diabetes include increased risk of congenital malformations involving the heart and central nervous system, macrosomia, intrauterine growth restriction, intrauterine fetal death, unexplained stillbirths, shoulder dystocia, operative intervention, birth trauma, and perinatal asphyxia.
- Babies born to diabetic mothers are at increased risk of neonatal metabolic complications such as hypoglycemia, hyperbilirubinemia, hypocalcemia and hypomagnesemia.
- Fourth International Workshop Conference on gestational diabetes mellitus (1997), recommended a selective screening strategy based on risk assessment for detecting gestational diabetes mellitus.
- Risk assessment should be done at the first prenatal visit.
- Screening for gestational diabetes mellitus can be done either by one step or two step approach.
- One step approach involves diagnostic OGTT (oral glucose tolerance test) without prior GCT (glucose challenge test).
- In the two step approach the first step is to subject all women to a glucose challenge test and then a selected few to OGTT.

16

Diabetes Mellitus with Pregnancy

- According to American Diabetes Association (2004) the criteria for diagnosis of overt diabetes during pregnancy include:
  - Random plasma glucose level >200 mg/dl and classic symptoms like polydipsia, polyuria and unexplained weight loss.
  - Fasting blood glucose >125 mg/dl.
  - Two or more abnormal values on 100 gm oral glucose tolerance test during pregnancy.
- The management of pregnancy in women with diabetes mellitus remains a challenging problem and a multidisciplinary team approach consisting of obstetrician, dietician, endocrinologist and pediatrician should be followed.
- In the preconception period woman should be counseled regarding need for regular follow up, evaluation of end organ involvement, review of drugs, lifestyle and dietary modifications and folic acid supplementation.
- Patient should be registered as early as possible and advised to attend antenatal clinic regularly. The frequency of follow up depends on the glycemic control and any coexisting obstetric complications.
- Self-monitoring of blood sugar is advocated (four to six times per day). The metabolic goal during pregnancy is premeal plasma blood glucose level of 70–105 mg/dl or 60-95 mg/dl of whole blood before meals and no higher than a plasma level of 130 mg/dl or whole blood level of 120 mg/dl at 2 hours postprandial.
- The HbA1c concentration should be monitored every 4 to 6 weeks with the goal of maintaining it at a normal level (< 6%).
- The diet should consist of 30 to 35 kcal/kg/day in the form of three major meals and two to three minor meals and the composition should be of 50-60% carbohydrates, less than 30% fat and adequate amount of dietary fiber.
- Insulin therapy is recommended when nutritional therapy fails to maintain self-monitored plasma fasting glucose <105 mg/dl and 2 hour post-prandial blood glucose < 130 mg/dl.
- Insulin dosage should be adjusted according to glycemic trends every 2 to 3 days as assessed by glucose profile.
- In insulin treated diabetics, elective delivery is indicated at 38 weeks with the primary intention of reducing the risk of stillbirth.
- Vaginal delivery is preferable unless there is an obstetric or medical contraindication.
- A strict glycemic control during labor is important to prevent neonatal hypoglycemia after birth.
- There is marked decrease in insulin requirement during the first 24-48 hours postpartum; hence the dose of insulin needs to be assessed carefully to prevent hypoglycemia.

- It is important to discuss contraception before discharging the patient from hospital. The ACOG recommends use of combined low dose OCPs in those diabetic women who do not smoke, are less than 35 years old, and who do not have hypertension or vasculopathy.

REFERENCES

1. Wild S, Roglic G, Green A, et al. Global prevalence of diabetes: Estimates for the year 2000 and projecting for 2030. Diabetes Care 2004; 27:1047-53.
2. Coustan DR. Gestational diabetes. In: National Institutes of Diabetes and Digestive and Kidney Diseases. Diabetes in America. 2nd edn. Bethesda, Maryland: NIDDK, 1995; NIH Publication No. 95-1468:703-17.
3. Moum KR, Holzman GS, Harwell TS, et al. Increasing rate of diabetes in pregnancy among American Indian and white mothers in Montana and North Dakota, 1989-2000. Matern Child Health J 2004; 8:71-76.
4. Engelgau MM, Herman WH, Smith PJ, German RR, Aubert RE. The epidemiology of diabetes and pregnancy in the US. Diabetes Care 1995; 18:1029-33.
5. Bhattacharya G, Awasthi RT, et al. Routine screening for gestational diabetes mellitus with glucose challenge test in antenatal patients. J Obstet Gynaecol India 2001; 51:245.
6. Ganguli RP, Raghavan SS, et al. A study of diabetes mellitus in pregnancy over 8 years. J Obstet Gynaecol India 1995; 45:27.
7. Goel N, Bathla S. Diabetes in pregnancy. Obstet Gynaecol Today 1999; 46:135.
8. Kumar A, Takkar D, Sunesh K. Diabetes complicating pregnancy. J Obstet Gynaecol India 1993; 43:27.
9. Maheshwari J, Mataliya MV, et al. Diabetes in pregnancy. J Obstet Gynaecol India 1989; 39:351.
10. Seshiah V, Balaji V, et al. Gestational diabetes mellitus in India. J Assoc Physicians India 2004; 52:707-11.
11. ACOG Practice Bulletin. Gestational Diabetes 2001; No 3(Sept) 525-37.
12. White P. Infants of diabetic mothers. Am J Med 1949; 7:609-16.
13. Expert Committee on the Diagnosis and Classification of Diabetes Mellitus. Report of the Expert Committee on the Diagnosis and Classification of Diabetes Mellitus. Diabetes Care 1997; 20:1183-97.
14. Albert K, Zimmett P. WHO consultation, definition, diagnosis and classification of diabetes mellitus and its complications, diagnosis and classification of diabetes mellitus. Diabet Med 1998; 15:539-53.
15. Lain KY, Calalano PM. Metabolic changes in pregnancy. Clinical Obstetrics and Gynaecology 2007; 50(4):938-48.
16. Ryan EA, Enns L. Role of gestational hormone in the induction of insulin resistance. J Clin Endocrinol Metab 1988; 67:341-47.
17. Buschard K, Buch I, Molsted-Pedersen L, et al. Increased incidence of true type 1 diabetic acquired during pregnancy. BMJ 1987; 294:275-79.
18. Chew E, Mills J, Metzger B, et al. Metabolic control and progression of retinopathy. National Institute of Child Health and Human Development Diabetes in early pregnancy study. Diabetes Care 1995; 18 (5): 631-37.
19. Rossing K, Jacobsen P, Hommel I, et al. Pregnancy and progression of diabetic nephropathy. Diabetologia 2002; 45(1):36-41.
20. Garner PR, D'Alton ME, Dudley DK, et al. Preeclampsia in diabetic pregnancies. Am J Obstet Gynecol 1990; 163(2):505-08.
21. Klein R, Klein BE, Moss S, et al. The Wisconsin epidemiologic study of diabetic retinopathy. Diabetic macular edema. Ophthalmology 1984; 91(12):1964-74.
22. Steth B. Does pregnancy accelerate the rate of progression of diabetic retinopathy? (Review). Current Diabetes Rep 2002; 2(4): 327-30.
23. Leguizamon G, Igarzabal ML, Reece A. Preconceptional care of women with diabetes. Obstet Gynaecol Clin N Am2007; 34:225-39.
24. Kitzmiller JL. Diabetes in women: Adolescence, pregnancy and menopause. In: Reece EA, Coustan DR, Gabbe SG, (Eds). 3rd edn. Philadelphia, PA: Lippincott Williams & Wilkins; 2004. 382-423.

16

25. Galerneau F, Inzucchi SE. Diabetes mellitus in pregnancy. Obstet Gynaecol Clin N Am 2004; 31:907-33.

26. Parker JA, Conway DL. Diabetic ketoacidosis in pregnancy. Obstet Gynecol Clin North Am 2007; 34:533-43.

27. Pitteloud N, Binz K, Caulfield, et al. Ketoacidosis during gestational diabetes: Case report. Diabetes Care 1998; 21:1031-32.

28. Carroll M, Yeomans ER. Diabetic ketoacidosis in pregnancy. Crit Care Med 2005; 33:S347-53.

29. Kucera J. Rate and type of congenital anomalies among offspring of diabetic women. J Reprod Med 1971; 7:61-70.

30. Fuhrmaun K, Reiher H, Semmler K, et al. Prevention of congenital malformations of infants of insulin dependent diabetic mothers. Diabetes Care 1983; 6:219-23.

31. Ylinen K, Aula P, Steinman UH, et al. Risk of minor and major fetal malformations in diabetes with high hemoglobin A1c values in early pregnancy. Br Med J (Clin Res Ed) 1984;289(6441):345-46

32. Khoury MJ, Becerra JE, Cordera JF, et al. Clinical epidemiologic assessment of pattern of birth defects associated with human teratogens: Application to diabetic embryopathy. Pediatrics 1989; 84(4):658-65.

33. Ballard JZ, Rosenn B, Khoury JC, et al. Diabetic fetal macrosomia; significance of disproportionate growth. J Pediatr 1993; 122(1): 115-19.

34. Robert MF, Neff RK, Hubbell JP, et al. Association between maternal diabetes and the respiratory distress syndrome in the newborn. N Engl J Med 1976; 294(7):357-60.

35. Expert Committee on the Diagnosis and Classification of Diabetes Mellitus. Report of the Expert Committee on the Diagnosis and Classification of Diabetes Mellitus. Diabetes Care 2000; 23(suppl 1):S4-S19.

36. Hunt KJ, Schullar KL. The increasing prevalence of diabetes in pregnancy. Obstet Gynaecol Clin North Am 2007; 34:173-99.

37. American Diabetes Association: Report of expert committee on diagnosis and classification of diabetes mellitus. Diabetes care 2004; 27(Supp): 5,2004

38. American Diabetes Association: Standards of medical care in diabetes. Diabetes care 2004; 27 (Supp 1): S15-35.

39. Kitzmiller JL, Buchanan TA, Kjos C, et al. Preconception care of diabetes, congenital malformations, and spontaneous abortions. Diabetes Care 1996; 19(5):514-41.

40. American Diabetes Association. Preconception care of women with diabetes. Diabetes Care 2004; 27 (Supp 1): S76-78.

41. Gutzin SJ, Kozer E, Mogel LA, et al. The safety of oral hypoglycemic agents in the first trimester of pregnancy: A meta-analysis. Can J Clin Pharmacol 2003; 10:179-83.

42. Diabetes control and complication Trial Research Group. Effect of pregnancy on microvasculature complications in diabetes control and complications trial. Diabetes care 2000; 23:1084-91.

43. Jerums G, Cooper M, Gilbert R, et al. Microalbuminuria in diabetes. Med J Aust 1994; 161(4):265-68.

44. Ekbom P, Damm P, Feldt-Raemussen B, et al. Pregnancy outcome in type 1 diabetic women with microalbuminuria. Diabetes Care 2001; 24:1739-44.

45. Schroder W, Heyl W, Hill-Grasshoff B, et al. Clinical value of detecting microalbuminuria as a risk factor for pregnancy induced hypertension in insulin treated diabetic pregnancies. Eur J Obstet Gynaecol Reprod Biol 2000; 91(2):155-58.

46. Biesenbach G, Stoger H, Zazgernik J. Influence of pregnancy on progression of diabetic nephropathy and subsequent requirement of renal replacement therapy in female type 1 diabetic patients with impaired renal function. Nephrol Dial Transplant 1992; 7:105-09.

47. Satks MI, Ootiz E, Daniels GH, et al. Subclinical thyroid disease: Scientific review and guidelines for diagnosis and management. JAMA 2004; 291:228-38.

48. Frecmark M, Levitsky L. Screening for celiac disease in children in Type 1 diabetes: Two views of the controversy. Diabetes Care 2003; 26:1932-39.

49. Hagay Z, Reece EA. Diabetes mellitus in pregnancy. In: Reece EA Hubbins JC (Eds). Medicine of the Fetus and Mother. 2nd edn. Philadelphia:Lippincott-Raven:1999; 1008-09.

50. Gabbe SG, Graves CR. Management of diabetes mellitus complicating pregnancy. Obstet Gynaecol 2003; 102(4):857-68.

51. Jovanovic-Peterson L, Peterson C. Pregnancy in the diabetic woman – Guidelines for a successful outcome. Endocrinol Metab Clin North Am 1992; 21:433-56.

52. American College of Obstetricians and Gynaecologists: Diabetes and pregnancy. Technical Bulletin No.200, December 1994.

53. Jovanovic-Peterson L (Ed). American Diabetes Association: Medical Management of Pregnancy Complicated by Diabetes, 2nd edn. Alexandria, VA, ADA, 1995.
54. Langer O. Oral antihyperglycemic agents for the management of gestational diabetes mellitus. Obstet Gynaecol Clinic N Am 2007; 34:255-74.
55. Langer O, Conway DL, Berkus MD, et al. A comparison glyburide and insulin in women with gestational diabetes mellitus. N Eng J Med 2003; 343(16):1134-38.
56. Langer O, Conway DL, Berkus MD, Xenakis EM-J, Gonzalez O. A comparison of glyburide and insulin in women with gestational diabetes mellitus. N Engl J Med 2000; 343:1134-38.
57. Powers AC. Diabetes mellitus. In: Kasper DL, Braunweld E, (Eds). Principles of Internal Medicine, 16th edn. McGraw Hill 2005; 2173-77.
58. Jovanovic L, Mille JI, Knopp RH, et al. The National Institute of Child Health and Human Development. Diabetes in early pregnancy study group. Declining insulin requirement in the late first trimester of diabetes pregnancy. Diabetes Care 2001; 24:1130-36.
59. Gabbe SG, Carpenter LB, Garrison EA. New strategies for glucose control in patients with Type 1 and Type 2 Diabetes Mellitus in Pregnancy. Clin Obstet and Gynaecol 2007;50(4):1014-24.
60. Hirsch IB. Insulin analogues. N Eng J Med 2005; 357:174-83.
61. Hagay Z, Reece EA. Diabetes mellitus in pregnancy. In: Reece EA, Hobbins JC (Eds). Medicine of the Fetus and Mother, 2nd edn. Philadelphia: Lippincott-Raven: 1999; 1068-69.
62. Gabbe SG, Graves LR. Management of diabetes mellitus complicating pregnancy. Obstet Gynaecol 2002; 102(4):857-68.
63. Spencer K, Crossley JA, Aitken DA, et al. The effect of temporal variation in biochemical markers of trisomy 21 across the first and second trimesters of pregnancy on the estimation of individual patient-specific risks and detection for Down's syndrome. Annals Clin Biochem 2003; 40:219-31.
64. Graves LR. Antepartum fetal surveillance and timing of delivery in the pregnancy complicated by diabetes mellitus. Clin Obstet and Gynaecol 2007; 50(4):1007-13.
65. Pietryga M, Brazer J, Wender-Ozegowska E, et al. Placental Doppler velocimetry in gestational diabetes mellitus. J Perinatal Med 2006; 34:108-10.
66. Hawkins JS, Case BM. Labour and delivery management for women with diabetes. Obstet Gynaecol. Clin N Am 2007; 34:323-334.
67. Bonlnain M, Sten C, Irion O. Elective delivery in diabetic pregnant women. Cochrane Database Syst Rev 2001; 2:CD001997.
68. American College of Obstetricians and Gynaecologists. Pregestational Diabetes Mellitus. ACOG Bulletin Report No.60. Washington, DC: 2005.
69. Kaushal K, Gibson JM, Railton A, et al. A protocol for improved glycemic control following corticosteroid therapy in diabetic pregnancies. Diabet Med 2003; 20:73-75.
70. Lowy C. Medical management of pregestational diabetes. In: Assche FA van (Ed). Diabetes and Pregnancy. European Practice in Gynaecology and Obstetrics. Elsevier 2004; 7:76-77.
71. Acker DB, Barss VA. Obstetrical complications. In: Brown FM, Hove JW (eds): Diabetes Complicating Pregnancy. The Joslin Clinic Method Wiley Liss 2nd edn. 1995; 156-59.
72. Kjos SZ, Brehanan TA. Postpartum management, lactation and contraception. In: Reece EA, Consten DR, Garbe SG (Eds). Diabetes in Women; 3rd edn. Philadelphia: Lippincott, Williams and Wilkins. 2004; 441-42.
73. WHO. Breastfeeding and maternal medication: Recommendations for drugs in the eleventh WHO model list of essential drugs 2002.
74. Hale TW, Kristensen TH, Hackett LP, et al. Transfer of Metformin into human milk. Diabetologia 2002; 45:1509-14.
75. Metzger BE, Buchanan TA, Cousten DR, et al. Summary and recommendations of the 5th International Workshop Conference on Gestational Diabetes Mellitus. Diabetes Care (in press).
76. Kjos SZ, Brehanan TA. Postpartum management, lactation and contraception. In: Reece EA, Cousten DR, Garbe SG (Eds). Diabetes in Women, 3rd edn. Philadelphia: Lippincott, Williams and Wilkins: 2004; 447.
77. WHO. Hypoglycemia of the newborn: Review of the literature. 1997.
78. Dabalea D, Knowler WC, Pettitt D. Effect of diabetes in pregnancy on offspring: Follow-up research in the Pima Indians. J Mat Fet Med 1993; 9:83-88.
79. Stride A, Shepherd M, Frayling TM, et al. Intrauterine hyperglycemia is associated with an earlier diagnosis of diabetes in HNF-1α gene mutation carriers. Diabetes Care 2002; 25:2287-91.

16

Diabetes Mellitus with Pregnancy

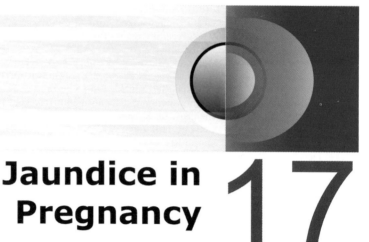

Jaundice in Pregnancy

17

Chitra Raghunandan

INTRODUCTION—MAGNITUDE OF PROBLEM

Jaundice in pregnancy is characterized by yellow discoloration of sclera, conjunctiva, skin and mucosa associated with rise in serum bilirubin above 1.2 mg/dl. Jaundice may be due to pregnancy specific conditions like obstetric intrahepatic cholestasis, acute fatty liver of pregnancy, HELLP syndrome and hyperemesis gravidarum or it may be due to coincidental causes like viral hepatitis.

There is a global variation in the incidence of this medical disorder. It is more often seen in developing countries than developed countries and affects 4 to 9 per 1000 women. Jaundice and pregnancy is a deadly combination that results in high maternal (30%) and perinatal mortality (61.76%).[1] At Lady Hardinge Medical College and Associated Hospitals, which is a tertiary care referral center, it has been among top of the list of causes of maternal deaths and is found to cause 29% of all maternal deaths.[2] An ICMR task force study reported anemia and jaundice as the most prevalent indirect causes of maternal deaths (17.4%) in seven districts of Uttar Pradesh.[3] In a study on 107 pregnant women with jaundice, maternal mortality was 19.7% and perinatal mortality was 35.4%.[4] Maternal mortality of 20.2% and perinatal mortality of 24.6% has been reported due to jaundice from South India.[5] Ching CL reported maternal mortality of 0-1.1% in pregnancy with liver disease in a recent study from Southwest Wales.[6] Of all types of viral hepatitis, hepatitis E in third trimester causes the highest mortality (30- 45%).[7-9] The maternal deaths are caused by hepatic encephalopathy, disseminated intravascular coagulopathy, acute hepatorenal failure, gastric hemorrhage and postpartum hemorrhage.

The anatomic and physiologic changes that accompany pregnancy alter physical findings and liver biochemistry. Yet, normal pregnancy does not significantly affect liver metabolism or function.

Anatomic Changes

Pregnancy does not affect the liver size and in the third trimester, the uterus displaces the liver superiorly and posteriorly. Therefore, a palpable liver in pregnancy suggests significant hepatomegaly and underlying liver disease. Spider angiomas, palmar erythema and peripheral edema are findings that usually suggest chronic liver disease but they can occur in pregnancy due to high levels of circulating estrogen.

Histologic Changes

Histologic changes in liver include nonspecific findings like lymphocytic infiltration in portal areas and increase in glycogen and fat.

Physiological Changes of Pregnancy

These include increase in plasma volume by 20% and increase in cardiac output by 30-50%. This increase is shunted to the placenta, with the hepatic blood flow being unaltered. This results in a proportional decrease in cardiac output being delivered to liver by 10% leading to reduction in the clearance of various compounds from blood especially during the latter half of pregnancy.

Liver Functions in Pregnancy

The liver in the human body performs important functions of protein synthesis, its metabolism and excretion. It also inactivates a large number of metabolites. Normal pregnancy may affect these functions and may interfere and overlap with alterations brought about by liver diseases.
1. Alteration in serum proteins include
   - Total serum proteins decrease by 20%.
   - Serum albumin decreases. This is due to the dilutional effect of increased plasma volume and also due to increased catabolism.
   - Serum globulin levels show slight decline.
   - Serum fibrinogen and coagulation factors vii, viii, ix, x increase.
   - Prothrombin time (PT) is unchanged.
   - Serum ceruloplasmin and serum transferrin increase.
   - Hormone binding proteins of thyroxine, corticosteroids, folate, vitamin D and testosterone increase.
2. Serum bilirubin is slightly reduced.
3. Serum alkaline phosphatase levels increase and is maximum in the third trimester. The increase is up to 2-4 times the normal, but if it is more than

17

Jaundice in Pregnancy

four times the normal it is usually indicative of pathology. It normalizes in 2-3 months postdelivery. The rise in alkaline phosphatase is mainly of placental origin.

4. Serum alanine (ALT) and aspartate (AST) levels are not altered, but increase during labor and normalize in 1-2 days postpartum.
5. 5' nucleotidase is significantly raised.
6. Gamma-glutamyl transpeptidase is slightly decreased.
7. Serum lipid alterations include an increase in triglycerides and VLDL. Cholesterol increases up to 2 times the normal.

CAUSES OF JAUNDICE IN PREGNANCY

The causes of jaundice in pregnancy can be either unique to pregnancy or coincidental with pregnancy. Table 17.1 gives the various causes.

WORK UP OF A PREGNANT WOMEN WITH JAUNDICE

Jaundice in pregnancy is a manifestation of a wide/spectrum of liver diseases with a large number of diagnostic possibilities. It has adverse fetomaternal effects, hence it is important to have awareness of typical clinical presentations and the course of disease in various clinical conditions so that a reasonable presumptive diagnosis can be made and optimum management is carried out.

AN APPROACH TO CLINICAL DIAGNOSIS

History Taking

The patient may present with vague upper abdominal discomfort and pain, fatigue, malaise, low grade fever, loss of appetite, nausea, vomiting followed by appearance of jaundice, clay-colored stools, pruritus, swelling of feet, headache, diminished urine output, blurring of vision and altered sensorium. It is important to assess socioeconomic status, geographic location, water supply, etc. Daily dietary intake needs to be assessed correctly. Menstrual date obstetric performance including period of gestation and any other clinical history associated with pregnancy needs to be enquired. Past history of jaundice, liver disease, gallstones and related surgery, drug intake and blood transfusion needs to be taken in detail.

Table 17.1: Causes of jaundice during pregnancy		
Liver diseases unique to pregnancy	Coincident occurrence of liver disease in pregnancy	Liver diseases probably related to pregnancy
Hyperemesis gravidarum	Hemolysis	
Acute fatty liver of pregnancy	Acute viral hepatitis	Biliary tract abnormalities
Preeclampsia /Eclampsia / HELLP syndrome	Cholelithiasis	Budd Chiari syndrome
Intrahepatic cholestasis of pregnancy	Drug induced	

Clinical Examination

General physical and systemic examination includes looking for:
- Level of consciousness and response to verbal commands
- Vital signs including temperature, pulse, blood pressure
- Icterus of skin, sclera, conjunctiva
- Presence of anemia, rash, bleeding diathesis
- Swelling of feet.

Per abdomen examination should include looking for enlarged tender liver, ascites, enlarged spleen, venous distention, bruit or rub and reduced liver dullness.The uterine size including fetal presentation and fetal heart sound should be assessed.

Initial Laboratory Tests

a. Hematological investigations
   - Hb, TLC, DLC, platelet count, peripheral smear
   - Prothrombin time, APTT.
b. Biochemical liver function tests
   - Total bilirubin (direct/indirect)
   - Serum ALP, AST/ALT
   - Serum total protein, albumin: globulin ratio.
c. Other tests
   - Urine examination – Albumin, sugar, bile pigment, bile salts and microscopy
   - Serum cholesterol
   - Blood sugar fasting
   - Serum creatinine, serum uric acid, serum electrolytes.
d. Immunological tests include.

Serum viral markers
- Hepatitis A-Hep A antibodies (IgM+IgG)
- Hepatitis B-HBsAg, HB Core Ab, HBV DNA, HBe Ag, HBeAb
- Hepatitis C-Hep C Ab
- Hepatitis E-Hep E Ag/Ab
- HIV, HSV, CMV, EBV

Differential Diagnosis of Liver Diseases is Carried Out on the Basis of:

- Timing, nature and course of disease
- Liver function tests
- Hematological tests
- Immunological tests.

Liver function tests may overlap in a wide range of abnormalities, but help in arriving at a clinical diagnosis, in assessing adequacy of treatment and in evaluating the course of disease.

Special Investigations

- Radioimaging including ultrasound which can diagnose fatty liver, cholelithiasis and subcapsular hemorrhage. While CT scan, MRI, selective angiography and Doppler studies are required in special situations.
- Liver biopsy and histopathology can be only done if coagulation profile is not deranged. Technical difficulties due to displacement of liver by enlarged uterus need to be kept in mind.

SPECIFIC CONDITIONS

Acute Fatty Liver of Pregnancy (AFLP)

It is defined as acute hepatic failure in the absence of other causes like viral hepatitis, intrahepatic cholestasis etc. It is referred to as acute yellow atrophy of liver in pregnancy, acute fatty metamorphosis of liver and reversible peripartum liver failure. It is a rare, but a potentially lethal disease and manifests usually in third trimester of pregnancy but may sometimes present after delivery.[10] It presents as an episode of fulminant hepatic failure. It is associated with high maternal (18-75%) and fetal mortality (23-90%).

Incidence

AFLP is reported to occur in 1 in 7000-15000 pregnancies. It is more common in primipara and associated with preeclampsia, multiple pregnancy and a male fetus. It is reported to recur in subsequent pregnancies.[11]

Etiology

Its exact etiology is not known. Molecular biology suggests AFLP may be the result of mitochondrial dysfunction. Mothers may be heterozygous carriers of long chain hydroxylacylco-enzymeA dehydrogenase (LCHAD) deficiency, resulting in a relative insufficiency of the oxidation pathway of fatty acids to meet the high energy demands of the maternal fetal unit during the advanced pregnancy. Children of these patients had homozygous deficiency of LCHAD and had Reye's syndrome. The fatty acids from the fetal liver traverse the placenta and overwhelm the mother's mitochondrial capacity for fatty acid oxidation.[12] Estrogens increase markedly in third trimester and suppress the mitochondrial oxidation and increase VLDL production by the liver. The distinctive histological feature is infiltration of centrilobular hepatocytes with microvesicular fat.

Diagnosis

Polydypsia with or without polyuria is a prominent early symptom. Diuresis is due to abnormally high levels of vasopressinase. It should be differentiated from postpartum diuresis due to normal shifts in volume. Anorexia, nausea, vomiting are also seen. Fatigue, malaise, headache and altered mental status may occur. Jaundice is seen in 90% of cases. Right upper quadrant pain, pruritus and ascites occur in 50% cases. Hepatic encephalopathy may occur later in the disease. Preeclampsia is present in 50-100% of cases in pregnancy affected with homozygous LCHAD deficiency.[13] It is complicated by upper GI bleeding due to coagulation abnormalities, acute renal failure, pancreatitis and hypoglycemia. Clinical improvement occurs 1-4 weeks after delivery. Abnormalities in laboratory investigations include.

- Hyperbilirubinemia occurs upto 5-15 mg/dl and is mostly conjugated.
- ALT shows moderate elevation but is usually< 1000 IU/ml.
- Alkaline phosphatase is increased to 3-4 times the normal but is nonspecific.
- Prolonged prothrombin time and PTTK.
- Decrease in serum fibrinogen.
- Hypoglycemia.
- Hyperuricemia.
- Increased blood urea nitrogen and ammonia levels.
- Leukocytosis upto 20,000-30,000 with shift to left.
- Blood smear show hemolytic features-fragmented RBC's in DIC. Platelets are usually normal but may be low due to DIC or overlap with HELLP syndrome.

Imaging of the liver with USG, CT scan or MRI demonstrate fatty liver in 30-50% cases. Changes are best proven by comparing the CT scan during the illness with that done several months later after resolution of the disease.Thus imaging may help to confirm the diagnosis in retrospect but may not be helpful in acute failure.[14]

Liver biopsy is the gold standard but is not required for diagnosis and it is also not feasible due to deranged coagulation profile. Rarely it is required to differentiate it from viral hepatitis as AFLP requires termination of pregnancy. Histopathological examination shows foaming cytoplasm in the hepatocytes in centrilobular zones due to microvacuolar fat deposition. No inflammation or necrosis is seen. Diagnosis is by clinical presentation and laboratory parameters. The liver function tests deteriorate with rapidity in aggressive phase of disease, which is often diagnostic as it is not observed in intrahepatic cholestasis or HELLP syndrome.

Differential Diagnosis

a. Fulminant viral hepatitis— It is usually associated with ALT >1000, marked jaundice and normal uric acid levels.
b. Toxemia of pregnancy with hemolytic jaundice and HELLP syndrome—
   Abdominal pain, nausea and vomiting are common in both the conditions.
   Recovery occurs gradually in most patients following delivery. The initial sign of recovery is decrease in prothrombin time. Full clinical and laboratory recovery occurs over 1-4 weeks. Even after delivery, the disease

may progress and starts resolving only after a few days but no recovery has been reported without resorting to immediate delivery. Complete recovery of liver function occurs after delivery. Recurrence may occur in future pregnancy in those with deficiency of LCHAD. Complications include GI bleeding, ARDS, renal failure, DIC and pancreatitis.

Management Options

- It is mainly supportive and is directed towards management of liver insufficiency and complications.
- The optimal management is prompt delivery that improves maternal and fetal prognosis. However this requires critical evaluation of the patient and a multidisciplinary approach. Once maternal condition is stabilized and blood products are made available induction of labor can be done.
- Transfer to high dependency unit with one to one nursing care is preferred
- FFP, platelet and blood transfusion are required to correct coagulopathy.
- Maintain normoglycemia by IV glucose.
- Monitor liver function by repeated glucose and PT values.
- In severe cases with fulminant hepatic failure, liver transplantation is the only alternative. Hence close liason with an advanced gastroenterology department which has a transplantation unit is required.
- In case of deranged coagulation, avoid episiotomy and regional anesthesia in case of cesarean section.
- Transfer to intensive care unit after delivery.

AFLP has been associated with significant maternal and fetal mortality. Maternal mortality is due to hepatic encephalopathy, DIC, ARDS, renal failure, acute pancreatitis, hypoglycemia and postpartum hemorrhage. Recent reviews of case series have however reported improved outcome for mother and baby. Fetal mortality is 27% and is due to prematurity and fetal death.[15] Babies may have deficiency of LCHAD and need to be screened. However, if the baby has LCHAD deficiency, the recurrence of AFLP in mother is 15-25% in subsequent pregnancy. Prenatal diagnosis is possible in next pregnancy by chorionic villous sampling or by amniocentesis, if previous baby is affected.[16] Relationship of HELLP and AFLP is controversial. Common high-risk factors are onset in late third trimester, primiparity and multiple pregnancy. Fatty change may occur in HELLP syndrome and it may be both macro and microvesicular, not characteristically central in location, periportal hemorrhage and fibrin deposition is seen.

Intrahepatic Cholestasis of Pregnancy

Intrahepatic cholestasis of pregnancy is also known as recurrent jaundice of pregnancy, cholestatic jaundice of pregnancy, jaundice of late pregnancy, hepatosis of pregnancy, idiopathic jaundice of pregnancy and icterus gravidarum. The preferred term used is intrahepatic cholestasis of pregnancy

(IHC) as jaundice is mostly absent in patients with this disease. It is characterized by cholestasis which manifests mainly by pruritus during the second or third trimester of pregnancy and by definition, disappears spontaneously after delivery. It frequently recurs in subsequent pregnancies.[17]

Incidence

It occurs in 1-2/1000 pregnancies and accounts for 20-50% of all causes of jaundice in pregnancy. Its prevalence is 0.2%- 0.6% in France and UK, 2-4% in Spain and 4% in Chile.[18]

Etiology

The pathogenesis of IHC involves pregnancy hormones which affect the gallbladder function resulting in slowing or stopping of the flow of bile. This leads to build up of bile acids in the liver, which can spill into the blood stream. Its occurrence in some pregnant women suggests hereditary hepatic sensitivity to estrogens leading to exaggerated liver response to estrogens.

The factors influencing the occurrence of this condition can be:

- Hormonal – IHC of pregnancy is more common in multiple pregnancies. It may be due to high estrogen levels.
- Genetic – Mutation in the hepatocellular phospholipids transporter MDR3 is present in 15% of the cases with IHC. A familial predisposition is also seen and it is more common in those whose mother or sister had cholestasis.[19]
- Nutritional factors–selenium deficiency.
- Previous liver damage–it predisposes to IHC.

Diagnosis

Symptoms of IHC typically manifest in third trimester of pregnancy but can occur as early as 10 weeks of gestation. Pruritus is the most dominant and most disturbing clinical feature and is seen in 70% cases of IHC in the third trimester. It occurs particularly on the hands and feet and is more severe at night. Dark colored urine occurs shortly after the onset of pruritus. Severe pruritus can lead to insomnia, fatigue, depression and other mental disturbances.[20]

Jaundice is seen in 10% of cases. It is usually mild and develops one to four weeks after pruritus. Right upper quadrant pain, biliary colic, nausea , anorexia, vomiting, fever and arthralgia are absent. Urinary tract infection may be associated, therefore it should be actively sought for in a patient with IHC. Physical examination reveals evidence of scratching and rarely slightly tender hepatomegaly may be present.

- Rise in serum bile acids is the earliest and the most consistent change. There is a 10-100 fold rise in serum cholic acid. Chenodeoxycholic acid also increases but less than serum cholic acid. Therefore ratio of cholic acid to chenodeoxycholic acid is high. Fasting serum total bile acid concentration is a specific test for diagnosis of cholestasis during pregnancy.[21] The rise may occur upto 15 weeks after the onset of pruritus. Therefore, repeat testing is required if pruritus persists.
- Alkaline phosphatase increases above the normal elevation but is not much helpful in diagnosis.
- 5' nucleotidase increases 2 fold.
- ALT and AST increase mildly, it is important to rule out viral hepatitis when the rise is excessive.
- Hyperbilirubinemia occurs in 20% of women and is almost exclusively direct reacting. Bilirubin levels are usually between 2-5 mg/dl.
- Serum cholesterol increases 2-4 times. Triglyceride levels may be normal or increase to about 2 fold above normal. Phospholipid and LDL levels also increase.
- Prothrombin time is usually normal unless there is malabsorption.
- Decrease in excretion of urinary estriol glucuronide.
- A new marker of hepatocellular damage (GST α- glutathione-S-transferase α) helps in differenciating between pruritus gravidarum and obstetric cholestasis much before the rise in bile salts and transaminases. It rises in IHC, 9 weeks before rise in bile salts and transaminases.[22]

Diagnosis

- Fasting serum bile acid is more than 10 micro mol/L and there is increase in liver transaminases.
- Serum viral markers are negative.
- Resolution occurs within 2-3 weeks after delivery.
- Liver failure and hepatic encephalopathy do not occur, if liver failure sets the diagnosis of IHCP must be reviewed.
- Absence of other diseases causing pruritus and jaundice.

IHC is a diagnosis of exclusion and is confirmed by resolution of the symptoms and biochemical abnormalities postpartum.

Imaging of liver by USG is not helpful in diagnosing IHCP, but can rule out extrahepatic biliary obstruction. Gallstones may be seen which are usually asymptomatic.

Liver biopsy is usually not required for diagnosis. It may be rarely required to exclude parenchymal liver disease. Biopsy shows dilated centrilobular bile canaliculi and bile plugs but these changes are not diagnostic of IHCP. Inflammation, necrosis or bile duct injury is not seen.

Jaundice usually disappears within weeks following delivery. Pruritus can be a distressing symptom. It begins to decline a few hours after delivery and usually disappears in a few days following delivery. Pruritus as a rule persists longer than jaundice. Biochemical abnormalities normalize in a few weeks following delivery. If biochemical abnormalities persist for more than 3 months after delivery, investigations to rule out chronic liver disease (chronic hepatitis, primary biliary cirrhosis (PBC), primary sclerosing cholangitis (PSC) must be carried out.[23]

IHCP leads to an increased cesarean section rate (25-36%). PPH occurs in 20-22% cases (due to prolonged prothrombin time). There is a risk of developing gallstones subsequent to pregnancy. There is also a risk of recurrence in next pregnancy and with usage of oral contraceptive.[24] Therefore these women should avoid estrogen containing OCPs.

The risk of preterm delivery is 15-60%. Perinatal mortality is 35-70/1000 live births. Intrauterine fetal death occurs in 0.4-4.1%. cases. Fetal distress occurs in one-third of cases. Fetal bradycardia occurs in 14% and MSL in 35% cases. Hence, close fetal monitoring is warranted. These outcomes are more likely if disorder begins early in pregnancy.[25] Higher fetal complications are seen with fasting serum bile acid level of > 40 μmol/l and severe pruritus at diagnosis.

Management Options

1. Ursodeoxycholic acid (UDCA): It relieves distressing pruritus by decreasing the concentration of bile acids in the blood and it also improves biochemical abnormalities. It is given in a dose of 10-20 mg/kg/d. It acts by improving impaired hepatocellular secretion by mainly posttranscriptional stimulation of canalicular expression of key transport proteins. It also restores the impaired maternal-placental bile acid transport across the trophoblast. It is well-tolerated. UDCA at first increases fasting bile acids therefore if UDCA is given follow up should be done with serum transaminases.[26]

2. Corticosteroids: Dexamethasone in a dose of 12 mg/d for 1 week, improves biochemical abnormalities but does not improve pruritis. However it is less effective as compared to UDCA.[27]

3. S.adenosyl methionine: It has recently been seen to improve pruritus. It decreases the negative effects of estrogen on bile acid secretion.

4. Cholestyramine: It binds to bile acids in the gut and relieves pruritus. It increases the risk of vitamin K deficiency thus increasing the risk of PPH. Therefore monitoring of prothrombin time is essential with the use of this drug. Side effects are nausea, anorexia and bloating.

5. Vitamin K: It is administered in the dose of 10 mg daily.

Liver function tests and prothrombin time should be repeated every week. Fetal surveillance is done with biweekly NST. Conventional antepartum testing does not predict fetal mortality as sudden fetal death is due to acute hypoxia. Therefore, delivery has been recommended at 37-38 weeks when lung maturity has been established, as continuation of pregnancy is associated with a risk of IUD. However those with jaundice (Serum bilirubin >1.8 mg%) termination of pregnancy should be done at 36 week.

Differential Diagnosis

The various conditions with a similar presentation are skin disease specifically dermatosis of pregnancy, Hodgkin's disease, polycythemia rubra vera, hyperemesis gravidarum (1st trimester), acute fatty liver of pregnancy, preeclampsia(2nd/3rd trimester), Primary biliary cirrhasis, viral hepatitis, autoimmune hepatitis, and drug induced hepatitis.

Preeclamptic Liver Disease: HELLP Syndrome

Preeclampsia is a multisystem disorder leading to proteinuria and hyperuricemia and when liver involvement is severe it leads to manifestations of HELLP syndrome, i.e. hemolysis, elevated liver enzymes and low platlets. It generally occurs in the later half of pregnancy, usually the third trimester. In 30% cases it may have its onset or be recognized clinically after delivery. It occurs in 10-15% of all cases of preeclampsia and has high maternal mortality of upto 25%.[4]

Pathogenesis

It involves vasospasm of the vascular system. In liver, segmental vascular spasm leads to vascular injury, release of thromboplastins with consequent platelet aggregation and fibrin deposition. Decreased liver perfusion leads to endothelial damage, hemorrhage and hepatocellular necrosis.

Clinical Features

Right upper quadrant, epigastric or right sided chest pain may occur. Not all patients diagnosed with this disease have hypertension and proteinuria at the time of presentation. One-third present with just hypertension and proteinuria. Nausea, vomiting and generalized edema may be there.

Laboratory changes

LFT changes are mostly suggestive of hepatocellular damage.

- Serum bilirubin may be normal or slightly increased. Clinical jaundice occurs rarely if severe hemolysis occurs.

- AST and ALT show a modest elevation but can sometimes be high (upto several thousand) suggestive of viral hepatitis.
- PT is usually normal unless DIC occur.
- Fibrinogen levels are normal.
- Platelets are low < 1 lac/dl.
- Peripheral smear shows features of hemolysis which is usually subclinical
- LDH is increased.

Liver biopsy shows unique features but biopsy is not needed to confirm the diagnosis. There is spotty involvement of liver. Periportal hemorrhage and fibrin deposition, peliotic collection of red cells and necrosis of hepatocytes, steatosis and neutrophilic infiltration adjacent to areas of hemorrhage is seen. There is no correlation between the severity of the histologic involvement and the degree of abnormality of aminotransferases and platelet count.

Course

Delivery is indicated for fetal and maternal indications. After delivery most women recover and platelet count returns to normal within 7 days. Failure to deliver the patient can lead to eclampsia , extension of the liver disease and hepatic hematoma or rupture.[28]

Differential Diagnosis

1. Viral hepatitis — Serology can be useful to differentiate but requires time. History of various risk factors for hepatitis is present and hypertension is absent.
2. Acute fatty liver of pregnancy— It is difficult to exclude this as it is often associated with preeclampsia but unlike HELLP syndrome there is true hepatic failure leading to coagulopathy, hypoglycemia and encephalopathy in AFLP.
3. Various other causes of thrombocytopenia
   a. Thrombotic thrombocytopenic purpura (TTP)- Involvement of CNS and renal system may mimic HELLP syndrome but hypertension is absent and fever is present
   b. Idiopathic thrombocytopenic purpura (ITP)
   c. Antiphospholipid antibody syndrome
   d. Incidental thrombocytopenia of pregnancy.

Management

- Stabilize maternal condition
- Control hypertension
- Antiseizure prophylaxis with magnesium sulfate.

17

Jaundice in Pregnancy

- Correct coagulopathy
- CT or USG if subcapsular hematoma is suspected
- Assessment of fetal wellbeing.

Definitive therapy is delivery as conservative therapy is associated with risks of eclampsia, abruptio placentae, pulmonary edema, renal failure, maternal and perinatal death. Delivery is indicated in all irrespective of gestational age. In case of fetal immaturity, delivery can be carried out after 48 hours following steroid administration under close maternal and fetal monitoring.

Mode of Delivery

Vaginal delivery is preferred. In cases where cesarean section is contemplated following points are to be taken care of:

- General anesthesia is administered if platelet count < 75,000/mm^3.
- 10 units of platelets should be arranged prior to surgery if platelet count is < 40,000/mm.^{3}
- Leave vesicouterine peritoneum (bladder flap) open.
- Secondary closure of skin incision or a subcutaneous drain is placed.
- Postoperative transfusions as indicated.
- Intensive monitoring for 48 hours postpartum.
- Dexamethasone therapy (10 mg I/V every 12 hours) until postpartum resolution of disease occurs.

Prognosis

The maternal mortality is 2% and perinatal mortality is 33%. The risk of recurrence in subsequent pregnancies is 25%.[29] Clinical features and abnormal LFT resolve rapidly in puerperium. There is no evidence of permanent liver damage after recovery from this disorder.

Hyperemesis Gravidarum

Hyperemesis gravidarum is characterized by intractable nausea and vomiting resulting in dehydration and ketosis and may lead to liver dysfunction. Hyperemesis is the extreme of the spectrum of morning sickness. It is more common in obese, nulliparous women and in twin pregnancy. Its prevalence varies between 3/1000 to 1/100. The exact etiology remains uncertain. The various factors implicated include psychological, hormonal and genetic factors, abnormal gastric motility, specific nutrient deficiencies, alterations in lipid levels and changes in autonomous nervous system.There may be high density *Helicobacter pylori* infection in these cases.[30]

Clinical Features

Its onset is in the first trimester usually by 10-12th week of gestation and resolves by 20th week in most cases. In 15-20% it continues till third trimester and in 5% till delivery. The symptoms include persistent nausea and vomiting, dehydration, ketosis, weight loss of more than 5% of body weight, electrolyte derangements like hypokalemia and metabolic alkalosis. Rarely, Wernicke encephalopathy and severe malnutrition may occur. Hyperthyroidism, hyperparathyroidism and hypercalcemia may also occur.

Liver Involvement

Abnormality in liver enzymes occur in 50% of the patients. ALT is the most sensitive test and may increase upto 1000 IU/ml. Mild hyperbilirubinemia can also occur. The exact etiology is not clear. Liver biopsy shows necrosis with cell dropout, steatosis, centrilobular vacuolization and bile plugs.

Differential Diagnosis

It includes various gastrointestinal disorders like gastroenteritis, hepatitis, pancreatitis and cholelithiasis, diabetes mellitus, psychological disorders and drug toxicity.

Course

Improvement in symptoms and laboratory abnormalities occur with supportive therapy and this condition mostly resolves by 20th week of gestation.

Acute Viral Hepatitis in Pregnancy (AVH)

Viral hepatitis is the most common cause of jaundice in pregnancy. This serious infection in pregnancy leads to high maternal morbidity and mortality. It is caused by hepatitis viruses A, B, C and E apart from CMV, HSV and HIV viruses. HEV and HBV are usually the most damaging, however, host immune status, malnutrition and virulence of viruses may alter the course of disease. The acute manifestation of these viral infections is similar but they differ in terms of viral structure, modes of transmission, epidemiology and their propensity to lead to chronic hepatitis and liver cancer.[31]

In a study done at tertiary level hospital from Delhi; a total of 220 patients of AVH with pregnancy were treated from 2003–2005. The Table 17.2 gives the distribution of various types of hepatitis. HEV was the most common. There were 91 patients (40%) of fulminant hepatic failure and 27% maternal deaths.[7] Various types of viral hepatitis in pregnancy are described in Table 17.2.

17

Jaundice in Pregnancy

Table 17.2: Types of viral hepatitis in pregnancy	
Total patients AVH	220
HEV	133(60%)
HBV	72(33%)
HCV	11(5%)
HAV	1(0.7%)
Coinfection(HDV+HBV) (HBV+HEV)	3(1.3%)

Hepatitis A

It is a global disease. Outbreaks occur frequently in areas of crowding or poor sanitation. It is caused by a Picorna virus and transmitted through orofecal contamination. The incubation period is 15-40 days. It is a self limiting condition but may occasionally lead to fulminant hepatitis. It does not lead to a chronic carrier state and there is no risk of increased severity in pregnancy. The clinical condition is characterized by initial period of fever, anorexia, nausea, malaise, fatigue and weight loss. Jaundice appears in the second week of disease. It is characterized by palpable hepatomegaly and liver function abnormalities with elevated ALT or alanine aminotransferase, Higher the enzymes the more severe is the liver disease. The viruses are not teratogenic in nature and there is negligible risk of fetal transmission. There may be increased risk of preterm birth with hepatitis A.[32]

Hepatitis B

It is endemic in Asia and Africa. India has 40-50 billion chronic HBV infected subjects. Prevalence of hepatitis B in pregnant women worldwide is 2.5-15%, whereas in India it is 0.2-7.7%.[33] In Lady Hardinge and associated hospitals, incidence was 0.6% in 6000 pregnant women screened. Hepatitis B is caused by a DNA virus. It leads to acute hepatitis and may also have serious sequelae in the form of cirrhosis and hepatocellular carcinoma.

Hepatitis B infection is transmitted through blood, blood products and sexual contact. It can coexist with HIV infection. Health personnel, homosexual, hemophiliacs, intravenous drug abusers are particularly prone to the hepatitis B infection. The infection is often chronic and asymptomatic and diagnosed during prenatal screening of women.[34] There is infrequent transplacental transmission of viral infection to fetus. The vertical transmission of infection is mainly in the peripartum period with infected vaginal secretions as well as breast milk. Women with HBsAg and HBeAg transmit infection to fetuses but those with presence of anti Hbe antibody are not infective.[35] Babies should be administered active and passive immunization shortly after birth with hepatitis B immunoglobulin and a three dose Hepatitis B recombinant vaccine. High risk women can be given vaccination during pregnancy. The infants though asymptomatic may develop chronic carrier state in 80-85% cases if not immunized.[36]

As with hepatitis A, risk of prematurity is increased. In acute infection, there may be transplacental transmission. 10% of fetuses may be infected in first trimester but in 80-90% cases, infection occurs in third trimester.

Hepatitis C

The infection carries a very high risk of chronic liver disease. The prevalence of hepatitis C infection in pregnancy is 2.3 – 17%. It can rarely cause acute fulminant hepatitis. After infection with hepatitis C virus, anti hepatitis C antibodies are not detected for long periods. Even if anti hepatitis C antibody are present, 86% cases are still infected with virus.[37] There are no major perinatal effects. Vertical transmission is said to occur in 3-6% cases especially if it is a persistent disease. Currently, there are no vaccines or immunoglobulins and there is no method to prevent fetal transmission at birth.

Hepatitis E

It is enterically transmitted. It is associated with epidemic out breaks of jaundice. Pregnant women are seen to be more susceptible to HEV and the incidence of fulminant hepatic failure is higher in pregnant than in non-pregnant women. HEV is endemic in India and causes acute viral hepatitis in sporadic and epidemic settings. The attack rates during epidemic are 3-30% amongst young adults with mortality >1% due to fulminant hepatic failure . Maternal mortality is > 21% in third trimester.[8] There is high vertical transmission through transplacental route. There is increased fetal loss due to abortions, stillbirths and neonatal deaths.[38]

Hemolytic Jaundice

Excessive destruction of red blood cells results in hyperbilirubinemia which is mainly due to the rise in unconjugated bilirubin. There are no changes in the level of transaminases on investigation. The cause of hemolytic anemia should be investigated and treated and these include thalassemia, sickle cell disease, hereditary spherocytosis, etc.

About 50% of pregnant women may experience worsening of jaundice. The serum transaminases and the reticulocyte counts remain normal. In Crigler-Najjar syndrome, there is absence of UDP transferase due to autosomal dominant trait that results in severe unconjugated hyperbilirubinemia and jaundice which may be seen at birth.

Dubin Johnson syndrome (autosomal recessive) and Rotor syndrome are similar conditions caused by mutations in multidrug resistance associated proteins that result in the failure of transfer of bilirubin across hepatocytes. The jaundice is usually mild and fluctuating.

Extrahepatic Biliary Obstruction

A rare cause of jaundice in pregnant women is cholelithiasis. There is usually a history of biliary colic, fever, jaundice and recurrent episodes of acute cholecystitis. USG of the upper abdomen will be helpful in diagnosing gallstones, distended gallbladder or hepatobiliary canaliculi.

Congenital Hyperbilirubinemia

In this condition there is either defective conjugation of bilirubin as in Gilbert's disease caused by deficiency of UDP transferase. This familial benign disease is probably due to a gene mutation. It is usually asymptomatic or there may be intermittent jaundice.

Liver Involvement in Drug Reactions

Medicinal agents can produce various types of hepatic injury by several mechanisms. Hepatic injury may lead to acute syndromes that resemble viral hepatitis, fatty liver of pregnancy and obstructive jaundice, as well as to a number of chronic syndromes. Acute liver damage relates, at least in part, to the apparent mechanism of injury. Hepatic injury induced by large single overdose of intrinsically toxic drugs (e.g. acetaminophen, ferrous salts) develops within 24 to 72 hours of intake and usually is accompanied by renal failure. Regular intake of some toxic drugs leads to slowly evolving chronic disease. Liver damage due to hypersensitivity-type idiosyncrasy usually appears after 1 to 5 weeks of taking the drug unless there has been previous exposure in which case it is accompanied by systemic features that are hallmarks of hypersensitivity. Hepatic injury attributable to metabolic idiosyncrasy may appear after weeks to months of taking the drug and usually presents without systemic features. Liver injury caused by drugs may mimic almost any kind of liver disease.

Clinical Findings

These include gastrointestinal symptoms like nausea, vomiting and abdominal pain, cholestatic liver injury with jaundice and pruritus or severe inflammatory and cirrhotic liver damage with signs of liver failure, encephalopathy and cerebral edema.

Common drugs causing severe liver injury are anabolic steroids, oral contraceptives, antitubercular and antifungal agents, nonsteroidal antiinflammatory drugs, antiemetics, chlorthiazides, antidepressants, methyldopa, cimetidine, ranitidine, penicillin, acetaminophen and antiarrhythmics. Drug reactions produce an array of hepatic lesions that mimic all known hepatobiliary diseases. The morphological changes vary from hepatitis, cholestasis, fatty liver, granulomatous hepatitis, periportal inflammation to fibrosis with cirrhotic alterations and vascular lesions and tumors. The prerequisite for specialized treatment of drug-induced adverse hepatic reactions is establishing the diagnosis which is obtained by a thorough medical history taken by an experienced physician with a special emphasis on drug or toxin exposure. Clinical criteria, for the diagnosis, are based on appearance of the disease, regression of symptomatology when the treatment is interrupted and recurrence when it is administered again.

The diagnosis may be confirmed by liver biopsy. A definite treatment may be available in only a minority of cases. Therefore, the main aim is to prevent chronic liver damage through early diagnosis and cessation of treatment and substitution with another drug. Increase in the serum concentration of aminotransferases might be the only biochemical disturbance and it might be overlooked if not investigated. Histological criteria may suggest the possibility of a drug induced cause and may help in establishment of a correct diagnosis.

MANAGEMENT OF LIFE-THREATENING HEPATIC FAILURE

- Aggressive multidisciplinary management.
- Patent airway/breathing should be ensured.
- Hemodynamic equilibrium should be maintained.
- Metabolic disturbances should be corrected.
- Coagulation defects should be corrected with fresh frozen plasma and platelet.
- Stabilization may be followed by termination of pregnancy.
- High risk labor management is needed.
- Postpartum hemorrhage, mainly traumatic variety, should be prevented and controlled fast.

The differential diagnosis of abrupt onset of disease with abdominal pain, jaundice, bleeding disorder and encephalopathy is given in the table on the next page.

Differential Diagnosis

Features	AFLP	HELLP	AVH
Symptoms	Nausea, vomiting, abdominal pain, jaundice, coma	Asymptomatic nausea, vomiting, abdominal pain, jaundice	Nausea, vomiting, abdominal pain, coma
Other features	High BP, edema, proteinuria-50%	High BP, edema, proteinuria	Normal BP
Hematological investigation			
a. Platelet	Normal	Low	Normal
b. PT, PTTK	Prolonged	Normal	Prolonged
c. Hemolysis	Nil	Present	Rare
d. Leucocytosis	Marked	Nil	variable
LFT	2-10 mg/d	1-6 mg/dl	10-30 mg/dl
a. S. bilirubin	l < 1000	< 500	500-3000
b. SGOT	Low	Normal	Normal/Low
c. S. fibrinogen			
S. glucose	Low	Normal	Normal
S. uric acid	High	High	Normal
S. ammonia	High	Normal	High
Liver biopsy (if possible)	Centrilobular fat particles	Periportal hemmorage with necrosis, fibrin deposition	Multilobular hepatic cell necrosis and collapse
Viral markers	Negative	Negative	Positive
Treatment	Prompt delivery with FFP	Control of BP,` convulsions prompt delivery with platelets	Control of coagulation defects, delivery for obstetric indications

KEY POINTS

- Jaundice in pregnancy is not uncommon and is the leading indirect cause of maternal mortality in tertiary care centers and it has serious fetal implications.
- It may be caused by several factors in pregnancy and it needs thorough clinical examination and investigations for accurate diagnosis and treatment.
- In the developing countries the commonest cause of jaundice is viral hepatitis mostly as a water borne disease due to hepatitis A or E virus. Hepatitis B and hepatitis C is found in endemic areas and are often transmitted by blood and blood products.
- Improved sanitation, safe drinking water, good personal hygiene and food habits, safe disposal of human excreta are some control measures.
- Detection of carriers of HBV infection during antenatal period and neonatal immunization is beneficial.
- Acute fatty liver is peculiar to pregnancy and leads to sudden hepatic failure and high material mortality. An intensive care, multidisciplinary approach

is needed along with the termination of pregnancy after correction of coagulopathy.

- Intrahepatic cholestasis of pregnancy is associated with maternal symptoms of intense pruritus and mild jaundice. It carries substantial fetal risks and warrants termination of pregnancy at 37-38 weeks.
- Preeclampsia is associated with liver dysfunction and HELLP syndrome.
- Clinical suspicion of liver disease before or after onset of jaundice, early diagnosis of its carriers, prompt referral to higher centers, adequate supportive measures, correction of coagulopathy and whenever required, a prompt decision for termination of pregnancy may go a long way in improving maternal and fetal outcome.
- Counseling is needed for women regarding future pregnancies.

REFERENCES

1. Tripti N, Sarita A. Fetomaternal outcome in jaundice during pregnancy. J Obstet Gynaecol India 2005; vol 55(5):424-27.
2. Trivedi SS, Goyal U, Gupta U. A study of maternal mortality due to viral hepatitis. J Obstet Gynaecol India 2003; 53: 551-53.
3. Gupta N , Kumar S, Saxena NC, Nanden D, Saxena BN Maternal mortality in seven districts of Uttar Pradesh –ICMR task force study. Ind J of Public Health, 2006; 50(3):173-8.
4. Rathi U, Bapat M, Rathi P, Abraham P, Effect of liver disease on maternal fetal outcome-Prospective study. Ind J of Gastroenterol 2007; 26 : 59-63.
5. Harish K, Nithe R, Harikumar R, Sunil Kumar K, Vaighese T, Steeden NS. Prospective Evaluation of liver function tests in pregnancy Trop, Gastroenterol 2005; 26:188-92.
6. Ching CL , Morgan M , Hainsworth J, Kinghan JGC. Prospective study of liver dysfunction in pregnancy in Southwest Wales .Gut 2002;51:876-80.
7. Patra S, Kumar A, Trivedi SS, Puri M, Sarin SK. Maternal and fetal outcome in pregnant women with acute hepatitis E virus infection. Ann Intern Med 2007;147(1):28-33.
8. Banali VS, Sandun V, Parikh F, Murvgesh M, Ranika P, Ramesh VS, Saridharan M, Sattar, Kannat S, Dalal A ,Bhatia SJ. Outcome of acute liver failure due to acute hepatitis E in pregnant women. Ind J of Gastroenterol 2007; 26: 6-10.
9. Benival M, Kumar A, Kar P, Shane J B, Jilani N. Prevalence and severity of acute viral hepatitis and fulminant hepatitis during pregnancy; A prospective study. Ind J Med Microbiol 2003;21:(3):184-85.
10. Alfred B. Liver and biliary tract diseases, medical disorders of pregnancy 330-52.
11. Castro MA, Fassett MJ, Reynolds TB, et al. Reversible peripartum liver failure; A new perspective on the diagnosis treatment and causes of acute fatty liver of pregnancy Am J. Obstet Gynaecol1999;181: 389-95.
12. Mansouri I, Fromehtry D, Durand E. Assessment of prevalence of genetic metabolic defects in AFLP. J. Hepatology 1996; 25: 781-83.
13. Tyni T, EKRolenE, Pikho H. Pregnancy complications are frequent in LCHAD deficiency. AmJ. Obstet Gynaecol 1998; 178: 603-08.
14. Castro MM, Duzoovarian JG, Colletti PM. Radiological studies in AFLP, a review of literature and 19 new cases. J Reprod, Med 1996;4:839-43.
15. Fagan EA. Disorders of liver. In Swiet M (Ed). Medical disorders in Obstetric Practice, 4th edn. Blackwell Science, 2002; 282-345.
16. Ibdah JA, Bennett MJ, Rinaldo P, et al. A fetal fatty-acid oxidation disorder as a cause of liver disease in pregnant women. Engl J Med 1999;340:1723-31.
17. Riely CA, Bacque Y. Intrahepatic cholestasis of pregnancy. Clin Liver Dis 2004;8:167-76.
18. Pusl T, Bevers U. Intrahapatic Cholestasis of pregnancy, Orphanet J Rare Dis 2007; 2;26.
19. Lamment F, Marshall HU, Glantz A, Matern S. Intrahepatic cholestasis of pregnancy: Molecular pathogenesis, diagnosis and management. J Hepatol 2000; 33:1010-12.

17

Jaundice in Pregnancy

20. Bewers U, Pusl T. Intrahepatic cholestasis of pregnancy— A heterogenous group of pregnancy related disorder. Hepatology 2006; 43: 647-49.
21. Laatikainen T, Tulenheimo A. Maternal serum bile acid levels and fetal distress in cholestasis of pregnancy. Int J Gynaecol Obstet 1984;22:91-94.
22. Joutsiniemi T, Leino R, Timonen S, Pulkki K, Ekblad U. Hepatocellular enzyme Glutathione S-transferase alpha and Intrahepatic cholestasis of pregnancy.Acta Obstet Gynaecol Scand 2008;87(12):1280-84.
23. Kenyon PA, Girling JC. Obstetric cholestasis progress in obstetric/gynaecology, 2004,16:37-55.
24. Heinonen S, Kirkinen P. Pregnancy outcome in intrahepatic cholestasis of pregnancy. Obstet Gynaecol 1999;94: 189-93.
25. Kondrackiene J, Bevers O, Zalin K, Eviav Z ,Tauschl HD, Ginactas L. Predictors of preterm delivery in patients with Intrahepatic cholestasis of pregnancy. World J Gastroenterol 2007;13(46):6226-30.
26. Glantz A, Marshall HU, Lambert F, Mattssor LA. IHC—A randomised controlled trial comparing dexamethasone and UDCA. Hepatology 2005;42:1399-1405.
27. Kondrackiene J, Bevers O, Kupeirskas L. Efficacy and safety of UDCA vs cholestyramine in IHC of pregnancy. Gastroenterol, 2005;129:894-901.
28. Tank PD, Nadanwar YS, Mayadeo NM. Outcome of pregnancy with severe liver disease Int J Gynaecol Obstet; 2002 (1):27-31.
29. Chabbra S, Qureshi A, Dalta N. Perinatal outcome with HELLP/HELLP complicating hypertensive disorders of pregnancy –An Indian rural experience. J Obstet Gynaecol 2006;206:531-33.
30. Bagis T, Gumirdule Y,Kayasalenk F, Endoscopy in hyperemesis gravidarum, Int J Gynae Obstet 2002;79:105.
31. Mathew Jaundice in pregnancy: Obstetrics and Gynaecology for Postgraduates, Insted. Jaypee Brothers Medical Publishers (P) Ltd. 993;73-77.
32. J Kenneth, Cunninghan G, Alexander M, Bloom J, Steven L, et al. Pregnancy complications. Williams Manual of Obstetrics 22nd edn. Tata McGraw Hill;332-36.
33. Gill HH, Majumdar PD, Dhurijibhoy KR, Desai HG.Prevalence of hepatitis, Be antigen in pregnant women and patients with liver disease, J Assoc Physicians India 1995;43:247-48.
34. Jonas MM, Reddy RK, DeMedina M, Schiff ER. Hepatitis B infection in a large municipal obstetrical population:Characterisation and prevention of perinatal transmission. Am JGastroenterol 1990;85:277.
35. Beasley RP, Hwang LY, Lin CC, et al. Incidence of hepatitis B virus infections in preschool children in Taiwan. J Infect Dis 1982; 146:198.
36. Delaplane D, Yogev R, Crussi F, Shulman ST. Fatal hepatitis B in early infancy: The importance of identifying HBsAg-positive pregnant women and providing immunoprophylaxis to their newborns.Pediatrics1983;72:176.
37. Conte D, Fraquelli M, Prati D, et al. Prevalence and clinical course of chronic hepatitis C virus (HCV) infection and rate of HCV vertical transmission in a cohort of 15,250 pregnant women. Hepatology 2000;31:751-55.
38. Singh S, Mohanty A, Joshi Y K, Deka D, Mohanty S, Panda SK. Mother to child transmission of Hep E virus infection .Indian J Paediatrics 2003;70:37-39.

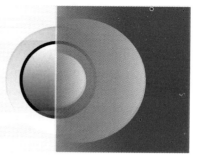

Heart Disease in Pregnancy 18

Monika B Nagpal, Shalini Malhotra

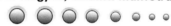

INTRODUCTION

Cardiac disease is among the leading causes of maternal mortality during pregnancy. It complicates approximately 0.8% of pregnancies.[1] The various types of heart disease complicating pregnancy include congenital and acquired defects. Rheumatic heart disease accounts for most of the heart disease in pregnancy in developing countries compared to congenital heart disease in the developed countries. Due to an increasing number of successful surgical corrections of congenital defects, a larger proportion of women are reaching child bearing age. Significant hemodynamic alterations occur during the course of normal pregnancy to supply blood to the fetoplacental unit. Such cardiovascular adaptations are well-tolerated by healthy women but the same can significantly compromise women with abnormal or damaged hearts. These women are at increased risk of complications such as heart failure, arrhythmias, thromboembolism, angina, hypoxemia, infective endocarditis, pulmonary edema, stroke and sudden cardiac death. The care of pregnant women with heart disease requires a multidisciplinary approach involving the obstetrician, cardiologist and anesthetist. These women should preferably be seen in an antenatal cardiac clinic to minimize the number of visits and maximize care. Knowledge of the pregnancy associated risks and complications specific to each type of heart disease allow the physician to choose management that optimizes the chance for good pregnancy outcome. This chapter reviews the current literature on the diagnosis and management of pregnancy complicated by various types of cardiac lesions.

Normal pregnancy entails significant changes in cardiovascular physiology. These changes create hemodynamic burden on a normal maternal heart and may cause symptoms and signs similar to those of heart disease. But women with preexisting cardiac disease may become symptomatic during this period and show clinical deterioration. The plasma volume begins to rise as early as 5 to 6 weeks of gestation secondary to the estrogen and progesterone induced relaxation of smooth muscle that increases the capacitance of the venous bed. It continues to increase until midpregnancy when it is 50% higher than the prepregnancy levels. On the other hand the red blood cell volume increases only by about 25-30%, resulting in physiologic anemia. Cardiac output increases by 40-50% by midpregnancy, by a further 30% during active labor and by 45% during the second stage of labor. The increase in cardiac output is achieved by increase in stroke volume and heart rate and remains constant from midpregnancy to term. Heart rate increases by 10-20 beats per minute by third trimester and may explain the increased risk of arrhythmias during pregnancy. The stroke volume increases by 30-50% by the end of second trimester. The peripheral vascular resistance falls by about 20% due to relaxation of smooth muscles on the arterial side as a result of progesterone, circulating prostaglandins, endothelial nitric oxide and low resistance vascular bed of placenta. The systemic arterial pressure falls during the second trimester. The reduction in diastolic pressure is more than the reduction in systolic pressure leading to a widening of pulse pressure. The colloid oncotic pressure decreases throughout gestation. Also, there is an accompanying increase in capillary pressure which favors peripheral edema formation especially in late pregnancy, complicating the diagnosis of cardiac decompensation. The same mechanism also makes the pregnant women particularly susceptible to pulmonary edema. The hypercoagulability of pregnancy may pose additional problems for women with prosthetic valves. In late pregnancy the pressure of the gravid uterus on the IVC in supine position may cause a reduction in venous return to the heart and a consequent fall in stroke volume and cardiac output called the supine hypotension syndrome. Pregnant women should therefore be advised to rest in the left lateral position.

During labor the uterine contractions pump an additional 300-500 ml of blood with each contraction, further augmenting the cardiac output. Also, the cardiac output during this time is influenced by the maternal position, pain, anxiety, maternal vascular volume and the method of pain relief. Immediately following delivery the central blood volume may drop as result of blood loss but the relief of caval compression coupled with autotransfusion from the contracting uterus produce further increase in cardiac output and can cause decompensation in the immediate postpartum period. These changes rapidly decline to prelabor values within one hour of delivery. Most of these changes revert to prepregnancy levels by two weeks postpartum, as there is loss of placental circulation, the peripheral vascular resistance increases and at the same time extravascular fluid is mobilized. Thus there are several periods during pregnancy when the risk of severe cardiac dysfunction is maximal before midpregnancy, between 28 to 32 weeks and in the peripartum period.

PRECONCEPTION COUNSELLING

A thorough evaluation of the woman with preexisting heart disease is ideally initiated before pregnancy. The issues to be addressed include:
- Optimal timing for conception.
- Completion of diagnostic procedures before hand.
- To establish baseline functional status of heart.
- Discontinuation of teratogenic drugs like ACE inhibitors.
- The risk of pregnancy based on her specific cardiac lesion.
- The possibility of optimizing her cardiac status by medical or surgical means.
- Any additional risk factors and the likely complications.
- The risk of having a child with same or different cardiac lesion.
- Her physical ability to care for a child after delivery.

For each patient, the prepregnancy cardiovascular status should be established and used as a reference for assessing any pregnancy-related cardiac changes. Although useful for categorizing symptoms this classification scheme does not necessarily prognosticate pregnancy outcome. However, this scheme can be used to assess changes in cardiac function and any change in classification during pregnancy even from Class I to Class II can be worrying and should prompt a thorough evaluation and aggressive management. The NYHA classification of heart disease is given in the Table 18.1.

Table 18.1: New York heart association cardiac functional classification
Class I- No limitations of physical activity; ordinary physical activity does not cause undue fatigue, palpitation, dyspnea or anginal pain.
Class II- Slight limitation of physical activity; ordinary physical activity results in fatigue, palpitation, dyspnea or anginal pain.
Class III- Marked limitation of physical activity; less than ordinary activity causes fatigue, palpitation, dyspnea or anginal pain.
Class IV- Inability to perform any physical activity without discomfort; symptoms of cardiac insufficiency or anginal syndrome may be present, even at rest; any physical activity increases discomfort.

It is important to counsel the women of the increased risk of maternal mortality due to certain cardiac lesions before she conceives. In general those with primary or secondary pulmonary hypertension, aortic coarctation with valvular involvement and Marfan's syndrome with aortic involvement carry a very high risk of maternal mortality and should be counseled to avoid pregnancy. The classification scheme which stratifies the mortality risk according to the type of lesion is given in Table 18.2.

Table 18.2: Risk categories of cardiac lesions in pregnancy

Low Risk (0-1%)

- Atrial and ventricular septal defects previously repaired or without pulmonary hypertension
- Pulmonary or tricuspid disease
- Mitral valve prolapse
- Patent ductus arteriosus
- Corrected congenital heart disease without residual cardiac dysfunction
- Mitral stenosis:NYHA Class I and II
- Bioprosthetic valve
- Fallot tetralogy, corrected

Moderate Risk (5-15%)

- Mitral stenosis Class III or IV or with AF
- Aortic stenosis
- Artificial valve
- Moderate to severe systemic ventricular dysfunction
- History of peripartum cardiomyopathy with no residual ventricular dysfunction
- Coarctation of aorta
- Tetralogy of Fallot; uncorrected or with residual disease
- Previous myocardial infarction
- Marfan's syndrome with normal aorta

High Risk (25-50%)

- Pulmonary hypertension
- Coarctation of aorta, complicated
- Marfan's syndrome with aortic involvement
- History of peripartum cardiomyopathy with residual ventricular dysfunction

Any additional risk factors which might worsen the outcome like anemia, thyrotoxicosis, etc. should be evaluated and corrected before conception to optimize the fetomaternal outcome. These women should also be counseled that risk of cardiovascular complications like heart failure, arrhythmias, thromboembolism, angina, hypoxemia, infective endocarditis, pulmonary edema, stroke or sudden cardiac death are increased if they had prior cardiac events like heart failure, arrhythmia, transient ischemic attack or stroke. Some other predictors for cardiac complications are NYHA class III or more or cyanosis, valvular and outflow tract obstruction; aortic valve area < 1.5 cm^2, mitral valve area < 2 cm^2 or left ventricular outflow tract peak gradient > 30 mm Hg and ejection fraction < 40%.

The risk of the congenital heart disease in the baby in a woman with congenital heart disease varies from 3 - 50% depending on the specific lesion in the mother.[2] Risk increases if the previous sibling or the father is also affected. In conditions such as Marfan's syndrome with autosomal inheritance there is a 50% risk of recurrence in the offspring.

The physiological changes of normal pregnancy may mimic or mask a cardiac problem making an accurate diagnosis of heart disease difficult. Also, many of the potentially significant cardiac lesions may be previously asymptomatic. Nonetheless, the diagnosis of heart disease and the specific cardiac lesion are essential so that the level of maternal and fetal risk can be determined and a therapeutic plan is developed.

History

The common findings encountered during the course of a normal pregnancy include fatigue, decreased exercise capacity, lightheadedness, syncope, palpitations, breathlessness on exertion and sometimes at rest. These changes are related to the weight gain, physiological anemia, mechanical compression of gravid uterus on IVC and the diaphragm and the overall hyperdynamic changes of pregnancy. But if the patient presents with progressive dyspnea or orthopnea, nocturnal cough, hemoptysis, recurrent attacks of syncope or chest pain, a thorough investigation for heart disease is warranted. It is also essential to enquire about the history of rheumatic fever, cyanosis during early childhood, family history of congenital heart disease, history of palliative or corrective surgery and history of sudden death in family members.

Physical Examination

The hyperdynamic circulation of pregnancy causes alterations in the physical findings in the cardiovascular system which mimics heart disease. The common findings in a normal pregnancy include distended neck veins, brisk and displaced left ventricular impulse, palpable right ventricular impulse, loud S1, exaggerated splitting of S2, third heart sound, midsystolic soft ejection type murmurs over the sternal borders or the pulmonary area. Any other murmur or additional heart sounds like fourth heart sound, ejection click, opening snap, mid or late systolic click suggest heart disease. Other clinical findings suggestive of heart disease include presence of cyanosis, clubbing, persistent neck vein distention, systolic murmur grade 3/6 or greater, diastolic murmur, cardiomegaly, persistent arrhythmia, persistent split second sound, features of pulmonary hypertension.

Laboratory Evaluation

1. *ECG:* Some common pregnancy induced changes include QRS axis deviation, small Q and inverted P waves in Lead III, sinus tachycardia and premature atrial/ventricular beats. Significant arrhythmias or heart block should be evaluated for underlying heart disease.

18

Heart Disease in Pregnancy

2. *Chest radiography:* The amount of radiation received by the fetus during a maternal chest X-ray is minimal and it should not be withheld if clinically indicated. Straightening of the left heart border, horizontal position of the heart and prominent lung markings are some of the changes which are seen in normal pregnancy.
3. Echocardiography is the investigation of choice to exclude/confirm or monitor structural heart disease in pregnancy. There is no radiation hazard, it is noninvasive and the information provided allows an accurate diagnosis. Transesophageal echocardiography is also safe and it can provide better visualization of left atrium and mitral valve. Some normal changes seen during pregnancy include enlargement of all cardiac chambers and mild physiologic regurgitation of mitral, tricuspid and pulmonary valves.

MANAGEMENT

General Principles

Antenatal

Between 15-52% of cardiac abnormalities are first diagnosed during pregnancy during routine antenatal examination or due to symptoms precipitated by the physiological changes of pregnancy.[3] Thus the cardiovascular system of all pregnant patients should be thoroughly evaluated in the first antenatal visit with a high index of suspicion. Once the diagnosis of heart disease is confirmed by appropriate investigations, the patients' functional cardiac status should be established according to the NYHA classification system. These women are evaluated for risk of maternal cardiac complications which include pulmonary edema, symptomatic arrhythmias, stroke, transient ischemic attack, congestive heart failure, thromboembolism and sudden cardiac death. The predictive indicators of complications include NYHA classification > II or cyanosis, previous arrhythmia, ejection fraction < 40 %, restrictive or hypertrophic cardiomyopathy, mitral stenosis with valve area of ≤ 2 cm^2, aortic stenosis with valve area ≤ 1.5 cm^2 or peak left ventricular outflow tract gradient >30 mm Hg. The presence of two or more of the above enlisted factors predict a cardiac complication rate of 66% as compared to only 30% when one factor is present and 3% when none of the factors is present at the beginning of pregnancy. Women with cardiac disease should avoid strenuous activity. They should be seen every two weeks in the antenatal clinic with special focus on the weight gain, vitals and signs or symptoms of cardiac failure. These women are instructed to avoid contact with persons with respiratory infections and report if there is any evidence of infection. Other factors which increase the risk of heart failure including anemia, obesity, hypertension, arrhythmias and hyperthyroidism should be identified and vigorously treated. They should be advised to avoid smoking and drug abuse. Medical management of the women's cardiac condition should be optimized and surgery is best avoided during pregnancy but failure of medical management and significant risk of recurrence of pulmonary edema are justifiable indications for surgery. There is increased risk of premature labor and intrauterine growth restriction in these women. Fetal assessment of growth should be monitored and fetal echocardiogram is performed between 18-22 weeks. Antenatal testing for fetal wellbeing is started at 32-34 weeks and the frequency of testing depends upon the maternal functional class. They should receive RHD (Rheumatic heart disease) prophylaxis. Also, endocarditis prophylaxis is indicated when a planned procedure likely to produce bacteremia is contemplated. The indications for hospitalization include:

- NYHA class III/IV irrespective of period of gestation.
- NYHA class I/II at 38 weeks for safe confinement.
- Symptoms and signs suggestive of complications.
- When patients on oral anticoagulants are switched over to heparin, i.e. from six weeks or earlier to twelve weeks and again at 36 weeks till delivery.

Spontaneous onset of labor is awaited in these women and induction of labor is reserved for obstetric reasons.

Labor and Delivery

During labor the mother should be nursed in a semirecumbent position with lateral tilt to avoid aortocaval compression and possible hypotension. Intermittent oxygen inhalation is provided. Fluid balance necessitates careful and expert attention as these women may easily develop pulmonary edema. Adequate pain control can be achieved with parenteral analgesics or epidural analgesia. However, it is important to avoid hypotension when establishing regional anesthesia. Maternal vital signs are monitored for features of congestive heart failure, pulmonary edema or any other cardiac complication. Continuous electrocardiographic monitoring may be used to detect arrhythmias. Invasive hemodynamic monitoring may be used in high-risk conditions as it facilitates a more rational use of fluid therapy, diuretics and inotropes. Progress of labor is monitored by maintaining a partogram and looking for the frequency, duration and intensity of uterine contractions and close fetal surveillance is kept. The number of per vaginum examinations is restricted to reduce the risk of infection. Intrapartum antibiotic prophylaxis against bacterial endocarditis should be used when bacteremia is suspected, in patients with prosthetic valves, previous bacterial endocarditis or complex cyanotic congenital heart disease (Fallot's transposition of great arteries) and surgical systemic/pulmonary shunts. Various antibiotic regimens to be used in patients with heart disease are described in Table 18.3. Endocarditis prophylaxis is also recommended in patients with acquired valvular disease, hypertrophic cardiomyopathy, mitral valve prolapse with mitral regurgitation and other congenital cardiac malformations. Vaginal delivery is preferred for patients with cardiac disease as

18

Heart Disease in Pregnancy

hemodynamic fluctuations and blood loss are more common with cesarean delivery. Also, cesarean section increases the risk of infection, thromboembolism and postoperative complications. Cesarean delivery should be reserved for standard obstetric indications. Operative vaginal delivery may be used if the second stage of labor is unduly prolonged and to avoid excessive bearing down efforts by the mother. Careful management of third stage of labor is very important in these patients. Concentrated oxytocin infusion is used in the third stage of labor unless the patient is in cardiac failure.

Postnatal

The immediate postpartum period is critical for these patients. During the first 48-72 hours significant fluid shifts occur and features of decompensation can appear, so careful monitoring of pulse, blood pressure, respiratory rate and urine output is required. It is important to discuss contraception with these women to avoid unwanted or unplanned pregnancies in the future. Barrier methods can be used but the efficacy is unreliable. Combined oral contraceptives are contraindicated in conditions where thrombosis is a risk. Progesterone only contraceptives are safe and have fewer side effects. Permanent sterilization should be offered if family is complete.

Table 18.3: Antibiotic regimens for women with heart disease

1. Standard regimen—Ampicillin, 2g IV or IM, plus gentamicin, 1.5 mg/kg iv (to a maximum of 120 mg) 30 min before delivery, followed by 1 g ampicillin iv or im or 1 g *amoxycillin po* 6 hour later;
2. Penicillin allergic standard regimen—Substitute vancomycin, (1g iv over 1-2 hour)

SPECIFIC LESIONS

Congenital Heart Disease (CHD)

With the relative decline of rheumatic heart disease especially in the developed world, this group now represents majority of women with heart disease during pregnancy. Asymptomatic acyanotic women with simple defects usually tolerate pregnancy easily. Whereas women with cyanotic lesions fare poorly. These women are at increased risk of having a baby with congenital heart disease for which genetic counseling and fetal echocardiography is recommended at 18-22 weeks.

Left to Right Shunts

Atrial Septal Defect (ASD)

It is the second most common congenital cardiac lesions among adults after bicuspid aortic valve. Ostium secundum type accounts for 70% of all ASDs and is more common in women. Most are asymptomatic until third or fourth decade. The defect should be repaired if discovered in adulthood.Complications of uncorrected lesions are more common after 40 years of age and include[4] supraventricular arrhythmias, paradoxical emboli following right ventricular heart failure, pulmonary hypertension and mitral regurgitation caused by mitral leaflet prolapse in 15 %. These complications should ideally be identified before pregnancy and managed appropriately. Pulmonary hypertension if present before pregnancy is a contraindication to conception. Pregnancy and labor are generally tolerated well but acute blood loss is tolerated poorly as it can increase systemic vascular resistance and the left to right shunt leading to a precipitous fall in left ventricular output, blood pressure, coronary blood flow and even cardiac arrest. Epidural analgesia is preferred during labor as it reduces the systemic vascular resistance and the left to right shunt. Early ambulation is encouraged in the postpartum period to reduce the risk of deep vein thrombosis and paradoxical embolization. The risk of having a baby with congenital heart disease varies from 3-10%.[5,6]

Ventricular Septal Defect

It is an uncommon lesion in adults as most are identified and repaired in childhood and small defects close spontaneously. Repaired defect usually do not present with problems. Maternal morbidity in an uncorrected lesion depends on the size of the lesion and presence and severity of pulmonary artery hypertension. In general, if the defect is smaller than 1.25 cm,[2] pulmonary arterial hypertension and congestive heart failure do not develop. Complications include congestive heart failure, pulmonary artery hypertension, paradoxical systemic embolization and bacterial endocarditis. These women should be evaluated prepregnancy for PAH and if present, pregnancy is discouraged. Pregnancy is usually well-tolerated. It is advisable to avoid hypotension during labor which can lead to shunt reversal. Risk of congenital heart disease in the baby varies from 6-10%.

Pulmonary Artery Hypertension (PAH) and Eisenmenger Syndrome

PAH is extremely dangerous in pregnancy and is associated with high maternal mortality (50%). It can be primary or secondary. Primary type is a rare idiopathic condition which occurs in the absence of intracardiac or aortopulmonary shunt. It is more common in women and mean survival from diagnosis is 2 years. The criteria for diagnosis of primary PAH include MPAP (Mean Pulmonary Arterial Pressure) > 25 mm Hg at rest or > 30 mm Hg with exertion in the absence of heart disease, chronic thromboembolic disease, underlying pulmonary disease or other secondary causes. Secondary PAH can be due to a number of cardiac, respiratory or embolic causes. Eisenmenger physiology occurs when the increased pulmonary vascular blood flow due to left to right shunt produces a right sided pressure greater than the left side and hence reversal of shunt occurs and subsequently cyanosis develops. The pulmonary vascular resistance in PAH is fixed and cannot fall in response to pregnancy and consequently pulmonary blood flow cannot increase resultant refractory hypoxemia. Elective termination of pregnancy carries a 7% risk of mortality and hence the importance of avoiding pregnancy, permanent sterilization should be offered to these women. If pregnancy is encountered termination should be offered. Treatment of pregnant women who are symptomatic requires a multidisciplinary care and includes limitation of activity, avoidance of supine position in late pregnancy, diuretics, supplemental oxygen, elective admission for bedrest, vasodilator and thromboprophylaxis with LMW heparin, and avoiding increase in pulmonary vascular resistance.[7] Use of calcium channel blockers has been reported to improve outcome. Heparin is given in the dose of 5000/10000 IU subcutaneously twice daily. During labor these women are at the greatest risk of dying because of diminished venous return and right ventricular flow. Spontaneous labor is preferred but when indicated induction with PGE_2 gel and oxytocin can be used. Cesarean section is reserved for obstetric indication which is associated with increased risk of maternal morbidity and mortality. Epidural catheter is placed early in labor but it is important to avoid hypotension. Oxygen is given at 5-6 liters per min and spO_2 is monitored. Arterial line is established for frequent blood sampling. CVP catheter is inserted early in labor and an adequate preload is maintained. Intravenous prostacyclin and inhaled nitric oxide have also been used during labor as these drugs can cause vascular dilatation and inhibition of platelet aggregation and have been shown to improve oxygenation, decrease pulmonary vascular resistance and the risk of thromboembolism. Fluid shifts in the postpartum period because of excessive blood loss and right heart failure can result in sudden death.

CYANOTIC HEART LESIONS

Tetralogy of Fallot

This is the most common type of cyanotic congenital heart disease characterized by large subaortic VSD, subvalvular pulmonary stenosis, right ventricular hypertrophy and overriding aorta that receives blood from both right and left ventricles. The magnitude of shunt varies inversely with systemic vascular resistance. During pregnancy when systemic vascular resistance decreases the shunt increases and hypoxemia and cyanosis worsens leading to rise in hematocrit. Pregnancy in a woman with uncorrected lesion carries high risk of maternal (40%) and fetal (36%) mortality. Women who have undergone repair and in whom cyanosis does not reappear, do well in pregnancy. Complications include supraventricular tachycardia, right ventricular failure, pulmonary embolism, pulmonary hypertension and progressive right ventricular dilatation. Preconception evaluation includes assessment of right and left ventricular function, severity of pulmonary insufficiency and stenosis and consideration for repair of severe pulmonary insufficiency before pregnancy if appropriate. Certain risk factors that worsen the prognosis are prepregnancy hematocrit exceeding 65%, a history of congestive heart failure or syncope, cardiomegaly, right ventricular pressure exceeding 120 mm Hg or strain pattern on electrocardiogram or oxygen saturation < 80%. Epidural or spinal anesthesia should be avoided as any decrease in systemic vascular resistance can be life-threatening. Neonatal outcome is poor in patients with uncorrected lesion because of increased rates of spontaneous abortion, prematurity and growth restriction.[8] Congenital heart disease affects approximately 5% of infants, if mother has tetralogy of Fallot.

Transposition of Great Arteries

Complete transposition of great arteries is a congenital heart disease consisting of discordance between the ventricles and the great arteries in which the aorta arises from the right ventricle and the pulmonary artery originates from the left ventricle. This condition is not compatible with life without an additional congenital shunt lesion or surgical procedure like Mustard rerouting or arterial switch procedure. If the patient has undergone a Mustard operation the right ventricle supports the systemic circulation and it is less able to cope with demands of pregnancy and right ventricular dysfunction and/or atrial arrhythmias may occur.[9]

COARCTATION OF AORTA

Coarctation of aorta is a relatively uncommon condition as most of these conditions are corrected during childhood. Other cardiovascular abnormalities which may be associated with coarctation of aorta include bicuspid aortic valve (20%), aneurysm of the circle of Willis, intercostal arteries and distal aorta, PDA, ASD and Turner's syndrome. Unrepaired lesion can lead to maternal hypertension in the upper extremity but normal or reduced blood pressure in the lower extremity. Ideally if identified preconceptionally the lesion should be repaired and the patient should be thoroughly investigated for associated abnormalities and elective surgery considered accordingly as these associated abnormalities put the patient at risk of significant morbidity. The major complications in a pregnant patient with uncorrected lesion include congestive heart failure, subacute bacterial endocarditis of the bicuspid aortic valve, aortic dissection and rupture and cerebral hemorrhage from aneurysm in the circle of Willis. Maternal mortality has been reported to be 3-9% and fetal death as high as 20%. During pregnancy, hypertension is controlled by beta blockers. During labor and delivery, hypertension should be controlled and use of epidural analgesia is encouraged as it controls pain and reduces the systemic vascular resistance. Regarding the mode of delivery though it was previously thought that CS is best for these women, the current available evidence suggests that cesarean delivery should be limited to obstetric indications. The risk of congenital heart disease in the fetus if 4-7%.

MITRAL VALVE PROLAPSE

Mitral valve prolapse may be sporadic or inherited as a dominant condition in some families with variants of Marfan's syndrome. The prevalence of MVP is 2-4% in general population and it is almost twice more common in females. Here one or more mitral valve leaflets extend above the plane that separates atria and ventricles due to myxomatous degeneration of the valve leaflets, annulus or the chordae tendinae. Most women are asymptomatic and diagnosed incidentally on cardiovascular examination which reveals a midsystolic click with or without a midsystolic or late systolic murmur. Reliance on strict diagnostic criteria is essential. On echocardiography the mitral valve is seen prolapsing into the left atrium. Complications are rare as pregnancy induced hypervolemia improves the alignment of mitral valve but include severe mitral regurgitation, infective endocarditis, cerebral ischemia and embolism and sudden death. The risk of complications is increased if there is associated mitral regurgitation or valvular damage. These women should avoid caffeine, alcohol, tobacco and beta mimetic drugs. Symptomatic women are given beta blockers to reduce the sympathetic tone and relieve symptoms.

RHEUMATIC HEART DISEASE

Rheumatic heart disease develops after Group A beta hemolytic streptococcal infection of the throat. Rheumatic fever typically occurs at the age of 6 to 15 years. If myocarditis is present mitral regurgitation develops followed by development of mitral stenosis after a period of five years. The patients becomes symptomatic after 15-20 years depending on the severity of the lesion. The major Jones criteria for diagnosis of rheumatic fever include prior evidence of Group A streptococcal infection, carditis, polyarthritis, chorea, subcutaneous nodules and erythema marginatum. Minor criteria consist of fever, arthralgias, raised ESR and first degree heart block.

Mitral Stenosis

Mitral stenosis is the most common form of RHD in women. Symptoms include fatigue, dyspnea on exertion which progress to dyspnea at rest, paroxysmal nocturnal dyspnea and hemoptysis. Dizziness and symptoms of low cardiac output like syncope may also be present. The stenotic mitral valve impairs left ventricular filling and limits any increase in cardiac output. Chronic left atrial outflow obstruction leads to severe pulmonary venous congestion, pulmonary hypertension and later right ventricular failure. Pregnancy mediated cardiovascular changes especially increased intravascular volume and increased heart rate can exacerbate the impaired filling and lead to decompensation during pregnancy and especially during labor, delivery and puerperium. On physical examination, there is loud first heart sound, an opening snap and a low frequency diastolic murmur at the apex with or without presystolic accentuation. The murmur is best heard in the left lateral position with the bell of the stethoscope. Accentuated pulmonic component of the second heart sound and other features of pulmonary hypertension may be present. ECG is often normal, may indicate left atrial enlargement, right axis deviation, right ventricular hypertrophy and left atrial p-waves. Chest X-ray shows a small heart with prominent left atrial appendage and pulmonary congestion and edema. Echocardiography is used to define the valvular anatomy, degree of stenosis, associated regurgitation and other valvular anomalies and presence of pulmonary arterial hypertension.

Goals of management include optimizing the cardiac output, preventing tachycardia, avoiding decrease in systemic vascular resistance, and reducing the stress on right ventricle by minimizing increase in blood volume and avoiding situations in which pulmonary artery pressures are increased like hypercarbia, hypoxia or acidosis. Serious complications are more common in severe mitral stenosis (mitral valve area < 1 cm^2), moderate or severe symptoms prior to pregnancy and in those diagnosed late in pregnancy. Pulmonary edema can develop by tachycardia, injudicious use of fluids during third stage of labor leading to an increase in intravascular volume. A rapid heart rate in mitral stenosis prevents ventricular filling decreasing the time for left atrial emptying and cardiac output leading to increase in left atrial pressure and pulmonary edema. This leads to more tachycardia and a vicious cycle. Thus beta blockers are indicated if HR > 90 /min. Labor imposes an additional stress and CHF may develop for the first time during labor in a previously well-controlled patient. Hence, bedside cardiac monitoring is necessary. Also, central hemodynamic monitoring is required if the patient is class III or IV or valve diameter is < 2.5 cm^2. For pain relief, epidural analgesia can be used but care should be taken to avoid fluid overload. If general anesthesia becomes necessary, agents that produce tachycardia (atropine and ketamine) should be avoided.

Mitral Regurgitation

This lesion has various etiologies like rheumatic, floppy mitral valve in association with MVP (mitral valve prolapse), papillary muscle dysfunction and ruptured chordae tendinae. Due to the fall in systemic vascular resistance and reduced left ventricular afterload, this condition is well-tolerated in pregnancy. Women in NYHA Class I and II need to be managed by rest to prevent fatigue. If ventricular failure develops, it should be managed with digoxin, diuretics and afterload reduction. Any rise of blood pressure could worsen regurgitation and should be avoided.

Aortic Stenosis

Aortic stenosis can be congenital, rheumatic or due to age related calcification, with the most common cause in women of childbearing age being congenital bicuspid valve.Aortic stenosis of rheumatic origin is less severe in women of child bearing age group as it is a progressive condition.This usually occurs in conjunction with mitral valve disease. Pregnancy outcome depends on the degree of stenosis. Women with severe AS (aortic valve area < 0.7 cm^2, mean gradient > 50 mm Hg) should be advised to delay conception until after surgical correction. If a pregnant woman becomes symptomatic or is so when pregnancy is confirmed, bedrest and valve replacement should be considered. However, open heart surgery and cardiac bypass should be avoided due to 1.5% maternal mortality rate and 16-33% fetal mortality rates irrespective of gestational age.[10] Thus, aortic balloon valvuloplasty should be considered as a palliative procedure deferring valve replacement after delivery. Fluid management is the central component of intrapartum care as volume over load can lead to pulmonary edema and hypovolemia, that can cause sudden death. Patients should labor in lateral position to avoid aortocaval compression. Spinal and epidural blocks are contraindicated due to vasodilatory effect however, narcotic epidural can decrease the chance of hypotension.

Aortic Regurgitation

This regurgitant lesion of the aortic valve could have several etiologies like rheumatic, Marfan's syndrome or syphilitic aortitis.Pregnancy is well-tolerated as the increased heart rate of pregnancy causes decreased time for regurgitation and the decreased systemic vascular resistance promoting forward flow.The management principles are the same as any other heart lesions.

PROSTHETIC HEART VALVES

Many women with severe valvular heart disease now survive and become pregnant because of surgical valve replacement. The two types of valves are mechanical and bioprosthetic. Pregnancy in women with prosthetic heart valves is associated with a maternal mortality of 3-4%, fetal loss is common. Porcine tissue valves are safer during pregnancy as anticoagulation is not required but valvular dysfunction and heart failure are more common. Also they are not as durable as mechanical valves and generally require another valve replacement in 10-15 years. Pregnancy does not appear to shorten this interval. Prosthetic or mechanical valves are longer lasting but require anticoagulation for life. ACOG recommends full anticoagulation throughout pregnancy with prosthetic valves. Warfarin has the advantage of oral administration but carries the risk of fetal intracerebral hemorrhage and if continued during the period of organogenesis leads to warfarin embryopathy (6 % if used between 6-9 weeks). Another disadvantage is that anticoagulant effect cannot be readily reversed. Warfarin embryopathy is characterized by nasal hypoplasia and stippled epiphysis. Warfarin has also been found to increase the risk of miscarriage (32%) and stillbirth (7%). The risk is higher if the daily dose exceeds 5 mg/day. Also, since warfarin crosses the placenta it causes fetal anticoagulation and bleeding particularly if used within 2 weeks of labor. On the other hand, heparin does not cross the placenta and its effects are rapidly reversible but is associated with increased risk of valve thrombosis, embolic events and retroplacental hemorrhage. Unfractionated heparin needs to be administered parenterally, has a short duration of action, narrow therapeutic index and in high doses can lead to osteoporosis. Though low molecular weight heparins have been found to have better safety profile in pregnancy, these are not recommended as anticoagulants in patients with prosthetic heart valves as there have been reports of valvular thrombosis in women who have been apparently anticoagulated.[11, 12] Though the optimal agent for anticoagulation during pregnancy is not available, the most commonly used regime is to stop warfarin and give high dose unfractionated heparin from 6 to 12 weeks gestation to avoid warfarin embryopathy and then switch back to warfarin from 12 to 37 weeks. Near term warfarin is substituted by heparin till the onset of labor. The target INR for heparin is 1.5 to 2.5 while it is 2 to 3 for warfarin. Laboratory monitoring is done twice a week. Heparin is restarted 6 hours after normal vaginal delivery and 24 hours after cesarean section. Warfarin is started concomitantly and heparin stopped after 3 days. If a patient fully anticogulated with warfarin requires urgent delivery the effects are reversed with fresh frozen plasma and vitamin K and the effects of heparin are reversed with protamine sulfate.

PERIPARTUM CARDIOMYOPATHY

Peripartum cardiomyopathy is a global congestive heart failure characterized by dilatation of all four chambers of the heart, low cardiac output and pulmonary edema. The criteria used for diagnosis include:
1. Development of cardiac failure in the last month of pregnancy or within five months of delivery.
2. The absence of an identifiable cause for cardiac failure.
3. Absence of recognizable heart disease prior to last month of pregnancy.
4. Left ventricular systolic dysfunction demonstrated by classic echocardiographic criteria such as depressed shortening fraction or ejection fraction.
   Peripartum cardiomyopathy is a subset of dilated cardiomyopathy and is a diagnosis of exclusion. Women usually present with heart failure at the end of pregnancy or more commonly during puerperium. It occurs in 1 in 1300 to 1 in 15000 deliveries.[13] These women are generally older than 30 years of age, multiparous, with recognized risk factors like preeclampsia, gestational hypertension and multiple gestation. The pathogenesis is unknown and various immunologic and infective etiologies have been proposed. These women present

with signs and symptoms of congestive heart failure. ECG shows tachycardia and arrhythmias. Chest X-ray is consistent with cardiomegaly with varying amount of pulmonary infiltrates and pleural effusion. On echocardiography the left atrium and ventricle are seen to be enlarged, ejection fraction is less than 45% or fractional shortening less than 30% or both and an end diastolic dimension > 2.7 cm/m^2. The complications include life-threatening arrhythmias and pulmonary or systemic embolization.[14] Management consists of aggressive treatment of heart failure with bedrest, sodium restriction, diuretics, digoxin, prophylactic heparin and afterload reduction with hydralazine or another vasodilator. Immunosuppressive therapy with prednisolone and azathioprine has been used to improve left ventricular function. Cautious use of beta blockers can be done if tachycardia persists and cardiac output is preserved well. Those who are seriously ill need intubation and ventilation and use of ventricular assist device. Heart transplantation can be life saving in severe cases. 50% make spontaneous and full recovery and those who do not, a 85% mortality in 4 to 5 years is reported. Persistent cardiac dysfunction is seen in 45-90% of patients. The prognosis is poor. Maternal mortality is as high as 25-50%. The risk of recurrence in a subsequent pregnancy is close to 80%. It depends on normalization of left ventricular function within six months of delivery. Those women with severe myocardial dysfunction, defined as left ventricular diastolic dimension more than 6 cm and fractional shortening less than 21% are unlikely to regain normal cardiac function on follow up. Those in whom left ventricular function and size do not return to normal within 6 months and prior to a subsequent pregnancy are at significant risk of worsening heart failure (50%) and death (25%) or recurrent peripartum cardiomyopathy in next pregnancy. Pregnancy is strongly discouraged in women with prior history of peripartum cardiomyopathy and especially those with residual cardiac dysfunction. If pregnancy occurs termination should be offered to those with persistent echocardiographic abnormalities. However, if pregnancy is continued decreased activity and bedrest along with symptomatic treatment is given. During labor and delivery, these women have to be closely watched for congestive heart failure and pulmonary embolism. Pulmonary artery catheterization for hemodynamic monitoring may be considered. Vaginal delivery is preferred and cesarean section is reserved for obstetric indications. Postnatally these patients can be given ACE inhibitors for afterload reduction. Reliable contraception is provided.

HYPERTROPHIC CARDIOMYOPATHY

Most cases of hypertrophic cardiomyopathy are familial, inherited as autosomal dominant.It is characterized by left ventricular hypertrophy without chamber dialation.The older names for this condition like idiopathic hypertrophic subaortic stenosis and hypertrophic obstructive cardiomyopathy have been replaced as there is no left ventricular outflow obstruction in most cases.Women may be asymptomatic, especially if diagnosed because of family screening, or may experience syncope or "angina-like" chest pain. Pregnancy in asymptomatic women is well-tolerated while cases with severe symptoms or heart failure before pregnancy are at a risk of symptomatic progression, atrial fibrillation, syncope and maternal death.[15] Clinical risk factors for sudden death include a family history of sudden cardiac death, previous syncope and documented ventricular tachycardia.

MYOCARDIAL INFARCTION

The risk of myocardial infarction among women in the reproductive age group is 1 in 10000. Most occur in late pregnancy or in the peripartum period. They can occur due to atherosclerosis and thrombosis and vasospastic disease. No cardiac risk factors are present in 40% of the cases.[16] In rest of the cases the associated risk factors include—administration of oxytocic agents, drug abuse (crack cocaine), embolism due to mitral stenosis/ infective endocarditis, smoking, diabetes, obesity, hypertension and hypercholesterolemia. Diagnosis is usually difficult because the index of suspicion is low and physiologic changes during pregnancy may mimic symptoms. The patient presents with chest pain and on clinical examination there is pericardial friction rub and the diagnosis is supported by typical ECG changes. Troponin-I should be used to document acute MI because myoglobin and creatine kinase are increased two-folds during labor and delivery. Creatine kinase-MB isoenzyme is also used for the diagnosis of MI during pregnancy. Bedrest is given to minimize cardiac workload and myocardial oxygen consumption. Aspirin, nitrates, calcium channel blockers and beta blockers have been found to be safe during pregnancy. Coronary angiography and percutaneous transluminal coronary angioplasty and stenting all have been successfully performed in pregnancy. Pregnancy is a relative contraindication to thrombolytic therapy because of theoretical increased risk of maternal and fetal bleeding. Complications during pregnancy include congestive heart failure and arrhythmias. Risk of death is high if delivery occurs within 2 weeks of infarction.[17] Spontaneous vaginal delivery should be allowed. Cesarean section is empirically advocated in patients who start laboring within 4 days of acute MI. Epidural analgesia should be provided during labor and delivery along with supplemental oxygen and left lateral tilt position. Oxytocin infusion is used rather than ergometrine which can cause coronary artery spasm. Patients are advocated not to become pregnant for at least one year after acute MI. A prepregnancy cardiac evaluation should be done with echocardiography and stress testing and pregnancy can be planned cautiously if there is no residual cardiac dysfunction.

CARDIAC ARRHYTHMIAS

The incidence of cardiac arrhythmias increases during pregnancy as a result of hormonal changes, alterations in the autonomic tone, increased hemodynamic demand and mild hypokalemia, with the highest risk during

Heart Disease in Pregnancy

labor and delivery. Atrial and ventricular premature beats are frequently present during pregnancy and have no adverse effects on the mother or fetus and thus, require no further investigations. The most common arrhythmia seen during pregnancy is supraventricular tachycardia (SVT).[18] Atrial fibrillation and atrial flutter are rare. Early treatment, either with conversion to sinus rhythm or ventricular rate control is important because of the risk of thromboembolism and detrimental effect on the fetus. Initial treatment should be the vagal maneuver but 50% of SVTs do not respond to vagal maneuvers. Intravenous adenosine, propranolol and verapamil have been safely used for acute termination of SVTs. Ventricular tachycardia is uncommon during pregnancy but can be associated with preexisting heart disease. Initial therapy with lidocaine or procainamide should be considered in hemodynamically stable women. Amiodarone is contraindicated as it is associated with fetal hypothyroidism, growth restriction and prematurity. Beta-blockers can be used. Electrical cardioversion is safe in pregnancy and necessary in all women with tachyarrhythmias who are hemodynamically stable. Airway management is essential and supine position should be avoided.

KEY POINTS

- Cardiac disease is among the leading causes of maternal mortality during pregnancy and it complicates approximately 0.8% of pregnancies.
- The physiologic cardiovascular adaptations of pregnancy are well tolerated by healthy women but the same can significantly compromise women with heart disease.
- A thorough evaluation of the woman with preexisting heart disease is ideally initiated before pregnancy.
- For each patient, the prepregnancy cardiovascular status should be established and used as a reference in assessing any pregnancy-related cardiac changes.
- It is important to counsel the women about the risk of maternal mortality due to the specific cardiac lesion before conception.
- Any additional risk factors which might worsen the outcome like anemia, thyrotoxicosis, etc. should be evaluated and corrected before conception to optimize the fetomaternal outcome.
- The risk of the congenital heart disease in the baby in a woman with congenital heart disease varies from 3-50% depending on the specific lesion.
- The hyperdynamic circulation of pregnancy causes alterations in the physical findings in the cardiovascular system which can mimic heart disease.
- The clinical findings suggestive of heart disease include presence of cyanosis, clubbing, persistent neck vein distention, systolic murmur grade 3/6 or greater, diastolic murmur, cardiomegaly, persistent arrhythmia and persistent split second sound and require further investigation.

- These women should be seen every two weeks in the antenatal clinic with special focus on the weight gain, vitals signs or symptoms of cardiac failure.
- Women with cardiac disease should avoid strenuous activity and contact with persons with respiratory infections. Other factors which increase the risk of heart failure including anemia, obesity, hypertension, arrhythmias and hyperthyroidism should be identified and vigorously treated.
- Labor, delivery and postpartum are periods of hemodynamic instability and require intensive monitoring.
- Vaginal delivery is preferred for patients with cardiac disease as hemodynamic fluctuations and blood loss are more common with cesarean delivery.
- Intrapartum antibiotic prophylaxis against bacterial endocarditis should be used when bacteremia is suspected according to the recommendations.

REFERENCES

1. Siu SC, Sermer M, Colman JM, et al. Prospective multicenter study of pregnancy outcomes in women with heart disease. Circulation 2001;104:515-21.
2. Uebing A, Steer PJ, Yentis SM, Gatzoulis MA.Pregnancy and congenital heart disease. BMJ 2006;332(7538):401-06.
3. Steer PJ. Pregnancy and Contraception. In: Gatzoulis MA, Swan L, Therrian J, Pantley GA (Eds). Adult Congenital Heart Disease: A Practical Guide. Oxford: BMJ, 2005;16-35.
4. Pitkin RM, Perloff JK, Koos BJ, Beall MH.Pregnancy and congenital heart disease. Ann Intern Med 1990;112:445-54.
5. Burn J, Brennan P, Little J et al. Recurrence risks in offspring of adults with major heart defects: results from first cohort of British collaborative study. Lancet 1998;351:311-16.
6. Rose V, Gold RJ, Lindsay G, Allen M. A possible increase in the incidence of congenital heart defects among the offspring of affected parents. J Am Coll Cardiol 1985;6:376-82.
7. Van Mook WN, Peeters L Severe cardiac disease in pregnancy, part II: Impact of congenital and acquired cardiac diseases during pregnancy. Curr Opin Crit Care 2005;11:435-48.
8. Whittemore R, Hobbins JC, Engle MA. Pregnancy and its outcome in women with and without surgical treatment of congenital heart disease. Am J Cardiol. 1982;50:641-51.
9. Therrien J, Barnes I, Somerville J. Outcome of pregnancy in patients with congenitally corrected transposition of the great arteries. Am J Cardiol 1999;84:820-24.
10. Parry AJ, Westaby S. Cardiopulmonary by pass during pregnancy. Ann Thorac Surg 1996;61:1865-69.
11. Leyh RG, Fischer S, Ruhparwar A, Haverich A. Anticoagulation for prosthetic heart valves during pregnancy: Is low-molecular-weight heparin an alternative? Eur J Cardiothorac Surg 2002;21:577-79.
12. American College of Obstetricians and Gynecologists: Safety of Lovenox in Pregnancy. Committee opinion number 2002.
13. Veille JC. Peripartum cardiomyopathies: A review. Am J Obstet Gynecol 1984;148: 805-18.
14. Pearson GD, Veille JC, Rahimtoola S, Hsia J, Oakley CM, Hosenpud JD, Ansari A, Baughman KL. Peripartum cardiomyopathy: National Heart, Lung, and Blood Institute and Office of Rare Diseases (National Institutes of Health) workshop recommendations and review. JAMA 2000;283(9):1183-88.

18

15. Autore C, Conte MR, Piccininno M, Bernabo P, et al. Risk associated with pregnancy in hypertrophic cardiomyopathy. J Am Coll Cardiol 2002;40;1864-69.
16. Badui E, Enciso R. Acute myocardial infarction during pregnancy and puerperium: a review. Angiology 1996;47(8):739-56.
17. Roth A, Elkayam U. Acute myocardial infarction associated with pregnancy. Ann Intern Med 1996;125(9):751-62.
18. Sheikh All, Harper MA. Mycardial infarction during pregnancy: Management and outcome of two pregnancies. Am J Obstet Gynecol 1993;169(2 pt 1):279-83.
19. Tawam M, Levine J, Mendelson M, et al. Effect of pregnancy on paroxymal supraventricular tachycardia. Am J Cardiol 1992;72:838-40.

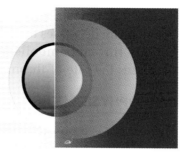

Thromboembolism in Pregnancy

19

Swaraj Batra, Sarita Malhotra

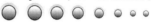

INTRODUCTION

Venous thromboembolism comprises deep vein thrombosis (DVT) or pulmonary thromboembolism or both and results in significant morbidity and mortality during pregnancy and puerperium. It occurs approximately in 1 in 1500 deliveries according to the western literature[1] and according to an Indian study, the incidence of antenatal DVT was reported as 0.1%.[2] The risk is lower for Asian and Hispanic women, higher for white and highest for black women. Postpartum DVT has been reported to occur 3 to 5 times more often than antepartum DVT and 3 to 16 times more frequently after cesarean section compared to vaginal delivery.[3] Venous thromboembolism is a leading cause of maternal mortality in western world and accounts for 17% of all maternal deaths.[1] Mortality is primarily due to massive pulmonary embolism. Most common source of pulmonary embolus is a thrombus embolising from deep veins of lower extremities. Pulmonary embolism can occur in up to 24% of untreated patients of deep vein thrombosis.[4] Risk of pulmonary embolism is greater with thrombosis of ileofemoral veins as compared to calf veins and the former is more common in pregnancy. The associated sequelae include pulmonary hypertension, right heart failure and post-thrombotic syndrome, manifesting as edema and skin changes, dependent cyanosis, associated varicose veins, recurrent thrombosis and leg ulcerations and deformities. These women may also suffer from poor pregnancy outcomes which include recurrent pregnancy losses, intrauterine growth restriction, stillbirths, early onset, severe preeclampsia and abruptio placentae.

Differential diagnosis includes superficial thrombophlebitis, calf muscle hematoma and ruptured plantaris tendon.

Diagnostic Tests

Diagnostic tests for evaluation are D-dimer assay, venous doppler ultrasound, magnetic resonance venography, CT and infrequently venography.

D-dimer

It is product of fibrin degradation formed by plasmin. Sensitivity and specificity reported in various studies is 85% to 97% and 35% to 45% respectively.[7]

Its utility in diagnosis of DVT in pregnant women is limited due to physiologically increased levels depending on duration of pregnancy.[8] Physiologically elevated levels make it difficult to assign normal cut-off values.

It may be useful in excluding the diagnosis of DVT in patients at low risk of DVT.

Doppler Venous Ultrasound

Real-time ultrasonography with color Doppler is the investigation of choice for diagnosis of DVT. It has been well studied for diagnosing DVT in pregnancy.[9] It is a safe, rapid and a noninvasive test, available at bed side and if necessary can be repeated. Noncompressibility of the venous lumen on ultrasound is the most accurate diagnostic criteria for venous thrombosis.[10] It's sensitivity for diagnosing distal venous thrombosis is 75-90%.

CT and MRI

CT and MRI are alternative modalities to establish the diagnosis of DVT and are indicated when there is a strong clinical suspicion of DVT and ultrasound findings are equivocal or negative.[11,12] Sensitivity and specificity of CT is similar to ultrasound.[2] However, routine use of CT is limited by risk of radiation exposure to the fetus. MRI has shown to be sensitive, specific and highly reproducible for the diagnosis of DVT in nonpregnant patients.[3] It has been rarely used for diagnosis of DVT in pregnant women. Diagnostic algorithm for DVT is shown in Flow chart 19.1.

Pulmonary Embolism (Flow chart 19.2)

Clinical Features

Early diagnosis is essential to improve maternal and fetal outcome. Signs and symptoms are not specific, they depend on the site of embolus and extent of right ventricle dysfunction.

Dyspnea, tachypnea, cough, pleuritic chest pain, hemoptysis, syncope, fever, anxiety and diaphoresis are the most common symptoms whereas tachycardia, cyanosis, hypotension and new murmur are the most common signs.

Flow chart 19.1: Diagnostic algorithm for DVT

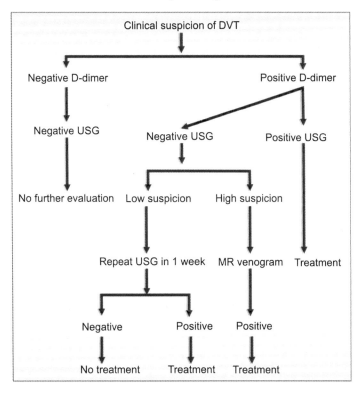

Flow chart 19.2: Diagnostic algorithm for suspected pulmonary embolism

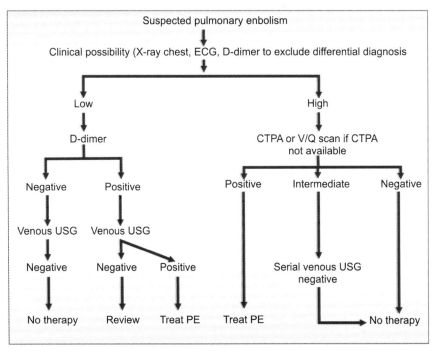

Thromboembolism in Pregnancy

When clinical suspicion is high, consideration should be given for empirical anticoagulation till work up is completed.

Differential diagnosis includes pneumonia, rib fracture and myocardial infarction.

Diagnostic Tests

Biochemical and radiological investigations are helpful in establishing the diagnosis are:

Arterial blood gas analysis

Hypoxia and hypocapnia may be present but a normal PO_2 does not exclude the diagnosis.

ECG

ECG changes are not specific.[13] ECG may show tachycardia, right axis deviation, P-pulmonale, nonspecific T-wave inversions and classic S wave in lead I, Q in lead III, T in lead III. Right axis deviation and right bundle branch block are suggestive of significant cardiac compromise. Up to 70-90% of patients have these ECG changes.

Chest X-ray

Chest X-ray can be abnormal in up to 85% of patients. Most common findings are atelectasis, pleural-based opacity and pleural effusion. Classic wedge shape infiltrate, decreased vascularity and enlarged right descending pulmonary artery are rare findings.[14] It is helpful in excluding other diagnoses with similar clinical presentation, e.g. pneumonia, pneumothorax, pleural effusion and pulmonary edema.

Echocardiography

Echocardiographic abnormalities of right ventricle function and size are seen with a large embolus. Typical findings are dilated and hypokinetic right ventricle and tricuspid regurgitation. Trans esophageal echocardiography may have better accuracy. Echocardiography helps in planning management, stratifying risk and delineating the prognosis.[15]

D-dimer

D-dimer assay is a sensitive (95%) but not a specific (25%) investigation in non-pregnant patients. Cutoff values are difficult to set up in pregnancy as levels are increased in pregnancy. The main diagnostic utility of D-dimer is to exclude the diagnosis in patients with low clinical suspicion.

Arteriography

Pulmonary arteriography for many years was the gold standard test for diagnosis of pulmonary embolism. This procedure is associated with morbidity and mortality primarily due to catheter placement and contrast injection. Complications like local hematoma, renal failure, respiratory failure and cardiac perforation can occur. At present it is rarely used for diagnosing pulmonary embolism.[16]

Ventilation and Perfusion Scan

It is a well established diagnostic modality in pregnant patients. It was the most frequently used test in these patients for establishing the diagnosis. Patients are categorized into different diagnostic probability categories, including high, intermediate, low, normal and indeterminate. In patients other than normal or high probability categories, further evaluation is required. Main drawbacks are that it is time consuming and sensitivity depends on the clinical suspicion, also there is risk of radiation exposure to the fetus and associated morbidity.[17]

CT Pulmonary Angiography (CTPA)

It has replaced other investigations for diagnosing pulmonary embolism. It is highly sensitive (94%) and specific (100%). In a systematic review of available studies the negative predictive value was reported to be very high (99.1%). Thus normal CT rules out the diagnosis of pulmonary embolism. It is easier to perform, readily available, does not require follow up imaging and can rule out other disorders with similar clinical presentations.

There is reluctance to use CT during pregnancy due to radiation exposure to the fetus. Winner-Muram in a recent study found that average radiation dose was higher with ventilation-perfusion V/Q scan as compared to CT in all trimesters of pregnancy. The average fetal radiation dose with CTPA is less than 10% of that with V/Q scanning during all trimesters of pregnancy.

In most recent guidelines from British Thoracic Society, CTPA is recommended as the initial imaging modality in pregnancy for diagnosing pulmonary embolism.[18] The drawbacks of CTPA over V/Q scan include high radiation dose to maternal breast tissue and if iodinated contrast is used, alteration of fetal thyroid function can occur.

MR Angiography

Newer generation of MRI have faster imaging acquisition time and this has made possible to visualize pulmonary vasculature. Initial studies are promising and have shown a high sensitivity and specificity.[19] There are no reported studies of its use in pregnancy at present and its role is yet to be established. Flow chart 19.2 depicts the diagnostic algorithm for suspected pulmonary embolism.

PROPHYLACTIC MEASURES

The patients should be classified as low risk, medium risk or high risk and should be managed accordingly (Table 19.2).

Thromboembolism in Pregnancy

Both mechanical and pharmacological methods are effective. Various preventive methods used are listed as below:

- Graduated compression stockings (TED stockings).
- Sequential pneumatic compression devices.
- IVC filters for prevention of pulmonary embolism.
- Low dose unfractionated heparin.
- Low molecular weight heparin.
- Adjusted dose warfarin.

The acquired risk factors can be reduced by measures like:

- Lifestyle changes and encouraging mild physical activity in pregnancy.
- Early detection of any risk factors: anemia, gestational hypertension, cardiac disease.
- Prompt management of infections and avoiding dehydration due to fever or hyperemesis gravidarum.
- Avoiding prolonged labor and immobility after delivery.
- Strict asepsis in all surgical procedures like instrumental delivery, episiotomy and cesarean section.

MANAGEMENT

Acute venous thromboembolism is a medical emergency and needs urgent therapy. Treatment of acute venous thromboembolism revolves around anticoagulants. Current guidelines for treatment during pregnancy are based on expert opinion rather than evidence from randomized trials.

Recent cochrane review concluded that at present there is insufficient evidence for making any recommendations for treatment and prophylaxis of VTE during pregnancy.[4]

Anticoagulants

Heparin
    Unfractionated heparin (UFH)
    Low molecular weight heparin (LMWH)
    Enoxaparin
    Nadoparin
    Dalteparin
    Reviparin
    Tinzaprin

Oral anticoagulants
    Warfarin

Unfractionated Heparin (UFH)

It is a mixture of polysaccharide chains ranging in molecular weight from 3000 to 30,000 daltons. It binds to AT-III and forms a complex which inhibits factors IIa, IXa and Xa.

Dose of heparin is based on body weight and standard nomograms are available. Periodic monitoring with Activated partial thromboplastin time (aPTT) is required to confirm the adequate dose (Table 19.3). Activated partial thromboplastin time (aPTT) of 1.5 to 2 times of normal or heparin level of 0.5 to 1.2 U/mL is required for therapeutic effect. It is not very sensitive as heparin resistance occurs due to increased fibrinogen and factor VIII. It is more useful to determine anti-Xa levels as a measure of heparin dose.

Advantage
1. Rapid reversal of anticoagulation, as it has a short half life.
2. Low cost.

Disadvantage
1. Monitoring is required.
2. Need of hospitalization for administration and monitoring.
3. Side effects like–bleeding, osteoporosis and heparin induced thrombocytopenia.
   Direct thrombin inhibitors like danaparoid and lepirudin (category B) can be used in heparin induced thrombocytopenia.

Low Molecular Weight Heparin (LMWHs)

LMWHs are produced by enzymatic or chemical depolymerization of UFH. LMWHs bind to AT-III and this complex selectively inhibits factor Xa.

Each LMWH is a distinct molecule and cannot be used interchangeably. In pregnancy enoxaparin and dalteparin have established safety profile. In small number of studies reviparin, tinzaparin and nadoparin have also been used.

Dosage of LMWH is according to body weight (Table 19.3).

In nonpregnant patients monitoring is not required as dose response is predictable. It is still controversial whether routine monitoring is required in pregnant patients due to altered pharmacokinetics. Monitoring is done by anti-Xa levels.

LMWHs are presently preferred over UFH for treatment of VTE unless there are cost constraints (Table 19.4).

Advantage

1. Lower incidence of side effects.
2. Monitoring is not required.

Disadvantage

High cost

Thromboembolism in Pregnancy

Table 19.2: Primary prophylaxis for congenital and acquired thrombophilias

Risk category	Disorders	Dose of anticoagulant
High	H/O Idiopathic DVT DVT in past pregnancy Antithrombin III deficiency Homozygous protein C Homozygous factor V Leiden Homozygous prothrombin 20210A	Therapeutic dose
Moderate	Heterozygous protein S Heterozygous G20210A Heterozygous factor V Leiden with family history of thrombosis	Prophylactic dose
Low	Single episode of DVT and no genetic risk factor Heterozygous factor V Leiden or Heterozygous G20210A with no family and personal history of thrombosis	Prophylactic dose

Oral Anticoagulants

Warfarin is a vitamin K antagonist. It inhibits production of factors II, VII, IX and X. It is listed as category D drug in pregnancy because of known teratogenic effects.

It crosses the placenta and if given between sixth and twelfth weeks of gestation it results in typical embryopathy consisting of short stature with stippled epiphysis, nasal hypoplasia, saddle nose and frontal bossing. In second and third trimesters the defects occur due to fetal hemorrhage and scarring and include dorsal midline dysplasia, Dandy walker malformation, midline cerebellar atrophy and ventral midline dysplasia with optic atrophy. It is also associated with still births and increased risk of fetal bleeding. The dose is adjusted to achieve an INR of 2.5 to 3.0.

Monitoring is required and done by INR (international normalized ratio). The patients who are on warfarin should have preconceptional counseling and should be switched to LMWH as soon as they conceive. In patients on warfarin due to cardiac valve replacement, warfarin should be restarted after 12 weeks as the risk of thromboembolism is higher with heparin. Warfarin is also considered in cases in which adequate anticoagulation is not achieved with heparin (refractory cases).

Management of Deep Vein Thrombosis (Flow chart 19.3)

The leg should be elevated and graduated elastic compression stocking should be applied to reduce edema. There is no requirement for bed rest in a stable patient on anticoagulant treatment with acute DVT. Mobilization with graduated

Drug	Therapeutic dose	Prophylatic dose	Side effects	Monitoring	Contra-indiactions	Reversal agents
Heparin	Loading dose is 80 to100 U/kg I.V. Maintainence dose is 14-18 U/kg/hr I.V. I.V. heparin is given for 7 to 10 days and switched over to S.C later· S.C. dosage is 2/3 rd of total IV dose.	5000U SC 12 hr	Bleeding (5-10%). Thrombocytopenia (5-30%) usually after 10 days of therapy. Osteoporosis (1-5%) usually after 2-3 months of therapy. Hypersensitivity <1%. Increase AST/ALT.	aPTT Platelet count	Active bleeding. History of HIT. Platelet count < 20,000. History of neurosurgery or ocular surgery in past 10 days. Intracranial bleed in past 10 days	Protamine Sulfate
LMWH	Enoxaparin 1mg/kg 12 hrly. Dalteparin 100U/kg 12 hrly.	Enoxaparin 40 mg S.C 12 hr Dalteparin 5000U S.C. OD	Bleeding. Thrombocytopenia. Increased AST/ALT.	anti-Xa Platelet count	Same as above	Partial reversal by protamine sulfate
Wafarin	Dosage according to INR Tablet 5mg	Dosage according to INR	Bleeding. Congenital anomalies (0-30%). Miscarriage (14-56%). Still birth (5-33%). Fetal bleeding (2%). Neurological sequel in neonates (14%).	INR	Same as above	Vitamin K Fresh Frozen plasma

19

Table 19.4: Comparison of heparin and LMWH

	Heparin	LMWH
Molecular weight	3000 to 30000 daltons	4000 to 6500 daltons
Route of administration	i.v. or s.c.	s.c.
Bioavailability	30% by s.c. route	92%
Half life	30 mins to 1hr for i.v., 1 to 2 hr for s.c.	4 to 6 hrs
Mechanism of action	Inhibits IIa, IXa and Xa	Inhibits Xa
Onset of action	Immediate if given i.v.	4 to 6 hrs
Duration of action	1 hr for i.v., 3 hr for s.c.	8 to 12 hrs
Monitoring	Required	Controversial in pregnancy
Monitoring method	aPTT	Anti-Xa
Side effects	More common	Less
Cost	Low	High

elastic compression stockings should be encouraged. If venous gangrene develops

Thromboembolism in Pregnancy

Flow chart 19.3: Management of deep vein thrombosis

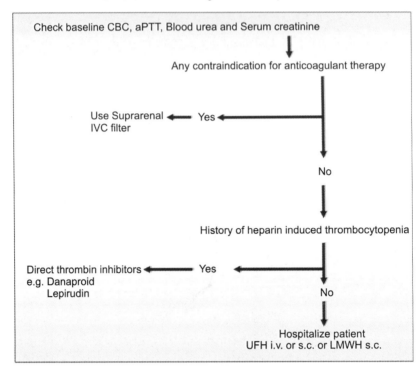

anticoagulation and limb elevation should be continued and consideration to surgical embolectomy or thrombolytic therapy should be given.

The delivery should be delayed if possible to allow maximum time for anticoagulation.

Temporary IVC filter should be considered in perinatal period in:
a. Women with iliac vein thrombosis to reduce risk of pulmonary embolism.
b. Women with proven DVT who have continuing PTE despite adequate anticoagulation.

UFH and LMWH are equally effective. Choice is determined by bleeding risk, medical history and affordability.The therapeutic dose should be continued throughout the pregnancy. It is not yet established whether the dose of heparin can be reduced after initial period of several weeks of therapeutic anticoagulation.

Management of Pulmonary Embolism (Flow chart 19.4)

Patients with pulmonary embolism need intensive care unit admission for management. In pulmonary embolism cardiac pulmonary stabilization is the first priority. The patient should be put in propped up position and high flow oxygen should be started immediately.

The management should be individualized based on the condition of the patient:

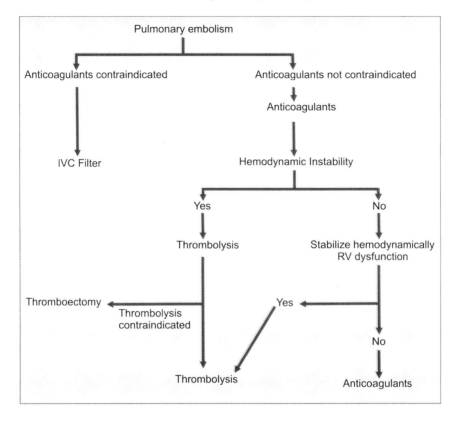

- Intravenous unfractionated heparin.
- Thrombolytic therapy.
- Thoracotomy and surgical embolectomy.
- Suprarenal placement of Greenfield IVC filter.
- Loading dose of heparin followed by infusion should be given. Loading dose should be omitted if thrombolysis has been given.
- The APTT should be measured 4-6 hours after loading dose, 6 hours after dose change and daily when in the therapeutic range.
- Thrombolytic therapy in pregnancy has been reported with streptokinase, urokinase and recombinant tissue plasminogen activator. It is contraindicated 24 hours before delivery and for 2 weeks postpartum. It should be reserved for women with severe pulmonary embolism with hemodynamic compromise. Associated maternal bleeding complications rate is in the range of 1-6% comparable to nonpregnant women. There are reports of fetal deaths but no maternal deaths have been reported.[5]
- Thoracotomy should only be undertaken in a patient not suitable for thrombolysis or is in a moribund state.

Thromboembolism in Pregnancy

Intrapartum Management of Patients Therapeutically Anticoagulated during Pregnancy

Patients at term require admission for further management. If the patient was on warfarin she should be switched to heparin after 36 weeks. It should be stopped as soon as patient perceives labor pains. For elective delivery, LMWH should be stopped 24 hours before induction of labor or cesarean section.

If the patient is on unfractionated heparin, at the spontaneous onset of labor or in case of emergency cesarean section, unfractionated heparin is discontinued and careful monitoring of aPTT is done. Protamine may be used for reversal of heparin effect, 1 mg of protamine neutralizes 100U of heparin. Protamine is routinely not used as anaphylaxis and bleeding can occur. Subcutaneous unfractionated heparin should be discontinued 12 hours before and intravenous should be stopped 6 hours before induction of labor or regional anesthesia.

Epidural and spinal anesthesia is not used when LMWH has been given in last 24 hours as permanent neurological deficit can occur due to hematoma formation. In women receiving therapeutic doses of LMWH, wound drains should be considered at cesarean section and skin incision should be closed with interrupted sutures to allow drainage of hematoma. Anticoagulation is restarted 8 to 12 hours after vaginal delivery and 18 to 24 hours after cesarean section.

Intrapartum management of patient's prophylatically anticoagulated during pregnancy includes discontinuation of heparin or LMWH at the onset of labor.

Anticoagulation is restarted 8 to 24 hours after delivery depending on the route of delivery.

Postpartum Management of Patients Anticoagulated During Pregnancy (Table 19.5)

Duration of anticoagulation in postpartum period depends on the indication of starting it. LMWH, UFH and warfarin are equally safe and effective in postpartum period. Choice of anticoagulant depends on patient preference. Both warfarin and heparin are safe in breastfeeding women. Warfarin should be avoided until third postpartum day in patients with high risk of hemorrhage. For switchover from heparin to warfarin daily INR should be checked after day 2 of therapy and subsequent doses should be titrated to maintain INR between 2-3. Treatment with heparin should be continued until the INR is greater than 2 on two successive days.

If the swelling persists after treatment of DVT, graduated elastic compression stocking should be worn on the affected leg for 2 years after the acute event to reduce the risk of post-thrombotic syndrome.

Oral contraceptives are contraindicated and the role of thromboprophylaxis in pregnancy is controversial if patient had developed DVT on oral contraceptives.

Table 19.5: Thromboprophylaxis during pregnancy and puerperium[20]

Risk*	Status of the patient	Prophylaxis
1.	Previous VTE (±thrombophillia) on long-term warfarin	Antenatal high prophylactic or therapeutic dose of LMWH and at least six weeks of postnatal warfarin
2.	Previous recurrent VTE not on long-term warfarin Previous VTE + thrombophilia Previous VTE + family history of VTE Asymptomatic thrombophilia	Antenatal and six weeks postnatal prophylactic LMWH
3.	Single previous provoked VTE without thrombophilia, family history or other risk factors Asymptomatic thrombophilia (except antithrombin deficiency, combined defects, homozygous FVL or prothrombin gene defect which come in high risk)	Six weeks of postnatal prophylactic LMWH±antenatal low dose aspirin

* 1. Very high risk 2. High risk 3. Moderate risk

KEY POINTS

- Venous tromboembolism is the leading cause of maternal mortality in western world.
- Pregnant and post-partum women are at increased risk of VTE.
- A high index of suspicion helps in early diagnosis and timely treatment.
- Women with thrombophilic disorders should be counseled about increased risk of thrombosis and adverse outcomes during pregnancy and offered prophylactic antepartum and postpartum anticoagulant therapy.
- Timely institution of therapeutic and prophylactic anticoagulation can prevent maternal morbidity and mortality.
- LMWHs are preferred anticoagulants unless there are cost constraints.

REFERENCES

1. Arkel YS, Ku DH. Thrombophilia and pregnancy: Review of the literature and some original data. Clin Appl Thromb Hemost 2001; 7(4):259-68.
2. Sonal Vora, Kanjaksha Ghosh, Shrimati Shetty, Vinita Salvi, Purnima Satoskar. Deep vein thrombosis in antenatal period in a large cohort of pregnancies from western India. Thrombosis Journal 2007;5:9-14.
3. Toglia MR, Nolan TE. Venous Thromboembolism during pregnancy: A current review of diagnosis and management. Obstet Gynecol Surv 1997;52:60-72.
4. Gates S, Brocklehust P, Davis LJ. Prophylaxis for venous thromboembolic disease in pregnancy and early postnatal period. Cochrane Database Syst Rev 2002;(2):CD001689.
5. Conard J, Hornellu MH, Samama MM. Inherited thrombophilia and gestational venous thromboembolism. Semin Thromb Hemost 2003;29:131-41.
6. Sandler D, Martin J, Duncan J, et al. Diagnosis of deep vein thrombosis: Comparison of clinical evaluation, ultrasound, plethysmography and venoscan with X-ray venogram. Lancet 1984;8405:716-19.

19

Thromboembolism in Pregnancy

7. Bounameaux H, De Moerloose P, Perrrier A, et al. Plasma measurement of D-dimer as diagnostic aid in suspected venous thromboembolism: an overview. Thromb Haemost 1994;71:1-6.

8. Francalanci I, Comeglio P, Liotta A, et al. D-dimer concentrations during normal pregnancy, as measured by ELISA. Thromb Res 1995;78(5)399-405.

9. Polak JF, Wilkinson DL. Ultrasonographic diagnosis of symptomatic deep vein thrombosis in pregnancy. Am J Obstet Gynecol 1991;165(3):625-29.

10. Kassai B, Boiseel J, Cucherat M, et al. A systematic review of the accuracy of ultrasound in diagnosis of deep venous thrombosis in asymptomatic patients. Thromb Haemost 2004;91:655-66.

11. Loud PA, Katz DS,Klippenstein DL, et al. Combined CT venography and pulmonary angiography in suspected thromboembolic disease: diagnostic accuracy for deep venous evaluation. AJR Am J Roentgol 2000;174(1):61-65.

12. Moody AR. Magnetic resonance direct thrombus imaging. J Thromb Haemost 2003;1(7): 1403-09.

13. Roger M, Makropoulos D, Turek M, et al. Diagnostic value of electrocardiogram in suspected pulmonary embolism. Am J Cadiol 2000;86:807-09.

14. Tapson V, Carroll B, Davidson B, et al. Diagnostic approach to acute venous thromboembolism. Clinical practice guidline. American Thoracic Society. Am J Respir Crit Care Med 1999;160:1043-66.

15. Come P. Echocardiographic evaluation of pulmonary embolism and its response to therapeutic interventions. Chest 1992;101:151S-62S.

16. Dalen J, Brooks H, Johnson L, et al. Pulmonary angiography in acute pulmonary embolism: Indications, technique and results in 367 patients. Am Heart J 1971;81:175-85.

17. Value of ventilation/perfusion scan in acute pulmonary embolism. Results of the prospective investigation of pulmonary embolism diagnosis(PIOPED). The PIOPED investigators. JAMA 1990;263:2653-59.

18. British Thoracic Society guidelines for management of suspected pulmonary embolism. Thorax 2003;58(6):470-83.

19. Moody AR. Magnetic resonance direct thrombus imaging. J Thromb Haemost 2003;1(7): 1403-09.

20. Thromboprophylaxis during pregnancy, labour and after vaginal delivery. RCOG, Guideline No. 37, 2004.

Thyroid Disorders with Pregnancy

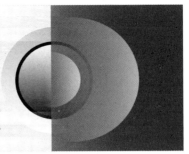

20

Kiran Aggarwal

INTRODUCTION

Thyroid disorder is a common endocrine disease second only to diabetes in the women of reproductive age group and can widely affect reproductive performance of a woman. It is difficult to make a diagnosis especially in pregnancy because physiological changes and symptoms of pregnancy are very similar to those of thyroid dysfunction.

This chapter highlights the normal maternal and fetal thyroid physiology in pregnancy, various thyroid dysfunctions and recommendations for their treatment and screening for thyroid disease in pregnancy.

MATERNAL PHYSIOLOGY

Thyroid gland is made up of follicles. Each follicle is a spherical structure lined by single layer of thyroid follicular cells and a lumen for storage of thyroglobulin.

Thyroid can maintain its iodine concentration by actively trapping it from the extra cellular pool. This function is potentiated by TSH (Thyroid Stimulating Hormone). This active uptake takes care of the dietary fluctuations of iodine. Iodide is oxidized to iodine by thyroid peroxidase and then incorporated into tyrosine residues of thyroglobulin in lumen. This iodide organification results in synthesis of mono-iodotyrosine and di-iodotyrosine. These are inactive compounds. Thyroid peroxidase couples these to form thyroxine (T4) and triiodiothyroxine (T3) which are the active hormones. T3 is three times more potent than T4 and most of it is produced by peripheral deiodination of T4.

Thyroid function is regulated by hypothalamus pituitary thyroid feedback mechanism. Thyroid stimulating hormone (TSH) is a glycoprotein with alpha and beta subunits. Alpha subunit is shared with other pituitary hormones but beta is unique and is somewhat related to the beta subunit of human chorionic gonadotropin.

TSH increases synthesis and release of thyroid hormones both thyroxine(T4)and triiodothyroxine (T3).

T3 and T4 are mostly protein bound in circulation and only small unbound portions are active. The binding proteins for thyroid hormones are thyroid binding globulin (TBG), albumin and transthyretin.

TBG has greatest affinity for T4 and T3 and 75% of the thyroid hormones are bound to it. Only 0.04% of T4 and 0.5% of T3 are free.

CHANGES IN THYROID PHYSIOLOGY DURING PREGNANCY (TABLE 20.1)

1. The high estrogen status of pregnancy increases the half-life of thyroid binding globulin (TBG) and decreases its clearance. TBG production begins to increase in first two weeks of pregnancy and reaches a plateau by 20 weeks of gestation. Thus total T4 and T3 production is increased during pregnancy to compensate for this rapid increase in extra thyroid pool of thyroxine.[1]
2. Increase in glomerular filtration rate from early first trimester of pregnancy causes increased renal loss of iodide.[2] This causes an increase in iodide requirement from diet. In iodine depleted areas it causes decrease in circulatory iodine.
3. Fetal thyroid activity starts in early second trimester. Transport of iodide to fetus causes further decrease in the maternal pool.
4. In dietary iodine deficiency thyroid increases its uptake of iodide from circulation and this may cause maternal hypothyroxinemia and enlargement of thyroid. Goiter may be seen in both mother and fetus.[1]
5. In iodine deficient areas, iodine deprived goiter may take up iodide preferentially over placenta thus causing cretinism in the child.

During first trimester fetus is dependent on maternal T4 and it is during this time that increasing total T4 necessitates a greater maternal requirement for iodine and in deficient states if maternal hypothyroxinemia occurs, it adversely affects fetal brain development. Fetal hypothyroidism and neonatal hypothyroidism may also occur.[3]

A part of beta subunit of hCG has thyrotropic activity. It may stimulate TSH receptors causing increase in free T4 levels and a decrease in TSH level by negative feed back mechanism, maximally seen at the end of the first trimester which is the time for peak circulating hCG.[4]

Increased thyroid binding globulin	Increased iodine requirement	Increased hCG
Increased plasma volume Increased total T4 and T3	Due to renal loss, transport to fetus requirement for increased maternal Pool of total T4 and T3 ↓ Increased iodine uptake by the thyroid gland 10-15% rise in the size of the thyroid gland	Increased free T4, Decreased TSH

ASSESSMENT OF THYROID FUNCTION IN PREGNANCY

In normal uncomplicated pregnancy minor fall in TSH and an increase in free T4 (fT4) concentration occurs in first trimester possibly because of hCG. This may be a mechanism to provide the fetus with T4 in first trimester before fetal thyroid activity is established in midtrimester.

Use of total T4 levels to asses the thyroid function at earlier gestational period is not useful. [5,6]

For assessing thyroid function in pregnancy, free T3 and free T4 and TSH should be analyzed rather than total values. For change of dose more importance is given to fT4 and fT3 levels as these reflect the actual thyroid status more accurately rather than TSH.

Direct free T4 assays are available which provide accurate estimates of free thyroid hormone concentration but the values should be adapted to trimester specific ranges.

Free T4 rises in first trimester and then it declines progressively during later gestational stages.[7] Serum TSH values are affected by thyrotrophic activity of circulating hCG particularly near the end of first trimester. TSH levels may be lowered to subnormal values but later on in pregnancy they gradually rise. By using classical non pregnant range of serum TSH (0.4-4.0 MIU/L) one may misdiagnose woman with increased TSH as normal and a woman as hyperthyroid with physiological fall in TSH.Lower normal limit of serum TSH decreases to 0.03 MIU/L in first and second trimester and to 0.13 in third trimester. Serum TSH levels above 2.5 MIU/L in first trimester and 3 MIU/L in second and third trimester may indicate a thyroid dysfunction.[8]

In hypothyroidism TSH may remain elevated despite normal fT4 and fT3 for sometime even after right dose of treatment and in hyperthyroidism TSH may remain suppressed once fT4 and fT3 return to normal for some time. Serum autoantibodies to the thyroid tissue like thyroid stimulating hormone (TSH) receptor stimulating antibodies found in Grave's disease and thyroid peroxidase antibodies found in autoimmune thyroiditis causing hypothyroidism and antibodies to thyroglobulin are also seen. They freely cross placenta and can be measured.

20

Thyroid Disorders with Pregnancy

The fetal thyroid gland develops at 5 weeks of pregnancy and begins concentrating iodine from 10-12 weeks onwards. Fetal free and total T3, T4, TSH and TBG can be detected in fetal blood from 12 weeks of gestation and increase with advancing gestation and reach adult levels by 36 weeks of gestation.[9] For first 10-12 weeks of pregnancy fetus is totally dependent on mother for thyroid hormones (T4). By end of first trimester hormone production starts, but fetus is dependent on mother for ingestion of enough iodide to make sufficient thyroid hormones.The fetal thyroid gland comes under control of fetal pituitary by 20 weeks of gestation. Maternal T3 and TSH do not cross placenta but maternal T4, thyroid stimulating hormone releasing hormone (TRH), iodine, thyroid receptor stimulating antibodies, antithyroid antibodies and antithyroid drugs cross the placenta readily. The peripheral conversion of T4 to T3 which accounts for most adult T3 is not active in fetus except in fetal brain.[10]

Human fetal brain has T3 receptors from late first trimester, whereas other tissues including liver, heart and lung have only T4 receptors throughout second trimester. Fetal brain T3 arises by conversion from T4 which is available only from the mother in the first trimester.[11]

Maternal T3 cannot cross placenta nor is taken up by the fetal brain which relies on it's own conversion from T4 to T3 so in areas of chronic iodine deficiency where maternal T4 is low but T3 is preserved, the fetal brain may be adversely affected .These are the areas where endemic cretinism occurs due to fetal thyroid dysfunction.[12]

IODINE NUTRITION IN PREGNANCY

Iodine deficiency causes goiter in adults and cretinism in newborns. It adversely affects reproductive performance in women. Neurological endemic cretinism is an important cause of mental retardation world wide which is preventable. Maternal iodine deficiency and hypothyroxinemia causes fetal hypothyroidism.[13] In areas of endemic iodine deficiency maternal findings are goiter in association with normal T3 and raised TSH. Neurological cretinism is common because fetal brain uses T3 from intracellular conversion of T4 to T3. This T4 is maternal, passed to the fetus during first trimester and maternal T4 production is impaired because of iodine deficiency.

Iodine administration to women before conception till second trimester helps in a long way in improving neurological status and protecting fetal brain.[14] Pre pregnancy iodine supplementation helps in improving the pregnancy outcome, reducing pregnancy loss and decreasing the stillbirth rate.

The recommended nurtrient intake for iodine in adults and children above the age of 12 years is 150 µg/day. Universal salt iodization is the most commonly used method to make sufficient iodine available. In pregnancy and breast feeding 200-300 µg/day of iodine is recommended.[15]

During lactation, thyroid hormone production returns to normal but iodine is efficiently concentrated by the mammary gland. Because breast milk provides approximately 100 μg of iodine daily to the infant, it is recommended that the breast feeding mother should continue to take 250 μg/day of iodine.

In countries or places without efficient salt supplementation programme, oral iodine supplement as potassium iodide 100-200 μg/day or incorporating it in multivitamin tablet especially for pregnancy should be done. In places where this is difficult orally, iodized oil containing 400 mg of iodine will take care of iodine requirement for one year period.[16]

Excess intake of iodine by mother causes suppression of thyroid hormone synthesis induced by high concentrations of intrathyroid iodine. Pregnant women should avoid taking cough remedies or eye drops with iodine because it will cause fetal hypothyroidism. Iodine intake during pregnancy and breast feeding should not exceed twice the daily recommended for iodine, i.e. 500 μg/day.

GESTATIONAL HYPERTHYROIDISM

Hyperemesis gravidarum is associated with high hCG levels but it's exact etiology is not known. 30-60% of patients with hyperemesis gravidarum have elevated free thyroid hormone concentration with suppressed TSH possibly due to thyroid receptor stimulating activity of hCG. A small portion of these patients have clinical hyperthyroidism called gestational hyperthyroidism.[17,18] Co-incidental Grave's disease may also be present. Gestational hyperthyroidism is characterized by elevated free T4 and T3 levels with suppressed TSH with variable evidence of clinical hyperthyroidism and absence of antithyroid antibodies. [19]

Most patients with gestational hyperthyroidism do not have obvious clinical symptoms of hyperthyroidism and spontaneous recovery of thyroid hormone levels to normal usually occurs. Close observation of clinical course, clinical symptoms and thyroid levels is needed. Antithyroid therapy to patient with symptomatic hyperthyroidism and severly elevated T4 and T3 should be given. Therapy often can be discontinued if hyperemesis subsides by mid gestation.

Subclinical Hyperthyroidism

Treatment of subclinical hyperthyroidism, that is TSH below normal with free T3 and T4 in normal pregnant range, has not been found to improve pregnancy outcomes and may risk unnecessary exposure of fetus to antithyroid drugs.[17, 18, 20,21]

HYPERTHYROIDISM

Hyperthyroidism is seen in 0.2% of pregnant women.[22] Thyrotoxicosis may be caused by:

- Grave's disease
- Toxic multinodular goiter
- Solitary toxic nodule
- Acute thyroidits (de Quervain's or postpartum)
- Subacute thyroiditis
- Well differentiated thyroid carcinoma
- Hyperfunctioning ovarian teratoma
- TSH producing adenoma
- hCG producing tumor

Grave's Disease

Grave's Disease is the most common cause of hyperthyroidism in the reproductive age group. It is characterized by diffuse hypertrophic and hyperplastic goiter, presence of IgG thyrotrophin receptor stimulating antibodies and other thyroid autoantibodies like antiperoxidase antibodies. Hyperthyroidism is there with presence of eye signs.

Postpartum Thyroiditis

It occurs after 10% of all pregnancies and may have a hyperthyroid phase in the initial one to two months followed by hypothyroid phase.[23] It may begin 6 weeks to 6 months after delivery and the woman may become pregnant again in this time frame and may be hypothyroid at the time of conception. Therefore sequential evaluation of thyroid functions is important because hypothyroidism is an important risk for fetal development.

Pregnancy and Hyperthyroidism

Clinical course of Grave's disease follows the levels of thyrotrophin receptor stimulating antibodies which increase in the first trimester, fall in the second and third trimesters and again rise in the puerperium. Disease may worsen in first trimester and puerperium.[24] Grave's disease remits in second and third trimesters and the doses of the antithyroid medications need to be reduced or discontinued in 30% of cases.[25] These changes reflect altered maternal immune state. Labor, cesarean section and infections may aggravate hyperthyroidism and even trigger thyroid storm.[26] Pregnancy does not influence long-term course of hyperthyroidism.

Effect of Hyperthyroidism on Pregnancy

If thyrotoxicosis is well controlled before and throughout pregnancy the outcomes for both mother and baby are generally good. Thyrotoxicosis may be associated with adverse outcomes for the mother as it increases the risk for hypertensive disease of pregnancy, pre-eclampsia, infections, thyroid storm and congestive cardiac failure. Cardiac failure is more common and occurs because of long-term myocardial effects of T4 and is precipitated by hypertension, infections and anemia.[27]

Fetal and neonatal risks of maternal hyperthyroid disease are related to the disease itself and or to the medical treatment of the disease. Inadequately treated maternal thyrotoxicosis is associated with an increased risk of miscarriage, growth restriction, premature labor, placental abruption and increased perinatal mortality.[28,29] In addition, over treatment of the mother with thionamides can result in iatrogenic fetal hypothyroidism.

Diagnosis of Hyperthyroidism

Thyrotoxicosis usually presents in late first and early second trimester. Clinical diagnosis of hyperthyroidism is difficult because symptoms like fatigue, anxiety, emotional lability, heat intolerance, sweating, warm extremities, etc. may also be reported by normal euthyroid pregnant patients. Failure to gain weight particularly in presence of a good appetite and presence of maternal tachycardia greater than 100 beats per minute which fails to slow with valsalva maneuver helps in the diagnosis. Symptoms that persist beyond 20 weeks gestation, symptoms that occur before onset of pregnancy and presence of thyroid stimulating antibodies suggest true hyperthyroidism. In early pregnancy if there are features suggestive of hyperemesis, hyperthyroidism and trophoblastic disease should be ruled out. Eye signs like exopthalmos and lid lag, significant goiter and presence of thyroid stimulating antibodies may indicate Grave's disease.The diagnosis is confirmed by elevated free T4 or free T3 levels with suppressed TSH level. The levels should be interpreted after keeping in mind the fluctuations of hormone levels in normal pregnancy. Thyroid receptor antibodies should also be measured.

MANAGEMENT

Pre-pregnancy

Patients with thyrotoxicosis may have hypomenorrhea and oligomenorrhea.[30] It is ideal to treat these patients before pregnancy is planned so that radioactive iodine if needed may be used or if surgery is needed it can be performed.

Patients who have received radioactive iodine should not conceive for four months after last treatment. It is contraindicated in pregnancy.[31] A euthyroid state of 3 months before conception is advisable. Well controlled thyrotoxicosis has a low risk of adverse obstetric outcome. Antithyroid medication should not be discontinued either pre-pregnancy or antenatally.

Antenatal Management of Hyper Thyroidism (Table 20.2)

Table 20.2: Therapeutic options for treatment of hyperthyroidism
Medical management
Thionamides like propylthiouracil, carbimazole and methimazole.
Beta blockers like propranolol.
Iodides
Radioactive iodine.
Surgery

Medical Therapy

This is usually the first treatment option. Lowest possible dose of medication should be used so that risk of fetal hypothyroidism is minimized.

The aim of the treatment is to maintain a euthyroid state and a free T4 level at the upper nonpregnant reference ranges.[32]

Antithyroid drugs thionamides like propylthiouracil (PTU), methimazole (MMI) and carbimazole are used during gestation. They inhibit thyroid hormone synthesis via reduction of iodine organification and iodotyrosine coupling. They also have an immunosuppressive effect reducing the titer of TSH receptor antibody.[33] Onset of action is delayed until preformed hormones are depleted which can take three to four weeks. Placental transfer kinetics appears to be similar for both PTU and MMI[34] and both cross placenta equally. The effect on fetal neonatal thyroid function appears to be similar for two agents. Available evidence suggests that methimazole may be associated with congenital anomalies like esophageal atresia and aplasia cutis. Propylthiouracil should be used as a first line drug if available especially during first trimester organogenesis. If propylthiouracil is not available or patient cannot tolerate propylthiouracil then methimazole may be prescribed.[35]

Dosage of drugs

Newly diagnosed patients should be given PTU 400 mg daily or carbimazole 40 mg daily for 4-6 weeks and then the dose can be reduced gradually.It takes 7-8 weeks after starting therapy for the patient to become euthyroid. The dose of the medication is titrated against maternal well-being and biochemical assessment of thyroid status.

Follow up

A well controlled patient should be seen at 4-6 weekly intervals, should be examined and thyroid functions performed but if newly diagnosed or if there is a relapse more frequent follow ups should be done.Patient should be followed in puerperium where increase in dosage may be needed.

Side effects

Drug induced agranulocytosis and hepatitis may occur which is idiosyncratic with propylthiouracil and dose related with carbimazole. Patients are asked

Management of High-Risk Pregnancy—A Practical Approach

to report sore throat and fever immediately. Total leucocyte count should be performed and if neutropenia is there, treatment should be discontinued. Nausea, vomiting and diarrhea may also occur. Drug rash and urticaria are seen in 1-5% of cases.

Beta blockers

Propranolol should be used for tremors or tachycardia.[36] It is used to treat symptoms of acute hyperthyroid disease and for preoperative preparation. There are no significant teratogenic effects of propranolol reported in humans or in animals.

Iodides.

Iodides should not be used as a first line therapy for women with Grave's disease but they could be used transiently if needed in preparation for thyroidectomy.

Radioactive iodine diagnostic tests or therapy is contraindicated during pregnancy and lactation. Fetal thyroid uptake of iodine commences after 12 weeks, exposure to maternal RAI (Radio active iodine) before the 12th week is not associated with fetal thyroid dysfunction.[37] Treatment after 12 weeks leads to significant radiation to the fetal thyroid, multiple instances of exposure causing fetal thyroid destruction and hypothyroidism have been reported.

Surgery

Subtotal thyroidectomy in pregnancy as therapy for maternal Graves' disease is considered if a serious adverse reaction to antithyroid therapy occurs, if very high doses of drugs are required, and in women who develop stridor, respiratory distress and dysphagia because of the disease. Surgery should be performed only when deemed to be medically necessary for the mother's health.[22] It is safest in the second trimester. Morbidity and mortality rates are increased when surgery is done in pregnancy.

Labor and Delivery

Thyroid storm is an uncommon life threatening crisis which requires immediate medical treatment. It carries a mortality of 10%. It is characterized by acute exacerbation of thyrotoxicosis in a patient of hyperthyroidism. It may get precipitated by labor, delivery, infection, anesthesia and withdrawl of antithyroid drugs.

Patient may present with extreme symptoms of thyrotoxicosis, pyrexia and changes in the mental state. There may be tachycardia, arrhythmias and cardiac failure. Gastrointestinal symptoms like nausea and vomiting may also be present. Diagnosis is clinical. Thyroid functions may be as in uncomplicated hyperthyroidism. Increased TLC, increased liver enzymes and hypercalcemia may also be seen.

Management of thyroid storm consists of supportive therapy like intravenous fluids, controlling infections, treating fever and removing precipitating factors. A large loading dose of 1000 mg of PTU is given followed by 150-300 mg 6 hourly. One to two hours after PTU Lugol's iodine 500 mg 6 hourly should be given to further inhibit release of thyroid hormones from the thyroid gland. Propranolol, digoxin, diuretics and steroids may be needed as required.

Prolonged maternal hypoxia and dehydration may affect fetus but cesarean section is dangerous in presence of fulminating thyroid storm. Correcting metabolic insult to the mother helps fetus to recover.

Postnatal

Breastfeeding is safe with a daily dose of propylthiouracil of 50-300 mg or less and carbimazole less than 15 mg daily for periods ranging from 3 weeks to 8 months.[38,39] 0.07% of maternal dose of PTU and 0.5% of carbimazole is excreted in breast milk.[40] No adverse effect on fetal thyroid function has been reported with these doses. Drugs should be given after feeding. Monitoring of the infant's thyroid function should be done. Graves' disease can flare postnatally and maternal antibodies may rise. In patients who have stopped taking medication during pregnancy, it may be needed to restart the drugs in 2-3 months after delivery.

Fetal Effects of Maternal Antithyroid Drugs

Antithyroid drugs (ATD) should be given to the mother ensuring that the fetal thyroid function is minimally affected. Serum level of propylthiouracil after ingestion varies in different individuals and also transplacental passage of antibodies also varies. Therefore fetal thyroid status is not strictly correlated with maternal antithyroid dosage.Current maternal thyroid status rather than antithyroid dose may be the most reliable marker for titration of therapy to avoid fetal hypothyroidism.[34] If the maternal serum free T4 concentration is either elevated or maintained in the upper third of the normal non pregnant reference range, serum free T4 levels are normal in more than 90% of the neonates.[21]

High doses of antithyroid medication may cause fetal hypothyroidism in 10-20% of patients on thionalamides but rarely goiter. Neonatal hypothyroidism usually resolves spontaneously by day 5 of life.[41] Umbilical cord blood sampling should be considered only if the diagnosis of fetal thyroid disease is not reasonably certain from the clinical data and the information gained would change the treatment.[32] The treatment for fetal hypothyroidism resulting from medical treatment of maternal Graves' disease includes decreasing or stopping maternal treatment and consideration of intra amniotic thyroxine. For fetal hyperthyroidism, treatment includes modulation of maternal antithyroid medication.

Fetal Effects of Hyperthyroiodism

Fetal or neonatal thyrotoxicosis can occur because of transplacental passage of maternal antibodies associated with Graves' disease though it is rare (0.05% of pregnancies).

Fetal thyrotoxicosis may lead to fetal tachycardia (>160 beats/min), fetal goiter, premature delivery, heart failure, hepatosplenomegaly, thrombocytopenia and IUGR.

To predict fetal thyrotoxicosis, maternal TSH receptor autoantibodies should be done at first trimester and at 6 months. If high titers are found in early pregnancy or if levels have not fallen with increasing gestation, fetal thyrotoxicosis should be suspected and fetal ultrasound is performed to look for evidence of fetal thyroid dysfunction which could include growth restriction, hydrops, presence of goiter, advanced bone age or cardiac failure.[42] Fetal thyrotoxicosis can be treated in utero by giving the mother increased doses of antithyroid medication and mother may be subsequently given thyroxine which does not cross placenta. In the neonate, thyrotoxicosis may cause jaundice, poor feeding and poor weight gain. Thyrotoxicosis in neonate is transient lasting only two to three months after delivery. Symptoms may be seen after two weeks postnatally if the mother is on medication at delivery because antibodies are cleared more slowly and drugs are cleared faster.

If high titers are found in late pregnancy then cord blood and neonatal sampling on days 3-4 and 7-10 for thyroid function tests should be performed. Symptomatic neonatal thyrotoxicosis should be treated. Management of Hyperthyroidism is pregnancy in summarised in Table 20.3.

20

Table 20.3: Management of hyperthyroidism in pregnancy

1. Maternal monitoring should include pulse, blood pressure and thyroid size. Levels of serum free T4 and serum free T3 and TSH should be done every 2-4 weeks. Dosage of antithyroid drugs should be changed accordingly.
2. In first trimester propylthiouracil is preferred to methimazole.
3. The treatment should consist of lowest dose of antithyroid drugs to maintain serum TSH concentrations between 0.1 and 0.4 mu /L. Patient may remain slightly hyperthyroid.
4. Antepartum fetal surveillance should be strictly done after 28 weeks.
5. If TSH receptor antibody titer is positive in early pregnancy fetal thyrotoxicosis should be ruled out.
6. If positive in late gestation neonatal thyrotoxicosis should be looked for.
7. Beta blockers like propranolol may be needed before surgeries like cesarean section.
8. Thyroid storm is a serious complication which occurs in labor and may cause maternal mortality.
9. The postpartum period should be carefully monitored as patient may worsen and the drugs may need to be started again or dose may need to be increased.
10. Surgery is indicated if patient is not able to tolerate antithyroid drugs or very high doses are needed.

The prevalence of overt hypothyroidism in pregnancy is 0.3-5% and of subclinical hypothyroidism is 2-3%.The various causes of hypothyroidism are:

- Autoimmune hypothyroidism.
- Hashimoto's thyroiditis.
- Iatrogenic hypothyroidism after: lithium, amiodarone, antithyroid drugs.
- Following treatment of hyperthyroidism with radioactive ablation or surgery.
- Following thyroid surgery for tumors.
- Iodine deficiency.
- Postpartum thyroiditis(transient).

Most common cause is autoimmune thyroiditis. Antibodies against thyroid peroxidase with atrophy, fibrosis and destruction of gland may be present. Antibodies against thyroid receptors may also be seen. Other causes of thyroid insufficiency include treatment of hyperthyroidism with radioiodine ablation or surgery. World wide most important cause of hypothyroidism is iodine deficiency affecting 1.2 billion individuals.

Hashimoto's thyroiditis is also an autoimmune thyroiditis with high titers of thyroid peroxidase autoantibodies where regeneration occurs after atrophy and goiter results.

Clinical Features and Diagnosis

There is an overlap of symptoms of normal pregnancy and hypothyroidism. Features which help in the diagnosis are cold intolerance, slow pulse rate, delayed tendon reflexes and dry skin. Others like drowsiness and constipation may also be seen. Many women are asymptomatic. In overt hypothyroidism increased TSH with reduced freeT4 concentration is seen. Subclinical hypothyroidism is manifested with elevated TSH but normal fT4. Results should be interpreted with pregnancy specific reference ranges. Thyroid peroxidase antibodies and thyroglobulin antibodies may be seen and their presence suggests autoimmune origin of the disease.[43] Serum TSH levels above 2.5 MIU/L in first trimester and 3 MIU/L in second and third trimester may already indicate subclinical hypothyroidism.[8]

Hypothyroidism and Pregnancy

Maternal Concerns

Hypothyroidism is related to decreased fertility. When hypothyroid patient becomes pregnant, there is an increased risk for early and late complications like abortion, anemia, gestational hypertension, placental abruption and postpartum hemorrhage.

These are seen more in overt hypothyroidism than with sub clinical hypothyroidism. Adequate thyroxine treatment decreases the risk of poorer obstetrical outcome.[44]

Fetal Concerns

Overt hypothyroidism is associated with premature birth, low birth weight and neonatal respiratory distress. Increase in gestational hypertension also increases neonatal risk.[45,46] In subclinical hypothyroidism, risk of preterm delivery increases.[47]

Neurological Development of the Fetus and the Neonate

Thyroid hormone is an important factor contributing to normal fetal brain development.[48,49] At early gestation when fetal thyroid is not efficient fetal hormone requirement is met with from transfer of maternal thyroid hormones to fetal compartment. T3 is required for fetal brain development which is made available by conversion of T4 received by fetus by maternal transfer, to T3 by deiodinases I and II present in fetal brain tissue.[50] Maternal hypothyroxinmia or maternal iodine deficiency at this time may cause mental retardation in the baby. A Dutch study[50] concluded that children born to mother with prolonged low T4 showed an 8-10 point deficit for motor and mental development.

Haddow et al in 1999[51] concluded that children of untreated hypothyroid women had IQ score seven points below mean IQ of children of healthy or thyroxine treated patients.

Cretinism (deaf mutism, spastic motor disorder, and hypothyroidism) is a distinct and severe form of brain damage caused by severe maternal iodine deficiency. Neonatal or fetal hypothyroidism as a result of transplacental transfer of maternal autoantibodies is extremely rare.[52]

Management

Pre-pregnancy

Thyroid disease should be suspected in patients with fertility and menstrual irregularities.

Woman with hypothyroidism should be counseled to delay pregnancy till good control of thyroid function has been achieved. If hypothyroidism has been diagnosed before pregnancy, adjustment of the preconception thyroxine dose should be done so that thyroid-stimulating hormone (TSH) level is not higher than 2.5 MIU/liter before pregnancy.

Antenatal

Patients who become pregnant with euthyroid state have a better outcome. Baseline thyroid function tests should be done as soon as possible. Levothyroxine is drug of choice for maternal hypothyroidism if the iodine nutrition status is adequate. The dose in pregnancy needs to be increased on an average by 30-50% above preconception dosage because of rapid rise in TBG levels because of estrogen, increased distribution volume of thyroid hormones, increased placental transport and metabolism of maternal T4.[44]

Patient on thyroxine preconceptionally need the dose to be altered at 4-6 weeks of gestation so that the euthyroid state is achieved.[44,53,19] If hypothyroidism has been diagnosed during pregnancy the functions should be normalized as soon as possible. Thyroxine doses should be titrated to rapidly reach and maintain serum TSH concentrations of less than 2.5 miu/l in first trimester and 3 miu/l in the second and third trimester. Monitor every 30 days till level normalises.[44,54] After this 6-8 weekly evaluation should be done.

Intrapartum

If adequately controlled, no extra measures are needed but large goiter may have anesthetic or surgical concerns.

Postnatal

After delivery dose in most patients needs to be decreased over a period of 4 weeks post partum. Patient with autoimmune etiology may develop post partum thyroiditis so monitoring should be done for at least six months post delivery.[44,54] The management of hypothyroidism in pregnancy is summarised in Table 20.4.

Table 20.4: Management of hypothyroidism in pregnancy
1. Baseline thyroid function tests to be done as soon as possible.
2. If thyroid functions show hypothyroidism in pregnancy, rapidly normalize the levels by starting thryroxine.to maintain serum TSH concentrations less than 2.5 miu/l in first trimester and 3 miu/l in second and third trimesters.
3. Repeat thyroid function tests every 4 weeks till controlled and then 6 weekly.
4. After delivery, dose may need to be decreased.

SUBCLINICAL HYPOTHYROIDISM (SCH)

This is characterized by serum TSH concentration above the upper limit of the reference range with a normal free T_4. It has been shown to be associated with an adverse outcome for both the mother and offspring.[47] Thyroxine treatment has been shown to improve obstetrical outcome, but has not been proved to modify long-term neurological development in the offspring. However, given that the potential benefits outweigh the potential risks, it is recommended that thyroxine replacement in women with subclinical hypothyroidism should be done.[51]

AUTOIMMUNE THYROID DISORDERS AND MISCARRIAGES

An association exists between thyroid antibodies and miscarriage in an unselected population but causality has not been established. Thyroid antibodies may simply serve as a marker for autoimmune disease in these patients.In euthyroid patients with recurrent miscarriages there may be an association between presence of thyroid antibody and miscarriage. Although a positive association exists between the presence of thyroid antibodies and pregnancy loss, universal screening for antithyroid antibodies, and possible treatment, cannot be recommended.

THYROID NODULES AND THYROID CARCINOMA

Thyroid nodules, solitary toxic nodules or adenomas are found in 2% of pregnant woman[55] and usually cause hyperthyroidism. Thyroid cancers are rare but most of them present as thyroid nodules. In iodine insufficiency pre-existing nodules are prone to increase in size during pregnancy. Thyroid function tests should be done for hypo or hyper thyroidism. Serum calcitonin levels may be useful for medullary carcinoma. Radionuclide scanning of thyroid is contraindicated in pregnancy which is used to distinguish cold (malignant) from hot (benign) nodules outside pregnancy. In pregnancy, diagnosis is dependent on ultrasound and fine needle aspiration biopsy.[56, 57] 5-20% of thyroid nodules in pregnancy are found to be malignant.

FNAC is done for any single dominant nodule larger than 1 cm,[58] and rapidly enlarging nodules.

Preconception

If patient comes before pregnancy thyroid nodule should be evaluated and treatment should be given before pregnancy. Pregnancy should be delayed for one year if radioactive iodine has been used because of risk of congenital anomalies.[59]

Pregnancy

Most of thyroid nodules are cytologically benign and don't need surgery. If suspicious or positive for thyroid carcinoma, gestational age, tumor stage and personal inclination of patient should be considered. If FNAC is highly suggestive of papillary or follicular or medullary carcinoma, surgery should be performed without interrupting pregnancy.[60]

In follicular neoplasm risk of malignancy is 10-15% and surgery can be delayed because it is minimally invasive and well capsulated. If the cytology is indeterminate one should wait till delivery. If nodule is found in third trimester further workup and treatment can be delayed until after delivery.[61] But surgery should be done if it is a rapidly growing lesion or if an anaplastic tumor is present.

Postnatal

Radioactive iodine can be used after delivery but breast feeding is contraindicated.

Postpartum thyroiditis is the occurrence of hyperthyroidism, hypothyroidism and/or hyperthyroidism followed by hypothyroidism in the first year postpartum in women without overt thyroid disease before pregnancy.Its incidence varies between 5-10% of pregnancies.[62] Postpartum thyroiditis (PPT) occurs almost exclusively in women who are thyroid antibody positive. The condition usually occurs 3-4 months postpartum but has been reported up to 6 months after delivery.[63] Lymphocytic infiltration of the gland is seen and these subjects have a subclinical autoimmune thyroiditis which exacerbates after delivery.It is believed to be caused by an autoimmunity induced discharge of preformed hormone from the thyroid which causes hyperthyroidism. Three months later it causes hypothyroidism as stores of preformed hormone are depleted and gland is destroyed. The thyrotoxic phase of postpartum thyroiditis is twenty times more common than postpartum Graves' disease. Symptoms during PPT are milder than Graves' disease. 95% of women with Grave's disease are TSH receptor stimulating antibody positive and may also present with a bruit and exophthalmos. In contrast to Graves' disease PPT is characterized by 0% radioactive iodine uptake.

Management

Most cases resolve spontaneously. In the hyperthyroid phase of the disease propranolol should be given to relieve symptoms. The duration of therapy does not exceed 2 months.

Treatment for women in hypothyroid phase depends on degree of the disease and plan to conceive. Asymptomatic patients not planning a pregnancy and whose TSH level is between 4-10 miu/l do not require intervention and should be evaluated again in 4-8 weeks time. Women with TSH between 4-10 miu/l who are either symptomatic or attempting to become pregnant should be treated with thyroxine. All women with levels of TSH above 10 miu/l should be treated with thyroxine.This dysfunction is transient but 20 to 64% of women may develop permanent hypothyroidism during long-term follow up.[64,65]

Women known to be thyroid peroxidase antibody (TPO-Ab)-positive should have a TSH performed at 3 and 6 months postpartum. Women with a history of PPT have a markedly increased risk of developing permanent primary hypothyroidism in the 5- to 10-year period following the episode of PPT. An annual TSH level should be performed in these women.

SCREENING FOR THYROID DYSFUNCTION DURING PREGNANCY

Universal screening is not recommended but the association of thyroid abnormalities and untoward outcomes during pregnancy and postpartum is impossible to ignore. Therefore aggressive case finding in high risk populations may provide an appropriate balance between inaction and screening the entire population.

Although the benefits of universal screening for hypothyroidism may not be justified by current evidence, in following groups of women targeted case findings should be done.

Targeted screening is recommended for women as listed below who have an increased incidence of thyroid disease and in whom treatment for thyroid disease if found, would be warranted.

1. Women with a history of hyperthyroid or hypothyroid disease, postpartum thyroditis or thyroid lobectomy.
2. Family history of thyroid disease.
3. Women with a goiter.
4. Women with thyroid antibodies.
5. Women with symptoms or clinical signs suggestive of thyroid under function or over function including anemia, elevated cholesterol and hyponatremia.
6. Women with type I diabetes.
7. Women with other autoimmune disorders.
8. Women with infertility should have screening with TSH as part of their infertility workup.
9. Women with prior therapeutic head or neck irradiation.
10. Women with a prior history of miscarriage or preterm delivery.

Screening should consist of a TSH measurement done before pregnancy when possible or at first prenatal visit and appropriate tests should be done accordingly.

KEY POINTS

- Thyroid disorders are common endocrine disorders in young women and difficult to diagnose clinically in pregnancy because of overlap of normal signs and symptoms of pregnancy with those of thyroid diseases.
- Human chorionic gonadotrophin has some thyrotrophic function, so it stimulates thyroid receptors causing increase in free T4 levels and decrease in TSH levels particulary in first trimester.
- For thyroid functions in pregnancy, free T4 T3 and TSH should be used and trimester specific range should be considered.
- During first trimester fetus is dependent on maternal T4 for its requirements as fetal thyroid is not active and maternal hypothyroxinemia or iodine deficiency at this time can affect fetal brain development.
- In pregnancy and lactation, 200-300 microg/day of iodine is needed.
- Medical treatment is of choice in hyperthyroidism. Propylthiouracil and methimazole both can be used but former is used in first trimester preferably.

Thyroid Disorders with Pregnancy

- In hyperthyroidism, maternal levels of free T4 should be maintained in the upper nonpregnant reference range with treatment.
- Both maternal and fetal hypothyroidism are known to have serious adverse effects on the fetus.
- Autoimmune thyroidits is the most common cause of hypothyroidism in pregnancy.
- If hypothyroidism is first detected in pregnancy rapid institution of thyroxine should be done to normalize thyroid levels otherwise neurological functions of the fetus are jeopardized.
- In subclinical hypothyroidism, treatment with thyronine improves obstetrical outcome.
- Fine needle aspiration cytology should be performed for single or dominant thyroid nodule larger than 1 cm in pregnancy.
- If these nodules are found to be malignant or rapidly growing, surgery should be offered in the second trimester without interrupting pregnancy.
- Women known to be thyroid peroxidase antibody positive should have a TSH performed at 3 and 6 months postpartum.
- Universal screening for thyroid disease is not recommended at present but case finding in the high risk group for thyroid dysfunction should be done.

REFERENCES

1. Glinoer D. The regulation of thyroid function in pregnancy: Pathways of endocrine adaptation from physiology to pathology. Endocr Rev 1997;18:404-33.
2. Glinoer D. The regulation of thyroid function during normal pregnancy: Importance of the iodine nutrition status. Best Pract Res Clin Endocrinol Metab 2004;18:133-52
3. Hetzel BS. Iodine deficiency disorders and their eradication. Lancet 1983;2:1126-29.
4. Pekonen F. Alfthan H, Stenman J-H, Ylikorkala O. Human chorionic gonadotrophin and thryroid function in early human pregnancy: Circadian variation and evidence for intrinsic thyrotropic activity of HCG. J Clin Endocrinol Metab 1988;66:853-56.
5. Demers LM, Spencer CA. Laboratory support for the diagnosis and monitoring of thyroid disease. National Academy of Clinical Biochemistry Laboratory Medicine Practice Guidelines. Washington, DC: National Academy of Clinical Biochemistry 2002.
6. Soldin OP, Tractenberg RE, Hollowell JG, Jonklaas J, Janicic N, Soldin. Trimester-specific changes in maternal thyroid hormone, thyrotropin, and thyroglobulin concentrations during gestation: Trends and associations across trimesters in iodine sufficiency Thyroid 2004;14:1084-90.
7. Kurioka H, Takahashi K, Miyazake K. Maternal Thyroid Function during pregnancy and puerperal period. Endocine J 2005;52:587.
8. Panesar NS, Li CY, Rogers MS. Reference intervals for thyroid hormones in pregnant Chinese women. Ann Clin Biochem 2001;38:329-32.
9. Thorpe-Beeston JG, Nicolaides KH, Felton CV, Butler J, McGregor AM. Maturation of the secretion of thyroid hormone and thyroid-stimulating hormone in the fetus. N Engl J Med 1991;324:532-36.
10. Santini F, Chiovato L, et al. Serum iodothyronines in the human fetus and the newborn: Evidence for an important role of placenta in fetal thyroid hormone homeostasis. J Clin Endocrinol Metab 1999;84: 493-98.
11. Bernal J, Pekonen FD. Ontogenesis of nuclear 3,5,3'-triiodothyronine receptor in the human fetal brain. Endocrinology1984;11:577-79.

12. Vulsma T, Gons MH, de Vijlder JJ. Maternal-fetal transfer of thyroxine in congenital hypothyroidism due to a total organification defect or thyroid agenesis. N Engl J Med 1989;321:13-16.
13. World Health Organization. Assessment of iodine deficiency disorders and monitoring their elimination: A guide for program managers, 2nd edn. 2001;7-8.
14. Cao XY, Jiang XM, et al. Timing of vulnerability of the brain to iodine deficiency in endemic cretinism. N EnglandJ Med 1994;331:1739-44.
15. Glinoer D. Fetomaternal repercussions of iodine deficiency during pregnancy. An update. Ann Endocrinol (Paris) 2003;64:37-44.
16. Chaouki ML, Benmiloud M. Prevention of iodine deficiency disorders by oral administration of lipiodol during pregnancy. Eur J Endocrinol 1994;130:547-51.
17. Goodwin TM, Montoro M, Mestman JH. Transient hyperthyroidism and hyperemesis gravidarum: Clinical aspects. Am J Obstet Gynecol 1992;167:648-52.
18. Tan JY, Loh KC, Yeo GS, Chee YC. Transient hyperthyroidism of hyperemesis gravidarum. BJOG 2002;109:683-88.
19. Rotondi M, Mazziotti G, Sorvillo F, Piscopo M, Cioffi M, Amato G, Carella C. Effects of increased thyroxine dosage pre-conception on thyroid function early pregnancy. Eur J Endocrinol 2004;151:695-700.
20. Casey BM, Dashe JS, Wells CE, McIntire DD, Leveno KJ, Cunningham FG. Subclinical hyperthyroidism and pregnancy outcomes. Obstet Gynecol 2006;107:337-41.
21. Momotani N, Noh J, Oyanagi H, Ishikawa N, Ito K. Antithyroid drug therapy for Graves' disease during pregnancy. Optimal regimen for fetal thyroid status. N Engl J Med 1986;315:24-28.
22. Burrow GN. The management of thyrotoxicosis in pregnancy. N Engl J Med 1985;313: 562-65.
23. Stagnaro-Green. A Clinical review 152: Postpartum thyroiditis. J Clin Endocrinol Metab 2002;87:4042-47.
24. Amino N, Tanizawa O, et al. Aggravation of thyrotoxicosis in early pregnancy and after delivery in Grave's disease. J Clin Endocrinol Metab 1982;55:395-401.
25. Mestman JH. Hyperthyroidism in pregnancy. Clin Obstet Gynecol 1997;40:45-64.
26. Sheffield JS, Cunningham FG. Thyrotoxicosis and heart failure that complicate pregnancy. Am J Obstet Gynecol 2004;190:211-17.
27. Glinowe D, Soto MF, Bourdux P, et al. Pregnancy in patients with mild thyroid abnormalities; Maternal and neonatal repercussions.J Clin Endocrinol Metab 1991;73:421-27.
28. Davis LE, Lucas MJ, Hankins GD, Roark ML, Cunningham FG. Thyrotoxicosis complicating pregnancy. Am J Obstet Gynecol 1989;160:63-70.
29. Millar LK, Wing DA, Leung AS, Koonings PP, Montoro MN, Mestman JH. Low birth weight and preeclampsia in pregnancies complicated by hyperthyroidism. Obstet Gynecol 1994;84:946-49.
30. Krasas G. Thyroid disease and female reproduction. Fertil Steril 2000;74:1063-70.
31. Drug and therapeutics bulletin: The practical management of thyroid disease in pregnancy. 1995;33:47-48.
32. The Endocrine Society. Management of thyroid dysfunction during pregnancy and postpartum: An Endocrine Society clinical practice guideline. Chevy Chase (MD): The Endocrine Society; 2007.
33. Ratanachaiyavong S, Mc Gregor AM. Immunosuppressive effects of antithyroid drugs. Clin Endocrinol Metab 1985; 14:449-66.
34. Mortimer RH, Cannell GR, Addison RS, Johnson LP, Roberts MS, Bernus. Methimazole and propylthiouracil equally cross the perfused human term placental lobule. J Clin Endocrinol Metab 1997;82:3099-3102.
35. Di GianantonioE, Schaefer C, Mastroiacovo PP, Cournot MP, Benedicenti F, Reuversm M, Occupati B, Robert E, Belemin B, Addis A, Arnon J, Clementi M. Adverse effects of prenatal methimazol exposure Teratology 2001;64:262-66.
36. Magee LA, Elran E, B ull SB, Logan A, Koren G. Risks and benefits of beta receptor blockers for pregnancy hypertension: Overview of randomized trials. Eur J Obstet Gynecol Repro Biol 2000;88:15-26.
37. Zanzonico PB. Radiation dose to patients and relatives incident to I^{131} therapy. Thyroid 1997;7:199-204.

38. Azizi F, Hedayati M. Thyroid function in breast-fed infants whose mothers take high doses of methimazole. J Endocrinol Invest 2002;25:493-96.

39. Momotani N, Yamashita R, Yoshimoto M, Noh J, Ishikawa N, Ito K. Recovery from fetal hypothyroidism: Evidence for the safety of breastfeeding while taking propylthiouracil. Clin Endocrinol (Oxf) 1989;31:591-95.

40. O'Doherty MJ, McElhatton PR, Thomas SHL. Treating thyrotoxicosis in pregnant or potentially pregnant women: The risk to the fetus is very low. BMJ 1999;318: 5-6.

41. Cheron RG, Kaplan MM, Larsen PR, et al. Neonatal thyroid function after propylthiouracil therapy for maternal Graves disease. N Engl J Med 1981;304: 525-28.

42. Luton D, Le Gac I, Vuillard E, Castanet M, Guibourdenche J, Noel M, Toubert ME, Leger J, Boissinot C, Schlageter MH, Garel C, Tebeka B, Oury JF, Czernichow P, Polak M. Management of Graves' disease during pregnancy: The key role of fetal thyroid gland monitoring. J Clin Endocrinol Metab 2005;90:6093-98.

43. Mandel SJ. Hypothyroidism and chronic autoimmune thyroiditis in the pregnant state: Maternal aspects. Best Pract Res Clin Endocrinol Metab 2004;18:213-24.

44. Davis LE, Leveno KJ, Cunningham FG. Hypothyroidism complicating pregnancy. Obstet Gynecol 1988;72:108-12.

45. Abalovick M, Gutierrez S, Alcaraz G, Maccallini G, Garoa A, Levalle O. Overt and Subclinical hypothyroidism complicating pregnancy. Thyroid 2002:12:63-68.

46. Allan WC, Haddow JE, Palomaki GE, Williams JR, Mitchell ML, Hermos RJ, Faix JD, Klein RZ. Maternal thyroid deficiency and pregnancy complications: Implications for population screening. J Med Screen 2000;7:127-30.

47. Casey BM, Dashe JS, Wells CE, McIntire DD, Byrd W, Leveno KJ, Cunningham FG. Subclinical hypothyroidism and pregnancy outcomes. Obstet Gynecol 2005;105: 239-45.

48. Calvo RM, Jauniaux E, Gulbis B, Asuncion M, Gervy C, Contempre B, Morreale de Escobar G. Fetal tissues are exposed to biologically relevant free thyroxine concentrations during early phases of development. J Clin Endocrinol Metab 2002;87:1768-77.

49. Iskaros J, Pickard M, Evans I, Sinha A, Hardiman P, Ekins R. Thyroid hormone receptor gene expression in first trimester human fetal brain. J Clin Endocrinol Metab 2000;85:2620-23.

50. Kester MH, Martinez de Mena R, Obregon MJ, Marinkovic D, Howatson A, Visser TJ, Hume R, Morreale de Escobar G. Iodothyronine levels in the human developing brain: Major regulatory roles of iodothyronine deiodinases in different areas. J Clin Endocrinol Metab 2004;89:3117-31.

51. Haddow JE, Palomaki GE, Allan WC, Williams JR, Knight GJ, Gagnon J, O'Heir CE, Mitchell ML, Hermos RJ, Waisbren SE, Faix JD, Klein RZ. Maternal thyroid deficiency during pregnancy and subsequent neuropsychological development of the child. N Engl J Med 1999;341:549-55.

52. Brown RS, Bellisario RL, Botero D, et al. Incidence of transient congenital hypothyroidismdue to maternal thyrotropin receptor-blocking antibodies in over one million babies. J Clin Endocrinol Metab 1996;81: 1147-51.

53. Alexander EK, Marqusee E, Lawrence J, Jarolim P, Fiscer GA, Larsen PR. Timing and magnitude of increases in levothyroxine requirements during pregnancy in women with hypothyroidism. N Engl J Med 2004;351:241-49.

54. Caixas A, Albareda M, Garcia-Patterson A, Rodriguez-Espinosa J, de Leiva A, Corcoy R. Postpartum thyroiditis in women with hypothyroidism antedating pregnancy? J Clin Endocrinol Metab 1999;84:4000-05.

55. Mazzaferri EL. Evaluation andmanagement of common thyroid disorders in women. Am JObstet Gynecol 1997;176:507-14.

56. Choe W, McDougall IR Thyroid cancer in pregnant women: Diagnostic and therapeutic management. Thyroid 1994;4:433-35.

57. Glinoer D. Thyroid nodule and cancer in pregnant women. Ann Endocrinol (Paris) 1997;58:263-67.

58. Hamburger J. I Thyroid nodules in pregnancy, Thyroid 1992;2:165-68.

59. Auala C, Navarro E, Rodriguez JR, et al. Conception after iodine-131 therapy for differentiated thyroid cancer. Thyroid 1998;8:1009-11.

60. Sam S, Molitch ME. Timing and special concerns regarding endocrine surgery during pregnancy. Endocrinol Metab Clin North Am 2003;32:337-54.
61. Tan GH, Gharib H, Goellner JR, van Heerden JA, Bahn RS. Management of thyroid nodules in pregnancy. Arch Intern Med 1996;156:2317-20.
62. Stagnaro-Green A. Recognizing, understanding and treating postpartum thyroiditis. Endocrinol Metab Clin North Am 2000;29(2):417-30.
63. Browne Martin K, Emerson CH. Postpartum thyroid dysfunction. Clin Obstet Gynecol 1997;40:90-101.
64. Lazarus JH Clinical manifestations of postpartum thyroid disease. Thyroid 1999;9:685-89.
65. Azizi F. The occurrence of permanent thyroid failure in patients with subclinical postpartum thyroiditis. Eur J Endocrinol 2005;153:367-71.

Thyroid Disorders with Pregnancy

during
thyroid
roiditis
Gynecol
85-89.
partum

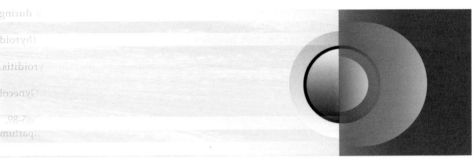

Renal Disease in Pregnancy

21

Suneeta Mittal, Pakhee Aggarwal

INTRODUCTION

Renal disease in pregnancy represents an alteration beyond physiological limits in renal structure and function that may result in a detrimental maternal and fetal or neonatal outcome. Renal disease may antedate pregnancy and may be exacerbated by the physiological alterations in pregnancy or it may arise *de novo* and progress during pregnancy. Management consists of a multidisciplinary team consisting of obstetrician, pediatrician, nephrologist and urologist.

To evaluate renal disorders in pregnancy, we should first know:
a. The effect of pregnancy on renal structure and function.
b. The effect of underlying renal disease on the outcome of pregnancy.

Effect of Pregnancy on Renal Structure and Function

Physiological adaptation to pregnancy include:[1-4]
- Increase in kidney size due to increased blood flow, such that they appear enlarged on ultrasound
- Dilatation of the renal collecting system
- Increased risk of pyelonephritis, especially in women with asymptomatic bacteriuria
- Increase in glomerular filtration rate (GFR) and renal plasma flow (RPF): GFR increases from the luteal phase of menstrual cycle by 10-20% and if pregnancy is established, reaches maximum in mid trimester (55%). Renal

blood flow reaches a maximum of 70-80% in mid trimester and falls to 45% above non pregnant levels at term.

- Fall in serum creatinine (20%) and serum urea levels, latter also due to reduced hepatic synthesis
- Proteinuria upto 200 mg in 24 hours is normal
- Fall in plasma albumin by 5-10gm/L
- Rise in serum cholesterol
- Gestational glucosuria due to reduced tubular re-absorption
- Bicarbonaturia due to metabolic acidosis compensating the respiratory alkalosis of pregnancy due to hyperventilation.
- Plasma osmolality falls by 10 mOsm/kg
- Increased plasma renin, erythropoietin and vitamin D levels.

Effect of Renal Disease on Pregnancy

The prognosis for feto-maternal outcome depends on the nature of renal disease, level of underlying renal impairment, degree of hypertension, other coexisting conditions like infection and proteinuria. Some diseases like renal scleroderma or polyarteritis nodosa contraindicate pregnancy as deterioration is the rule, while in others like systemic lupus erythematosus and mesangio-capillary glomerulonephritis deterioration may occur despite normal function prior to pregnancy.[5]

The diagnosis of pregnancy may be doubtful and confirmed late, as women with chronic kidney disease have irregular cycles and impaired fertility. In addition, blood hCG levels are usually elevated in the presence of renal failure making the diagnosis of pregnancy uncertain.

Specific renal diseases will be discussed subsequently, but certain features which are common to all renal pathologies in general include:[1]

1. Isolated mild renal dysfunction (Serum creatinine up to 1.5 mg%): Low risk of worsening during pregnancy.
2. Moderate dysfunction (Serum creatinine 1.5-2.4 mg%): Up to 40% may worsen in pregnancy and in about half of these the deterioration persists in the postpartum period.
3. Severe dysfunction (Serum creatinine > 2.5 mg%): 33-45% progress to end stage renal disease in the postpartum period.

The normal gestational increment in GFR is attenuated in women with moderate renal impairment and is absent in those with serum creatinine > 2.3 mg/dl (200 mmol/l).

Similarly, the gestational increase in blood volume and erythropoiesis is inversely related to the pre-conception serum creatinine.[4]

Chronic hypertension and pre-conception proteinuria usually worsen in the third trimester and may have an accelerated decline postpartum. Asymptomatic proteinuria (> 500 mg per day) detected in early pregnancy often reveals underlying renal impairment. Such women should be followed up postpartum until proteinuria disappears or a diagnosis is made.[2]

In terms of fetal prognosis, there is increased incidence of spontaneous abortions, preterm labor—both spontaneous and iatrogenic, low birth weight and growth restricted infants (secondary to hypertension and uremia), dehydration (due to osmotic diuresis caused by high blood urea levels), osteomalacia (due to maternal disturbance of calcium metabolism) and a higher perinatal mortality.[5] Fetal outcome also correlates with level of renal dysfunction:[1]

1. Mild dysfunction: overall good fetal outcome with 95% live birth rate, 20% preterm and 25% small for gestational age (SGA), 10% superimposed preeclampsia (SPE)
2. Moderate dysfunction: 7-16% perinatal mortality, 30-60% preterm delivery rate, 35% SGA, 40% SPE
3. Severe dysfunction: 73-86% preterm delivery, 43-57% SGA, 80% SPE

A cesarean section rate of around 60% is a consistent finding in most series with women who have markedly impaired renal function.[2]

GENERAL PRINCIPLES OF ANTEPARTUM MANAGEMENT

Management should ideally be in a tertiary care center. Initial baseline renal function helps in detecting the degree of renal impairment as well as superimposed preeclampsia. These tests include serum creatinine and its clearance, blood urea nitrogen, serum albumin and cholesterol, serum electrolytes, uric acid levels, SGOT and SGPT, LDH, prothrombin time, partial thromboplastin time, platelet count, 24 hour protein excretion, urine analysis for casts and culture.[6] These tests may detect renal insufficiency in an asymptomatic patient without known dysfunction, in which case infection, inflammation and renal toxic exposures, such as NSAID overdose or abuse should be ruled out.[1]

Maternal Surveillance

Folic acid 400 µg daily should be started periconceptionally and continued up to 12 weeks gestation. With pre-existing kidney disease, diagnosis of pregnancy should be confirmed by early ultrasound as it helps in accurate dating of the pregnancy.

Because of the risk for preterm delivery, an increased frequency of antepartum visits is recommended for women with renal dysfunction. Some authorities suggest 2-week intervals until 28 weeks and then weekly till delivery.[1] After baseline investigations serum creatinine can be repeated every 4 to 6 weeks. Proteinuria should be checked by dipstick at each visit. Notable increase in proteinuria should prompt testing for 24-hour urine protein.

Blood pressure (diastolic) less than 90 mm Hg is a reasonable target, although it should be maintained between 120/80 and 140/90 mm Hg throughout pregnancy. Women who are hypertensive at conception or in early pregnancy have a 10 times higher relative risk of fetal loss as compared to normotensive women with the same level of renal dysfunction.[4] Regarding antihypertensive agents calcium channel blockers, beta-blockers, and alpha-methyldopa are safe and can be continued if the patient is taking them pre-pregnancy. Thiazide diuretics may attenuate gestational plasma volume expansion and are associated with an increased risk of IUGR, thus they are better avoided. If a woman conceives on ACE inhibitors and angiotensin receptor blockers (ARB), although they appear safe up to six weeks gestation, they should be changed as soon as pregnancy is diagnosed, due to their teratogenic action at later gestations.[4]

Some authorities recommend prophylactic low-dose aspirin (50-150 mg/day) on confirmation of pregnancy to prevent glomerular capillary thrombosis, preserve maternal renal function and reduce the risk of pre-eclampsia.[4]

Pregnant women with proteinuria (>1 gm/24 hours), whether due to nephrotic syndrome or preeclampsia, are at increased risk of venous thrombosis and should receive thromboprophylaxis with low-molecular-weight heparin (LMWH)—enoxaparin 40 mg s.c. daily, until 6 weeks postpartum. Twice the non-pregnant thromboprophylaxis dose is required due to increased renal clearance of heparin in pregnancy.[3,4]

Fetal Surveillance

Fetal growth may be compromised in pregnancies complicated by renal disease, thus it is prudent to monitor it by ultrasonography every 2 weeks. Umbilical artery doppler can be used to detect compromise early in the growth restricted fetus. Monitoring of fetal wellbeing should start at 26 weeks gestation when the fetus begins to have a reasonable chance of survival outside the uterus.

Timing, mode and place of delivery is decided by the degree of fetal compromise and iatrogenic preterm delivery may be required.

Increasing proteinuria alone is not an indication for delivery, since after correction for prematurity, massive proteinuria (>10 gm/24 hours) has no significant effect on neonatal outcome.[4]

SPECIFIC RENAL PATHOLOGY IN PREGNANCY

Special problems associated with renal impairment influencing pregnancy outcome include:

1. Pre-eclampsia
2. Lupus nephritis
3. Glomerulonephritis and IgA nephropathy
4. Asymptomatic bacteriuria
5. Reflux nephropathy
6. Upper urinary tract obstruction
7. Acute renal failure/renal cortical necrosis

21

Renal Disease in Pregnancy

8. Diabetic nephropathy
9. Polycystic kidney disease
10. Renal calculi
11. Dialysis
12. Post renal transplant

Pre-eclampsia

The ultrastructural pathology characteristic of pre-eclampsia is, 'glomerular capillary endotheliosis', characterized by enlargement of the glomeruli with maintenance of normal amounts of stroma and cells. This affects the kidney both functionally and morphologically, causing increased protein excretion and decreased blood flow.[7]

More importantly, pre-eclampsia is more common in women who have underlying renal disease, especially when associated with chronic hypertension. In fact in one report, women who had gestational proteinuria or preeclampsia before 30 weeks' gestation were more likely to have underlying renal disease.[8] The diagnosis of pre-eclampsia may be difficult if there is chronic hypertension and proteinuria, as these two parameters usually worsen in late pregnancy. However, the presence of raised hepatic transaminases, thrombocytopenia and hyperuricemia support the diagnosis of pre-eclampsia.[2]

Lupus Nephritis

Pregnancy outcomes are favorable when SLE has been in remission for at least 1 year.

Best outcomes are seen in:[4]
• Women with quiescent lupus nephritis,
• Absent antiphospholipid (APL) antibodies,
• Normal or near normal renal function (serum creatinine < 1.4 mg/dl),
• Proteinuria < 500 mg/24 hours and
• Controlled hypertension for at least 6 months before conception

However, pregnancy or puerperium can provoke exacerbations of lupus. Paracetamol is the first-choice analgesic and antirheumatic agent in pregnancy. Non-steroidal anti-inflammatory drugs should be avoided in the third trimester as they may induce premature closure of the ductus arteriosus.[9] A flare of lupus nephritis during pregnancy usually needs treatment with intravenous methylprednisolone 500 mg daily for 3 days and an increase of oral prednisolone to around 60 mg daily. Azathioprine has also been safely used in pregnancy.[2] Steroid resistant and progressive lupus nephritis has been successfully treated during pregnancy with cyclophosphamide.[4]

Additional treatment includes antihypertensive medication to control blood pressure and thromboprophylaxis with low-dose aspirin and LMW heparin, especially in the presence of APL antibodies and proteinuria of >1 gm/24 hours.

Even though flares are more common postpartum, there is a consensus not to enhance steroid therapy prophylactically in the peripartum period in the absence of signs of disease activity. Flares of SLE are more common in pregnant women who have had more than three flares before pregnancy, have antiphospholipid antibodies, C3 hypocomplementemia and hypertension.[3] A relapse of SLE during pregnancy may be difficult to distinguish from pre-eclampsia, but the following should be kept in mind:[2,4]

- Features in favor of lupus: Consumption of complement (C3 and C4), active urinary sediment with hematuria and red cell casts, extra-renal manifestations affecting the skin and joints, rising titer of dsDNA antibodies.
- Features in favor of preeclampsia: Associated low platelet counts, elevated liver enzymes and uric acid.

Sometimes a renal biopsy may be required to distinguish between the two as the treatment options are very different.

There is increased risk of early pregnancy loss, IUGR, preterm delivery, pre-eclampsia and perinatal and maternal mortality. Women with anti-Ro and anti-La antibodies are at risk of having an infant affected by congenital lupus. Neonatal lupus may be associated with transient liver dysfunction (25%), congenital heart block (1-2%) or cutaneous lupus.

Glomerulonephritis

The histological type of primary glomerulonephritis (GN) does not affect pregnancy outcome as much as the clinical parameters of hypertension, proteinuria and reduced GFR.[2] Nevertheless, rarely a kidney biopsy may be required to settle the diagnosis and exclude a steroid responsive glomerular disease, especially if there is sudden renal impairment (serum creatinine >1.4 mg/dl) or new onset heavy proteinuria (> 5 gm/24 hours) or an active urinary sediment with red cell casts occuring before 30-32 weeks gestation in the absence of pre-eclampsia.[4] Some authorities however advise against a renal biopsy in pregnant women with a rapidly deteriorating renal function and swollen kidneys, severe preeclampsia or any kind of severe renal disease due to increased risk of complications.[10] IgA nephropathy is the commonest pattern of chronic primary glomerulonephritis in young people and therefore quite common in pregnant women. Pregnancy outcomes are not different significantly.[4] Acute nephritic syndrome is defined as the abrupt onset of hematuria, proteinuria, reduced glomerular filtration rate, salt retention and arterial hypertension. Nephrotic proteinuria is defined as protein excretion of 3.5 gm/24 hour or greater. Non-nephrotic proteinuria is protein excretion between 0.31 and 3.5 gm/24 hour.[11]

Asymptomatic Bacteriuria (ASBU)

About 5% of all pregnant women have asymptomatic bacteriuria. Untreated infection can ascend the urinary tract to cause acute pyelonephritis in 25% of these patients (about 1% of all pregnancies).

Clinical presentation is with backache, fever with chills and urinary symptoms. Most common pathogen is *E. coli* and 15-20% may have bacteremia with endotoxic shock.

Patients are often dehydrated from nausea and vomiting and require intravenous crystalloids. Impaired renal function, thrombocytopenia, hemolysis and ARDS are more common than in non-pregnant women.[2] Treatment involves intravenous broad spectrum antibiotics with gram negative cover until antibiotic sensitivity is determined. If patient does not respond within 48-72 hours, underlying structural abnormality must be excluded by ultrasound which can also help to exclude stones. Plain abdominal X-ray, single-shot intravenous pyelography is a sure way to identify calculi with minimal radiation exposure and may be done in suspicious cases. Following successful treatment, urine culture is repeated after 7-10 days and screening for infection is done every 4-6 weeks, as relapse is common. In addition, untreated bacteriuria has been associated with low birth weight infants. Acute pyelonephritis can trigger preterm labor, but the use of tocolytics, especially beta-mimetics should be judicious as it may precipitate pulmonary edema in patients with endotoxemia.

Reflux Nephropathy

It is characterized by renal scarring, reduced GFR, recurrent urinary tract infections (UTI), proteinuria and hypertension. Vesico-ureteric reflux (VUR) leading to reflux nephropathy is one of the most common renal disease in women of child-bearing age.[2] Acute pyelonephrits is twice as common in women with persistent VUR compared with those who have had spontaneous or surgical resolution of VUR.[4]

Certain guidelines have been proposed for management of reflux nephropathy in women planning conception.[12]

Preconception Counseling

- Consider surgical correction of reflux prior to conception in cases with recurrent episodes of upper urinary tract infection despite careful prophylaxis.
- Discourage pregnancy when the serum creatinine level exceeds 0.22 mmol/1 (2.5 mg/dl).
- There is considerable maternal morbidity when serum creatinine values exceed 0.16 mmol/l (2 mg/dl), especially when hypertension is also present.

Management of Pregnancy

- Every patient should be frequently screened (every 4-6 weeks) for bacteriuria and treated for urinary tract infection.
- Following one UTI, low-dose prophylactic antibiotics, chosen according to the sensitivity of the most recent urine culture, will reduce the risk of further UTI and may therefore preserve renal function.

- In women with impaired renal function, the following are required:
  i. Close cooperation between the obstetrician and the physician or the nephrologist
  ii. A monthly determination of the serum creatinine concentration, creatinine clearance, proteinuria and blood pressure
  iii. Active antihypertensive treatment
  iv. Treatment of anemia by subcutaneous recombinant erythropoietin
  v. Initiation of dialysis if serum creatinine > 0.4 mmol/1 (5 mg/dl) and/or blood urea > 20 mmol/l (120 mg/dl)
  vi. Reinforced fetal monitoring and preterm delivery when necessary, according to fetal status
  vii. Prolonged surveillance of maternal renal function and blood pressure after delivery.

Pregnancy is uneventful whenever renal function is normal or near normal and hypertension is absent at conception.

Upper Urinary Tract Obstruction

Ultrasonography of the renal pelvis at the end of first trimester provides a useful baseline. The right pelvi-calyceal system normally dilates by a maximum of 0.5mm each week from 6 to 32 weeks, reaching a maximum diameter of approximately 20 mm (90th centile), which is maintained until term. The left pelvi-calyceal system reaches a maximum diameter of 8 mm (90th centile) at 20 weeks gestation.[4] A repeat ultrasound scan is indicated whenever there is renal pain suggestive of obstruction, persistent infection or a rise in serum creatinine in a woman with a single kidney. Monitoring during pregnancy involves serial assessment of renal function, urine culture and blood pressure. Hydronephrosis can be managed symptomatically by insertion of pigtail catheter to drain the distended kidneys with good outcome.[13]

Acute Renal Failure/Renal Cortical Necrosis

Acute renal failure (ARF) in pregnancy is uncommon, occurring in only one of every 10,000 pregnancies.[14] Usually, it is associated with septic abortion, preeclampsia or uterine hemorrhage from placenta previa or placental abruption. Other rare causes may be hyperemesis gravidarum,[15] post streptococcal glomerulonephritis,[16] bilateral ureteral obstruction, cocaine associated rhabdomyolysis,[17] hemolytic uremic syndrome, thrombotic thrombocytopenic purpura, amniotic fluid embolism and disseminated intravascular coagulation. Abruption is reported to be the most frequent precipitating event in developed nations, however in our country septic abortion may be a more important cause. Acute tubular necrosis is a more likely diagnosis but renal cortical necrosis should be suspected if anuria persists for longer than a week. A definitive diagnosis can be made with renal biopsy. Selective renal angiography will also confirm the diagnosis.[2]

Renal failure has been classified as pre-renal, renal and post-renal in causation. Pre-renal ARF occurs due to hypovolemia and hypoperfusion, intrinsic renal failure occurs due to reno-vascular obstruction, diseases of glomeruli or renal vasculature, tubular necrosis and interstitial nephritis, while post renal failure is due to obstruction of the urinary tract. It is important to distinguish pre-renal from intrinsic renal azotemia as the former responds to a fluid challenge, while in the latter fluids should be restricted if kidney damage has already occurred. The rate of fluid replacement should be based on central venous pressure, hourly urine output and insensible losses. Low dose dopamine infusion and furosemide have been used to maintain renal flow and defer hemodialysis.

Pre-renal and renal failure can be distinguished by certain blood and urine parameters.[18]

Parameter	Pre-renal	Renal
Urine osmolality	> 500 mOsm/kg	< 350 mOsm/kg
Urinary sodium (mmol/L)	< 20	> 40
Urinary urea/plasma urea nitrogen ratio	> 8	< 3
Urinary creatinine/plasma creatinine ratio	> 40	< 20
Fractional excretion of Na (%)	< 1	> 1
Urinary sediment	Hyaline casts	Muddy brown granular casts

Hepatorenal Syndrome

It is defined as the development of renal failure in patients with severe acute or chronic liver disease in the absence of any identifiable cause of renal pathology. Hepatorenal syndrome is a diagnosis of exclusion. It is diagnosed only when all other causes of renal failure such as dehydration, nephrotoxic agents, sepsis and organic renal diseases have been excluded.[19]

Diabetic Nephropathy

It affects about 30% of all patients with insulin dependent diabetes mellitus. The characteristic glomerular lesion is Kimmelsteil Wilson lesion. Unlike the increased GFR of normal pregnancy, the hyperfiltration of early diabetic nephropathy is damaging to the glomeruli, as it is mediated by an increase in glomerular capillary pressure. Pregnancy in women with IDDM does not lead to an increased risk of diabetic nephropathy and established diabetic nephropathy with preserved renal function does not progress more rapidly in pregnancy. However, women with diabetic nephropathy and moderate to severe renal impairment have considerable maternal and fetal morbidity as a consequence of pregnancy.[2] Although ACE inhibitors are the standard drugs used outside pregnancy, their use in pregnancy is contraindicated. Microalbuminuria in early pregnancy increases during the third trimester and is associated with an increased incidence of pre-eclampsia and preterm delivery.[4]

Autosomal Dominant Polycystic Kidney Disease

Those who have normal renal function and blood pressure usually have a successful outcome of pregnancy. Complications during pregnancy can be severe hypertension, anemia, hemorrhage into the cysts and peritonitis. There is a 50% chance of their offspring being affected.

Renal Calculi

The most common nonobstetric cause of abdominal pain requiring hospitalization during pregnancy is renal colic.[20] Symptomatic renal calculi are more common in Caucasians compared with African-Americans and in multigravidae compared with primigravidae. Renal colic is also more common in the second and third trimesters.[4]

Despite renal tract dilatation, urinary stasis, partial obstruction and hypercalciuria, symptomatic renal stone disease is not more common in pregnancy. This is because inhibitors of stone formation such as magnesium, citrate and nephrocalcin (an acidic glycoprotein) are excreted in greater concentrations in the urine during pregnancy.[2] Physiological alkalinization of the urine during pregnancy usually prevents precipitation of uric acid and cysteine stones. Struvite stones are associated with infection rather hypercalciuria and have a higher frequency of urological surgery and contralateral stone formation.

A good history and physical examination can point towards renal calculi in the symptomatic patient. Specific points to be asked are: age at onset of stone disease, family members with stone disease, diet and medications, prior urinary tract infections, results of previous abdominal radiographs and other medical disorders or prior surgeries. Ultrasound can identify renal calculus in about 50% cases. In women with a normal ultrasound, plain X-ray KUB and single shot intravenous urogram (IVU) can identify the rest.

Indications for an IVU during pregnancy include:[20]
1. Symptoms of calculi unresponsive to conservative therapy.
2. A decline in renal function in association with symptoms of kidney stones.
3. Severely symptomatic pyelonephritis refractory to antibiotics, especially in a patient with a past history of nephrolithiasis.

Standard excretory urograms usually deliver less than 1.5 rad to the fetus. To decrease fetal radiation exposure, one should film only the involved side, shield the maternal pelvis and limit the number of films obtained.

To avoid even a small dose of radiation to the fetus, magnetic resonance urography has been used to differentiate physiological urinary tract dilatation and obstruction due to calculi.[4]

Up to 75% of pregnant women with renal stones will pass their stones spontaneously with conservative management, which consists of adequate hydration, antibiotics and pain relief with either pethidine or NSAID prior to the third trimester.

Specific indications for interventions during pregnancy include:[20]

1. Persistent infection proximal to an obstructing stone
2. Intractable pain
3. Renal colic precipitating premature labor that is refractory to drug therapy,
4. Worsening renal function with a persistent obstruction
5. Obstruction of a solitary kidney

The options are ureteral stenting (which requires X-ray guidance), percutaneous nephrostomy (which has to be maintained for the entire duration of pregnancy) and the most recent holmium laser lithotripsy, which delivers direct stone crushing energy up to within 0.5 mm of the laser fiber tip using a ureteroscope. This technique has been successfully and safely used in all stages of pregnancy.[4]

The increased frequency of UTI with symptomatic renal stones is associated with an increased risk of preterm rupture of membranes. UTIs associated with renal stones should be treated for longer time and followed up with antibiotic prophylaxis. During pregnancy, xanthine oxidase inhibitors for uric acid stones and D-penicillamine for cysteine stones should be avoided.[2]

Stone disease should always be evaluated postpartum using the following tests:[20]

- Serum calcium, phosphorus, uric acid, creatinine
- Spot urine for urinalysis and culture, pH
- 24 hour urine for creatinine, uric acid, calcium, phosphorus, oxalate, citrate
- Stone analysis (if stone is available)
- X-ray KUB and intravenous pyelography.

Patients on Dialysis

In the past, pregnancy was discouraged as fetal outcome was poor and maternal complications were almost universal. Today, almost 60% of reported pregnancies result in a live birth, although 80% of these are preterm (around 32 weeks) or small for gestational age. Urea crosses the placenta and a high fetal urinary urea causes osmotic diuresis, which leads to polyhydramnios and preterm labor. Premature rupture of membranes and maternal hypertension are other causes for preterm delivery.

Although the focus should be on contraceptive counseling, if an unintentional conception occurs, termination of pregnancy is no guarantee that the decline in renal function will be reversed.[4]

It is a common practice to begin dialysis in the pregnant woman before it becomes necessary for her health. In this circumstance, the normal hyper filtration of pregnancy is mimicked with daily dialysis.

Women on peritoneal dialysis are less likely to conceive than women on hemodialysis. Furthermore, as pregnancy progresses it is increasingly difficult for peritoneal dialysis to meet the physiological demands of pregnancy, and a switch to hemodialysis may be necessary. Frequent dialysis should aim to keep the pre-dialysis blood urea nitrogen (BUN) < 50 mg/dl (serum urea < 17 mmol/l). It will also reduce the need for large fluid shifts, which may compromise uteroplacental blood flow.[4] Daily dialysis reduces the fetal azotemic environment, prevents polyhydramnios, ensures optimal fluid and electrolyte balance and allows easier control of hypertension. If peritoneal dialysis is employed it often becomes difficult to tolerate large exchange volumes in late pregnancy. Thus, the volume of each exchange is reduced (say from 2-1.5 liters), and compensated by increased exchange frequency.[9] Hypokalemia may become a problem requiring potassium supplementation. Also, the dialysate sodium and bicarbonate levels should fall with the gestational reduction in these levels.[21]

No obvious superiority of peritoneal or hemodialysis in pregnancy has been demonstrated, although a recent study said that infant survival appears to be better in women who use continuous ambulatory peritoneal dialysis (CAPD) rather than hemodialysis. However, the numbers in the former group were small, therefore, pregnant women new to dialysis should start with CAPD, but those who are established on hemodialysis need not switch.[2] A recent analysis of pooled data showed no significant difference in the rate of successful delivery between patients on hemodialysis and those on peritoneal dialysis.[22]

Anemia and hemorrhage are common in the dialysis population. Like other pregnant women, dialysis patients should receive 1 mg folic acid daily over and above their usual supplement. Blood iron, total iron binding capacity and serum ferritin should be monitored monthly and the patient treated with intravenous iron and erythropoietin as needed. The dose of erythropoietin usually has to increase by 50-100% in pregnancy. It does not appear to cross the placenta and consequently, there have been no reports of teratogenicity or polycythemia in the infant.[21]

The long-acting erythropoietin stimulating protein darbepoetin has also been used in a transplant patient during pregnancy, but more information regarding its safety is needed before widespread use can be recommended.[4]

Post-transplant Patient

Ovarian dysfunction, anovulatory vaginal bleeding, amenorrhea, high prolactin levels, and loss of libido are the causes of infertility in women with chronic renal failure. After renal transplantation, endocrine function generally improves after recovery of renal function. Following transplantation, libido and fertility usually return rapidly to normal. Conception is usually not recommended in the context of severe renal impairment or dialysis-dependent renal failure.

The ideal method of contraception in transplant recipients should be individualized. Oral contraceptive pills interfere with the metabolism of some immunosuppressive agents and may also aggravate hypertension. There is increased risk of bacterial pelvic infection associated with the use of an intra-uterine devise. Barrier contraception is safe, effective and the method of first choice in this group of patients.[9]

Following kidney transplantation, there is experience worldwide in over 7000 pregnancies.[9] Pre-conception counseling with a transplant physician and obstetrician should be encouraged in all transplant recipients who are contemplating pregnancy. Approximately 20% of pregnancies will end in spontaneous abortion in early pregnancy, but of those that go beyond the first trimester, at least 90% will end successfully. These pregnancies are, however, more likely to be complicated by preterm labor (30-50%), preeclampsia (30-37%) and IUGR (20-33%).[4] The overall incidence of congenital anomaly is similar to the background population.

Criteria for Advising Pregnancy Post-transplantation:[9]

• At least 2 years post-transplantation
• Good general health
• Stable renal function with serum creatinine < 0.18 mmols/l (< 2 mg/dl)
• On maintenance immunosuppression regimen
• Absence of ongoing rejection episodes
• Blood pressure controlled (< 135/85 mm Hg)
• 24-hour protein excretion < 500 mg
• Drugs contraindicated in pregnancy have been withdrawn (e.g. angiotensin receptor blockers, mycophenolate mofetil)

A shorter interval between transplantation and conception is associated with an increased risk of very low-birth-weight infants and neonatal death. Perinatal outcome is good if renal function is preserved (creatinine clearance > 60-70 ml/min) and blood pressure is normal. However, hypertension in early pregnancy and impaired renal function are associated with a poor perinatal outcome and premature labor.[2]

A retrospective study on 23 post-transplant pregnancies in 15 patients from Croatia showed that patients with arterial hypertension in pregnancy, elevated serum creatinine level and bacteriuria, as well as those with conception occurring less than 2 years after transplantation, had a higher rate of therapeutic and spontaneous abortions, preterm deliveries and low birth weight infants.[23]

The common pregnancy complications in transplant recipients are infection, pre-eclampsia, premature delivery, premature rupture of the membranes, intrauterine growth retardation, low birth weight, gestational diabetes, and graft rejection.[24] Pregnancy does not appear to affect the rate of rejection.[21]

Kidney transplant recipients are also at higher risk for ectopic pregnancy because of previous surgical procedures and continuous ambulatory peritoneal dialysis. Owing to immunosuppression, prophylactic antibiotics are essential for all surgical interventions. During labor, the pelvic kidney seldom obstructs, therefore vaginal delivery should be the aim. Furthermore, the dose of steroids should be temporarily increased at this time.[2]

Human studies have reported that compared to a normal population, infants delivered by kidney transplant recipients have higher rates of low birth weight, prematurity, jaundice, respiratory distress syndrome and aspiration.[24]

Prednisolone at doses of 20 mg/d rarely causes problems for the neonate, as only small amounts cross the placenta (maternal: cord blood ratio is 10:1). Azathioprine crosses the placenta, but it is not converted to its active metabolite, 6-mercaptopurine by the immature fetal liver and appears to be safe. Women taking cyclosporin appear to have small for gestational age babies compared with women who take prednisolone and azathioprine. However, it is otherwise well tolerated in pregnancy with no increased risk of teratogenesis.[21]

The presence of azathioprine and cyclosporin in breast milk suggests that breast feeding should be discouraged.[2]

Commonly prescribed immunosuppressive drugs are given as follows[9]				
Drug	*Class*	*Use in transplant recipient*	*Maintenance dose*	*FDA category*
Prednisolone	Corticosteroid	Maintenance	5-10 mg/day	B
Methyl-prednisolone	Corticosteroid	Induction; acute rejection		B
Azathioprine	Purine antagonist	Maintenance	1.5-2 mg/kg/day	D
Mycophenolate mofetil	Purine antagonist	Maintenance; refractory rejection	1-2 g/day	C
Cyclosporine	Calcineurin antagonist	Maintenance	3-6 mg/kg/day (depending on serum levels)	C
Tacrolimus	Calcineurin antagonist	Maintenance; refractory rejection	0.1-0.2 mg/kg/day (depending on serum levels)	C
Rapamycin	Macrolide	Maintenance; refractory rejection	2-5 mg/day	C

KEY POINTS

- Gestational changes in renal physiology can both mimic and mask renal disease.
- Renal disease with preserved renal function carries a good prognosis for the mother and baby.
- In general, the worse the baseline renal function and more the associated complications (proteinuria, hypertension, UTI, poor glycemic control), the more likely is an adverse pregnancy outcome for the mother and fetus.
- Women with a baseline serum creatinine > 0.18 mmol/l (2 mg/dl) have a one in three chance of an accelerated decline in renal function that is unlikely to recover postpartum.

The disease is responsible for killing more women of reproductive age than all the combined causes of maternal mortality.[4] Exact data about the proportion of pregnant women with tuberculosis are unavailable in India. An increased obstetric morbidity has been reported in such women.[5] Studies have also suggested no unusual increase in preterm labor or other adverse pregnancy outcomes in treated cases of tuberculosis.[6,7]

CLINICAL PRESENTATION

About half to two-thirds of pregnant women with tuberculosis remain asymptomatic.[8] The clinical presentation of tuberculosis in the pregnant women is similar to that in the nonpregnant women. The symptoms are listed in Table 22.1.

Table 22.1: Symptoms of tuberculosis in pregnancy	
Common	*Less common*
Cough	Lethargy
Weight loss	Abdominal distension
Fever	Irritability
Hemoptysis	Skin lesions
Fatigue	Alteration in bowel habit

Nonspecific symptoms like lethargy, alteration in bowel habit or failure to gain weight simulate usual symptoms of pregnancy and cause delay in diagnosis.[9]

During pregnancy pulmonary tuberculosis is more common than extra-pulmonary tuberculosis. Only five to ten percent of pregnant women have extrapulmonary disease[8] and sites most commonly involved are lymph nodes, pleura, genitourinary tract, bones, joints, meninges and peritoneum.[10-13] Extra pulmonary tuberculosis is being seen more often because of HIV coinfection. In a recent retrospective study,[14] 53% of patients were diagnosed with extra pulmonary tuberculosis, 38% with pulmonary tuberculosis and 9% had both. The commonest reason for a delay in diagnosis was late presentation (52%), followed by nonspecific symptoms in 38%.

EFFECT OF PREGNANCY ON TUBERCULOSIS (TABLE 22.2)

Effect of pregnancy on tuberculosis was a matter of controversy since the days of Hippocrates.[15] Raised diaphragm during pregnancy was believed to cause atelectasis of basal lung regions.[16] In early 20th century, it was believed that pregnancy has deleterious effects on tuberculosis and induction of abortion was recommended.[10,17]

Now it is believed that TB gets flared up by the stress of pregnancy, especially if associated with poor nutritional status, immunodeficient state or co-existent diseases. There is also increased risk of development of postpartal TB during lactation, due to loss of protective antibodies in mother.[22] However,

Table 22.2: Studies showing effect of pregnancy on tuberculosis	
Study	*Effects*
1. Hedvall et al[18]	Equal number of women with tuberculosis benefited and worsened during pregnancy
2. March et al[19]	No relapse if adequately treated
3. Schaefer et al[20]	No difference in progression in pregnant and nonpregnant
4. Hamadeh et al[10] Good et al[21]	Small risk of relapse and progression in postpartum period

all this is still controversial and more studies are needed to support these hypothesis.

EFFECT OF TUBERCULOSIS ON PREGNANCY

The pulmonary and extrapulmonary forms of tuberculosis affect the pregnant women in same way as in nonpregnant state. With the advent of chemotherapy, most studies have demonstrated that TB does not increase complications of pregnancy and labor.[10,18] The effect of TB on pregnancy are spontaneous abortions, intrauterine death, premature labor, small for gestational age neonates, low birth weight and increased perinatal mortality. The various studies carried out to study the effect of tuberculosis on pregnancy are listed in Table 22.3.

Table 22.3: Studies showing effect of tuberculosis on pregnancy		
Study	*Year*	*Outcome*
1. Selikoff et al[23]	1965	Seven spontaneous abortions, nine antepartum and intrapartum fetal deaths
2. Schaefer et al[20]	1975	No increase in risk of prematurity
3. Jana et al[24]	1994	Two-fold increase in prematurity, small for gestational age and low birth-weight neonates, 6-fold increase in perinatal deaths
4. Maurya and Sapre[25]	1996	Four spontaneous abortions, two premature deliveries, one intrauterine death
5. Kothari et al[14]	2006	Two abortions, two preterm deliveries

The effect of TB on pregnancy depends on many factors like stage of pregnancy when treatment is started, site, type and extent of the disease, nutritional status of mother, presence of any concomitant disease, immune status, co-existence of HIV infection, availability of facilities for early diagnosis and treatment.

FACTORS DETERMINING EFFECT OF DISEASE ON FETOMATERNAL OUTCOME

1. Antituberculosis treatment
If antituberculosis treatment (ATT) is started early in pregnancy, the outcome is same as that in nonpregnant patients, whereas late diagnosis and care is

associated with 4-fold increase in obstetric morbidity and 9-fold increase in preterm labor.[5]

Maternal and fetal complications are more frequent in pregnant women with multiple drug resistant tuberculosis compared to those with drug sensitive disease.[21]

2. Extrapulmonary tuberculosis

The diagnosis of this condition is often delayed[11,12,26,27] and it is difficult to identify this type of tuberculosis with the use of radiological and bacteriologic evaluation.[28]

Biopsy and surgical intervention during pregnancy may not be possible because of the risk of preterm labor, poor accessibility of the lesions and anesthetic risk to the fetus.[29]

Effects of extrapulmonary tuberculosis on pregnancy[30] depend on the:
- Site, severity and duration of the disease.
- Occurrence of pregnancy-associated complications.

3. Multi-drug resistant tuberculosis (MDR-TB)

Pregnant mothers with MDR-TB have increased risk of maternal and neonatal complications as this is more advanced disease with extensive radiographic changes and longer sputum conversion times.

4. Incomplete or irregular treatment

5. Advanced lung disease

6. Poor maternal nutrition

7. Co-existence of HIV infection

CONGENITAL TUBERCULOSIS

Congenital tuberculosis is a rare entity and around 300 cases have been reported in literature.[31] The fetus may be infected by two ways:
1. Hematogenously through umbilical vein
2. Aspiration or ingestion of amniotic fluid that is contaminated by hematogenous dissemination of tuberculosis through placenta.

The primary focus develops in the liver which is the major site along with involvement of the periportal lymph nodes. The tubercle bacilli infect the lung secondarily. Alternatively, the fetus may have multiple primary foci in the gut or the lungs. Central nervous system involvement is rare.[32,33]

Cantwell et al[34] criteria for confirming fetal/neonatal tuberculosis comprises
   i. Demonstration of either primary hepatic complex or caseating hepatic granulomas on percutaneous liver biopsy at birth.
   ii. Presence of maternal genital tract/ placental TB.
   iii. Presence of lesions during first week of life by excluding postnatal transmission by a thorough investigation of all the contacts.

Congenital tuberculosis usually seen in second or third week of life has nonspecific symptoms and signs which are:[34]

- Respiratory distress and hepatosplenomegaly (most common)
- Fever and lymphadenopathy
- Abdominal distension
- Lethargy
- Irritability
- Ear discharge
- Skin lesions

A failure to obtain favorable response with broad spectrum antibiotics along with negative results for other congenital infections should lead to suspicion of congenital tuberculosis.

Diagnosis of congenital tuberculosis can be made by eliciting maternal history of exposure and a tuberculin skin test carried out in the newborn which may be negative initially but becomes positive within 4-6 weeks. The chest X-ray of these newborns is abnormal and 50% have a miliary pattern. It is not easy to obtain sputum from newborn however, tubercular bacilli can be easily cultured from gastric aspirates. Direct smears from the middle ear, bone marrow and tracheal aspirates may show acid-fast bacilli (AFB). The overall mortality for congenital TB is 38% in the untreated and 22% in the treated cases.[34,35]

Diagnosis

It is important to identify pregnant women with tuberculosis, as early diagnosis and treatment will result in better maternal and neonatal outcome.

History

A careful history is mandatory in high-risk cases in the antenatal period. It should include any history of exposure to the disease and presence of any symptoms. However, similarities of symptoms between tuberculosis and pregnancy should be kept in mind.

Chest Radiograph

In the past, routine chest X-ray was advocated to detect tuberculosis. As there is a risk of radiation exposure, the routine use of chest radiograph is not justified.

In case of suspicion of tuberculosis, a tuberculin skin test should be carried out. If tuberculin skin test is greater than 10 mm of induration, a chest radiograph should be obtained in asymptomatic patient with proper abdominal shielding preferably after first trimester.

Tuberculin Skin Test

In India where most of the population will have a tuberculin positive result, the routine use of this test remains questionable. There has also been some concerns about the sensitivity of tuberculin test during pregnancy and earlier reports suggested that tuberculin test sensitivity might be diminished in pregnancy.[36] However, well-controlled trials have found that there was no significant difference.[37]

Tuberculin test is deemed a safe and useful method for screening tuberculosis infection in pregnancy and should be used in women with:
- Symptoms and signs of tuberculosis
- Pregnant women with diabetes or HIV
- Women employed in hospitals, old age homes
- Prisoners
- Low socioeconomic status.

In women who are HIV positive, there may be diminished or negative tuberculin reaction and therefore, an area of 5 mm or greater induration in an HIV positive patient is considered positive.[38]

Microbiological Methods

Demonstrating *Mycobacterium tuberculosis* by Ziehl-Neelsen staining or culturing in sputum or any other material obtained from suspicious site confirms diagnosis. Bronchoscopy may be required if patient is unable to produce sputum.

Protocol for Diagnosis of TB in Pregancy under Revised National Tuberculosis Control Program (RNTCP)[39]

- Sputum examination is the preferred method for diagnosis of pulmonary tuberculosis.
- A chest skiagram (after shielding the abdomen) is done if all the 3 sputum smears are negative and symptoms persist despite giving antibiotics for 1-2 weeks.
- In the absence of positive smears and the presence of any radiographic abnormalities, it is medical officer's discretion to treat with ATT labeling the patient as a 'smear-negative' tuberculosis case.
- Routine hematology and Mantoux test are not included in this program.
- A pregnant woman with extrapulmonary tuberculosis has constitutional and specific organ-affection symptoms.
- Co-existence of HIV infection should specially lead to a thorough search for any extrapulmonary tuberculous focus.
- Investigations which are specific for the site are carried out for the establishment of specific diagnosis.

Treatment of Tuberculosis in Pregnant Women

Treatment with ATT should be initiated without delay when TB is diagnosed in pregnant women. The decision to treat tuberculosis in pregnancy must take into account the potential risks to mother and fetus from medication, and the benefits of adequate treatment to mother, fetus and community. It is widely considered that the benefits of treating tuberculosis in pregnancy outweigh any risk of treatment. The indications for treatment of active tuberculosis in pregnant women are the same as that for nonpregnant women.

In a study, overall teratogenic effects of isoniazid, rifampicin, streptomycin, and ethambutol, the first line ATT, were analyzed and none was found to be teratogenic, except streptomycin which causes ototoxicity in fetus.[40]

The same regimens are recommended for use in pregnancy as for the non-pregnant state with the exception of withholding streptomycin. Pyrazinamide should preferably be avoided in pregnancy.

Currently, an intermittent regimen (thrice weekly on alternate days) under the DOTS strategy of RNTCP is being increasingly used worldwide for the pregnant women having tuberculosis.[41]

In a retrospective analysis of 12,367 TB patients who were put on DOTS, there were 16 pregnant women suffering from either pulmonary or extrapulmonary form of disease, of these 25% had become pregnant while receiving ATT. All the 16 completed their treatment and overall drug tolerance was good. There were no adverse pregnancy outcome reported.[42]

First Line Drugs (Table 22.4)

Isoniazid (INH) (Pregnancy Category A)
It is a bactericidal drug, available data reveal that INH is safe during pregnancy and is recommended for use. Although it crosses the placental barrier, it is not teratogenic even when administered in the first trimester. Abnormalities have been reported in only 1% of infants born to mothers treated with isoniazid, which falls below the 1.2-6% incidence of fetal malformations cited in the population at large.[42] Side effects of isoniazid are cutaneous hypersensitivity, hepatitis, and peripheral neuropathy.

Hepatitis is a major side effect and risk of INH-induced hepatitis may be 2.5 times higher in prenatal patients than the general population,[43] although largely unconfirmed.[44] Addition of pyridoxine in a dose of 50 mg/day has been recommended during pregnancy to prevent neurotoxicity in the mother and fetus.[40]

Rifampicin (Pregnancy Category C)
It is a bactericidal drug. The rate of congenital malformations was 3.35% in infants whose mothers received rifampicin and included limb reduction, CNS lesions and hemorrhagic complications.[40] However, the incidence falls within the safety limits and hence rifampicin is also considered to be safe. It may cause nausea, vomiting and hepatitis.

Ethambutol (Pregnancy Category A)
Ethambutol is a bacteriostatic drug. It is recommended for use in pregnancy with a reported incidence of 2% malformations. Although, it was feared

that ethambutol might interfere with ophthalmological development of fetus, this was not observed in doses of 15-25 mg/kg body weight/day.[40] Major side effect is retrobulbar neuritis occurring in <1% of cases on a daily dose of 15 mg /kg.[44]

Pyrazinamide (Pregnancy Category C)
Pyrazinamide, a bactericidal drug used in most first line regimens, little is known about the safety of this drug during pregnancy. Although, some international organizations recommend its use, it is preferably avoided due to inadequate data on teratogenicity.[39] Pyrazinamide may produce gastrointestinal side effects, arthralgia, hyperuricemia and hepatitis.

Streptomycin (Pregnancy Category C)
Streptomycin is potentially teratogenic drug throughout pregnancy causing fetal malformations. It causes eighth nerve paralysis with deficits ranging from mild hearing loss to bilateral deafness.[45,46] It is not recommended for use in pregnancy. Streptomycin may commonly cause vertigo apart from ototoxicity and nephrotoxicity in mother.

Table 22.4: First line anti TB drugs used in pregnancy		
Anti-TB drug	*Mode of action*	*Recommended dose (mg/kg)*
Isoniazid (H)	Bactericidal	5 (4-6)
Rifampicin (R)	Bactericidal	10 (8-12)
Ethambutol (E)	Bacteriostatic	15 (15-20)
Pyrazinamide (Z)	Bactericidal	25 (20-30)

Second Line Drugs

With the emergence of MDR-TB and HIV associated TB, pregnant women may sometimes need to be treated with second line drugs, the data on safety of which are lacking.
- *Para-aminosalicylic acid (PAS)*: It was used in conjunction with INH and did not appear to increase the malformations in infants but causes gastrointestinal side effects, which were difficult to tolerate during pregnancy.
- *Ethionamide*: It is known to cause teratogenic effects in animals and is not recommended for use in pregnancy.[35]
- *Others*: Little is known about the safety of cycloserine, kanamycin, capreomycin and fluoroquinolones like ciprofloxacin and ofloxacin during pregnancy. There are no existing guidelines for the treatment of pregnant women with drug resistant tuberculosis and it has been suggested that elective abortion may be considered while treating a pregnant woman with MDR-TB.[21] If a woman insists on continuation of pregnancy, all the consequences should be discussed with her in detail. The management of pregnant tuberculous women with HIV is complicated due to involvement of drug reactions, so the regimens and drug dosages need appropriate adjustments.

Supportive Measures during Antitubercular Therapy

Along with ATT certain other measures need to be taken to optimize the outcome of treatment which include:

1. An intake of pyridoxine with isoniazid during the entire period of therapy to prevent peripheral neuropathy. It is being practiced under the RNTCP.
2. Prophylactic vitamin K administration to baby at birth for preventing hemorrhagic disease of the newborn.
3. Segregation of the mother from neonate if she has active and infectious disease (especially MDR-TB) and either is not likely to receive ATT due to maternal non-compliance or has received it only for less than 2 weeks prior to delivery.
4. Substitution of either protease inhibitors with another class of antiretroviral drugs or rifampicin with rifabutin in case of their coadministration.
5. Cautious addition of drugs in case multiple therapies need to be given during the coexistence of various diseases.
6. Examination of the contacts of the pregnant woman's household.
7. Necessary procedural interventions like pleural, pericardial or ascitic tapping, intercostal chest drainage tube, etc.[22]

Treatment of Tuberculosis in Lactating Women

The safety of breastfeeding if mother is on ATT is a very important issue. There is a general consensus that although small concentrations of antituberculosis drugs are excreted in breast milk, treatment for tuberculosis is not a contraindication to breastfeeding. Under RNTCP, breastfeeding of neonates is recommended regardless of the mother's tuberculosis status.

Several studies have measured the concentration of ATT drugs in breast milk.[47-50]

- INH concentration peaks three hours after ingestion and reaches a concentration of 16.6 mg/l with a 300 mg dose.[47]
- Rifampicin, has a peak milk concentration of 10-30 mg/l when given in a dose of 600 mg daily.[48]
- Streptomycin reaches a concentration of 1.3 mg/l in thirty minutes after injection of a 1 gm dose.[49]
- No information on the concentration of ethambutol in breast milk has been published.

The effect of these drugs gets minimized, if breastfeeding is done before taking the ATT and the next feed is substituted with formula preparation.

Supplemental pyridoxine should be administered to an infant on INH or if the breastfeeding mother is taking INH because pyridoxine deficiency may cause seizures in the newborn.

In general, mothers with fully drug susceptible pulmonary TB can continue breastfeeding their infants provided the infant has been given

22

Tuberculosis in Pregnancy

appropriate antimycobacterial cover, i.e. isoniazid, if no evidence of disease in the infant, or full treatment if active TB disease cannot be excluded.

INH Prophylaxis in Pregnant Women

- Preventive therapy with INH is very effective and there is no teratogenic risk in pregnant women treated with standard dosages for 6 to 12 months.
- However, there is a significant risk of hepatotoxicity, which is more during the postpartum period.[51]
- A baseline liver function tests should be done before starting prophylactic therapy and it is repeated every month.
- Pyridoxine should be given to these women to decrease the risk of isoniazid induced neuropathy.[43]
- In the areas with high endemicity for tuberculosis like India approximately 50% of adult population is tuberculin positive.[52] Therefore, the usefulness of isoniazid chemoprophylaxis in such areas is unclear.
- However, isoniazid prophylaxis is considered if:
  - Documented recent tuberculin conversion
  - Recent exposure to close contact with active tuberculosis
  - Immunosuppression
- Dose is 5 mg/kg body weight with a maximum dose of 300 mg/day.

Care of Newborn

- Tuberculin positive mother without active tuberculosis and pregnant woman with active pulmonary tuberculosis who is sputum negative during the last three months of gestation does not pose any risk to the newborn.
- However, if the mother is sputum positive or on ATT, the infant needs evaluation for active tuberculosis with chest radiograph and examination of gastric aspirate or sputum for AFB.
- If there is no evidence of active tuberculosis, the infant should receive INH prophylaxis for three months or until after the mother's sputum becomes negative for AFB and the baby is tuberculin negative.
- BCG vaccination may be postponed or done with INH-resistant BCG vaccine.
- If the infant is tuberculin positive, INH prophylaxis should be given for a total period of six months after ruling out active tuberculosis.[53]
- There is a recommendation that if the mother is suffering from MDR-TB, INH prophylaxis has no role and hence should not be given.
- In such cases, the infant should receive BCG vaccination which has been shown to have a protective effect.[54-56]
- BCG is contraindicated in HIV positive children.
  If tuberculosis is diagnosed and treated appropriately and early, the prognosis for both mother and child is excellent.

CONTRACEPTION

Rifampicin accelerates the metabolism of oral contraceptives and other drugs resulting in sub-therapeutic serum levels.[10] So, the reliability of oral contraceptive is decreased in women taking ATT.[57] All other contraceptive measures can be considered in postpartum women taking anti-tuberculosis treatment.

KEY POINTS

- Tuberculosis (TB) is a public health problem especially in developing countries and India accounts for 30% of the burden of all tuberculosis cases in the world.
- About half to two-thirds of pregnant women with tuberculosis remain asymptomatic.
- During pregnancy pulmonary tuberculosis is more common than extrapulmonary tuberculosis.
- TB gets flared up by the stress of pregnancy, especially if associated with poor nutritional status, immunodeficient state, or co-existent diseases.
- With the advent of chemotherapy, most studies have demonstrated that TB does not increase complications of pregnancy and labor.
- Sputum examination is the preferred method for diagnosis of pulmonary tuberculosis during pregnancy.
- A chest skiagram with shielding of the abdomen is done if all the 3 sputum smears are negative and symptoms persist despite giving antibiotics for 1-2 weeks.
- Co-existence of HIV infection should specially lead to a thorough search for any extra-pulmonary tuberculous focus.
- Treatment with ATT should be initiated without delay when TB is diagnosed in pregnant women.
- The same regimens are recommended for use in pregnancy as for the non-pregnant state with the exception of streptomycin which should not be given. Pyrazinamide should preferably be avoided in pregnancy.
- Currently, an intermittent regimen (thrice weekly on alternate days) under the DOTS strategy of RNTCP is being increasingly used worldwide for the pregnant women having tuberculosis.
- Small concentrations of antituberculosis drugs are excreted in breast milk but treatment for tuberculosis is not a contraindication to breastfeeding.
- Congenital tuberculosis is a rare entity and the fetus may be infected by hematogenous route or by aspiration or ingestion of contaminated amniotic fluid.
- The chest X-ray of these newborns is usually abnormal and 50% have a miliary pattern.
- The overall mortality for congenital TB is 38% in the untreated and 22% in the treated cases.

- If there is no evidence of active tuberculosis, the infant should receive INH prophylaxis for three months or until after the mother's sputum becomes negative for AFB and the baby is tuberculin negative.
- BCG vaccination may be postponed or done with INH-resistant BCG vaccine.
- If the infant is tuberculin positive, INH prophylaxis should be given for a total period of six months after ruling out active tuberculosis.

REFERENCES

1. Centers for Disease Control and Prevention (CDC). Trends in tuberculosis—United States, 2005. Morbidity and Mortality Weekly Report 2006;55(11):305-08.
2. World Health Organization; Research for Action: Understanding and controlling tuberculosis in India; 2000;12.
3. RNTCP Status Report. Central TB Division India 2008; New Delhi.
4. World Health Organization; World Health Report 1999;12368.
5. Figueroa-Damien R, Arredondo–Garcia JL. Pregnancy and tuberculosis: Influence of treatment on perinatal outcome. Am J Perinatol 1998;15:303.
6. Riley L. Pneumonia and tuberculosis in pregnancy. Infect Dis Clin North Am 1997;11(1):119.
7. Robinson CA, Rose NC. Tuberculosis: Current implications and management in obstetrics. Obstet Gynecol Surve 1996;51:115.
8. Wilson E, Thelin T, Dilts P. Tuberculosis complicated by pregnancy. Am J Obstet Gynaecol 1972;115:526-31.
9. Good JT Jr, Iseman MD, Davidson PT, Lakshminarayan S, Sahn SA. Tuberculosis in association with pregnancy. Am J Obstet Gynecol 1981;140:492-98.
10. Hamadeh MA, Glassroth J. Tuberculosis and pregnancy. Chest 1992;101:1114-20.
11. Govender S, Moodley SC, Grootboom MJ. Tuberculous paraplegia during pregnancy: A report of four cases. S Afr Med J 1989;75:190-92.
12. Kingdom JCP, Kennedy DH. Tuberculous meningitis in pregnancy. Br J Obstet Gynaecol 1989;96:233-35.
13. Brooks JH, Stirvat GM. Tuberculosis peritonitis in pregnancy: Case report. Br J Obstet Gynaecol 1986;93:1009-10.
14. Kothari A, Mahadevan N, Girling J. Tuberculosis and pregnancy—Results of a study in a high prevalence area in London. Eur J Obstet Gynecol Repro Biol 2006;126:48-55.
15. Carter EJ, Mates S. Tuberculosis during pregnancy. Chest 1994;106:1466-70.
16. Snider DE Jr. Pregnancy and tuberculosis. Chest 1984;86:115.
17. Vallejo JG, Starke JR. Tuberculosis and pregnancy. Clin Chest Med 1992;13:693.
18. Hedvall E. Pregnancy and tuberculosis. Acta Med Scand 1953;147:1-101.
19. De March P. Tuberculosis and pregnancy. Five to ten year review of 215 patients in their fertile age. Chest 1975;68:800-4.
20. Schaefer G, Zervoudakis IA, Fuch FF, David S. Pregnancy and tuberculosis. Obstet Gynecol 1975;46:706-15.
21. Good JT Jr, Iseman MD, Davidson PT, Lakshminarayan S, Sahn SA. Tuberculosis in association with pregnancy. Am J Obstet Gynecol 1981;140:492-98.
22. Arora VK, Rajnish G. Tuberculosis and Pregnancy. Ind J Tub 2003;50:13.
23. Selikoff IJ, Dorfmann HL. Management of tuberculosis. In: Rovinskey JJ, Gulmatcher AF, (Eds): Medical, surgical and gynecological complications of pregnancy. Baltimore: Williams and Wilkins 1965;111.
24. Jana N, Vasista K, Jindal SK, Khunnu B, Ghosh K. Perinatal outcome in pregnancies complicated by pulmonary tuberculosis. Int J Gynaecol Obstet 1994;44:119-24.
25. Maurya U, Sapre S. Tuberculosis and Pregnancy. J Obstet Gynecol India 1996;46:460-3.
26. Casper GR, Heath P, Garland SM. A pain in the neck in pregnancy: Cervical spinal tuberculosis. Aust N Z J Obstet Gynaecol 1995;35:398-400.
27. Schaefer G, Douglas RG, Dreishpoon IH. Extrapulmonary tuberculosis and pregnancy. Am J Obstet Gynecol 1954;67:605-15.

28. Extrapulmonary tuberculosis. Indian J Tuberc 1985;32:115-16.
29. Kochi A. The global tuberculosis situation and the new control strategy of the World Health Organization. Tubercle 1991;72:01-6.
30. Jana N, Vasishta K, Saha SC, Ghosh K. Obstetrical outcomes among women with extra pulmonary tuberculosis. N Engl Med 1999;341:645-49.
31. Armstrong L, Garay SM. Tuberculosis and pregnancy and tuberculous mastitis. In: Rom WN, Garay SM (Eds): Tuberculosis. Boston. Little Brown and Company 1996;689-98.
32. Gogus S, Uner H, Akcoren Z, et al. Neonatal tuberculosis. Pediatr Pathol 1999;13:299-304.
33. Hageman J, Shulman S, Schreiber M, et al. Congenital tuberculosis: Critical reappraisal of clinical findings and diagnostic procedures. Pediatrics 1980;66:980-84.
34. Cantwell MR, Shehab ZM, Costello AM, et al. Brief report: Congenital tuberculosis. N Engl J Med 1994;330:1051-54.
35. Ormerod P. Tuberculosis and pregnancy and the puerperium. Thorax 2001;56:494.
36. Finn R, St Hill C, Grovan A, et al. Immunological responses in pregnancy and survival of fetal homograft. BMJ 1972;3:150-52.
37. Present P, Comstock GW. Tuberculin sensitivity in pregnancy. Am Rev Respir Dis 1975;112: 413-16.
38. Bass JB Jr, Farer LS, Hopewell PC, et al. Treatment of tuberculosis and tuberculosis infection in adults and children. Am J Respir Crit Care Med 1994;149:1359-74.
39. Central TB Division; Managing the Revised National Tuberculosis Control Programme in your area–A training course; Modules 1-4, New Delhi: 2001;1.
40. Snider DE Jr, Layde PM, Johnson MW, Lyle MA. Treatment of tuberculosis during pregnancy. Am Rev Respir Dis 1980;145:494-98.
41. Anderson GD. Tuberculosis in pregnancy. Semin Perinatol 1997;21(4):328.
42. Arora VK, Sarin R. Revised National Tuberculosis Control Programme: Indian Perspective; Ind J Chest Dis Allied Sci 2000;42:21.
43. Snider DE, Caras GJ. Isoniazid associated hepatitis deaths: A review of available information. Am Rev Respir Dis 1992;145:494.
44. Brost BC, Newman RB. The maternal and fetal effects of tuberculosis therapy. Obstet Gynecol Clin North Am 1997;24(3):659.
45. Conway N, Bird BD. Streptomycin in pregnancy. Effects on fetal ear. BMJ 1965;2:260-63.
46. Robinson GC, Cambon KG. Hearing loss in infants of tuberculous mothers treated with streptomycin during pregnancy. N Engl J Med 1964;271:949-51.
47. Berlin C, Lee C. Isoniazid and acetylisoniazid disposition in human milk, saliva and plasma. Fed Proc 1979;38:426.
48. Vorherr H. Drug excretion in breast milk. Postgrad Med J 1974;56:97-104.
49. Fujimori H, Imai S. Studies on dihydrostreptomycin administered to the pregnant and transferred to their fetuses. Jpn Obstet Gynecol Soc 1957;4:133-49.
50. Snider DE Jr, Powell K. Should women taking antituberculous drugs breast feed? Arch Intern Med 1984;144:589-90.
51. Moulding TS, Redeker AG, Kanel GC. Twenty isoniazid associated deaths in one state. Am Rev Respir Dis 1989;140:700-05.
52. Gothi GD. Epidemiology of tuberculosis in India. Indian J Tuberc 1982;29:134-48.
53. Central TB Division, New Delhi. Tuberculosis: A Guide for Practicing Physicians. Revised National Tuberculosis Control Programme. Central TB Division, Directorate General of Health Services, Nirman Bhawan, New Delhi.
54. Kendig E. The place of BCG vaccination in the management of infants born of tuberculous mothers. N Engl J Med 1969;281:520-23.
55. Curtis H, Leck I, Bamford F. Incidence of childhood tuberculosis after neonatal BCG vaccination. Lancet 1984;1:145-48.
56. Young T, Hershfield E. A case-control study to evaluate effectiveness of mass neonatal BCG vaccination among Canadian Indians. Am J Public Health 1986;76:783-86.
57. Skolnick JL, Stoler BS, Katz DB, Anderson WH. Rifampicin, oral contraceptives and pregnancy. JAMA 1976;236:13.

22

Tuberculosis in Pregnancy

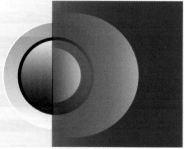

Epilepsy with Pregnancy 23

Monika Madaan

INTRODUCTION

Epilepsy is a common neurological disorder and has a prevalence of 5.25 per 1000 pregnancies.[1] During pregnancy 0.15 to 10% of women have seizures.[2] Managing epilepsy during pregnancy is to balance maternal and fetal risks associated with uncontrolled seizures against the potential teratogenic effects of antiepileptic drugs (AEDs). A rational approach requires knowledge of such risks as well as an understanding of effect of pregnancy on seizure control and on metabolism of AEDs.

EFFECT OF PREGNANCY ON EPILEPSY

Approximately one-third of women experience an increase in seizure frequency during pregnancy.[3] This is attributed to physiological changes and psychological stress associated with pregnancy. The control of epilepsy achieved before pregnancy directly affects the number of seizures occurring in pregnancy. The fewer the number of seizures occurring in 9 months before pregnancy, the lesser is the risk of seizures during pregnancy.[3]

The disposition of many AEDs may change during pregnancy, reflected by declining plasma drug concentrations. The causes are:
- Nausea and vomiting may cause missed doses.
- Gastrointestinal absorption decreases because of decreased intestinal motility and use of antacids.
- Increased hepatic and renal clearance of most AEDs.
- Expanded intravascular volume lowers serum drug levels.
- Decreased albumin levels in pregnancy leading to lower total drug levels.
- Poor compliance often due to fear of teratogenicity.

The reduction in drug levels caused by all the above factors is combated in part by the fact that decreased protein binding during pregnancy increases the serum levels of free drug.

These changes reverse in postpartum period resulting in prepregnancy drug levels.

EFFECT OF EPILEPSY ON PREGNANCY

Women with epilepsy have an increased risk of bearing children with congenital malformations that is approximately twice that of general population.[4]

Polytherapy with AEDs is associated with an increased risk of congenital malformations than monotherapy.[4] Available evidence does not suggest that epilepsy per se is associated with increase in risk of congenital malformations.[5]

Several of these drugs cause fetal hydantoin syndrome characterized by craniofacial anomalies (mildly dysmorphic face and fingers with stubby distal phalanges), fingernail hypoplasia, developmental delay, cardiac defects and facial clefts. Valproate and carbamazepine have been associated with neural tube defects specifically spina bifida.[6] Other factors may contribute to the risk including genetic predisposition, concomitant diseases like diabetes mellitus, occupational exposure to teratogens, excessive prepregnancy weight and various nutritional deficiencies.

Maternal folate deficiency has also been linked with neural tube defects and periconceptional folate supplementation reduces the risk. But it is still not proven that folate supplementation has a protective effect for women with epilepsy.

Data concerning the risk of congenital malformations associated with newer AEDs (gabapentin, lamotrigine, levetiracetam, oxcarbazepine, tiagabine, topiramate, zonisamide) are still limited.[7]

Dose dependent increased risk of congenital malformations is specifically seen with valproic acid which is associated with increased risk at doses above 800-1000 mg/day.[5] It is also associated with cognitive impairment and developmental delay in babies born to mothers with epilepsy.[8] Table 23.1 summarizes the congenital malformations associated with commonly used AEDs.[9]

Table 23.1: Congenital malformations associated with commonly used AEDs

Drug	*Teratogenesis*
Phenytoin	Fetal hydantion syndrome, craniofacial anomalies, fingernail hypoplasia, growth deficiency, developmental delay, cardiac defects, facial clefts.
Carbamazepine	Fetal hydantoin syndrome, spina bifida
Valproate	Neural tube defects
Trimethadione, paramethadione	Craniofacial anomalies, including cleft palate, V-shaped eyebrows, microcephaly, growth deficiency, mental retardation, speech disturbance, cardiac defects
Phenobarbital	Clefts, cardiac anomalies, urinary tract malformations
Lamotrigine	Theoretical – lowers fetal folate levels by inhibiting dihydrofolate reductase
Topiramate	Theoretical – has produced defects or abnormal pregnancy outcomes in all animals tested, even at low or therapeutic doses

Coagulopathy has been seen with drugs like phenobarbitone, primadone and phenytoin as they cause functionally defective neonatal vitamin K dependent clotting factors.[2,7,9,10]

MANAGEMENT

Preconception

The treatment of women with epilepsy has to be done in conjunction with a neurologist. Women who have been seizure free for more than 2 years can be considered for withdrawal of AEDs. In women where drug cannot be withdrawn the common treatment strategy is to use the appropriate AED as monotherapy in the lowest effective dosage throughout pregnancy, the objective being to use AEDs in such a way that seizures are avoided but with a minimized risk to the fetus, the newborn and the breastfed infant. Valproic acid should be avoided if possible. Any major change in the treatment of women with epilepsy should ideally be done before conception.

Folic acid supplementation in the dose of 5 mg/day should be started 3 months before conception.

Couple should be made to understand the importance of compliance regarding AEDs for seizure control and the associated risk of fetal congenital malformations.

Antenatal Management

- Regular intake of drug needs to be emphasized in the antenatal period to achieve optimal drug levels. Nausea and vomiting needs to be treated in the first trimester. Stress on adequate diet, sleep and refraining from activity that can provoke seizures should be given during each antenatal visit.
- Fetal evaluation: Screening for fetal anomalies can be done by Level II second trimester USG, maternal serum AFP levels, amniocentesis for AFP and acetycholinesterase.
- Role of monitoring drug levels is controversial: Some clinicians routinely measure serum AED levels during each trimester and during last month of pregnancy.[10] But some studies show no advantage of monitoring drug levels as they are unreliable because of altered protein binding.[11] Free drug levels although more helpful are not widely available, but drug levels may be measured if a woman throws a fit or if noncompliance is suspected.
- Role of administering vitamin K during last month of pregnancy is again controversial as it is not clear whether vitamin K crosses placenta or not.
- Durgs most commonly used in pregnancy are carbamazepine, valproic acid, phenytoin, phenobarbitone. Now newer AEDs have become widespread in patients with epilepsy like gabapentin, lamotrigine, levetiracetam, oxcarbazepine, tiagabine, topiramate, zonisamide.

But the alteration in the pharmacokinetics of these drugs during pregnancy has not been adequately studied and they have been classified under category C. Also there is little good quality evidence from clinical trials to support the newer monotherapy or adjunctive therapy over older drugs or to support the use of one newer AED in preference to another.

Intrapartum Management

Monitoring of patients with epilepsy during labor is same as that of normal pregnant women. Most patients can have normal vaginal delivery. Cesarean section is indicated in the following circumstances:
1. Patients refractory to treatment during third trimester.
2. Status epilepticus as it may cause fetal asphyxia and IUD.
3. Repeated absence or psychomotor seizures which limit maternal awareness and ability to cooperate.

If seizures occur during labor, lorazepam (a short acting benzodiazepine) is given intravenously in 2 mg boluses every 5 minutes. Diazepam 5-10 mg slow IV may also be used.

Postpartum Management

As physiological alterations caused by pregnancy revert postpartum, the drug levels increase. This may necessitate decreasing the drug levels to prepregnancy levels if the dose has been increased in pregnancy. Seizures occurring for the first time in postpartum period require complete evaluation to rule out intracranial hemorrhage, cortical venous thrombosis, infections and eclampsia. Neonates are given vitamin K 1 mg intramuscular to prevent coagulopathy. Breastfeeding is not contraindicated in women with epilepsy.

Contraception

Contraception counseling should be done for all women with epilepsy. Women should be explained that oral contraceptive failure may occur with phenobartitone, primadone, phenytoin and carbamazepine because of induction of hepatic microsomal enzymes which increases the metabolism of oral contraceptive pills.

ACOG has recommended oral contraceptive pills with 50 microgram of estrogens to be used in women with epilepsy on AEDs.

STATUS EPILEPTICUS

Status epilepticus is a medical emergency. In status epilepticus, seizures continue for more than 30 minutes or there are recurrent seizures without full recovery of consciousness between the seizures. Causes include uncontrolled epilepsy, eclampsia, encephalitis, meningitis, tumor, trauma, sudden drug withdrawal, metabolic derangements and cardiovascular disease. Effects of status epilepticus on mother and fetus are listed in Table 23.2.

Table 23.2: Effects of status epilepticus on mother and fetus

Maternal effects	—	Metabolic acidosis
	—	Acute renal failure
	—	Irreversible brain damage
Fetal effects	—	Fetal hypoxia and asphyxia
	—	Fetal death
	—	Preterm labor

Management

- Investigations to find the underlying cause are performed simultaneously. These include complete blood count, liver and kidney function tests, serum electrolytes, antiepileptic drug levels in blood and CSF analyses if indicated.
- ABC of resuscitation is followed. This involves:
  - Securing patient's airway
  - Supplemental oxygenation
  - Left lateral position
  - Intravenous fluids to avoid hypotension

Control of Seizures

For acute control of seizures, either lorazepam 2 mg intravenously repeated every 5 minutes or diazepam 5 to 10 mg intravenous is given. Simultaneously, phenytoin is started at a loading dose of 18 mg/kg in 100 ml normal saline given over ½ an hour. This regimen can control seizures in 75-85% of cases. In cases where seizures persist additional 5 mg/kg of phenytoin can be added. In refractory cases, last resort is to perform elective intubation.

KEY POINTS

- Management of epilepsy in pregnancy requires an understanding of optimal dose of AEDs for seizure control and their associated risk of fetal congenital malformation.
- Seizure control before pregnancy is as important as their control in pregnancy.
- The levels of many AEDs change (decline) during pregnancy and these changes revert postpartum necessitating change in drug dosage.
- Women with AEDs have twice the risk of fetal congenital malformation compared to general population.
- Polytherapy is associated with major risk of congenital malformation than monotherapy.
- Valproate is associated with dose dependent increase in risk of congenital malformation especially at doses above 800-1000 mg/day.
- Valproate is also associated with cognitive impairment and developmental delay in babies born to mothers on AEDs.
- Folic acid supplementation is must in women on AEDs.

- Changes in the dose of AEDs if required should be done before conception.
- Counseling of the couple regarding compliance of drugs and risk of teratogenicity must be done.
- Fetal evaluation for congenital malformation is a must in women on AEDs.
- Lorazepam or diazepam are the drugs of choice in women with seizures during labor or if the women goes into status epilepticus.

REFERENCES

1. Koehler P, Bruyn G, Pearee JMS. Neurological eponyms. Oxford University Press, New York 2000.
2. Brodie MJ. Management of epilepsy during pregnancy and lactation. Lancet 1990;426-7.
3. Yerby MS, Devinsky O. Epilepsy and pregnancy. Adv Neurol 1994;64:45-63.
4. Battino D, Tomson T. Management of epilepsy during pregnancy. Drugs 2007;67(18):2707-46.
5. Perucea E. Birth defects after prenatal exposure to antiepileptic drugs. Lancet Neurol 2005; 4(11):781-6.
6. Lindhort D, Omzigt JGC, Cornel MC. Spectrum of neural tube defects in 34 infants prenatally exposed to antepeileptic drugs. Neurology 1992;42:111-8.
7. Yerby MS. Clinical care of women with epilepsy: Neural tube defects and folic acid supplementation. Epilepsy 2003;44(Suppl 3):33-40.
8. Adab N, Nivie U, et al. The longer term outcome of children born to mothers with epilepsy. J Neurol Neurosing Psychiatry 2004;75(11):1575-83.
9. Pennell PB. Antiepileptic drug pharmakinetics during pregnancy and lactation. Neurology 2003;61:S35-S42.
10. Lander CM, Eadie MJ. Plasma antiepileptic drug concentrations during pregnancy. Epilepsia 1991;32:257.
11. Wilby J, Kainth A, et al. Clinical effectiveness, tolerability and cost effectiveness of newer drugs for epilepsy in adults : a systematic review and economic evaluation. Health Technol Assess 2005;9(15):1-157 iii-iv.

23

Epilepsy with Pregnancy

5. Economic factor: Women are mostly economically dependent on men. They have little control or negotiation power in their sexual relation (e.g. abstinence during menstrual period, condom use etc.) including marriage. Violence against women including rape, incest, assault by family members and friends make them more vulnerable to HIV infection. Social norms are that women are not supposed to know about sexual practices. They are less educated than men, especially in poverty striken communities and hence have no access to information about HIV.

6. Migration, poverty and gender inequality influence the rate of HIV infection in women.

HIV IN CHILDREN

Almost all cases of HIV infection in children (91%) are acquired by mother to child transmission (MTCT). As the mother usually gets the infection from the male partner, hence it is also called parent to child transmission (PTCT). Diagnosis of HIV serostatus in early pregnancy in women is of paramount importance because this can prevent the HIV transmission in the child by proper management.

Definition of Perinatal Transmission

It is vertical transmission of HIV from mother to child during pregnancy, labor, delivery or breastfeeding. Transmission by this route can be prevented if the disease is detected in time. Since 1994 when zidovudine (ZDV) was tried to reduce perinatal transmission more and more pregnant women are being tested during pregnancy (if not tested earlier).[2]

Not all fetuses of HIV positive mothers acquire the infection. The incidence varies from 15 to 48%. Hence it is important to know the factors which enhance the MTCT of HIV. The main determinants are given below:[3]

Factors Affecting MTCT of HIV

1. Maternal plasma viral load
2. Concurrent STI and other infections
3. Unprotected sexual intercourse
4. Maternal CD4 and lymphocyte count
5. Mother's neutralizing antibody status
6. Nutritional status
7. Smoking, illicit drug use
8. Ruptured fetal membranes
9. Operative procedures during vaginal delivery
10. Viral type
11. Placental barrier
12. Viral load in genital tract

13. Mode of delivery
14. Fetal factors
    - Genetic makeup
    - Prematurity
    - Duration of exposure to maternal secretions
    - Newborn immune response
15. Breastfeeding

Viral Load

Viral load in a pregnant woman is maximum just after infection (when body's immune response is not developed and hence virus replicates at a rapid pace) and in advanced stage of the disease. It can be diagnose by RNA HIV-I PCR or quantitative culture. In the current era of potent anti retroviral therapy (ART) knowledge of the base line viral load is very important. Transmission to the fetus is there at all concentrations but generally more concentration means more MTCT of HIV.

Concurrent RTI and STI

STIs especially with ulcers, e.g. syphilis, increases MTCT of HIV. Evidence is accumulating to suggest that malaria, tuberculosis, parasitic infestation (hookworm etc.), bacterial vaginosis and chlamydia trichomatis in pregnant women is associated with more MTCT of HIV. Hepatitis C with HIV in pregnancy doubles the MTCT of HIV. It disturbs dynamics of immune transmission. HIV and Hepatitis B increase the transmission from 16% to 26%. Herpes simplex virus (HSV) is also associated with more MTCT of HIV.

Unprotected Sexual Intercourse

Unprotected sexual intercourse during pregnancy increases the risk of transmission to the fetus. Use of spermicides, e.g. Nanoxinone disrupts the membranes of cells in the lining of the vagina making HIV virus to enter easily. Traditional practices like douching with lime juice, etc. may damage the vaginal lining increasing the susceptibility to acquire HIV infection.

Maternal CD4 and Lymphocyte Count

It is an independent predictor of prenatal transmission risk. There is inverse relation, i.e. lower the CD4 and lymphocyte count more is MTCT of HIV.

Maternal Neutralizing Antibody Status

Maternal neutralizing monoclonal HIV antibodies may have a protective effect, preventing MTCT of HIV.

Nutritional Status of the Mother

Malnutrition may increase MTCT of HIV. There is weakness in epithelial integrity of the placenta and genital tract and hence associated accelerated transmission of HIV infection. The trace element zinc is involved in many immunologic impairments and may reduce circulating T lymphocytes of HIV patient. More studies are underway to define the role of zinc in the vertical transmission of HIV from mother to child. Low vitamin A level during pregnancy is seen to be associated with more MTCT of HIV.

Use of Illicit Drugs

Smoking and alcohol consumption may have direct effect on the integrity of placenta. They may adversely affect the developing immune system in the fetus thus increasing MTCT of HIV.

Status of Fetal Membranes

Both amnion and chorion when intact reduce MTCT of HIV. A correlation between the time elapsed from rupture of membranes to actual delivery affects the rate of MTCT of HIV. If the membranes are ruptured for more than 4 hours the transmission rate doubles.

Operative Procedures

Procedures like episiotomy, forceps or ventouse delivery, fetal scalp blood sampling, amniocentesis, or umbilical blood sampling increase MTCT of HIV.

Type of Virus

The biological phenotype of virus may influence the transmission risk. Monocyte macrophage tropic (M-Tropic) maternal virus is reported to be more likely to be transmitted than maternal isolates of T cell tropic phenotype.

Placental Barrier

Breaches in the placenta may be associated with mixing of maternal and fetal blood cells as in chorioamnionitis, cigarette smoking and use of illicit drugs. These are associated with increased MTCT of HIV.

Viral Load in Genital Tract

Increased viral load in the cervix and vagina will have more MTCT of HIV.

Mode of Delivery

It depends on many factors like viral load, whether the woman is on any treatment etc. If the pregnant women is on highly activate anti retroviral therapy (HAART) throughout pregnancy the MTCT is less than 2% (1.2-1.5%). In such cases, vaginal delivery is indicated as cesarean section will not reduce MTCT of HIV any further and there will be morbidity and mortality of the operation. But if the pregnant women is not properly covered with ARV drugs elective cesarean section at 38-39 weeks is to be done. If the woman is on ARV and the viral load is more than 1000 copies/ml then also elective cesarean section is done. *After rupture of membranes* the advantage of reducing MTCT of HIV by caesarean section is lost. Hence emphasis on 'elective' cesarian section.

Fetal Factors

Susceptibility to HIV infection may be different for different fetuses due to separate genetic make up.

Maturity

Immunological maturity is parallel to the fetal maturity because of CD4+ expression. In preterm neonates the MTCT of HIV is 3.7 times more than a term neonate.

Duration of Exposure to Maternal Secretions

MTCT is directly proportional to duration of exposure of maternal secretions. It is more with the first twin than second twin (26% versus 13% respectively).

Newborn Immune Response

Immune response to HIV has a role in averting MTCT of HIV by cell mediated immunity in the fetus or newborn. It may play a crucial role in protection or clearance of infection.

Breastfeeding

There is HIV I in both cellular and acellular components of breast milk. There is a 30% independent risk of MTCT of HIV by breastfeeding by HIV infected mother or wet nurse. Therefore, complete avoidance of breastfeeding is the surest way to avoid MTCT of HIV through breastfeeding.

The risk of transmission depends on the period of breastfeeding, maternal viral load, HIV disease status (early or terminal stage) associated breast abscess or cracked nipples and exclusive or mixed feeding. It may not be feasible to stop breastfeeding in women belonging to lower socioeconomic status in developing countries. If the mother is not knowledgeable enough and cannot afford top feed the infant may die of diarrhea and other diseases. Hence UNICEF and WHO have recommended exclusive breastfeeding for a shorter duration (6 months). Mixed feeding is avoided as there is more MTCT of HIV with mixed feeding.

Timing of in utero transmission from mother to the fetus is not clear. Most acquire infection at the time of delivery and rest through breastfeeding. Intrauterine transmission has been documented by identification of HIV in aborted products placental tissue, fetal blood samples and amniotic fluid.

Kourtis and associates found that 20% of transmission occurs before 36 weeks, 50% before delivery, 30% during delivery and 30% through breast milk in postpartum period.[4] Hence protection at all levels is essential to prevent MTCT of HIV. MTCT of HIV cannot be prevented unless the HIV serostatus of the pregnant mother is known. Most of the HIV positive pregnant women do not know their HIV status and hence are at high risk of transmitting the virus to their offsprings. They miss the opportunity to prevent MTCT of HIV and of getting life saving treatment for themselves. Ideally, HIV testing is to be done before pregnancy. If positive the partner is also tested. Sero discordant couples with women positive and male partner negative (or vice versa) may be seen. If positive, improve her health, identify risk factors (RTI, STI) and treat them. She is also treated with ARV drugs so that her viral load is suppressed maximally before pregnancy and hence reducing her chances of MTCT of HIV. Any side effects with these drugs can be observed and replaced by other drugs prior to pregnancy. In preconception counseling, besides investigations and treatment, the women are asked to stop smoking and consuming alcohol and illicit drugs. Advice of safe sexual practices is given including correct and consistent use of condom. She is vaccinated against Hepatitis B (if not vaccinated before).The sexual partner is also clinically examined and appropriate care is given.

Diagnosis

Centers for Disease Control (CDC) in America has recommended that all pregnant women be tested for HIV as early as possible, and in high-risk groups repeat HIV test is performed at 36 weeks of pregnancy.[5] Early diagnosis of HIV in the pregnant woman can prevent MTCT of HIV by ARV therapy and other interventions, therefore the need for early diagnosis. Before testing for HIV pre-test counseling is done in which important points like: What is HIV, how does it spread, how to reduce risky behavior etc. are covered and confidentiality is assured. Pretest counseling can be done in groups. After pretest counseling the woman is offered the test for HIV detection.[6] If she agrees (opts in) her blood sample is drawn. If she refuses – (opt out) her blood sample is not drawn but she is given all antenatal and postnatal services available. The counselor may go into the causes of opting out and address them with empathy and eventually may turn her round for 'opting in' to get the test done. The common test performed is serological test for detection of viral specific antibodies by ELISA (Enzyme linked immunosorbant assay). Three different ELISA kits are used on the serum samples, to diagnose an asymptomatic woman (strategy III of NACO of India). The pregnant woman is called on a subsequent day to collect the report. The importance of collecting the report is emphasized. Before handing over the report, one to one posttest counseling is done. The report is confidential and not told to any one except her without her permission. When she comes in labor in odd hours with no previous testing, then rapid test can be offered on whole blood which takes less time and immediate treatment can be started if positive. The confirmation is done in the morning of next working day from the same blood sample by confirmatory tests like Western Blot or Immuno Fluorescence Assay (IFA). If positive the mother and the neonate can be started on HAART or any other therapy and if negative the drugs are stopped. This rapid testing and immediate treatment will reduce MTCT of HIV from 25% to 9-13%.

Barriers to knowing the HIV serostatus in pregnant women

- Lack of knowledge of the importance of knowing the women's HIV status in prevention of MTCT of HIV.
- Unmet needs; There are less resources (Counselors, technicians) for testing in big government hospitals. Half of the patients are unbooked hence come without testing in labor any time of the day. Rapid HIV antibody testing facilities are not available on a 24 hour basis in all labor rooms and nurseries.

Interventions Aimed at Decreasing MTCT of HIV

Primary Prevention

Prevention of unintended pregnancy is a very important and cost effective primary preventive measure. Since more than 25% pregnancies are unintended as many HIV positive pregnancies can be averted by contraception. Overall attention to increase contraceptive choices will be an effective strategy. Safe sexual behaviors, promotion of use of condoms (male and female condoms), teaching negotiation skills, dual protection, early diagnosis and treatment of RTI, STI and other infections will go a long way in preventing HIV.

Secondary Prevention

The broad principles are an early testing of the pregnant woman for HIV and giving her the option of medical termination of pregnancy (MTP) if positive. If she wants MTP, safe MTP services are provided and if she wants to continue pregnancy all available care is given.

General measures: General examination is done. Any deficiency in diet is addressed to, as well-nourished women will pass less viral load to the fetus. Any infection e.g. STI, RTI, tuberculosis, etc. if present should be treated. Screening for Hepatitis B, Hepatitis C and cancer cervix should be done.

HIV in Pregnancy

Obstetric measures: She is advised to discontinue smoking, drinking alcohol and using illicit drugs. Unless essential, fetal umbilical blood sampling should not be done. Artificial rupture of membrane is to be avoided as far as possible. Fetal scalp blood sampling to be reserved for dire cases. Chorioamnionitis is to be prevented, and if present to be treated. Systematic birth canal cleaning has been attempted with betadine, chlorhexidine, etc. Vaginal gel which kill the HIV virus are under research. If possible, episiotomy and operative vaginal delivery should be avoided. Cord should be clamped immediately after birth. Give bath to the neonate just after delivery, before any vaccination. All these measures play a very important role in prevention of MTCT of HIV to a great extent.

Immunological measures: As is evident from different publications, maximum transmission of HIV to the neonate is at or around the time of delivery. Hence, a combination of active and passive immunization will be effective in prevention of this transmission (as is seen in Hepatitis B infection). Till date, vaccination i.e. active immunization is still a dream. But passive protection using HIV IgG is under investigation. Protocols to test neutralizing monoclonal antibodies are in the developing stage.

Antiretroviral (ARV) drugs: ARV drugs are given to prevent MTCT of HIV and treating mother for her disease. Zidovudine (ZDV) was the first drug to be tried (ACTG 076) for decreasing MTCT of HIV in 1994 and it was a long therapy. Then short course of ZDV was tried in Thailand. Nevirapine (NVP) as a single dose (HIV/NET 012) is being propagated by NACO in India.[7] However, all monotherapy treatments are fraught with the danger of developing resistant strains of HIV. Recent trend is towards multidrug therapy. The ARV drugs act by reducing MTCT of HIV by multiple mechanisms detailed as follows:

1. Lower maternal viral load in blood and genital secretions. Thus leaving less number of viruses to cross the placenta and infect the foetus.
2. Some of drugs cross the placenta and enter the fetus giving adequate systemic levels of drug in fetus. This gives pre-exposure prophylaxis to the fetus during it's passage through the birth canal of the mother.
3. Post exposure prophylaxis by giving ARV drugs to the neonates after birth. Thus antepartum, intrapartum and postpartum ARV therapy is essential to reduce MTCT of HIV. But besides lowering viral load, there are other mechanisms which are not yet well understood.

MANAGEMENT

Antepartum Management

The management of HIV positive pregnant woman is a team approach by a counsellor, obstetrician, physician, psychiatrist and pediatrician.

On her first antenatal visit, besides routine history, any history of antiretroviral (ARV) drug therapy in the past or present, any symptoms of opportunistic infection is elicited.

A general examination is done. If she opts for MTP, safe MTP services are provided. Universal precautions sould be observed like hand washing, using gloves, gown, mask, boots, and eye glasses, etc. (Fig. 25.1).

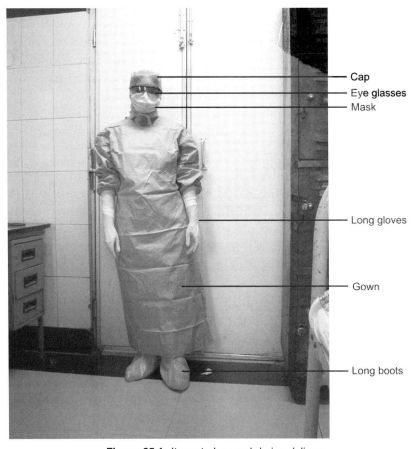

Figure 25.1: Items to be used during delivery

After MTP, all used instruments, gloves, linen should be kept in 0.5% bleech solution for 10-20 minutes (decontamination) before washing and further processing. The blood on the floor and table is to be flooded with 0.5% bleach solution and cleaned after 20-30 minutes.

The routine antenatal check up is done. If she has come in first trimester besides routine blood group testing screening for other STIs is done by VDRL and HBsAg test. Tests for *Chlamydia trachomatis*, *Neisseria gonorrhea* and bacterial vaginosis are carried out. She must also be screened for Hepatitis C and opportunistic infections (OI), e.g. Pneumocystis jiroveci pneumonia (PCP), Mycobacterium avium complex (MAC) and cancer cervix. Screening for diabetes mellitus is done at 24-28 weeks of pregnancy as protease inhibitor drugs cause hyperglycemia and diabetic ketoacidosis. A baseline CD4 count is done and repeated every 3 months. If possible, plasma HIV RNA is done initially and repeated every 2 months and finally at

36 weeks (to decide about mode of delivery). First trimester ultrasound is required for exact dating of pregnancy.

Hemoglobin should be checked from time to time for development of anemia as ZVD causes anemia. Liver functions tests (LFT) are performed as a baseline before starting on protease inhibitors (PI). Follow-up with LFT and electrolytes is required from time to time and monthly in last trimester. Also assess the need for support care like psychological support , home support etc. Second trimester ultrasound is performed to know about the growth of the fetus and any detectable congenital abnormality.

Start counseling about contraceptive choices from early pregnancy so as to prevent next pregnancy.

Antiretroviral (ARV) Therapy

It is tailored according to the needs of the pregnant woman in different situations in consultation with physician. The various factors influencing the ARV therapy include—period of gestation, whether the pregnant woman requires it for her own health or only for prophylaxis against MTCT and the risks, toxicity and resistance of different drugs. Inform the pregnant mother about the benefits and risks of ARV drugs. She should be counseled about the effects of these drugs in the first trimester of pregnancy if the woman comes for antenatal check up in that period. Antenatal administration of ARV drugs reduces plasma HIV/RNA to undetectable levels which lowers the perinatal transmission of HIV to very small percentage.[8] She is explained about the necessity of consistent use of these drugs for prevention of emergence of resistant strains and optimizing prevention of MTCT. CDC recommends ARV medication to all pregnant women irrespective of CD4 count, viral load and even to those who do not require it for themselves (i.e. CD4 count more than 350/ml and low viral load). She is also assessed for the need of prophylaxis against opportunistic infections (OI) e.g. PCP, MAC, etc. Use of steroids for lung maturity is not contraindicated even with low CD4 counts.

Monotherapy is to be avoided as it causes resistance to ARV drugs. Whenever feasible and affordable combination regimens are more effective and avoid emergence of resistant strains of HIV. However highly active anti-retroviral therapy (HAART) is the best. A combination of two nucleoside reverse transcriptase inhibitors (NRTIs) and one non nucleoside reverse transcriptase inhibitors (NNRTIs) or protease inhibitor (PI) (2 TRTIs+1 NNRTIs/sPI) are given with at least one drug which crosses the placenta like Zidovudine.[9]

The physiological changes during pregnancy like increase in gastro-intestinal transit time, increased water and fat content of body, decreased plasma proteins, increased cardiac output, increased blood flow to the liver and kidney, increased sodium absorption by kidney and alteration in liver enzymes along with the fetus should be taken into account while considering the toxicity of ARV drugs in a pregnant woman. The drugs to be avoided during pregnancy are efavirenz (EFV), stavudine (d4T) and didanosine (dd1) combination, zalcitabine and renofovir. No ARV drug is category A, they are either B, C, or D category.

ARV in Different Situations

1. If the pregnant woman does not require ARV medicine for herself but for prophylaxis of perinatal transmission, the drugs are started after first trimester of pregnancy usually at 28 weeks of gestation to prevent any teratogenic effect during pregnancy. Timing of initiating the treatment can be individualized. It may be started earlier in cases where chances of preterm delivery may be more, like in women with past history of preterm delivery, multiple pregnancy, etc. The combination of Zidovudine(ZDV), Lamivudine (3TC) and Abacavir (ABC) is started. Of these ZDV and 3TC are NRTIS and ABC is protease inhibitor. Pharmacokinetic profile of these three drugs show acceptable toxicity during pregnancy. Instead of a PI, viracept (Nelfinavir) can be given. ZDV alone as monotherapy can be given if viral load is less than 1000 copies per ml in women who do not agree to combination therapy. In women on ARV in addition to CD4 count and plasma HIV RNA copies, glucose challenge test is done at 24-28 weeks as protease inhibitors (PI) may cause hyperglycemia and diabetic ketoacidosis.[10]

2. In pregnant woman not requiring ARV medicine for themselves but who had the drugs for prophylaxis in last pregnancy, drug resistance test should be done. ARV drugs are given from second trimester onwards after basic investigations.

3. If she is receiving HAART before pregnancy it should be continued even in first trimester because the benefit of treatment to mother is more than potential fetal risk. Stopping drugs may increase the viral load which will deteriorate mother's condition and increase MTCT of HIV. These drugs should be prescribed in special centers under the supervision of HIV physician. Replace EFV, d4T, dd1 and renofovir with less toxic drugs and use ZDV as a component, whenever feasible.

4. If she has come in labor without any diagnosis and ARV medication. Do rapid testing for HIV from whole blood and keep a sample for further testing. If positive, start the treatment immediately, give HAART. Do the confirmatory test as soon as possible by Western blot or immunofluorescent assay (FAI). If she is positive the therapy is started and she is further evaluated. If found to be negative the treatment is stopped.

5. If she is a diagnosed HIV positive case and reports during labor, give NVP 200 mg and start ZDV drip.

6. If results of rapid test come after delivery and the mother is positive give ZVD to the neonate within 6-12 hours of birth and continue for 6 weeks. Evaluate the mother and manage accordingly.

7. Associated hepatitis B (HBV) in HIV positive women should be treated for HIV but ZDV is avoided. The definitive treatment of HBV is only given after delivery with pegylated interferon alpha (as it is contraindicated during pregnancy). The neonate gets hepatitis B immunoglobulin (HBIG) and first dose of hepatitis B vaccine within 12 hours of birth. Second and third doses are given at 1 month and 6 months of age respectively.
8. Associated hepatitis C (HCV) with HIV positive pregnancy. These women cannot be given ribavirin and pegylated interferon alpha during pregnancy, but can be administered after delivery. After birth, the infant is tested for HCV RNA between 2 and 6 months of age and for HCV antibodies after 15 months of age.

Mode of Delivery

It is individualized for each woman. If the woman is already on HAART and the HIV RNA is less than 1000 copies/ml she can be allowed vaginal delivery. If her membranes have ruptured, treatment is given according to the duration of rupture of membranes, plasma HIV RNA level, ARV drugs used recently, and clinical condition. After rupture of membranes the advantage of cesarean section in lowering MTCT of HIV is lost. Moreover, HIV positive women have more complications during cesarean section especially sepsis.[11] Blood less cesarean section, in which the uterus is opened with a staple gun which cuts and prevent bleeding at the same time is shown to have less chances of MTCT of HIV. If woman has incomplete cover of ARV drugs, advise elective cesarean section at 38-39 weeks.

HIV positive pregnant women after 36 weeks of pregnancy not receiving any ARV therapy should be started on ARV medication and counseled for elective cesarean section at 38-39 weeks.

Care during delivery: Giving NVP in a pregnant woman in labor who had HAART throughout pregnancy is not recommended as it gives no extra advantage.

During cesarean section or normal vaginal delivery a drip of ZDV is started 3 hours before surgery. If d4T was a component of antenatal ARV drugs it should be stopped before giving ZDV as they are pharmacologically antagonists. Continue all other drugs, which were being used antenatally in this patient. Oral NVP 200 mg can be given in patients who have suboptimal prophylactic ARV drugs. With NVP, 3TC 150 mg BD orally and ZDV are also given in labor. ZDV infusion is given at the rate of 2 mg/kg first hour then 1 mg/hour till delivery. Blood sample of the woman is taken for testing for viral load. It will guide whether to continue ARV drugs after delivery or not

Procedures like artificial rupture of membranes, fetal scalp blood sampling, episiotomy and operative vaginal delivery (forceps or ventouse) are avoided unless strongly indicated. Local cleaning of vagina is done. Antibiotics are given after cesarean section.

The umbilical cord is clamped as early as possible. Methergine is not used with protease inhibitors (PI) as it can cause exaggerated vasoconstriction response, however, prostaglandin F_2 alpha, misoprostol or oxytocin can be used.

Care of the Neonate at Birth

The neonate should be bathed promptly after birth before giving any injections (e.g. hepatitis B vaccination or vitamin K injection etc). Detailed physical examination is done.

A baseline complete blood count and serum chemistry is done. Anemia should be monitored with ZDV treatment. If possible a PCR test for HIV I is done. It is repeated after 14-21 days 1-2 months, 4-6 months after birth. In a non breastfed infant if HIV PCR is negative at 6 months of age the child is 99% not infected. A final test of HIV antibody at 18 months of age gives final diagnosis. No breastfeeding is advised if the mother can sustainably afford top feed with all hygeinic conditions.

Prophylactic ARV medicines are given to the neonate. Give NVP 2 mg/kg orally within 72 hours of birth as advised by NACO. Also add (if available) ZDV and 3TC 2 mg /kg BD orally for 7 days after birth to reduce NVP resistance or give only ZDV orally depending on period of maturity of the neonate. If the neonate is more than 35 weeks give ZDV 2 mg/kg orally (1.5 mg/kg IV) every 6 hours till 6 weeks. If less than 35 weeks 2 mg/kg body weight orally (or 1.5 mg/kg IV) every 12 hours advance to 8 hourly at 2 weeks of age till total 6 weeks after birth. In 30 weeks or less maturity the neonate is given 2 mg/kg/body weight of ZDV orally (or 1.5 mg/kg IV) 12 hourly till 4 weeks of age then give 8 hourly till 6 weeks of age.

At discharge both mother and neonate must be referred for ongoing care to appropriate centers. She is educated about ARV prophylaxis of the neonate and contraceptive counseling. Need of safe sex is emphasized.

After delivery screen for cancer cervix, emphasize the need of healthy eating habits, mental health check up and de-addiction of ilicit drug, smoking and alcohol uptake. Need for treatment is assessed and also look for support services.

The infant is given prophylaxis against *Pneumocytis jiroveci* pneumonia after 6 weeks of age.

Stopping ARV Drugs

The various indications for stopping ARV drugs are when there is serious toxicity, hypertension in pregnancy, during surgery, patient's request and when drug is not available. The drug is also stopped in the mother if it was started for only prophylaxis for MTCT of HIV. Abrupt stopping of all drugs will lead to virtual monotherapy of long acting drugs and development of resistant strains because different drugs have different half life. Continue NRTI for period of 7 days after stopping NNRTI, i.e. stop NNRTI first then continue NRTI for 7 days.

Contraception

She can use almost all methods of contraception if clinically well. She is advised to always use condom (male or female) **consistently** and **correctly** to prevent further transmission of HIV, for protection from STI and for contraception.[12]

IUCD both copper and hormone bearing can be used. An IUCD already in place need not to be removed unless it gets infected later on or she develops AIDS. Pelvic inflammatory disease is not significantly more common in these women (According to WHO criteria).

Dual method means using condom with other methods like IUCD or hormonal methods. Oral contraceptive drug levels may be decreased by NVP, retonavir, amprenavir and fosamprenavir as they expedite metabolism but use of condoms will make up for this. NET_EN or depo-medroxy progesterone acetate (DMPA) does not significantly alter the levels of ARV drugs as the hormone is absorbed in the blood before being metabolized by the liver.[13] The dose of emergency contraceptive is not to be increased. Spermicides are not to be used. Diaphragm is a good method but protection against HIV and other STI is not very good. Women can be counseled for sterilization as a permanent method of contraception.

Except condom no other method of contraception can prevent transmission of STI/HIV.

Effect of HIV on Pregnancy

Spontaneous premature delivery is noted in some women at a CD4 count below 30%. Low apgar score, still birth and IUGR are also seen. Low CD4 count corresponds to postpartum endometritis. Wound infection is more common in postpartum period.

Effect of Pregnancy on HIV Disease Progression

No major effect is seen in otherwise asymptomatic HIV positive women. Morbidity and mortality (though CD4 count falls during pregnancy) is not increased by pregnancy. Chances of acquiring HIV during pregnancy are higher possibly due to hormonal influence or immunosuppression in pregnancy.

Therefore, it is concluded that knowing HIV serostatus of pregnant women is very important in prevention of MTCT of HIV. Contraception also plays a very vital role in avoiding MTCT.

- There are two types of HIV viruses viz. HIV-1 and HIV-2. HIV-1 is associated with higher mother to child transmission (MTCT) rate (20-35%) compared with 0.4% with HIV-II.
- It is estimated that in our country 2 adults get infected every minute and 0.5 million young people, 2, 30, 000 women and 30,000 children get infected every year.
- Women are more vulnerable to acquire this infection than men due to many factors.
- Almost all cases of HIV in children (91%) are acquired by mother to child transmission (MTCT).
- Not all fetuses of HIV positive mothers acquire the infection. The incidence varies from 15 to 48%. Transmission by this route can be prevented if detected in time.
- Centers for Disease Control (CDC) in America has recommended that all pregnant women be tested for HIV as early as possible, and in high-risk groups repeat HIV test is performed at 36 weeks of pregnancy
- It is important to know the factors which enhance the MTCT of HIV.
- Most acquire infection at the time of delivery and rest through breast-feeding.
- ARV drugs are given to prevent MTCT of HIV and treating mother for her disease
- Giving NVP in a pregnant woman in labor who had HAART throughout pregnancy is not recommended as it gives no extra advantage
- Prophylactic ARV medicines are given to the neonate. NVP 2 mg/Kg orally within 72 hours of birth is advised by NACO.
- There is 30% independent risk of MTCT of HIV by breastfeeding by HIV infected mother or wet nurse.
- UNICEF and WHO have recommended exclusive breastfeeding for a shorter duration (6 months). No mixed feeding is advised as there is more MTCT of HIV with mixed feeding.
- At discharge both mother and neonate must be referred for ongoing care to appropriate centers.

REFERENCES

1. Salhan S. Women and HIV infection including mother to child transmission. In Salhan S (Ed): Women and HIV. Jaypee Brothers Medical Publishers (P) Ltd, New Delhi: 2003;92.
2. Conner EM, Sperling RS, Gelber R, et al. Reduction of maternal infant transmission of HIV type with Zidovudine treatment. New England J of Med 1994;331:1173.
3. Salhan S. Mother to Child Transmission of HIV. In Salhan S (Ed): Textbook of Obstetrics 2007;334.
4. Kourtis AP, Bullory M, Nesheim SR. Understanding the timing of HIV transmission from mother to infant. JAMA 2001;285:709.
5. CDC revised recommendations for HIV testing for adults, adolescents and pregnant women in health care setting MMWR 2006;55 (RR-14)1.

25

HIV in Pregnancy

6. Salhan S. Voluntary counseling and testing and its rationate for HIV infection. Women and HIV. Jaypee Brothers Medical publishers (P) Ltd, New Delhi: 2003;49.
7. Moodley D, Moodley J, Coovadia H, et al. A mulli center randomized controlled trial of neverapine versus a combination of zidovudine and lamivudine to reduce intrapartum and early postpartum MTCT of HIV type I. J Infect Dis 2003;167:725.
8. Pubic Health Service Task Force recommendations for use of ARV drugs in pregnant HIV infected woman for maternal health and interventions to reduce perinatal HIV transmission in USA July 2008.
9. http://AIDS info.nih.gov.
10. Tang JH, Sheffield JS, Grimes J, et al. Effect of protease inhibitor therapy on glucose intolerance in pregnancy. Obstet Gynecol 2006;107(5):1115.
11. Panburana P, Phaupradit W, Tantisirin O, et al. Maternal complication after CS in HIV infected pregnancy women. Aust NZJ Obstet Gynecol 2003;43(2):160.
12. World Health Organization (WHO). Reproductive choices and family planning for people living with HIV Counselling tool. Geneva WHO, 2006.
13. Cohn SE, Park JG, Watts DH, et al. DMPA in women on ART effective contraception and lack of clinically significant interactions. Clin Pharmacol Ther 2007;81(2):222.

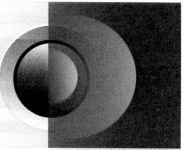

Obesity and Pregnancy 26

Evita Fernandez

INTRODUCTION

Obesity, defined as a body mass index above 30 kg/m^2, is the major public health issue of our time. The World Health Organization describes obesity as: One of the most blatantly visible, yet most neglected, public-health problems that threaten to overwhelm both more and less developed countries.

The effect of adiposity is evident in nearly every aspect of a woman's reproductive life. This could present as a metabolic or a reproductive complication. Obesity is known to be associated with serious obstetric complications. This article will review the obesity-related adverse pregnancy outcomes and discuss the most appropriate steps in the care of an obese mother, through her pregnancy.

Obesity is usually defined epidemiologically using the body mass index (BMI), weight related to height, where > 30 kg/m^2 is considered as obese and > 40 kg/m^2 as morbidly obese. A BMI of 18–25 kg/m^2 is considered a healthy weight with 26–29 kg/m^2 identified as overweight.

In pregnancy, BMI is calculated using pre-pregnant weight. If this is unknown, the first weight measurement at prenatal care is used.[1] The BMI is an imprecise estimate of body fat. It does not consider the difference in lean body mass between individuals of the same height and weight, or differences in the distribution of body fat (waist circumference and waist-hip ratio) which are important determinants of the risk of disease.[2]

A recent study in the UK showed that 1:5 women booking for antenatal care in 2002–2004 were obese.[3] In the most recent confidential enquiry into maternal deaths in the UK[4] report (2000-2002), 35% of all women (n = 78) who died were obese compared with 23% of the general maternal population. This means a dramatic rise from 16% reported in 1993.

Indian Scenario

In December 2008, The Hindu newspaper featured an article, where a study done in Puducherry and Tamil Nadu revealed that obesity was high among rural population (22%) compared with the national data of 7%. Abdominal obesity was high.

BASIC BIOLOGY OF ENERGY BALANCE

We are an obesogenic society. There is a drastic reduction in physical activity, increase in sedentary leisure activities (TV/home theater), and increase in use of labor-saving devices.

Fat consumption, overall, via fast food outlets, together with carbonated drinks has increased phenomenally all over the globe. These energy-dense foods are less satiating and more likely to cause "passive over-consumption".[5, 6] There is an established link between these products, weight gain and development of type 2 diabetes.[5]

Women who are obese are two to three times more likely to develop hormone-dependent malignancies, including breast, ovarian and endometrial cancer, and have menstrual irregularities, often in association with PCOS. Younger and more deprived individuals are the most likely to be affected. People of South Asian origin may be susceptible to diabetes and other metabolic consequences of obesity at lower BMI and waist circumference measurements than white populations.[7]

OBESITY AND FERTILITY

A high BMI is related to a lower livebirth rate and a higher incidence of early pregnancy loss among women achieving IVF/ICSI conceptions.[8] There is also an impaired response to ovarian stimulation, especially when there is central deposition of fat.

For every BMI unit above 29 kg/m^2, the probability of pregnancy was reduced by 4% compared with women with a BMI between 21-29 kg/m^2. Very obese women (BMI 35-40) had a probability of pregnancy that was between 26-43% lower than women with BMI between 21-29 kg. The National Institute for Health and Clinical Excellence (NICE) Fertility Guideline, published in 2004, gave recommendations based on BMI as shown in Table 26.1.[9]

- Women with a BMI > 29 kg/m^2 should be informed that they are likely to take longer to conceive.
- Women with a BMI > 29 kg/m^2 and who are NOT ovulating should be informed that losing weight is likely to increase their chance of conceiving.
- Dietary restriction and exercise together will lead to weight loss and more pregnancies.

OBESITY-RELATED ADVERSE OUTCOMES IN PREGNANCY

Obesity has a major impact on pregnancy. There are major maternal complications associated with obesity during pregnancy.[10]

Miscarriages

Obesity is associated with increased risk of first trimester miscarriages, both in women with polycystic ovaries and those with normal ovarian morphology. The incidence of spontaneous miscarriages has been reported to rise as insulin resistance increases. It has been suggested that in these women, insulin sensitizing agents such as metformin reduce miscarriage rates.[11] The risk of miscarriage before the first liveborn child is 25-37% higher in obese women.[12] With a BMI > 30 kg/m^2, there is a four-fold increased risk of miscarriage in women undergoing fertility treatment.[13]

Fetal Anomalies

There is conflicting evidence regarding the association between congenital fetal malformation and obesity. However, two case-control studies have demonstrated a significant increase in neural tube defects (NTD), defects of the central nervous system, the great vessels in the heart, the ventral wall and intestinal defects[14] in obese women.

Glazer et al in another study concluded that, for every incremental unit increase in BMI, the risk of NTD is increased by 7%, three-fold increase in omphalocele, two-fold increase in cardiac anomalies, especially septal defects and multiple defects among the overweight and obese group.[15] The reasons are poorly understood. One hypothesis suggests an association with undetected type 2 diabetes in early pregnancy or lower circulating levels of folate.[16]

Congenital malformation is more common when the mother has pre-existing type 2 diabetes. In UK, an abnormality rate of 6.1% was found with type 1 diabetes but 12.2% with type 2 diabetes.[17]

Hypertensive Disease

O' Brien et al in a systematic review have demonstrated a consistently strong positive association between maternal pre-pregnancy BMI and the risk of pre-eclampsia.[18] The risk doubled with each 5–7 kg/m^2 increase in pregnancy BMI. Waist circumference greater than 80 cm, measured at 16 weeks gestation,

26

Obesity and Pregnancy

was found to be predictive of pregnancy induced hypertension (PIH) (odds ratio of 1.8 (95% CI 1.1–2.9) and pre-eclampsia, odds ratio 2.7 (95/CI 1.1-6.8).

Obesity and Gestational Diabetes

A BMI of > 30% is considered a risk factor for development of GDM.[19] In a large prospective population-based Swedish study (151025 women) the implications of inter-pregnancy weight gain were strikingly obvious[20] (Table 26.2).

One possible unifying hypothesis is that there may be a syndrome of insulin resistance, low grade inflammation, dyslipidemia and an alteration in systemic microvascular function. This is similar to the metabolic syndrome observed among those with coronary heart disease and/or diabetes. Stewart et al[21] demonstrated that obese women have a pro-inflammatory phenotype, with impaired microvascular function, from early in pregnancy.

Approximately 1–3% of women, compared to 17% of obese women develop GDM during pregnancy.[22] A tight control of blood sugar levels does reduce the risk of macrosomia. Apart from a strict dietary regime, insulin therapy is required more often in obese women with gestational diabetes, than in lean women.[23]

Mothers who develop GDM have a 50% higher risk of developing diabetes during their lifetime[24] with this risk increasing in obese women.[25] Therefore for the obese woman with GDM, pregnancy is a wake-up call for a lifestyle change in terms of exercise, weight loss and in reducing the risk for vascular disease in the long-term. Obese mothers with GDM have twice the risk of delivering children with chromosomal defects.[26]

Table 26.2: Weight gain between pregnancies: Change in risk of GDM	
Baseline BMI 23, and weight gain	*Risk of GDM*
Gains 3 kg: 1 unit increase in BMI	30%
Gains 6 kg : BMI 29 (overweight)	100%
Gains 8 kg : BMI 31 (obese)	200%

Thromboembolic Complications

The Royal College of Obstetricians and Gynecologists report on maternal deaths concluded that obesity is the most common risk factor for thromboembolism. Pregnancy increases the risk of venous thrombo-embolism because of venous stasis, changes in blood coagulability (hyper-coagulable) and damaged vessels. Low molecular weight heparin is effective as a thrombo-prophylactic agent.[27]

Several studies have shown that obese patients have a higher plasma concentration of all prothrombotic factors (Fibrinogen, VWF and Factor VII) especially with central fat distribution. Therefore, venous thromboembolism remains the leading cause of maternal mortality in the obese group.

Respiratory Complications

Sleep apnea and asthma are associated with obesity in pregnancy. Sahota, et al have shown an increased rate of snoring, sleep-related apnea and 4% oxygen desaturation in obese pregnant women compared to non-obese pregnant women.[28]

A neck circumference of 40.5 cm or more is associated with episodes of disrupted breathing recurring up to 30 times a night. Sleep apnea leads to pulmonary hypertension, right heart failure, drug resistant hypertension, stroke and arrhythmias.

Infections

Genital tract, wounds and urinary tract infections are all significantly more common in women who are obese or overweight.[29]

INTRAPARTUM ISSUES

Obese women have higher rates of induction of labor (10.3 versus 7.9%).[30] The incidence of failed induction was found to be higher. There is a higher cesarean section rate in nulliparous obese women, than in lean women (20.7% in the control group versus 33.8% in obese group and 47.4% in the morbidly obese; p>0.01).[31] There is a higher rate of obstetric complications among obese women[32] (Table 26.3).

The frequency of both elective (8.5 versus 4%) and emergency cesarean section (13.4 versus 7.8%) is almost doubled for very obese women compared with the normal BMI group. Sheiner et al in a large study of 126080 deliveries, after excluding women with diabetes and hypertensive disease, found a three-fold increased risk of failure to progress in the first stage and almost a trebling of CS rate from 10.8 to 27.8% (OR 3.2) among obese women when compared with the normal BMI group[33] (Table 26.4).

Table 26.3: Obstetric complications among obese women

Complications	BMI > 30	Normal BMI	P value
Operative vaginal delivery	11.4	8.4	< 0.001
Shoulder dystocia	1.8	1	< 0.021
3rd and 4th degree laceration	27.5	26.3	< 0.001

Table 26.4: Body mass index under cesarean section

BMI	Cesarean section
Normal BMI	20.7%
Obese group	33.8%
Morbidly obese	47.4%

The increase in cesarean section rate may be due to the increased incidence of large-for-gestational-age infants, suboptimal uterine contractions and increased fat deposition in the soft tissues of the pelvis leading to dystocia during labor.

Vaginal Birth After Cesarean Section

In a study of 1213 women, obese women were 50% less successful when attempting a trial vaginal delivery after a cesarean section, compared with underweight women.[34]

POSTPARTUM ISSUES

Deep venous thrombosis, endometritis, postpartum hemorrhage, prolonged hospitalization, wound infection and dehiscence are seen with increased frequency in obese women.[35]

Skin Incision and Wound Infection

Wall et al reported an overall wound complication rate of 12.1% with a vertical skin incision having a higher incidence (34.6 versus 9.4%). The transverse incision is reported to have a more secure closure, less fat dissection and less postoperative pain. However, the warm moist area underneath the pannus is a potential site for infection. During surgery, the retraction of the large pannus for better accessibility of the operative field, may compromise the maternal cardiopulmonary system.[36]

A vertical skin incision allows better visualization with less physical exertion by the assistant, decreases operative time with decreased blood loss. However, the vertical skin incision should be closed using a "mass closure" technique with either a permanent/delayed absorbable monofilament suture. Allaire AD et al in a randomized study (n = 76) concluded that a subcutaneous drainage in women with more than 2 cm subcutaneous fat can reduce the incidence of postoperative wound complications.[37]

Postpartum Hemorrhage

The risk of postpartum hemorrhage rises with increasing BMI. In the puerperium, endometritis, postpartum hemorrhage (PPH) prolonged hospitalization and wound infections are more frequent in obese women. It is 30% more frequent with moderate obesity and 70% more frequent with morbidly obese women.[38]

Difficulties

Difficulty in ultrasound imaging is a worrying consequence of maternal obesity. A 14.5% reduction in visualization of organs was observed in obese women when compared with lean women.

The inability to obtain an interpretable external cardiotocograph tracing in obese woman, makes intrapartum monitoring difficult. The labor or operating table needs to be adequate. Experienced personnel trained to lift and transfer obese individuals are a specific requisite.

OBESITY AND ANESTHESIA

Obese mothers present difficulties for anesthetists. Blood pressure recording may be inaccurate, peripheral intravenous access is difficult to obtain and the risks of failed epidurals is higher. Intubation may also pose a problem. Respiratory complications such as aspiration and pneumonitis are increased.[35]

The obese mother may require to be monitored postpartum in a high dependency unit and at times in an intensive care unit. The support of an anesthesia team, especially trained and who are aware of the complications of obesity, is essential.[35]

LACTATION

Lactation is not very well established in obese mothers. The newborn does not latch on because of positioning difficulties. There is a decreased response to suckling in terms of serum prolactin levels.

The newborn is often given formula feeds which in turn lead to childhood obesity. Maternal obesity is associated with a reduction in breastfeeding frequency.[39]

COST IMPLICATIONS

Galtier-Dereure et al in a prospective study of 435 women, found the average cost in terms of antenatal care and duration of hospital stay was five times higher in women with a high pre-pregnancy BMI. The duration of stay was also 3.9 to 6.2 fold higher.[40]

IMPLICATIONS FOR THE FETUS OF OBESE MOTHER

Short-term

Macrosomia

Pre-pregnancy BMI is a strong positive predictor of birth weight. The odds ratio for an obese mother delivering a large-for-dates infant is 1.4-1.8.[41] Macrosomia in turn increases the risk of shoulder dystocia, birth injury and the incidence of low Apgar scores and perinatal death. Kristen et al found a higher incidence of cesarean section (25.8%) among the macrosomic group (> 4 kg) compared with the general population (13.1%) P < 0.0001. This was a 3-year retrospective analysis of infants weighing > 4 kg.[42]

Fetal hyperinsulinemia and an increased energy flux to the fetus, (secondary to increased amino acids in insulin-resistant individuals) may explain the increased frequency of large-for-gestational-age infants seen in women who are obese but not diabetic.

Stillbirths

One cohort study by Kristensen J et al found that maternal obesity was associated with almost a three-fold increased risk of stillbirth (OR 2.8, 95% CI 1.5-5.3) and neonatal death (OR 2.6, 95% CI 1.2–5.8) compared with women of normal weight.[42]

NICU Admissions

In a retrospective analysis, Galtier-Dereure et al found the percentage of infants requiring NICU admissions was 3.5 times higher when maternal obesity was present.[43] Lower Apgar scores have been reported in the neonates of obese mothers, when compared with those of lean mothers.[41]

The higher incidence of DM and GDM in the obese population may contribute to this effect in view of the need for glycemic control in these infants. Birth trauma due to macrosomia may also increase the rate of perinatal morbidity in these infants.

Long-Term Fetal Implications

Intrauterine programming has long-term effects in the adult life of the fetuses of mothers with a high BMI. Forsen et al found an increased risk of coronary heart disease among men whose mothers had a high BMI in pregnancy. The direct effects of maternal obesity on fetal programming are under-researched.[44]

LONG-TERM IMPLICATIONS FOR THE MOTHER

Obese women who gain weight during pregnancy are at risk of retaining this additional weight in the long-term. This can lead to increased mortality and morbidity from coronary heart disease, diabetes, hypertension, stroke, cancers. All of this may also be associated with poor self esteem and a negative self image, thus leading to poor mental health.[45]

Diabetes

Many women with gestational diabetes have type 2 diabetes which is first recognized in pregnancy. Obesity, especially central obesity, is more common in GDM and type 2 diabetes. South Asians have a higher prevalence of GDM, higher risk of type 2 diabetes, at a lower BMI than whites.[46]

Women are less likely to address their type 2 diabetes (compared with type 1 diabetes) before pregnancy; possibly because they are unaware that they have it or because the pregnancy is unplanned.[47]

GDM is a major risk for later type 2 diabetes, the risk being greatest for women who are obese. The most rapid occurence of type 2 diabetes following GDM is in the first five years after delivery, after correcting for ethnicity.[48]

MANAGEMENT OF OBESITY IN PREGNANCY

The obese mother must be considered a high risk and should be managed in a perinatal center where a multidisciplinary approach can be offered.

Recommendations for Maternal Weight Gain in Pregnancy: A systematic review in the year, 2000 by the California School of Public Health, confirmed that pregnancy weight gain within the 'Institute of Medicine' range is associated with the best outcome for both mothers and infants.[49] (Table 26.5)

In pregnant women, a weight gain of 10 kg is statistically associated with the best obstetric outcome. A weight gain in pregnancy over 9 kg is more likely to be retained when not pregnant.[50]

Table 26.5: A suggested protocol for management

Pre-pregnancy BMI	Recommended weight gain (kg)	Recommended weight gain (lb)
Underweight, <19.8	12.5 - 18	28–40
Normal, 19.8–24.9	11.5 - 16	25–35
Overweight, 25–29.9	7–11.5	15–25
Obese, > 29.9	At least 6.8 (higher limit not specified)	At least 15 (higher limit not specified)

Pre-pregnancy

- Advise weight loss and aim to bring BMI between 20–25 kg/m^2
- Fertility treatment should not be offered if BMI > 35 kg/m^2
- Folate supplement (5 mg if BMI > 40 kg/m^2).

At Booking

- Calculate BMI.
- Provision of specific information concerning maternal and fetal risks in pregnancy.
- Dietary advice to all obese women (BMI > 30).
- Suggest diet but not weight loss.
- Early ultrasound to confirm dating and detailed anomaly scan.

Antenatal Care

- Uterine artery Doppler screening at 18 weeks.
- Offer low dose aspirin if risk factors for pre-eclampsia are present.
- Screen for GDM in all overweight and obese mothers.
- Regular antenatal visits with blood pressure checks.
- Anesthesia review.

- Anticipation of problems and effective preparation in terms of equipment, monitoring and personnel.
- If BMI > 40 kg/m^2, assess the ability for hip abduction to allow vaginal delivery and allow McRoberts' maneuver for shoulder dystocia.

Operative Intervention

- Regional anesthesia unless contraindicated.
- General anesthesia if required should be delivered with tracheal intubation and controlled ventilation.
- Experienced operators.
- Graduated compression stockings, hydration and early mobilization after any operative delivery.
- Thromboprophylaxis and adequate dose of anticoagulants for an appropriate duration is recommended.
- Postoperative care including close monitoring, early mobilization and chest physiotherapy in a high-dependency setting may be appropriate.
- Judicious use of neuraxial, oral and intravenous opioid for postoperative pain.
- Beware of increased risk of infections.

Postnatal Advice

- Advise on long-term risks of obesity, hypertension and diabetes
- Suggest weight loss prior to next pregnancy
  While significant weight loss before pregnancy is rarely practical, guidance to minimize weight gain during pregnancy and to achieve weight loss after delivery should be offered on an urgent basis.

KEY POINTS

- Obesity is growing health epidemic.
- The pregnancy in obese mother must be considered a 'high-risk pregnancy' that needs multidisciplinary care. She is at an increased risk of almost every complication of pregnancy.
- Obese mothers are more likely to develop metabolic syndrome later on in life thus posing a significant health and economic burden worldwide.
- Greater awareness is needed by the health professionals who can target obese women of childbearing age, education and advice being the key factors.
- Preventing obesity needs a change in thinking—a societal change. There is an urgent need for active partnership between government, science, business and civil society.

REFERENCES

1. Andreasen KR, Anderen ML, Schantz AL. Obesity and Pregnancy. Acta Obstet Gynecol Scand 2004;83:1022-29.
2. Yusuf S, Hawken S, Ounpug S, Bautista L, Franzosi MG, Commerford P, et al. Obesity and the risk of myocardial infarction in 27000 participants from 52 countries: a case–control study. Lancet 2005;366:1640-49.
3. Kanagalignam MG, Forouhi NG, Greer IA, Sattar N. Changes in booking body mass index over a decade: Retrospective analysis from a Glasgow Maternity Hospital. Br J Obstet Gynaecol 2005;112:1431-33.
4. Confidential Enquiry into Maternal and Child Health. Why Mothers Die? 2000-2002. The Sixth Report. London; RCOG Press; 2004;2000-02.
5. Pereira MA, Kartashov AI, Ebbeling CB, Van Horn L, Slattery M, Jacobs DR, et al. Fast-food habits, weight gain, and insulin resistance (the CARDIA Study): 15-year prospective analysis. Lancet 2005;265:36-42.
6. Ludwig DS, Peterson KE, Gortmaker SL. Relation between consumption of sugar-sweetened drinks and childhood obesity: A prospective, observational analysis. Lancet 2001;357:505-08.
7. World Health Organization. The Asia-pacific Perspective: Redefining Obesity and its Treatment, Australia: Health Communications Australia, 2000.
8. Linsten AM, Pasker-de Jong PC, de Boer EJ et al. Effects of subfertility cause, smoking and body weight on the success of IVF. Hum Reprod 2005;20:1867-75.
9. National Institute for Clinical Excellence. Fertility: Assessment and treatment for people with fertility problems. Clinical Guideline. London: RCOG Press, 2004.
10. Castro L, Avina R. Maternal Obesity and Pregnancy Outcomes. Curr Opin Obstet Gynecol 2002;14:601-06.
11. Stewart FM, Ransay JE, Greer IA. Obesity, impact on obstetric practice and outcome. The Obstetrician and Gynaecologist 2009;11:25-31.
12. Hamilton-Fairlers D et al. Association of moderate obesity with a poor pregnancy outcome in women with polycystic ovary syndrome treatment with low dose gonadotrophin. Br J Obstet Gynaecol 1992;99:128-31.
13. Clark AM et al. Weight loss in obese infertile women results in improvement in reproductive outcome for all forms of fertility treatment. Hum Reprod 1998;13:1502-5.
14. Waller DK et al. Are obese women at higher risk for producing malformed offspring? Am J Obstet Gynecol 1994;170:541-48.
15. Glazer NL et al. Weight change and the risk of gestational diabetes in obese women. Epidemiology 2004;15:733-37.
16. Werler MM et al. Pre-pregnant weight in relation to risk of neural tube defects. JAMA 1996;275:1089-92.
17. Brydon P et al. Pregnancy outcome in women with type 2 diabetes mellitus needs to be addressed. Int J Clin Pract 2000;54:418-19.
18. O' Brien TE, Ray JG, Chau WS. Maternal body mass index and the risk of pre-eclampsia: A systematic overview. Epidemiology 2003;14:368-74.
19. National Institute for Health and Clinical Excellence. Diabetes in pregnancy. Management of diabetes and its complications from pre-conception to the postnatal period. Nice Clinical Guideline 63, London. NICE;2008 (www.nice.org.uk/Guidance/CG63).
20. Villamor E, Cnattingius S. Interpregnancy weight change and risk of adverse pregnancy outcomes: A population-based study. Lancet 2006;368:1164-70.
21. Stewart FM, et al. Longitudinal assessment of maternal endothelial function and markers of inflammation and placental function throughout pregnancy in lean and obese mothers. J Clin Endocrinol Metab 2007;92:969-75.
22. Linne Y, et al. Effects of obesity on women's reproduction and complications during pregnancy. Obes Rev 2004;137-43.
23. Comtois R, Seguin MC, Aris-Jilwan N, Couturier M, Beauregard H. Comparison of obese and non-obese patients with gestational diabetes. Int J Obes Relat Metab Disord 1993; 17:605-08.
24. Linne Y, Barkeling B, Rossner S. Natural course of gestational diabetes mellitus: long-term follow-up of women in the SPAWN Study. BJOG 2002;109:1227-31.

26

Obesity and Pregnancy

25. Schranz AG, Sarona, Ventura C. Long-term significance of gestational carbohydrate intolerance: a longitudinal study. Exp Clin Endocrinol Diabetes 2002;110:219-22.
26. Kral JG. Preventing and treating obesity in girls and young women to curb the epidemic. Obes Res 2004;12:1539-46.
27. Drife J. Thromboembolism. Br Med Bull 2003;67:177-90.
28. Sahota PK, Jain SS, Dhand R. Sleep disorders in pregnancy. Curr Opin Pulmon Med 2003;9:477-83.
29. Sebire NJ, Jolly M, Harris JP, et al. Maternal obesity and pregnancy outcome: A study of 287213 pregnancies in London. Int J Obes Relat Metab Disord 2001;25:1175-82.
30. Usha Kiran TS, Hemmadis S, Bethel J, Evans J. Outcome of pregnancy in a woman with an increased body mass index. BJOG 2005;112:768-72.
31. Weiss JL, et al. Obesity, obstetric complications and caesarean delivery rates: A population based screening study. Am J Obstet Gynaecol 2004;190:1091-97.
32. Kabiru W, Raynor BD. Obstetric outcomes associated with increase in BMI category during pregnancy. Am J Obstet Gynecol 2004;191:928-32.
33. Sheiner E, et al. Maternal obesity as an independent risk factor for caesarean section delivery. Paediatr Perinat Epidemiol 2004;18:196-201.
34. Juhas G, et al. Effect of BMI and excessive weight gain on success of vaginal birth after caesarean delivery, Obstet Gynecol 2005;106:741-46.
35. Stephansson O et al. Maternal weight, pregnancy weight gain and the risk of antepartum stillbirth. Am J Obstet Gynecol 2001;184:463-69.
36. Perlow JH. Obesity in the obstetric intensive care patient. In: Foley N. Strong T (Eds): Obstetric Intensive Care: A Practical Manual. Philadephiam, PA: WB Saunders Co 1997; 77-90.
37. Allaire AD, et al. Subcutaneous drain Vs. Suture in obese women undergoing caesarean delivery. A prospective, randomized trial. J Reprod Med 2000;45:327-31.
38. Sebire NJ, et al. Maternal obesity and pregnancy outcome: A study of 287213 pregnancies in London. Int. J Obes Related Metab Disord 2001;25:1175-82.
39. Rasmussen KM, Kjolhede CL. Pre-pregnant overweight and obesity diminish the prolactin response to suckling in the first week postpartum. Pediatrics 2004;113:465-71.
40. Galtier-Dereure, et al. Obesity and pregnancy:complications and cost. Am J Clin Nutr 2000;71(Suppl 5):12425-83.
41. Edwards LE, et al. Pregnancy complications and birth outcomes in obese and normal–weight women: effects of gestational weight change. Obstet Gynecol 1996;87:389-94.
42. Kristen J, et al. Prepregnancy weight gain and the risk of stillbirth and neonatal death. BJOG 2005;112:403-08.
43. Galtier-Dereure, et al. Weight excess before pregnancy: complications and cost. Int J Obes Relat Metab Disord 1995;19:443-48.
44. Forsen T, et al. Mother's weight in pregnancy and coronary heart disease in a cohort of Finnish men: follow-up study. BMJ 1997;315:837-40.
45. Morin KH. Obese and nonobese postpartum women: Complications, body image, and perceptions of the intrapartal experience. Appl Nurs Res 1995;8:81-7.
46. Department of Health. National Sevice Framework for Diabetes. Standards. London. www.dh.gov.uk/publications&statisitics/
47. Boulot P et al. Diabetes and Pregnancy Group, France. French multicentric survey of outcome of pregnancy in women with pregestational diabetes. Diabetes care 2003;26: 2990-93.
48. Kim C, Newton KM, Knopp RH. Gestational diabetes and the incidence of type 2 diabetes: a systematic review. Diabetes Care 2002;25:1862-68.
49. Abrams B, Altman SL, Pickett KE. Pregnancy weight gain: still controversial. Am J Clin Nutr 2000;71:1233S-42S.
50. Greene GW et al. Postpartum weight change: how much of the weight gained in pregnancy will be lost after delivery? Obstet Gynecol 1998;71:701-07.

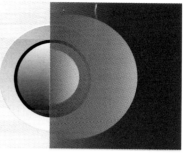

Gynecological Diseases in Pregnancy

27

Smiti Nanda

LEIOMYOMAS AND PREGNANCY

Introduction

The incidence of uterine myomas during pregnancy ranges from 0.09-3.9%.[1,2] The reason for this low incidence is that the majority of pregnancies occur within the age group below that of the development of fibroids. However, recently, as more and more women are delaying child bearing, the incidence of fibroids is likely to increase.[3]

The clinical diagnosis of uterine myoma in pregnancy is not always easy unless the myoma is discrete. During early pregnancy, the apparent asymmetrical enlargement of the uterus may be the only noticeable finding. Later on, uterus may appear larger than period of gestation besides irregular and asymmetrical enlargement.[3]

Ultrasound establishes the diagnosis more accurately. The ultrasound criteria for diagnosis of myoma in pregnancy are as follows: [4,5]

1. Size >3 cm.
2. Spherical shape.
3. Distortion of myometrial contor.
4. Different acoustic structure from myometrium.
5. Speckled pattern of internal echoes increasing in density with increased ultrasound sensitivity.
6. No enhancement of echoes behind the mass.
7. Color-flow Doppler showing splaying of blood vessels around the mass.

Changes in Myomas during Pregnancy

Until recently, it was believed that fibroids increase in size during pregnancy in response to hormonal stimulation. Recent studies have demonstrated that approximately eighty percent of fibroids remain of the same size or even decrease during the course of pregnancy. The fibroids that increase in size during pregnancy mostly grow in first trimester.[3]

Red degeneration or carneous degeneration occurs in 5-8% of myomas, mostly seen during the second half of pregnancy. The pathophysiology is unclear; however, following theories are identified to account for this phenomenon: (1) primary rupture of arteries in the tumor (2) venous obstruction at the periphery of tumor.[1]

The signs and symptoms are variable and include localized pain, tenderness, low grade fever, premature labor, moderate leucocytosis and peritoneal friction rub. Other causes of abdominal pain such as abruption, pyelonephritis, ureteric calculus, appendicitis and adnexal torsion must be ruled out.[1,6] The treatment is conservative, i.e. rest, hydration and analgesics.

Effect of Myoma on Pregnancy

The impact of myoma on pregnancy depends on the size, number and location of myoma.[10] The overall risk of complications is 71% with a complication rate of 10-40% in antepartum period. The complications that can occur are summarized below:[7]

Pregnancy Loss

Uterine fibroids increase the risk of miscarriage and are a cause of recurrent pregnancy loss; however, not all fibroids pose equal risk. Large submucosal fibroids are consistently associated with recurrent pregnancy loss. Several mechanisms that have been suggested are distortion of cavity, compression of underlying endometrium leading to its dysfunction, distortion of its vascular architecture, failure of development of uteroplacental circulation, increased uterine contractility and altered placental oxytocinase activity with the latter two causing disruption of placenta.[7]

Preterm Labor

Increased risk of preterm labor has been reported with fibroids larger than 3 cm. Uteri with fibroids are suggested to be less distensible, which leads to preterm labor in a way similar to congenital mullerian abnormality of the uterus. Also, decreased oxytocinase activity in the gravid uterus with fibroid may result in a localized increase in oxytocin levels and predisposition to premature contractions.[7]

Premature Rupture of Membranes

The association between PROM and fibroids is not well established. The greatest risk of premature rupture of membranes seems to be in women having retroplacental fibroid; however, some studies have reported no increase in risk.[7]

Placental Abruption

Submucosal and retroplacental fibroids with volumes greater than 200 ml (corresponding to 7-8 cm diameter) have the highest risk of abruption. The explanation for increased risk for abruption in the setting of uterine fibroids is likely related to decreased placental perfusion and decidual necrosis.[7]

Pain

It is the most frequent complication of fibroids in pregnancy with 5-15% of women requiring hospitalization at some point during antenatal period. This risk for pain increases with size and is especially high in fibroids larger than 5 cm in diameter. Fibroid pain is likely to result from ischemia and necrosis with release of prostaglandins. Most patients are admitted for pain in the relative absence of symptoms like nausea and vomiting, leucocytosis and pyrexia.

The management of fibroid pain includes rest, hydration and pain control with a standard analgesic or if necessary narcotic analgesia. Although, ibuprofen resulted in dramatic reduction in length of hospital stay compared to narcotic analgesia, it is not recommended beyond 32 weeks because of the possibility of premature closure of ductus arteriosus, neonatal pulmonary hypertension, oligohydramnios and platelet dysfunction.[1,6,7]

Placenta Previa

The presence of fibroid was thought to predispose to placenta previa; however, no such relation has been proved.[3]

Preeclampsia

No significant increase was noted in prevalence of preeclampsia in association with fibroids but women having multiple fibroids are more likely to develop preeclampsia than those with single fibroid. The increased risk is due to disruption of trophoblastic invasion, which leads to inadequate uteroplacental vascular remodeling.[8]

Fetal Anomalies

The fetal anomaly commonly associated with fibroid uterus is caudal dysplasia. Limb reduction defects, congenital torticollis and head deformities are also associated. The risk is found to be 2 times greater than normal patients. [9-11]

Malpresentations

Large submucosal fibroids, by distorting the shape of the cavity, have been consistently associated with malpresentations, however, increased prevalence is also noted with multiple fibroids or retroplacental fibroid or lower segment fibroids.[2,4,7,12,13]

Dysfunctional Labor

The disruption in the coordinated spread of contractile wave leads to dysfunctional and prolonged labor.[14,15]

Obstructed Labor

Cervical fibroid or fibroid very low in the uterine cavity may, however, remain below the presenting part and may threaten to obstruct labor. The anterior fibroid has a far better opportunity of being drawn up out of the pelvis after the onset of labor than a posterior tumor which tends to get trapped within the pelvis.[3]

Cesarean Delivery

Cesarean delivery rates are increased due to factors such as an increased risk of malpresentations, dysfunctional labor and placental abruption.[3]

Postpartum Hemorrhage

Pathophysiologically, uterine fibroids may predispose to postpartum hemorrhage by decreasing force and coordination of uterine contractions, which leads to uterine atony. When the placenta happens to be situated over a fibroid, there is often a defective decidual reaction so that it is liable to be morbidly adherent placenta. Very rarely, a fibroid situated at the fundus of the uterus may, for mechanical reason, precipitate uterine inversion.[3]

Infection in the Postpartum Period

Other Complications

Less common complications like spontaneous hemoperitoneum, DIC, incarceration of uterus behind sacral promontory leading to urinary retention and rarely acute renal failure is also seen.[2]

MYOMECTOMY AND PREGNANCY

Antenatal Myomectomy

Although, every effort should be made to avoid surgery during pregnancy, indications for myomectomy may include intractable fibroid pain that is refractory to rest, hydration and NSAIDs or narcotic analgesia. Subserosal pedunculated fibroids can be removed if the stalk is 5 cm or less in thickness.[3]

Myomectomy during Cesarean Section

Since a term uterus receives about 17% of the cardiac output, myomectomy at the time of cesarean section is associated with significant hemorrhage and has been discouraged traditionally. A few cases of myomectomy at the time of cesarean section have been reported in the recent literature; however it appears safe for pedunculated fibroids mainly. Nonpedunculated fibroids may be associated with severe hemorrhage. The decision to proceed with myomectomy should be approached with caution.

CERVICAL CANCER IN PREGNANCY

Introduction

Pregnancy and prenatal care offer an excellent opportunity to implement screening for premalignant disease, especially in women who do not seek routine health care . Whereas, the incidence of invasive cancer ranges from 1 in 1000 to 1 in 10,000 pregnancies,[16] the incidence of preinvasive cancer is 1 in 750,[17] depending on the type of population studied. However, cervical cancer remains the most common malignancy diagnosed during pregnancy. Approximately 30% cervical cancers are diagnosed during child-bearing age with 3% of cervical cancers diagnosed during pregnancy and only 0.05% of all pregnancies are complicated by cervical cancers.[18]

The physiological changes in the lower genital tract secondary to pregnancy may cause specific alterations that may make screening a challenge; but the effectiveness of papanicolaou smear and colposcopy in the detection of preinvasive and early invasive disease is well proven. Pregnancy does not alter the rates of false negative results significantly, however, diagnostic difficulties in interpretation of a smear do occur.[19] Recommendation for Pap smear screening includes screening at first prenatal visit and again at 6 weeks postpartum.[20]

Diagnostic Pitfalls associated with Pap Smear in Pregnancy[19]

1. The exaggerated ectropion in pregnancy exposes the glandular epithelium to the harsh vaginal environment, making inflammatory changes more common on smear. *Candida* and *Trichomonas* are the most common organisms in the smear.
2. The exposure of endocervical epithelium to acidic pH increases the number of foci of squamous metaplasia, giving an erroneous impression of dysplasia.
3. Decidualization of the cervix and endocervix has been reported. Cytologically, the decidual cells can be confused with normal parabasal cells and high grade dysplastic cells. Decidual cells tend to be polygonal to round with sharp cytoplasmic borders having vacuolated, basophilic cytoplasm and large hypochromatic centrally placed nuclei with prominent nucleoli. Dysplastic cells rarely have nucleoli and have clumped chromatin.

27

4. Trophoblast cells, typically seen as multinucleated giant cells, can be shed and picked up by Pap smear which should be differentiated by the presence of βHCG on immunohistochemistry from low grade dysplasia, viral infection (HPV or HSV) or any granulomatous condition (tuberculosis).

5. Arias Stella reaction related cells (9% of pregnancies) are seen as small, loosely cohesive cells in a clean (nondesmoplastic) background exhibiting high nuclear-to-cytoplasmic ratio with eccentric nuclei and prominent cherry red nucleoli. These mimic high-grade adenocarcinoma, which is verified on biopsy.

The use of abrasive endocervical sampling device such as the Cytobrush has a theoretical risk of significant hemorrhage or pregnancy-related complication and its use has been controversial. The point of controversy remains between the chance of detection and complication.[19]

Due to immunosuppression, the prevalance of HPV and its sequelae may increase during pregnancy. Studies suggest increased incidence of high cancer risk viruses—HPV type 16, 18, 31, 35, 45, 51, 32 and 56 as compared with non-pregnant women.[21]

Diagnosis

Diagnosis of a cervical cancer during pregnancy can be delayed because symptoms of invasive cervical cancer (vaginal spotting, discharge, postcoital bleeding and pain) are mistaken for those of pregnancy complications,[22] subtle preinvasive or early invasive cancer is mistaken for an ectropion, cervical decidualization, or other exaggerated changes of pregnancy.[18,23] The need for speculum examination for every abnormal bleeding or discharge occurring in the pregnant woman is obvious, and a cervical smear should be taken.[22]

PREINVASIVE CANCER

Guidelines for Managing Abnormal Pap Smear

For pregnant patients with high grade squamous cell intraepithelial lesions, it is recommended that colposcopic examination should be performed by clinicians with experience in pregnancy-induced cytological changes. High-grade disease or malignancy should be biopsied. Unsatisfactory colposcopic findings require repeat examination after 6-12 weeks. Postdelivery, repeat cytology and colposcopy should generally be delayed for at least 6 weeks.

The management of abnormal cytology during pregnancy has changed dramatically during the last 3 decades. The goal of evaluation remains timely diagnosis and planning of treatment for invasive carcinoma of cervix. Low-grade lesions are apt to regress in 36-70% cases. The regression rates for high-grade lesions vary from 30-40%. Therapy for preinvasive carcinoma, therefore, can be postponed to postpartum period, so biopsy is avoided. The use of cone biopsy has been significantly reduced by diligent application of colposcopy. Cone biopsy is necessary when colposcopy is unsatisfactory.

Cone biopsy cannot be considered therapeutic during pregnancy owing to the high incidence of positive margins and residual disease on postpartum evaluation.[19] The diagnostic accuracy of colposcopy is 99% and complication rate less than 1%.[24] During pregnancy it is easy to perform as the transformation zone is better exposed due to physiological eversion. Colposcopy is a safe and reliable method for evaluating pregnant patients with abnormal cervical cytological findings.

CIN-I: It is important, however, not to treat or perform a diagnostic excisional procedure on women who are pregnant unless invasive cancer is present or of significant concern (high risk).

CIN-II and III: Unless invasive cancer cannot be ruled out, high grade disease detected during pregnancy is generally followed until postpartum because of the low risk of progression to invasion and the potential to regress postdelivery. Follow up is generally by cytology and colposcopy every 8-12 weeks and 6 weeeks postpartum. The relative increase in immune response postpartum and the decrease in hormonal influences that promote progression, result in regression in 69% cases.

Role of Conization in Pregnancy

It is reserved only for cases with high suspicion of invasive cancer.[25] Classical conization in pregnancy can be disastrous, resulting in significant hemorrhage (>500 ml) necessitating vaginal packing, transfusion, hospitalization, miscarriage, fetal loss and increased perinatal death rates. If absolutely indicated, a cone biopsy is best performed between 14 and 20 weeks with or without cervical cerclage.[20]

Colposcopy in Pregnancy

The challenges of performing an adequate colposcopic examination in pregnancy are increased friability caused by relative eversion of the columnar epithelium, cevical distortion from a low riding fetal head, early effacement, and obstruction of visualization by the mucus plug.[17,18] Special considerations for colposcopy in pregnancy are as follows:[25]
- Expert colposcopist should perform the evaluation.
- Unsatisfactory examinations may be satisfactory in 6-12 weeks or by 20 weeks.
- Limit biopsy to worst area.
- Prepare for increased biopsy site bleeding.
- Re-evaluate lesion with Pap smear or colposcopy every 8-12 weeks.
- Perform repeat biopsy only if lesion worsens.
- Recommend excisional biopsy only if concerned about invasive cancer.

Among patients with the disease, approximately 1% to 3% are pregnant at the time of diagnosis.[26] The diagnosis of cancer evokes a multitude of feelings ranging from denial and disbelief to anxiety and anger. The management of such patients can present difficult ethical, emotional and social considerations for the patient, fetus and the health care team.[27]

Diagnosis and Evaluation

Pregnancy represents an ideal time for cervical cancer screening. A pelvic examination including visual inspection of the cervix, cervical cytology from the ectocervix, and bimanual examination is a routine part of prenatal care. Accurate determination of the extent of cancer is more difficult during pregnancy because induration of base of broad ligaments may be less prominent during pregnancy. Such induration in nonpregnant women characterizes tumor spread beyond the cervix.[21]

Symptoms are variable and pregnancy can mask some of the common symptoms. More than 70% are asymptomatic during presentation. The recognition of the cancer cervix in pregnancy may be missed through attributing vaginal bleeding directly to pregnancy- threatened abortion in early pregnancy and placenta previa or accidental hemorrhage in the later months. Vaginal discharge and pain are some of the nonspecific and less common symptoms.[22,28]

The initial step in the evaluation of the cancer cervix is Pap smear. When the lesion is visible, biopsy should be performed. This is the only gynecological malignancy that is clinically staged. Staging procedure as proposed by International Federation of Gynecology and Obstetrics (FIGO) are general physical examination, systemic examination, per speculum examination, per vaginum examination, chest radiograph, cystoscopy and proctoscopy. Other diagnostic modality such as MRI may be useful in assessing tumor volume and the extent of disease. MRI is a safe and noninvasive modality to assess tumor extent and volume in pregnant patients with cervical cancer. In addition, it may be used to monitor tumor response during and after radiation treatment and may help to guide the physician in selection of therapy and follow up care in these patients. Pregnant patients with cervical cancer should be staged according to the most recent FIGO staging system.[16]

Management

Treatment varies for each patient depending on the stage of disease and duration of pregnancy and the woman's desire to continue the pregnancy. Counseling and treatment include a multidisciplinary approach (ACOG, 2002). Treatment for microinvasive disease diagnosed by cone biopsy follows guidelines similar to those for intraepithelial disease. In general, continuation of pregnancy and vaginal delivery are considered safe and definitive therapy is provided postpartum.[21]

Invasive cancer demands relatively prompt therapy. During the first half of the pregnancy, immediate treatment may be advisable. During the later half of pregnancy, a reasonable option is to wait for not only fetal viability but also fetal maturity. There are issues regarding the safety of a planned delay in treatment. With recent advances in neonatal care the definition of fetal viability has been lowered. The survival of neonates born at earlier gestations has improved with steroids, surfactant and contemporary neonatal intensive care. Antepartum steroids should be given to enhance fetal lung maturity. Accurate dating of pregnancy is important to determine the timing of delivery. Delivery should be considered as soon as fetal viability can be expected with minimal anticipated neonatal morbidity.[16]

Mode of Delivery

Cesarean section is the recommended mode of delivery although studies suggest that survival after vaginal delivery is not significantly different from after abdominal delivery.

Other concerns include hemorrhage and obstructed labor associated with vaginal delivery in pregnant patients with cervical cancer. Episiotomy site recurrences may be associated with high mortality. Recurrences at the episiotomy site most likely occur from direct tumor spillage and implantation during vaginal delivery. Owing to these concerns, cesarean delivery should be the mode of delivery.

Pregnant women diagnosed with cervical cancer in the first or second trimester who require immediate treatment with radiation should be allowed to deliver vaginally. Hysterotomy during the second trimester usually requires a vertical uterine incision and can result in large blood loss. Thus, in patients in whom a planned delay in treatment is not possible, radiation should be given without exposing the patients to the high morbidity associated with hysterotomy.[16]

Surgical Treatment

Radical hysterectomy and lymphadenectomy are widely accepted as the preferred therapy for early stage cervical cancer (stage I and IIA) in pregnant and nonpregnant women. Pregnant women are most likely to benefit from surgical treatment because of their young age as the ovarian function can be preserved.[16]

Except for the increased blood loss in conjunction with cesarean section, the studies reported that the outcome of radical hysterectomy with the fetus *in situ* or after cesarean delivery did not differ significantly from that of radical hysterectomy in the nonpregnant state. There were also no differences in operative morbidity and major complication rates. Thus, the surgical management of cervical cancer complicating pregnancy seems to be safe and effective, with morbidity rates comparable with those for nonpregnant patients.[16]

Before 20 weeks gestation, radical hysterectomy can usually be performed with the fetus *in situ*. If the fetal age is >20 weeks or if better visualization is needed, the fetus can be delivered via hysterotomy through a fundal incision or classic cesarean section prior to hysterectomy. The lower uterine segment and the cervix should be avoided during fetal delivery.[16]

Intraoperatively, surgery should not be abandoned on the basis of enlarged pelvic and para-aortic lymph nodes because node hypertrophy can occur with pregnancy alone. Physiologic decidual cell reactions in lymph nodes, as a result of pregnancy, can be confusing, and histological evaluation should be carefully performed.[16]

Radiation Treatment

Treatment for stage IIB and higher stages cervical cancer is usually limited to radiation therapy. In addition, woman at high risk for surgical morbidity and mortality should also be treated primarily with radiotherapy. When the fetus is viable, delivery should be performed via cesarean section prior to the initiation of therapy. If the fetus is not viable, external beam radiation therapy can be started prior to delivery. The mean radiation dose at which abortion occurs is 34 Gy. Thus, teletherapy is a safe and effective modality for evacuating the uterus prior to brachytherapy. If spontaneous abortion does not ensue, curettage is performed.[16]

RETROVERSION OF THE GRAVID UTERUS

Of all the displacements of gravid uterus, retroversion is the most important, for the reason that certain serious complications can occur if spontaneous correction does not occur. One in every ten women has a retroverted uterus.[3] Though, it is not uncommon for a normally placed uterus to become retroverted during early pregnancy by mechanical reasons, i.e. increased weight of the uterus, however, in majority of cases, this condition results from occurrence of conception in a uterus which is already retroverted or retroflexed.

Clinical Features

In majority of cases of uterine retroversion, no symptoms occur because spontaneous correction takes place soon after the 12th week of pregnancy when gravid uterus grows out of pelvis. Only if this rectification fails to occur, symptoms are produced due to incarceration of uterus.[30]

There is pelvic discomfort and low sacral pain. The prominent symptom is retention of urine. Usually, the onset is gradual. The initial symptom is frequency of micturition passing on to retention of urine and then overflow incontinence. Mechanical pressure upon the bladder neck and elongation of the urethra resulting from upward displacement of the cervix and stretching of the anterior vaginal wall are the obvious reasons for the retention.[29,30] Edema in the region of bladder neck adds its effect to those of mechanical compression and neuromuscular incoordination.[3]

Because of urinary retention, the bladder may become enormously distended and its wall much thickened due to true hypertrophy and edema.[29] Rupture of bladder either spontaneously or following manual rectification is extremely rare. Overdistention of bladder predisposes to cystitis, pyelitis and pyonephrosis.

Bowel disturbance may occur with persistent constipation. Rarely, uterus continues its development in abnormal position, giving rise to anterior sacculation. This may persist until term. More commonly abortion takes place if the displacement remains uncorrected.

Diagnosis

Marked disturbance of bladder functions in association with three or four months of pregnancy should raise the suspicion of retroverted gravid uterus.[30] On abdominal examination, an overdistended bladder reveals itself as a soft swelling, reaching well above the umbilicus in extreme cases. Any doubt can be dispelled by passing the catheter. On per vaginal examination, there is forward bulging of the posterior vaginal wall due to retroverted uterus and the direction of vaginal canal is altered so that it passes from below upwards and a little forwards instead of upwards and backwards. Secondly, cervix is felt high up behind the pubic symphysis. Often the posterior lip alone can be reached and sometimes cervix is inaccessible to touch. Bimanual examination after emptying the bladder will reveal that swelling felt through posterior vaginal wall is the gravid uterus. Per rectal examination will allow complete palpation of the displaced uterus. Diagnosis can be confirmed with ultrasound which helps exclude extrauterine pregnancy, ovarian cyst or a posterior wall fibroid.

Differential Diagnosis

Extra uterine pregnancy, especially if the sac has ruptured and there is pelvic hematocele. But in this condition, one usually gets a history of acute abdominal pain and/or blood-stained vaginal discharge, the retention of urine is seldom so complete, there is often rectal tenesmus, adnexa is tender on palpation, and the cervix is seldom displaced upwards so much.

An ovarian cyst, or more commonly a posterior wall fibroid, may cause trouble in diagnosis.

Treatment

In the absence of symptoms, no attempt should be made to correct the retroversion discovered on routine vaginal examination in early pregnancy. Because uterus as a rule corrects itself in majority of cases and secondly manipulation especially a difficult one may induce abortion.[29,30] Postural treatment by exaggerated Sim's position is encouraged. Frequent bladder evacuation and abstinence from intercourse to avoid risk of miscarriage is advocated.

In cases presenting with bladder symptoms, treatment must not be delayed. Best method of treatment is bedrest in semi prone or exaggerated Sim's position and indwelling catheter to keep the bladder empty. In most of cases, uterus undergoes spontaneous correction within 24-48 hours. Very rarely, if it fails, manual reposition should be tried by pushing the fundus upwards and forwards with two fingers in the vagina. Manipulation is done in genupectoral (knee-chest) or Sim's position. The advantage of Sim's position is that it does not preclude the administration of anesthesia should this be necessary. While pushing the fundus, pressure should be made more to one side to avoid sacral promontory. A finger in the rectum usually succeeds where vaginal manipulation fails. If an anesthetic is administered, manipulation will often succeed after being employed unsuccessfully without it.[30] Even when manipulation fails initially, it may succeed after a few days of bedrest.

OVARIAN TUMOR/ADNEXAL MASS IN PREGNANCY

Incidence and Diagnosis

Ovarian mass of any type can complicate pregnancy. The incidence of tumor and cyst varies depending on the age group studied and frequency with which prenatal sonography is used. The average incidence of ovarian mass is 1 in 1000 in pregnancy. Two to five percent of these masses are malignant. Most common ovarian tumors are cystic. With the widespread use of routine prenatal ultrasound, the finding of an adnexal mass in pregnancy is an increasingly common occurrence.[21,31]

Most adnexal masses removed during pregnancy are either mature teratomas or cystadenomas.[32] The histological distribution in pregnancy is, however, different from that seen in general population, partly because pregnant women are relatively young and have a higher incidence of germ cell tumors. The distribution is as depicted in Table 27.1.[33-35]

Table 27.1: Distribution of adnexal masses removed during pregnancy	
Histologic profile	Incidence (Percentage)
Cystadenoma	33
Dermoid	27
Parovarian cyst	12
Functional cyst	14
Endometrioma	3
Benign stromal	2
Leiomyoma	1.5
Luteoma	0.5
Miscellaneous	3
Malignant	4
Germ cell tumor	33-40
Epithelial tumor	33-53
Gonadal stromal cell tumor	9-20

The majority of ovarian cancers associated with pregnancy are diagnosed at an early stage, i.e. when the disease is still confined to ovary.[33]

Symptoms

Symptoms of adnexal mass are variable. Most masses are asymptomatic at the time of presentation. The discovery of adnexal masses is mostly during routine ultrasound examination in early pregnancy.[35] Sometimes, it is possible to discern a groove between the fundus of gravid uterus and an ovarian cyst if the patient is placed in head down Trendelenberg's position (Hingorani's sign).[36] The most common presenting complaint is pain due to torsion, rupture or intracystic hemorrhage. Torsion occurs mostly during the puerperium when rapid changes in the anatomical relations of the pelvic viscera combined with lax abdominal musculature favor twisting. Second trimester is another period during which the chances of torsion are increased as uterus becomes an abdominal organ and intestinal peristalsis can initiate torsion. Large cysts can lead to malpresentation, obstructed labor and increased risk of cesarean delivery.[35,36]

The most important risk is miscarriage and premature delivery which may be induced by surgical removal. They can also cause pressure symptoms, especially when they are large.[35]

Management

Management depends upon symptoms, gestational age, size and characteristics of the mass. Small simple ovarian cysts < 6 cm are managed conservatively. Surgery is usually indicated if:
1. Malignancy is suspected that is, complex masses with increased flow on Doppler ultrasound or ascites.
2. Acute complications like—torsion, rupture or intracystic hemorrhage develop.
3. Size of tumor is likely to cause difficulty—obstruction, malpresentation and prematurity.
4. A size > 6 cm persists during second trimester.[37-39]

Elective surgery is delayed until the second trimester, a time associated with reduced risk of spontaneous abortion, hormonal independence of the corpus luteum of pregnancy and resolution of functional cysts. The procedure should ideally be performed at 18-20 weeks of gestation preferably under general anesthesia. Once the neoplasm is identified at surgery, the other adnexa should be examined for pathology. In the majority of cases the adnexal mass is benign. A simple cystectomy should be attempted as primary therapy. A frozen section should be obtained and decision is taken accordingly. Elective surgery for an adnexal mass any time during pregnancy increases the risk of pregnancy loss and the likelihood of intrauterine growth restriction (IUGR) and preterm delivery.[34,36]

While performing a laparotomy for an adnexal mass, the surgeon must take into account a number of variables when selecting the type of incision (i.e vertical vs transverse). In general, if malignancy is suspected, or if uterine manipulation is to be minimized, a vertical incision is best. Other considerations include a prior scar, body habitus, obstetric issues and the patient's wishes.

Laparoscopy or Laparotomy?

The data on laparoscopy during the first and second trimesters of pregnancy indicate that it is as safe as laparotomy. Small series of laparoscopic procedures to manage an adnexal mass during pregnancy suggest that this approach is most applicable during the first and early second trimester to manage masses <10 cm in diameter, particularly when adnexectomy is planned. Laparoscopy may be considered "minimally invasive" because it reduces manipulation of the pregnant uterus during adnexal surgery.

Follow-up with Tumor Markers

Several researchers have reported elevations of maternal serum CA 125 values during normal pregnancy. Serum CA 125 values are highest during the first trimester, levels as high as 1250 U/ml have been reported. Serum CA 125 values decrease during the late first trimester and remain below 35 U/mL until delivery. However, within 1 hour after a term delivery the CA 125 values transiently rise and decrease rapidly thereafter.

Serum alpha-fetoprotein (AFP) levels have been used as a tumor marker for the follow-up of patients with germ cell malignancies. It is routinely measured at approximately 16 to 20 weeks of gestation to screen for neural tube defects. Marked elevations of maternal AFP levels have resulted in the antenatal diagnosis of germ cell tumors in asymptomatic pregnant women.

Lactic dehydrogenase (LDH) has been used as a marker for gonadal and extragonadal dysgerminomas. With the exception of preeclampsia, LDH values change little with pregnancy and the puerperium. In both cases, the LDH values closely correlate with the clinical activity of disease.[35]

REFERENCES

Myomas and pregnancy

1. Phelan JP. Myomas and pregnancy. Obstet Gynecol Clin North Am 1995;22:801-05.
2. Coronado GD, Marshall LM, Schwartz SM. Complications in pregnancy, labor and delivery with uterine leiomyomas: A population based study. Obstet Gynecol 2000;95:764-69.
3. Donald I. Local abnormalities. In: Practical obstetric problems; 5th edn. London, Lloyd Luke Ltd 1979;256-83.
4. Kessler A, Mitchell DG, Kuhlman K, et al. Myomas vs. contraction in pregnancy: Differentiation with color Doppler imaging. Journal of Clinical Ultrasound 1993; 21:241.
5. Winer-Muram HT, Muram D, Gillieson MS. Uterine myomas in pregnancy. Journal of the Association of Canadian Radiologists 1984;35:168.

6. Cunningham FG, Leveno KJ, Bloom SL, Hauth JC, Gilstrap III LC, Wenstorm KD. Abnormalities of the reproductive tract. In: Williams Obstetrics 22nd edn. New York, McGraw-Hill 2005;962-64.
7. Ouyang DW, Economy KE, Norwitz ER. Obstetric complication of fibroids. Obstet Gynecol Clin North Am 2006;33:153-69.
8. Roberts WE, Fulp KS, Morrison JC, et al. The impact of leiomyomas on pregnancy. Aus NZ J Obstet Gynecol 1999;39:43-47.
9. Graham JM, Miller ME, Stephan MJ, et al. Limb reduction anomalies and early in utero limb compression. J Pediatr 1980; 96:1052-56.
10. Romero R, Chervenak FA, De vore G. Fetal head deformation and congenital torticollis associated with uterine tumor. Am J Obstet Gynecol 1981;141:839-40.
11. Matsunga E, Shiota K. Ectopic pregnancy and myoma uteri: Teratogenic effects and maternal characteristics. Teratology 1980;21:61-69.
12. Rice JP, Kay HH, Mahony BS. The clinical significance of uterine leiomyomas in pregnancy. Am J Obstet Gynecol 1989;160:1212-16.
13. Hasan F, Arumugam K, Sivanesaratnam V. Uterine leiomyomata in pregnancy. Int J Gynecol Obstet 1990;34:45-48.
14. Vergani P, Ghidini A, Stobelt N, et al. Do uterine myomas influence pregnancy outcome. Am J Perinatol 1994;11:356-58.
15. Szamatowics J, Laudanski T, Bulkszas B, et al. Fibromyomas and uterine contraction. Acta Obstet Gynecol Scand 1997;76:973-76.

Cervical cancer in pregnancy

16. Sood AK, Sorosky JI. Invasive cervical cancer complicating pregnancy: How to manage the dilemma. Obstet Gynecol Clin North Am 1998;25:343-52.
17. Brown D, Buran P, Kaplan KJ, et al. Special situations: abnormal cervical cytology during pregnancy. Clin Obstet Gynecol 2005;48:178-85.
18. Nguyen C, Montz FJ, Briston RE. Management of stage I cervical cancer in pregnancy. Obstet Gynecol Surv 2000;55:633-43.
19. Connor JP. Noninvasive cervical cancer complicating pregnancy. Obstet Gynecol Clin North Am 1998;25:331-42.
20. Muller CY, Smith HO. Cervical neoplasia complicating pregnancy. Obstet Gynecol Clin North Am 2005;35:533-46.
21. Cunningham FG, Leveno KJ, Bloom SL, Hauth JC, Gilstrap III LC, Wenstorm KD. Neoplastic diseases. In: Williams Obstetrics 22nd edn. New York, McGraw-Hill 2005;1257-74.
22. Myerscough PR. Tumours and Extragenital Infections complicating Pregnancy, Labour and the Puerperium. In: Munro Kerr's Operative Obstetrics 9th edn. New York, Macmillan Publishing Co Inc 1977; 342-86.
23. Lishner M. Cancer in pregnancy. Am Oncol 2003;14(suppl-3):31-36.
24. Hacker NF, Berek JS, Lagasse LD, et al. Carcinoma of the cervix associated with pregnancy. Obstet Gynecol 1982;59:735.
25. Wright Jr TC, Con JT, Massad LS, et al. Consensus guidelines for the management of women with cervical cytological abnormalities–JAMA 2002;287:2120-29.
26. Donegan WL. Cancer and Pregnancy. Cancer J Clin 1983;33:194.
27. Jones WB, Shingleton HM, Russell A, et al. Cervical carcinoma and pregnancy: A national pattern of care study of the American College of Surgeons. Cancer 1996;77:1479.
28. Sood AK, Sorosky J, Krogman S, et al. Surgical management of cervical cancer complicating pregnancy: A case control study. Gynecol Oncol 1996;64:294.

Retroversion in pregnancy

29. Myerscough PR. Retroversion and other displacements of the gravid uterus. In: Operative obstetrics by Munrokerrs; 9th edn. New York, Macmillan Publishing Co Inc 1977;387-97.
30. Percival R. Abnormal pregnancy. In: Holland & Brews Manual of Obstetrics; 13th edn. London, Churchill Livingstone 1976;246-53.

Gynecological Diseases in Pregnancy

31. Waalen J. Pregnancy poses tough questions for cancer treatment. J Natl Cancer Inst 1991; 83;900.

32. Beischer NA, Buttery BW, Fortune DW, et al. Growth and malignancy of ovarian tumours in pregnancy. Aust N Z Obstet Gynecol 1971;11:208.

33. James DK, Steer PJ, Weiner CP, Gonik B. Malignant Disease. In: High risk pregnancy. 3rd edn. Philadelphia Elsevier 2006;1163-73.

34. Creaseman WT, Rutledge F, Smith JP. Carcinoma of the ovary associated with pregnancy. Obstet Gynecol 1971;38:111.

35. Boulay R and Podczaski E. Ovarian cancer complicating pregnancy. Obstet Gynecol Clin N Am 1998;25:385-98.

36. Hingorani Vera. J Obstet Gynaec Brit Cwlth 1966;73:897.

37. James DK, Steer PJ, Weiner CP, Gonik B. Nonmalignant Gynecology. In: High risk pregnancy. 3rd edn. Philadelphia Elsevier 2006;1248-58.

38. Whitecar P, Turner S, Higby K. Adnexal masses in pregnancy: A review of 130 cases undergoing surgical management. Am J Obstet Gynecol 2000;182:503-05.

39. Platek DN, Henderson CE, Goldberg GL. The management of a persistent adnexal mass in pregnancy. Am J Obstet Gynecol 1995;173:1236-40.

Management of High-Risk Pregnancy—A Practical Approach

Critical Care Issues in High Risk Obstetric Patient

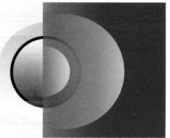

28

Satinder Gombar, K.K. Gombar, Nidhi Bhatia

INTRODUCTION

The management of critically ill pregnant and early postpartum patient presents challenges to the intensive care team due to disease states unique to pregnancy, concurrent anatomic changes in the mother and altered cardiopulmonary physiology of mother and fetus. Obstetric admissions to the intensive care unit (ICU) are uncommon, comprising less than 1% of ICU admissions. Outcome is influenced by the precipitous deterioration which can occur and the equally rapid recovery which may follow delivery. ICU mortality rate of obstetric patients is generally 2 to 3%.[1] In general, admissions to ICU are based on the need for specialized care which is not available in the regular wards. Pregnant and postpartum patients requiring invasive hemodynamic monitoring, intensive respiratory care and an increased level of nursing care are mainly transferred to the ICU. Once the patient is in ICU, the critical care should focus on various aspects of disease processes and the effect of treatment on mother and fetus.

OBSTETRIC CASES REQUIRING CRITICAL CARE

The patients are admitted to ICU for obstetrical as well as non obstetrical causes (Table 28.1). The most common ICU diagnoses in these cases are obstetric hemorrhage in 26 to 33%; hypertensive disorders, especially preeclampsia, in 21 to 42%; respiratory failure in 10%; and infection in 10% of obstetric admissions. Disorders specific to pregnancy such as preeclampsia and amniotic fluid embolism may also lead to respiratory failure in pregnancy.[1]

Table 28.1: Causes of admission to ICU in obstetric cases	
Obstetrical causes	*Nonobstetrical causes*
Hypertensive diseases: • Preeclampsia • Eclampsia Maternal hemorrhage: • Placental abruption • Placenta previa • Uterine rupture • Postpartum hemorrhage Sepsis: • Septic abortion • Puerperal sepsis Amniotic fluid embolism Peripartum cardiomyopathy	Sepsis Respiratory failure Trauma Aspiration Pneumonitis Adult Respiratory Distress Syndrome Chronic hypertension Disseminated intravascular coagulation Endocrine disorders Cardiovascular diseases Nonobstetric hemorrhage Pulmonary embolism Intracranial hemorrhage Status asthmaticus Hepatic encephalopathy

OVERVIEW OF THE PROBLEM

Admission of an obstetric patient to an ICU in developed countries occurs in roughly 2– 4/1,000 deliveries. During the last 15 years, several reports from a variety of centers all over the world have described the characteristics and treatment of critically ill pregnant or puerperal women. The studies report significant variations in patient populations, definition of major morbidity, ICU admission criteria, usage rates, outcomes and treatment. Differences in access to health care in different set-ups make comparisons of standard of care and recommendations for improvement difficult.[2]

Usually, women are young and frequently primipara. In general, for most obstetric patients, rapid recovery follows correction of the acute insult. This is reflected in that most women are admitted to an ICU for < 48 hours. Expectedly, this is shorter than the mean length of stay in the nonpregnant population. The most common reasons for ICU admission are preeclampsia-related complications and postpartum hemorrhage. Lapinsky et al in their retrospective study reported that obstetric complications accounted for 71% of obstetrical ICU admissions; the remaining 29% had medical conditions not related to pregnancy but which may have been aggravated by pregnancy. The most common obstetric diagnosis was preeclampsia and its complications, accounting for 40% of all ICU transfers.[3]

However, maternal mortality continues to be high in India and in other developing countries. In a recent study from a tertiary care hospital in India, Irene et al reported a mortality rate of as high as 43%. Severe anemia, postcesarean problems puerperal sepsis, pregnancy induced hypertension, eclampsia, and cortical vein thrombosis were the main reasons for ICU admissions while renal failure, coagulopathy and respiratory dysfunction were the main organ failures. All women required ventilatory support. 43.63% (24/55) women died, most of them due to multi-organ dysfunction.[4]

Cardiovascular System

Circulatory changes during pregnancy include:

- An increase in maternal blood volume which is almost 40% above baseline by 30th week. This increase is due to 20-40% increase in the red cell mass and 40-50% increase in plasma volume, also resulting in dilutional anemia.
- Cardiac output is increased by 30-40% due to increase in both stroke volume and heart rate, and reaches its maximum value by 32 weeks after which there is only a slight increase. The increase in stroke volume is due to an increase in pre-load secondary to an increased venous return and to a decrease in afterload secondary to fall in systemic vascular resistance (SVR). The fall in SVR is attributable to increased synthesis of prostacycline and to arteriovenous shunting to the low resistance placental bed which lacks autoregulation.
- Aortocaval compression by the gravid uterus is extremely important; in fact, in late pregnancy, the inferior vena cava may be completely obstructed in the supine position, and venous return occurs through azygous, lumbar, and paraspinal veins.

28

Clinical Implications

When the maternal circulation is compromised, compensatory vasoconstriction occurs, and uteroplacental perfusion is reduced, leading to rapid fetal hypoxia and acidosis. For this reason, evidence of fetal distress such as fetal bradycardia may be a sign of maternal deterioration. For the team of intensivist and obstetrician, fetal heart monitoring provides crucial information about both the maternal and fetal conditions. Secondly, because of the cardiovascular changes, patient can also bleed extensively and lose almost 35% of her blood volume before the normally recognizable physical signs, such as tachycardia and hypotension and other signs of hemodynamic instability can be identified.

Respiratory System

Pulmonary changes in normal pregnancy are as follows:

- Changes in lung volume and capacity: Elevation of the hemidiaphragm occurs due to enlarging uterus especially during the last trimester, leading to decrease in functional residual capacity (FRC) by as much as 20% of prepregnant values. Total lung capacity remains unchanged but minute ventilation increases by 45% primarily due to increase in tidal volume (V_T) thus decreasing the expiratory reserve volume and functional residual capacity (FRC). As such these changes make critical closing capacity (CC) come very near to FRC. There is no change in lung compliance, but chest wall compliance is reduced. Reduction in FRC leads to increase in ventilation perfusion mismatch resulting in hypoxemia.

Heparin does not cross the placenta and has not been shown to be teratogenic. Warfarin is associated with a distinct syndrome of developmental defects and should be avoided, especially in early pregnancy.

Radiation Exposure

Radiography is often essential in diagnosis and management of critically ill patient, but in pregnant patient one must be concerned about radiation exposure to the fetus. The risks to fetus of death, malformation, or later childhood cancers depend on gestational age at the time of exposure and the amount of radiation delivered. In the first few weeks of pregnancy radiation doses of 10 centigrays (cGy) may cause fetal death. The risk of malformations is much increased at doses above 15 cGy. A chest roentgenogram exposes the maternal lungs to approximately 0.5 cGy and the shielded fetus to much less ionizing radiation. Abdominopelvic CT scans deliver a larger radiation dose, between 5 and 10 cGy, to the fetus. Therefore plain films necessary for diagnosis and safe care of the pregnant patient should be obtained without undue concern over fetal exposure.[18]

DIAGNOSIS AND MANAGEMENT OF SOME COMMON CRITICAL CONDITIONS IN OBSTETRIC PATIENTS

Hypertensive Disorders of Pregnancy

Pregnancy induced hypertension (PIH) occurs in 5% of all pregnancies and is characterized by hypertension with proteinuria or edema or both occurring after 20th week of gestation. Eclampsia implies the occurrence of convulsions in a pregnant woman suffering from PIH.

Severe preeclampsia is characterized by one or more of the following:
- Blood pressure more than or equal to 160/110 mm Hg
- Proteinuria more than 5 gm/24 hours
- Oliguria less than 500 ml/24 hours
- Headache, visual disturbances, epigastric pain, pulmonary edema or cyanosis
- Platelet count below 100 000/mm^3

Preeclampsia is a procoagulant and proinflammatory state caused by placental hypoperfusion. Impaired invasion of the uterine spiral arteries by trophoblast prevents the normal increase in blood flow to the placenta. The placenta secretes antagonists to vascular endothelial growth factor and placental growth factor. Locally, there is endothelial release of the vasoconstrictor thromboxane, activation of platelets, reduction in nitric oxide and vascular sensitivity to angiotensin. In addition, inflammatory cytokines such as interleukin-6 and tumor necrosis factor are released resulting in placental hypoperfusion.[1,2,6,15]

Blood volume is characteristically reduced and viscosity is increased. In addition there is decrease in renal blood flow and glomerular filtration rate, central nervous system irritability and hyperreflexia. Adequate oxygenation, urine output and normal blood pressure are typical therapeutic goals in the management of critically ill ICU patients, even more so in preeclampsia. The care of critically ill obstetric patients with PIH may require intervention for management of hypertension, seizures, volume replacement of the contracted intravascular compartment, improve circulation to uterus, placenta and kidneys, correct electrolytes, acid base balance and decrease central nervous system irritability. Definitive treatment is delivery of the fetus and placenta.[1,2]

Control of Hypertension

The blood pressure in preeclampsia is variable and can fluctuate on a minute-to-minute basis. Blood pressure should be measured manually using standard aneroid sphygmomanometer because automated blood pressure monitors are unreliable in women with preeclampsia Therapy should be directed towards lowering blood pressure so as to limit further development of vasogenic cerebral edema and subsequent ischemia. The aim is to prevent cerebral hemorrhage and hypertensive encephalopathy. Control of hypertension is best achieved by α methyldopa, hydralazine.

Control of Seizures

Magnesium sulfate ($MgSO_4$) is the anticonvulsant drug of choice because it is effective for prevention and treatment of seizures. The drug is administered in a dose of 2 gm to 4 gm as slow intravenous bolus, followed by 1 gm to 2 gm/hour (Table 28.5). The possibility of magnesium toxicity is to be kept in mind. However, when using the cited dosage regimen in the absence of renal insufficiency, therapy can be monitored safely by measurement of the patellar reflexes and respiratory rate. In case of overdose, first ensure adequate ventilation, then 1 gm of 10% calcium gluconate can be given over a 10-min period.[2]

Only when seizures continue, despite administration of a second bolus, should diazepam or thiopental be given intravenously. Intubation then becomes necessary to protect the airway and ensure adequate oxygenation. Further seizure activity should be managed by ventilation and muscle relaxation.

Table 28.5: Magnesium sulfate for prevention and treatment of eclampsia

1. Loading dose: 4-6 gm diluted in 100 mL of intravenous fluid administered over 15–20 minutes
2. Maintenance dose of 1-2 gm/hour in 100 mL of intravenous maintenance infusion
3. Serum levels should be maintained between 4-7 mEq/L (4.8-8.4 mg/dL or 2–4 mmol/L)
4. Discontinue infusion 24 hours after delivery or last convulsion

The hemodynamics of severe PIH vary among patients. Increased cardiac output with normal systemic vascular resistance to decreased cardiac output with poor left ventricular function and markedly increased systemic vascular resistance may be seen. Most oliguric PIH patients who require invasive monitoring have low ventricular filling pressures, increased systemic vascular resistance, and hyperdynamic ventricular filling pressures, coupled with contracted plasma volume. Monitoring with a pulmonary artery catheter may be helpful in severe PIH with pulmonary edema, refractory oliguria or unremitting hypertension requiring continuous infusion of antihypertensive agents. These patients should be carefully monitored in the postpartum period because of fluid shifts and centralization of blood volume, they are more susceptible to pulmonary edema.

HELLP Syndrome

A syndrome of hemolysis, elevated liver enzymes and thrombocytopenia (HELLP) occurs in a subset of patients. The only cure for a patient with PIH having HELLP syndrome is delivery and appropriate component therapy. The acute cerebral complications of preeclampsia, such as intracranial hemorrhage or massive cerebral edema, account for > 75% of such fatalities, particularly in the presence of HELLP syndrome. Management of the HELLP syndrome includes corticosteroid therapy for fetal lung maturation, antepartum corticosteroids have been shown to increase platelet count. Plasma exchange has been advocated in patients with severe HELLP syndrome (platelet count below 50,000/mm^3) that does not resolve postpartum. Improvement in antenatal and intensive care has reduced the prevalence of and death attributable to eclampsia in western countries in the past decade.[1]

Pulmonary Edema

It complicates 3% of cases of preeclampsia and usually occurs postpartum Respiratory failure occurs in the setting of fluid overload, hypoalbuminemia and decreased colloid oncotic pressure and increased pulmonary capillary hydrostatic pressure. Pulmonary edema may develop in severe preeclampsia complicated by cardiopulmonary arrest, hypertensive crisis, disseminated intravascular coagulation, acute renal failure and cerebral edema. Delivery is indicated for severe maternal organ failure, placental abruption or gestation over 34 weeks.[1,2] The topic is discussed in detail in the respective chapter .

Maternal Hemorrhage[2,6,19]

Haemorrhage during pregnancy may be massive and is frequently associated with coagulation failure. Most often initial care is provided in the labor and delivery suite, but continued bleeding and resuscitation may require ICU care. The common causes of hemorrhagic shock in pregnant patients are:

Abruptio placentae: It is the premature separation of placenta occuring in 0.5% to 1% of deliveries and carries a mortality of 35%. Presenting signs and symptoms include vaginal bleeding, pain abdomen, uterine tenderness and fetal distress. Significant maternal or fetal distress requires an emergency cesarean section. Otherwise, vaginal delivery may be attempted with continuous fetal monitoring. The sequelae of severe abruption is hemorrhage out of proportion to the presenting symptoms, disseminated intravascular coagulation (20-40%), acute renal failure (1-4%) and major organ necrosis (Sheehan syndrome, liver failure).

Placenta previa: This is the implantation of the placenta in lower uterine segment. Vaginal bleeding in placenta previa is usually painless. Parturients who present prior to term are managed with transfusion and bedrest whenever possible until fetal maturity is demonstrated. Perinatal hypoxia is a real danger to both premature and mature infants. Uterine bleeding at the time of surgery or in the postpartum period can be severe because of poor contractility, or if the placenta has grown into the myometrium and becomes abnormally adherent (placenta accreta). In severe cases with major blood loss, ICU management is essential.

Uterine rupture: This condition is rare (0.02%-0.08%) and usually occurs in patients in active labor. Bleeding into the peritoneal cavity may result in little vaginal bleeding. Initial clinical presentation is hypotension and bradycardia with severe abdominal pain. The sudden onset of fetal distress and an unusual abdominal mass are characteristic findings. Prompt operative intervention is necessary and a cesarean hysterectomy may be required.

Postpartum hemorrhage: Bleeding following delivery usually results from uterine atony, but may reflect trauma, coagulopathy, or retained products of conception. Management entails uterine massage, oxygenation, and certain prostaglandins or ergot alkaloids. If pharmacological methods fail, surgical intervention is necessary.

Management

- The patients at risk should be identified early as circulatory impairment may be life threatening. in this relatively young patient population.
- Maternal monitoring should include arterial pressure, ECG, urinary output, arterial oxygen saturation, blood gas analysis, serum chemistry and coagulation profile.
- The establishment of appropriate venous access and in undelivered patient immediate correction of fetal distress is mandatory. Fetal distress correction should be achieved by placing the mother in left lateral position, increasing the inspired concentration of oxygen, using intermittent positive pressure breathing, correcting maternal hypotension and discontinuing oxytocin.

Critical Care Issues in High Risk Obstetric Patient

In hemorrhagic shock, it is essential to position the patient in left lateral position to ensure that venacaval obstruction does not worsen already diminished venous return.

- Immediate volume resuscitation with crystalloid or colloid should be undertaken to restore the circulating blood volume until blood is available.
- Uterotonic agents, such as oxytocin, are used in the management of uterine atony in PPH. This synthetic nonapeptide is a first-line agent because of the paucity of side effects and the absence of contraindications. Methylergonovine, an ergot alkaloid, is used as a second-line uterotonic agent in the setting of massive postpartum hemorrhage due to atony.
- Injectable prostaglandins may also be used when oxytocin fails. Prostaglandin E_2 and prostaglandin F_2 alpha stimulate myometrial contractions and have been used for refractory hemorrhage due to uterine atony. A major contraindication to the use of PGF_2 alpha is asthma, and there is a considerable risk for myocardial infarction, when used in the presence of severe hypovolemia, due to coronary artery spasm.[2]
- Evidence for coagulopathy should be sought early and appropriate blood component therapy be instituted.
- Recombinant activated factor VII has recently shown to be an adjunctive hemostatic measure for the treatment of severe obstetric hemorrhage. Based on the mechanisms of action, circulating factor VII is active after it binds to tissue factor, which is exposed at sites of vessel injury. This complex initiates coagulation on activated platelet surfaces adhering to the site of injury and resulting into formation of a localized fibrin clot. The drug can be administered in obstetric cases with life-threatening hemorrhage, even in the presence of disseminated intravascular coagulation. A dose of 90-200µg/kg seems to be appropriate.[2,19]

Sepsis

Septic shock is an important cause of hypoperfusion in obstetrics and accounts for 15% of the maternal deaths. Septic shock is a subset of systemic inflammatory response syndrome (SIRS) and usually occurs due to bacterial, viral, fungal, rickettsial or parasitic infection. The common causes of sepsis in obstetrics include septic abortion, intrauterine fetal death, puerperal sepsis, chorioamnionitis, etc.[1]

The diagnosis of septic shock may be obscured by the normal hemodynamic changes seen during pregnancy. The most useful clinical signs of sepsis like tachycardia, hypotension and low systemic vascular resistance are present in both pregnant and septic states. The extreme values and/or rapid changes in hemodynamic parameters usually point towards infection. The untreated and unresolved sepsis may progress to adult respiratory distress syndrome and disseminated intravascular coagulation (DIC) due to uncontrolled pulmonary capillary leak and derangement in the coagulation cascade.[1,2]

The immediate management of critically ill septic patient involves:
- Restoration of intravascular volume
- Restoration of tissue perfusion
- Restoration of oxygen delivery

General Considerations

- Early goal-directed therapy for sepsis should not be delayed until the admission to the ICU but should begin as soon as septic shock is diagnosed.
- Broad spectrum antibiotics covering likely pathogens based on site of infection, host factors and culture sensitivity should be started early, preferably within 1 hour of the diagnosis of severe sepsis or septic shock
- Multiple-organ failure is a strong predictor of mortality in patients with sepsis with ARDS.
- Oxygen and mechanical ventilation should be instituted early for successful outcome.
- A typical fluid challenge of 1-1.5 liters over 15-20 minute should be considered, but some patients may not be able to tolerate intravenous fluids because of myocardial depression, associated with some cases of septic shock.
- Vasopressors such as dopamine (5-20 µg/kg/min) or norepinephrine (0.5-30 µg/kg/min) may be required. The use of dobutamine (5-25 µg/kg/min) is beneficial in patients with myocardial depression.
- Metabolic acidosis, if severe (pH < 7.2), must be corrected to achieve desired results with inotropes and vasopressors.
- Pulmonary artery catheterization may help not only in managing fluids based on intra-cardiac filling pressures but also myocardial depression.
- There is no definitive role of corticosteroids in the management of septic shock.
- Activated protein C (Drotrecogin α), a circulating anticoagulant with anti-inflammatory properties, has been shown to reduce mortality rate in patients with severe sepsis with high Acute Physiology and Chronic Health Evaluation II score and high risk of death but this has not been studied specifically in pregnancy.[1,20]
- Strict glycemic control is recommended in critically ill patients, particularly in patients with sepsis. Blood glucose levels should be maintained below 150 mg/dl. The goals of tighter control may be especially prudent in obstetric patients.
- Early Goal Directed Therapy:[21] Goals during first 6 hours are to maintain
  A. Central venous pressure: 8-12 mm Hg
  B. Mean arterial pressure ≥ 65 mm Hg
  C. Urine output ≥ 0.5-1 mL/ kg/hour

D. Central venous (superior vena cava) or mixed venous oxygen [SvO$_2$] saturation $\geq 70\%$

E. If central venous or mixed venous O$_2$ sat < 70% after CVP of 8-12 mm Hg then transfuse packed RBCs to increase hematocrit by 30% and give dobutamine to maximum 20 mg/kg/min

F. Begin intravenous antibiotics within first hour of recognition of severe sepsis.

Acute Respiratory Distress Syndrome (ARDS)

ARDS can occur in obstetric patients as a complication of pneumonia, aspiration, sepsis and amniotic fluid embolism. ARDS during pregnancy is often initiated by potentially reversible or self limiting disease processes. Thus, it potentially carries a greater chance for resolution of the underlying disease and perhaps a greater chance for recovery from ARDS as well. Physiological consequences are hypoxemia, decreased compliance and pulmonary hypertension.

Diagnostic criteria:
1. Acute onset of respiratory distress (tachypnea)
2. Presence of predisposing condition
3. Bilateral opacities on chest radiograph
4. PaO$_2$/FiO$_2$< 200 mm Hg
5. PCWP $\leq$ 18 mm Hg or no evidence of left atrial hypertension.

Respiratory system compliance may already be reduced in pregnant patients near term because of upward displacement of the diaphragm, so measurements of end-inspiratory (plateau) pressure may be elevated even without severe ARDS. The management in pregnant patients is similar to the nonpregnant population with ARDS.The essential support in patients with ARDS is mechanical ventilation using low tidal volumes (6 ml/kg), limited maximum plateau pressures to 30 cm H$_2$O to minimize ventilator induced lung injury (VILI), with positive end expiratory pressure (PEEP). Additional strategies like prone positioning are not feasible in pregnancy. Although there are no studies of utilization of low tidal volumes in treatment of pregnant patients with acute lung injury the proven efficacy of this mode of ventilation in nonpregnant patients with ARDS provides strong support for its universal use. The goal of low tidal volume therapy is to avoid overdistention of the lung and because total lung capacity varies little between the pregnant and nonpregnant state, it is reasonable to use this method of determining tidal volume. It is important to maintain maternal arterial PCO$_2$ in its usual range of 28-32 mm Hg. Permissive hypercapnia is not an attractive option for ventilating the pregnant patient. Transfer of CO$_2$ across the placenta is dependent on a PCO$_2$ difference of approximately 10 mm Hg between fetal and maternal umbilical veins. This difference remains fairly constant over a wide range of CO$_2$ tensions. Therefore, maternal hypercapnia quickly results in fetal respiratory acidosis, a factor that limits the use of permissive hypercapnia.[22]

Nitric oxide has been utilized in the treatment of ARDS in nonpregnant patients, but there is still no consensus on whether inhaled NO improves clinical outcome as defined by oxygen requirements, ventilator days, or mortality.[22]

Trauma

Trauma in pregnancy is common and complicates 6 to 7% of pregnancies. Maternal injury has been associated with an increased incidence of spontaneous abortion, premature labor, abruptio placentae, fetomaternal hemorrhage and intrauterine fetal demise.

The physiologic and anatomic changes that occur during pregnancy alter the type of injuries seen and the maternal response to accompanying blood loss. The increase in blood volume that accompanies gestation may improve tolerance for hemorrhage but may significantly delay the appearance of signs until severe shock is manifested. As fetal well being depends on uterine blood flow, moderate decreases in maternal cardiac output and blood pressure, which are insufficient to cause maternal shock, may be detrimental to the fetus. As the uterus grows and becomes an abdominal organ, it becomes more vulnerable to direct trauma.

The initial concerns in the management of these patients are establishment of a patent airway, functional breathing and adequate circulation. Standard fluid and blood resuscitation should be used to restore circulating blood volume, keeping in mind the requirement of an increased blood volume in pregnancy. If possible, the pregnant patient should be transported and cared for lying on the left side, to improve venous return to the heart. If thought necessary, peritoneal lavage may be performed.

Mother and fetus should have continuous monitoring. It is important that the fetus has cardiotocographic monitoring because fetal demise is much more common than maternal death.[1,2,6]

The definitive therapy rendered to the pregnant trauma victim should mirror that given to those who are not pregnant. Because of increased vascularity around the uterus, pelvic fractures should be aggressively stabilized. Special consideration should be given to cesarean section in situations of fetal distress and in states of refractory maternal shock. Removal of the fetus may be life saving to the child and to the mother and the increase in venous return after delivery may improve resuscitative efforts.

Pulmonary Embolism

Venous thromboembolism (VTE) is an important cause of maternal morbidity and mortality especially in the immediate postpartum period. Specific changes related to pregnancy favor the development of venous thrombosis: venous stasis, endothelial injury, and hypercoagulability. The clinical findings of pulmonary embolism include dyspnea and chest pain. As in nonpregnant women, a massive pulmonary embolism may present with shock attributable

28

Critical Care Issues in High Risk Obstetric Patient

to embolic obstruction to right ventricular cardiac output. The hypotension with elevated right ventricular wall tension may lead to coronary ischemia and further impair myocardial function.[1]

Although measurement of serum D-dimer, a breakdown product of fibrin, has been applied to exclude pulmonary embolism, levels are generally increased in the postpartum period and so this test is not as useful in pregnancy. A chest radiograph should always be performed to assess for an alternative diagnosis, particularly pneumonia. The ventilation/perfusion (V/Q) lung scan has been the traditional initial test for pulmonary embolism during pregnancy. Pulmonary angiography has been considered the gold standard for the diagnosis of pulmonary embolism for patients with suspected pulmonary embolism and nondiagnostic noninvasive tests. Echocardiography may be useful in supporting the diagnosis and in guiding therapy of massive pulmonary embolism. Right ventricular dilation and hypokinesis, paradoxical septal motion and compression of the left ventricle may be observed in major pulmonary embolism.

Right ventricular failure may occur attributable to the embolic obstruction and may require hemodynamic support. Hypotension is first addressed by positioning the patient in the left lateral decubitus position, so that compression of the inferior vena cava may be relieved and venous return improved. Intravenous fluids should be administered. Vasopressors should be administered to achieve adequate maternal perfusion; although uterine artery vasoconstriction may occur, improving maternal circulation will enhance vital organ perfusion. Dopamine has been used as an effective vasopressor during pregnancy and may be required in the setting of massive pulmonary embolism.[1,2]

For treatment of pulmonary embolism, heparin is administered during pregnancy because it does not cross the placenta, in contrast to warfarin, which can cause fetal hemorrhage and malformations. Low molecular weight heparin or intravenous unfractionated heparin may be used. Low molecular weight heparin is advantageous in terms of fixed dosing and lack of monitoring, potentially lower incidence of heparin-induced thrombocytopenia and decreased risk of osteoporosis in women who must continue heparin throughout the pregnancy. Warfarin is administered for postpartum anticoagulation. Anticoagulation for pulmonary embolism is generally administered for 6 months and should include 6 weeks postpartum.[23]

Thrombolytic therapy with tissue plasminogen activator may be administered for massive pulmonary embolism with hemodynamic compromise.[24]

Pulmonary Edema

The gravid patient undergoes physiological changes in pregnancy which alter fluid balance in the lung predisposing to development of pulmonary edema. In the presence of usual predisposing causes of ARDS such as infection, aspiration and hypotension secondary to hemorrhage, pulmonary edema is usually characterized by increased capillary permeability. In patients with pre-eclampsia leading to pulmonary edema, there is considerable uncertainty regarding the underlying mechanisms leading to alveolar flooding. Oliguric pre-eclamptic patients may present with elevated systemic vascular resistance but have normal or decreased intravascular volume. In addition, patients with elevated systemic vascular resistance may have depressed cardiac function, which produces increased pulmonary capillary wedge pressures.

Uncertainty concerning the mechanism leading to development of pulmonary edema in an obstetric patient hampers decision making in management. As a result, invasive hemodynamic monitoring is advised when alveolar flooding does not respond to initial therapy. In addition to pulmonary edema and other usual indications for Swan-Ganz cardiac catheterization, specific obstetric-related indications include pregnancy-induced hypertension complicated by oliguria, the need for rapid antihypertensive therapy, Class 3 or 4 cardiac disease during labor or delivery, amniotic fluid embolism, and pulmonary hypertension complicating delivery.

WHAT IS THE OBSTETRICIAN–GYNECOLOGIST'S ROLE IN THE CARE OF A PATIENT IN A CRITICAL CARE UNIT?

When obstetric patients are transferred to the ICU, regardless of the primary caregiver, patient care decisions must be made collaboratively between the intensivist, obstetrician and neonatologist and should involve the patient, her family, or both. Obstetric input in the care of the postpartum ICU patient may include evaluation of vaginal or intra-abdominal bleeding evaluation of obstetric sources of infection, duration of specific therapies such as magnesium for eclampsia prophylaxis and feasibility of breastfeeding, especially compatibility of various medications with breastfeeding. There may be issues related to surgical interventions, including reexploration of the abdomen or reclosure of abdominal or vaginal incisions. Multidisciplinary care is essential for the critically ill obstetric patient. When a pregnant patient is transferred to the ICU, members of the care team should assess the anticipated course of her condition or disease, including possible complications and set parameters for delivery, if appropriate. The plan should be clear to the medical team and to the patient's family and to the patient herself if she is able to understand.[8]

CARDIOPULMONARY RESUSCITATION IN PARTURIENTS[25,26]

Causes of cardiopulmonary arrest during peripartum period include venous thromboembolism, pregnancy-induced hypertension, sepsis, amniotic fluid embolism, hemorrhage, trauma, and cardiac disease. Pregnant patients may have preexisting cardiac disorders, myocardial infarction or peripartum cardiomyopathy as causes of cardiopulmonary arrest. During cardiopulmonary resuscitation (CPR) in an obstetric patient, blood flow is less than 30% of normal blood flow. Significant changes in maternal anatomy and physiology associated with pregnancy limit the effectiveness of standard CPR regimens:

1. Altered airway anatomy: The more anterior and cephalad larynx, friable tissues, enlarged breasts obesity all contribute to increased incidence of failed intubation.
2. Altered respiratory mechanics: Increased oxygen consumption, decreased FRC and chest compliance lead to precipitous drop in arterial and venous oxygen tension.
3. Circulatory changes: Significant changes in maternal cardiovascular physiology cause a 35-50% increase in resting cardiac output and a decrease in arterial blood pressure.
4. Successful resuscitation in late pregnancy is difficult because the gravid uterus acts like an abdominal binder producing an increase in intrathoracic pressure, diminished venous return and obstruction to forward flow of blood into the abdominal aorta, especially in the supine position. In addition, the gravid uterus accounts for 10% of cardiac output and this massive shunting of blood may hinder efforts at CPR.[25]
5. Aortocaval compression: Aortic compression by the gravid uterus causes decrease in renal and uterine blood flow. Inferior vena caval compression results in decreased venous return to the heart leading to hypotension, bradycardia and decrease in cardiac output in supine position.

Modifications in Emergency Cardiac Care for the Parturients

1. During CPR aggressive airway management with prompt intubation is important.
2. During CPR closed chest massage is not very effective due to aortocaval compression in supine position, hence uterus should be manually displaced to the left with a wedge at an angle of 27º.
3. Perform chest compressions higher on the sternum, slightly above the center of the sternum. This will adjust for the elevation of the diaphragm and abdominal contents caused by the gravid uterus.
4. Aggressive restoration of circulatory volume should be carried out
5. Defibrillation: No modifications in dose or pad position are required. Defibrillation shocks transfer no significant current to the fetus. Always remove any fetal or uterine monitors before shock delivery.
6. "4-minute rule": If the fetus is thought to be viable and maternal resuscitation is unsuccessful, cesarean **delivery should be started within 4 minutes of cardiac arrest** and accomplished within 5 minutes to optimize maternal and fetal survival. Delivery will immediately relieve the uterine compression and improve venous return and allow more effective chest compressions.
7. The maternal oxygen reserve is limited; a delay of 6-9 min may lead to irreversible brain damage. Fetal oxygen reserve is approximately 2 min.

8. Advanced cardiac life support (ACLS Drugs): Current recommendations are that ACLS protocols be followed in pregnancy as they are in nonpregnant individual. Vasopressor agents such as epinephrine, dopamine, and vasopressin will decrease uterine blood flow. Resuscitative drug like atropine can cause fetal tachycardia and sodium bicarbonate given in large doses can cause fetal intracerebral bleeding, thus these drugs should be used judiciously. There are however, no alterations to using all indicated medications in recommended doses. The mother must be resuscitated even if the chances of fetal resuscitation vanish.[26]

In conclusion, critical care of obstetric patients should focus on both maternal and fetal welfare in any intervention or management decision. The presence in ICU of a young patient with viable pregnancy or postpartum with a neonate demands many skills. The critical care clinician must be knowledgeable about the physiological changes and distinctive complications and illnesses in a critically ill obstetric patient.

KEY POINTS

- The obstetric patient poses exceptional challenges in the intensive care unit. Knowledge of the physiologic changes of pregnancy and specific pregnancy-related disorders is necessary for optimal management.
- Approximately 75% of obstetric ICU patients are admitted to the unit postpartum.
- Intensive care unit diagnoses may include preeclampsia, including the HELLP syndrome, maternal hemorrhage, pulmonary embolic disease, amniotic fluid embolism, respiratory infection, the acute respiratory distress syndrome and sepsis. Hemorrhage and hypertension are the most common causes of admission from obstetric services to intensive care.
- Scoring systems such as the APACHE II or the SAPS score accurately predict hospital mortality among obstetric patients admitted to the ICU for medical reasons but perform poorly in predicting deaths from patients admitted purely for obstetric reasons.
- Treatment of sepsis should not await admission to an ICU but should begin as soon as septic shock is diagnosed.
- Decisions about care for a pregnant patient in the ICU should be made collaboratively with the intensivist, obstetrician, and neonatologist.
- Necessary medications should not be withheld from a pregnant woman because of fetal concerns.
- Necessary imaging studies should not be withheld out of potential concern for fetal status, although attempts should be made to limit fetal radiation exposure during diagnostic testing.
- Cesarean delivery should be considered for both maternal and fetal benefit approximately 4 minutes after a woman has experienced cardiopulmonary arrest in the third trimester.

Critical Care Issues in High Risk Obstetric Patient

- The admission rate to intensive care and the problems faced by critically ill parturients may be reduced by improving the management of hypertensive disease during pregnancy and by reducing the prevalence of hemorrhagic complications by emphasis on early detection and anticipation.
- A delay in the correction of hypovolemia, in diagnosis and treatment of impaired coagulation and in the surgical control of bleeding are the avoidable factors in most maternal mortality cases caused by hemorrhage.

REFERENCES

1. Shapiro J M. Critical Care of the Obstetric Patient. J Intensive Care Med 2006; 21: 278.
2. Zeeman GG. Obstetric critical care: A blueprint for improved outcomes. Crit Care Med 2006 Vol. 34, No. 9 (Suppl.) :(S208–S214).
3. Lapinsky S E, Kruczynski K, Seaward GR, Farine D, Grossman RF. Critical care management of obstetric patient. Can J Anaesth 1997; 44: 3, p 325-29.
4. Irene Y V, Kaur V, Kaur G, Andappan A, Afzal L. Critical care in obstetrics - scenario in a developing country J Obstet Gynecol India Vol. 58, No. 3 : May/June 2008,217-20.
5. Ross A: Physiological changes of pregnancy. In Birnbach DJ, Gatt SP, Datta S (Eds): Textbook of Obstetric Anaesthesia. New York, Churchill Livingstone,2000 pp 31-45.
6. Birnbach DJ, Browne IM. Anesthesia for Obstetrics. In Miller RD (Ed): Miller's Anesthesia, 6th edn. Philadelphia, Elsevier, 2005, pp 2307-42.
7. Gabbe SG, Niebyl JR, Simpson JL, Galan H, Goetzl L, Jauniaux ER, et al (Eds). Obstetrics: Normal and problem pregnancies. 5th edn. Philadelphia (PA): Churchill Livingstone Elsevier;2007.
8. ACOG Practice Bulletin. Clinical management guidelines for obstetrician–gynecologists. Critical Care in Pregnancy. February 2009;113:2, part 1,p 443-50.
9. Guidelines for intensive care unit admission, discharge, and triage. Task Force of the American College of Critical Care Medicine, Society of Critical Care. Crit Care Med 1999; 27:633-38.
10. Aggarwal AN, Sarkar P, Gupta D, Jindal SK. Performance of standard severity scoring systems for outcome prediction in patients admitted to a respiratory intensive care unit in North India. Respirology 2006;11:196-204.
11. Knaus W A, Draper E A. APACHE II: A severity of disease classification system. Crit Care Med 1985; 13: 818-29.
12. Vasquez DN, Estenssoro E, Héctor S. Canales HS, Reina R, María G, Saenz MG, Das Neves AV, María A, Toro MA, Loudet CI. Clinical Characteristics and Outcomes of Obstetric Patients Requiring ICU Admission. Chest March 2007 vol. 131 no. 3 718-24.
13. Tempe A, Wadhwa L, Gupta S, Bansal S, Satyanarayana L. Prediction of mortality and morbidity by simplified acute physiology score (SAPS II) in obstetric ICU admissions. Indian J Med Sci 2007; 61:179-85.
14. Shoemaker WC. Routine clinical monitoring in acute illnesses. In Shoemaker WC, Velmahos GC, Demetriades D (Eds): Procedures and monitoring for the critically ill. Philadelphia: Saunders Elsevier; 2002, p 155-66.
15. Santos AC, Braveman FR, Finster M. Obstetric Anesthesia. In Clinical Anesthesia (Eds): Barash PG., Cullen B F.; Stoelting R K. 5th edn. 2006 Lippincott Williams & Wilkins. p 1153-80.
16. Pilbeam SP. Oxygenation and acid-base evaluation. In Pilbeam SP, Cairo JM, (Eds): Mechanical ventilation-Physiological and clinical applications. 4th edn. Philadelphia (PA): Churchill Livingstone Elsevier; 2006, p1-11.
17. Marino PL. Parenteral Nutrition In Zinner R (Ed): The ICU book. 3rd edn. Pennysylvania, Williams & Wilkins; 2004, 754-65.
18. Critchlow JF. Obstetric problemc in the Intensive Care Unit. In Irwin RS,Cerra FB,Rippe JM (Eds): Irwin and Rippe's Intensive Care Medicine. 4th edn, Philadelphia, Lippincot-Raven;1999,p1950-57.

19. Kjaer K,Cappielo E. Peripartum hemorrhage. In Yao FF (ed), Yao & Artusio's Anesthesiology: Problem oriented management, 6th edn, Philadelphia, Lippincott Williams & Wilkins, 2008, 881-903.
20. Dellinger RP, Carlet JM, Masur H, et al. Surviving sepsis campaign guidelines for management of severe sepsis and septic shock. Crit Care Med. 2004; 32:858-71.
21. Rivers E, Nguyen B, Havstad S, et al. Early goal-directed therapy in the treatment of severe sepsis and septic shock. N Engl J Med 2001; 345:1368-77.
22. Campbell LA, Klocke RA. Implications for the Pregnant Patient Am. J. Respir. Crit. Care Med 2001;163(5):1051-54.
23. Bates SM, Greer IA, Hirsh J, et al. Use of antithrombotic agents during pregnancy. The seventh ACCP conference on antithrombotic and thrombolytic therapy. Chest. 2004; 126: 627S-644S.
24. Buller HR, Agnelli G, Hull RD, et al. Antithrombotic therapy for venous thromboembolic disease. The seventh ACCP conference on antithrombotic and thrombolytic therapy. *Chest*. 2004; 126:401S-428S.
25. Dabbous A , Souki F .Cardiac Arrest In Pregnancy M.E.J. Anesth 19 (2), 2007.
26. AHA task force guidelines Part 10.8. Cardiac Arrest Associated with Pregnancy: Circulation; 2005, 112:150-63.

28

Critical Care Issues in High Risk Obstetric Patient

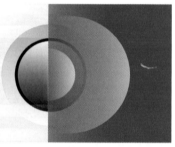

Drugs in Pregnancy

29

Pikee Saxena

INTRODUCTION

The use of drugs in pregnancy requires special attention. There are many issues which must be considered prior to the administration of a drug during pregnancy. It is clear that any drug or chemical substance administered to the mother may cross the placenta unless it is destroyed or altered during this process. Transplacental transport is established at about 8th week of gestation and is dependent on molecular weight and lipid solubility of the substance. It is therefore important to determine the rate and extent of transfer sufficient to result in significant concentration within the fetus.

Number of drugs prescribed during pregnancy should be restricted to a minimum, with the lowest effective dose given for the shortest time. Drugs should be prescribed in pregnancy only if the benefits outweigh the risks.[1-3] Drugs should be given after enquiring about the last menstrual period and should be avoided especially in the first trimester of pregnancy as this is a critical period and drugs have the greatest potential to cause gross malformations during organogenesis in the first trimester.The time period between day 35 to day 55 from last menstrual period is most crucial because prior to day 35 all cells are totipotent, so any insult before day 35 will result in either a missed abortion or has no effect on the growing embryo. Most women who become pregnant do not consult a doctor until six weeks of gestation, by which time organogenesis is well under way for the central nervous system, ears, and eyes. This must be taken into account when prescribing drugs to any woman of childbearing age, many of whom may be unaware that drugs may harm the fetus even before pregnancy has been diagnosed and some of whom will have unplanned pregnancies. These women should also be targeted to ensure that the beneficial effects of folate supplements in reducing fetal abnormalities are fully realized.

The effects of the drugs on fetal development are not only an issue for the mother but sometimes drug intake by sexually active men, is excreted in their semen and may cause fetal problems. Low doses of 5-alpha reductase inhibitors such as finasteride[4] given to husbands of sexually active women during pregnancy can cause abnormalities of the external genitalia of the male offspring. Griseofulvin also appears in the semen, and men should be advised not to try to father a child within six months of treatment.

There is another concern that relates to unknowns. Many pregnant women are turning to herbal remedies and dietary supplements, believing that they might be safer than synthetic drugs. But since there is often even less safety information about the effects of these remedies in general and especially in pregnant women, this represents a risk of unknown magnitude.

Concern related to the effect of a drug on both mother and fetus used by pregnant women is not new. In 1979, the United States Food and Drug Administration (FDA)[5] introduced a classification of fetal risks due to pharmaceuticals (Table 29.1). The United States FDA has the following definitions for the pregnancy categories:

Table 29.1: United states FDA pharmaceutical pregnancy categories	
Pregnancy Category A	Well-controlled studies have failed to demonstrate a risk to the fetus in the first trimester of pregnancy (and there is no evidence of risk in later trimesters), e.g. Multivitamins
Pregnancy Category B	Animal reproduction studies have failed to demonstrate a risk to the fetus and there are no adequate and well-controlled studies in pregnant women; or animal studies which have shown an adverse effect, but adequate and well-controlled studies in pregnant women have failed to demonstrate a risk to the fetus in any trimester, e.g. Penicillins
Pregnancy Category C	Animal reproduction studies have shown an adverse effect on the fetus and there are no adequate and well-controlled studies in humans, but potential benefits may warrant use of the drug in pregnant women despite potential risks, e.g. Aminoglycosides, Trimethoprim
Pregnancy Category D	There is positive evidence of human fetal risk based on adverse reaction data from investigational or marketing experience or studies in humans, but potential benefits may warrant use of the drug in pregnant women despite potential risks, e.g. Carbamazepine, Phenytoin
Pregnancy Category X	Animal or human studies have demonstrated fetal abnormalities and/or there is positive evidence of human fetal risk based on adverse reaction data from investigational or marketing experience, and the risks involved in use of the drug in pregnant women clearly outweigh potential benefits, e.g. Thalidomide, Methotrexate.

TERATOGENICITY

Teratogens are agents which act during embryonic and fetal development and result in permanent alteration of form or function. The mechanism of teratogenicity is as described in Table 29.2.

Teratogenic Drugs[6,7] are drugs which have potential to develop congenital anomalies in the fetus when administered to a pregnant woman.

Criteria for Establishing Teratogenicity

- The defect must be completely characterized
- The agent must cross placenta
- Exposure must occur during the critical period
- Cause and effect must be biologically plausible
- Epidemiological studies must be consistent.

Table 29.2: Mechanism of teratogenicity[5-7]	
Disruption of folic acid metabolism	Hydantoin, valproic acid
Formation of oxidative intermediates	Carbamazepine, phenobaribitone
Fetal genetic composition or genetic mutation	Thalidomide, methotrexate
Chaotic gene expression due to homeobox regulatory genes	Retinoic acid, valproic acid

DRUGS WITH PROVEN TERATOGENIC POTENTIAL

Some of the drugs with proven teratogenic potential and their effects on the developing fetus include:[6-9]

1. Angiotensin Converting Enzyme Inhibitors: Renal damage in the fetus especially during 2nd and 3rd trimester.
2. Carbamazepine: Neural tube defects if administered during the first trimester.
3. Cocaine: Contraindicated in all trimesters. Can lead to various congenital anomalies.
4. Anticancer drugs: Cyclophosphamide, cytarabine, methotrexate, etc. Various congenital malformations can result if given during the 1st trimester.
5. Diethylstilbestrol: Vaginal adenosis and clear cell vaginal adenocarcinoma in pubertal girls exposed to diethylstilbestrol during pregnancy.
6. Ethanol: Fetal alcohol syndrome.
7. Etretinate and Isotretinoin: High risk of multiple congenital anomalies especially of CNS, face, ear and other organs.
8. Iodide: Congenital goiter, hypothyroidism.
9. Lithium: Ebstein's anomaly.
10. Phenytoin: Fetal hydantoin syndrome.
11. Tetracycline: Discoloration and defects of teeth and altered bone growth.
12. Thalidomide: Phocomelia.
13. Valproic acid: Neural tube defects.
14. Warfarin: CNS and facial abnormalities.

TOCOLYTICS

These are drugs which are used to suppress premature labor when delivery would result in premature birth. Preterm delivery is a major cause of perinatal morbidity and mortality. Tocolytic agents are effective in reducing the likelihood of delivery within 48 hours, but do not reduce the overall risk of preterm delivery. Consideration should be given for the administration of tocolytics[10-13] to all women experiencing preterm labour when there is a need to delay delivery in order to:

- Permit in-utero transfer to a tertiary perinatal center for multidisciplinary management (obstetrician, neonatologist, anesthetist); and/or to
- Gain up to 48 hours to allow for the administration and effect of corticosteroids to enhance pulmonary maturity.

Several factors may contraindicate delaying birth with the use of tocolytic medications:[12]
- Fetus is older than 36 weeks gestation.
- Fetus is in acute distress or has died (or has a fatal anomaly).
- Cervical dilation is equal to or greater than 4 centimeters.
- Presence of Chorioamnionitis or intrauterine infection.
- Mother has severe pregnancy-induced hypertension, eclampsia, active vaginal bleeding, is cardiac disease or any other condition which warrants termination of pregnancy.
- Heavy vaginal bleeding during pregnancy which may cause risk to mother or fetus.

Commonly used tocolytic drugs, their mechanism of action and their doses:[12,13]

1. β Agonists: These agents act on β adrenergic receptors to cause smooth muscle relaxation.
   - Ritodrine: Loading dose 30 to 350 mcg/minute IV or 10 mg 2 hourly to 10-20 mg 4-6 hourly orally
   - Salbutamol: Dose 10 to 50 mcg/minute
   - Terbutaline: Dose 250 mcg S/C every 1 to 6 hours or by intravenous infusion started at 2.5 to 5 µg/min and increased every 20 minutes by increments of 5 µg/min to a maximum of 25 µg/min.
   - Isoxsuprine: Dose 0.5 to 1 mcg/min IV infusion to 10 mg I/M 8 hourly followed by 10-20 mg orally 8 hourly.
2. Magnesium sulfate: Magnesium ions reduce uterine contractility by displacing calcium ions, thus reducing excitation of the muscle.
   Dose 4 gm IV over 5-10 min or in 200 ml of normal saline to be given slowly over 20 minutes followed by 1-2 gm/hour intravenously.
3. Calcium channel blockers
   - Nifedipine: It is a calcium channel blocker that inhibits both prostaglandin and oxytocin induced contractions resulting in uterine relaxation.

Drugs in Pregnancy

Dose 10-20 mg oral stat followed by 20-40 mg 4-6 hourly not exceeding 160 mg/day

4. Atosiban: It is an oxytocin antagonist and thus inhibits uterine contractions.

   Dose: One bolus dose 0.9 ml (6.75 mg) is given IV during one minute; high dose infusion 24 ml/h (300 μg/min) during the first three hours; low dose infusion 8 ml/h (100 μg/min) up to 45 hours.

5. Indomethacin: It blocks the pathway for stimulation of uterine muscle contractions as it is a prostaglandin inhibitor.

   Dose 100 mg loading dose per rectum followed by 50 mg orally 6 hourly

6. Glyceryl trinitrate: It is a nitric oxide donor and causes smooth muscle relaxation *via* the metabolite nitric oxide (NO) which acts as a second messenger to increase calcium ion uptake.

   Dose 5-10 mg transdermal patch is applied to abdominal skin and repeat dose in 1 hour if contractions persist (maximum dose 20 mg in 24 hours).

Adverse Effects[12,13]

Salbutamol

- Maternal side effects: Tremor, anxiety, nausea, palpitations, chest pain, dyspnea or vomiting.
- Fetal and neonatal side effects: Fetal tachycardia, RDS, intracranial hemorrhage.

Terbutaline

- Maternal side effects: Pulmonary edema, cardiac or cardiopulmonary arrhythmias, myocardial ischemia, hypotension and tachycardia.
- Fetal and neonatal side effects: Fetal hyperinsulinemia, hyperglycemia, myocardial and septal hypertrophy, myocardial ischemia and tachycardia.

Ritodrine

- Maternal side effects: Metabolic hyperinsulinemia, hyperglycemia, hypokalemia, antidiuresis, altered thyroid function, physiologic tremors, palpitations, nervousness, nausea or vomiting, fever and hallucinations.
- Fetal and neonatal side effects: Neonatal tachycardia, hypoglycemia, hypocalcemia, hyperbilirubinemia, hypotension, and intraventricular hemorrhage.

Isoxsuprine

- Maternal side effects: Severe allergic reactions (rash; hives; difficulty in breathing; tightness in the chest; swelling of the mouth, face, lips, or tongue); chest pain; fast or irregular heartbeat and severe or persistent dizziness.

- Fetal and neonatal side effects: Fetal tachycardia, hypocalcemia, hypoglycemia, ileus and hypotension at high doses.

Magnesium Sulfate

- Maternal side effects: Flushing, lethargy, headache, muscle weakness, diplopia, dry mouth, pulmonary edema and cardiac arrest.
- Fetal and neonatal side effects: Lethargy, hypotonia, respiratory depression and demineralization with prolonged use.

Calcium Channel Blockers

- Maternal side effects: Flushing, headache, dizziness, nausea and transient hypotension. Caution should be used in patients with hypotension. In addition, concomitant use of calcium channel blockers and magnesium sulphate is potentially harmful and can result in cardiovascular collapse.
- Fetal and neonatal side effects: None noted as yet.

Atosiban

- Maternal side effects: Cardiac arrhythmias, muscular paralysis, central nervous system and respiratory depression in mother.
- Fetal and neonatal side effects: Cardiac arrhythmias, muscular paralysis, CNS and respiratory depression.

Indomethacin

- Maternal side effects: Nausea and heartburn.
- Fetal and neonatal side effects: Constriction of ductus arteriosus, pulmonary hypertension, reversible decrease in renal function with oligohydramnios, intraventricular hemorrhage, hyperbilirubinemia and necrotizing enterocolitis.

Glyceriye Trinitrite

- Maternal side effects: Headache, flushing, hypotension and tachycardia.
- Fetal and neonatal side effects: Tachycardia and asphyxia.
  Combining tocolytic drugs potentially increases maternal morbidity and should be used with caution.

CORTICOSTEROIDS

Both topical and systemic corticosteroids are used for a variety of autoimmune and inflammatory conditions like eczema, psoriasis and asthma. Topical and inhaled steroid therapy during pregnancy for other diseases is not associated with any risks for the child even though small amounts of the steroids are

Drugs in Pregnancy

absorbed. Recent meta-analysis suggests a small but significant association between use of systemic corticosteroids during the first trimester and oral clefts. This is consistent with results of animal studies. No similar evidence exists for topical or inhaled corticosteroids, probably because of much lower systemic exposure.

Liggins and Howie[14] were the first to describe the beneficial effects of antenatal corticosteroids (ANCS) on lung maturity in preterm neonates. Use of ANCS have been associated with a decrease in Respiratory Distress Syndrome (RDS) related mortality and morbidity in infants < 34 weeks of gestation. Additionally long term follow up studies have ruled out any harmful effect on the lungs, growth and development.[14,15] The national institute of health consensus statement (1995) endorsed the use of ANCS and since then, this has become standard practice in the management of preterm labor (< 34 weeks of gestation).

Beta-agonists should be used to delay delivery for 24 to 48 hours in order to administer corticosteroids to promote fetal lung maturation. Maternal corticosteroid is administered by giving two doses of 12 mg betamethasone 24 hours apart or four doses of 6 mg dexamethasone intramuscularly 12 hours apart. The effect of treatment is optimal if the baby is delivered between 24 hours to 7 days after the start of treatment. Although it seems that the effect on lung maturity can be sustained effectively by repeated courses of ANCS, use of multiple courses may cause potential side effects of steroids on the fetal hypothalamic-pituitary-adrenal (HPA) axis, future growth and development. A retrospective analysis of 710 infants enrolled in the North American Thyrotrophin-Releasing Hormone Trial,[16] has shown that more than 2 courses of ANCS was associated with a small decrease in fetal growth and lower plasma cortisol levels at 2 hours of age but no change in head circumference or neonatal mortality. Therefore more than one course of ANCS is not recommended.[17]

Cochrane Database Systematic Review, 2008 compared different corticosteroids and regimens for accelerating fetal lung maturation for women at risk of preterm birth. They concluded that dexamethasone has some benefits compared with betamethasone such as less intraventricular hemorrhage, although perhaps a higher rate of NICU admission (seen in only one trial). Apart from a suggestion from another small trial that the intramuscular route may have advantages over an oral route for dexamethasone, few other conclusions about optimal antenatal corticosteroid regimens were made.

ANTIEMETICS

Antiemetic Drugs used in Pregnancy[1,3]

Nausea is a common complaint during pregnancy especially during the first trimester. It generally subsides after first trimester and does not require any medication but sometimes it becomes excessive and may cause dehydration and electrolyte imbalance. In such cases it becomes essential to treat the condition vigorously. Table 29.3 gives the doses and safety profile of commonly used antiemetics in pregnancy.

Table 29.3: List of commonly used antiemetics				
Drugs	*Dose*	*Max dose*	*Adverse effects*	*Safety in pregnancy*
Dopaminergic antagonists				
Metoclopramide	10 mg po or IV tds	30 mg	Dystonia, extrapyra-midal effects, Sedation	Not established
Prochlorperazine	5 mg po/PR tds or 12.5 mg IM/IV tds	35-50 mg	Dystonia, extrapyramidal effect, Sedation	Use with caution
Domperidone	25 mg PR, 10-20 mg po tds	60 mg	Extrapyramidal reactions rare	Use with caution
Antihistamines				
Promethazine	25 mg po tds	100 mg	Sedation	Use with caution
Pheniramine	43.5 mg ½ tab po tds	130 mg	Sedation	Use with caution
Dimenhydrinate	50 mg po tds	150 mg	Sedation	Use with caution
Anticholinergics				
Doxylamine	10 mg (+10 mg Vitamin B6)	—	Sedation	May be given
	1bd during day and 2 HS	40 mg	—	
5HT3 receptor antagonists				
Ondansetron	2-8 mg tabs or po/IV tds	32 mg	Constipation	May be given
Nutritional supplement				
Pyridoxine (Vitamin B_6)	10-30 mg orally for up to 3 week	—	Numbness, tiredness, low sensorium	May be given

DRUGS FOR BRONCHIAL ASTHMA

A joint committee of the American College of Obstetricians and Gynecologists (ACOG) and the American College of Allergy, Asthma and Immunology (ACAAI)[18] was recently convened to provide guidance for physicians on asthma management of pregnant patients, particularly with regard to the use of newer asthma and allergy medications. The committee's recommendations included:

- A stepped approach, beginning with inhaled β2-agonists for mild, intermittent asthma and including inhaled cromolyn for mild persistent asthma; inhaled corticosteroids for moderate persistent asthma and inhaled plus oral corticosteroids for severe persistent asthma (Table 29.4).
- Use of either beclomethasone or budesonide if inhaled corticosteroids are initiated during pregnancy.
- Consideration of inhaled salmeterol instead of or in addition to, theophylline for asthma that is not controlled by inhaled corticosteroids.
- Avoidance of oral decongestants during the first trimester.

In general, the committee preferred inhaled medications (because they have fewer systemic effects) and time-tested drugs (because of greater experience with their use during pregnancy). Physicians are advised to limit the use of medication as much as possible during the first trimester, although birth defects related to most asthma drugs are uncommon.

Table 29.4: Step therapy for chronic asthma during pregnancy			
Category	Frequency/severity of symptoms	Pulmonary function (untreated)	Step therapy
Mild intermittent	Symptoms not > twice/ week; nocturnal symptoms < twice/ month, brief exacerbations, asymptomatic between episodes	Normal > 80% pulmonary function between episodes	Inhaled β 2-agonists as needed
Mild persistent	Symptoms > twice/week but persistent not daily; nocturnal symptoms > twice/ month; exacerbations affect activity.	80%	Inhaled cromolyn; continue inhaled nedocromil; substitute inhaled beclomethasone/ budesonide if not adequate
Moderate persistent	Daily symptoms; nocturnal symptoms >once/week; exacerbations affect activity	60%-80%	Inhaled beclomethasone or budesonide continue inhaled salmeterol, add oral theophylline and/or inhaled salmeterol for patients inadequately controlled by medium-dose inhaled corticosteroids
Severe persistent	Continual symptoms; limited activity; frequent nocturnal symptoms; frequent acute exacerbations.	Less than 60%	Treatment as described above, plus oral corticosteroids

Safety in Pregnancy[3,5,18]

Inhaled Steroids

Beclomethasone, 2-5 puffs 6-12 hourly for asthma and/or 2 sprays in each nostril 12 hourly to control allergic rhinitis. May be used safely during pregnancy and lactation in usual doses.

Oral Steroids

Prednisone, short courses of 40 mg/day in single or divided doses for 1 week and then taper over 1 week. If prolonged therapy is necessary, a single morning dose of prednisone on alternate days may help to minimize side effects. Intake of steroid tablets for a long time may increase the risk of cleft palate in the baby.

Cromolyn Sodium

Mast cell stabilizer, 2 puffs 6 hourly for asthma and/or 2 sprays in each nostril 6-12 hourly to control allergic rhinitis. May be used safely during pregnancy and lactation in usual doses.

Inhaled Beta Agonists

Two puffs every 4 hours as needed. No adverse effect has been seen in the fetus during pregnancy and lactation in usual doses.

Theophylline

Oral sustained-release preparations to reach serum concentrations of 8-12 µg/mL. Despite widespread use no harmful effects on unborn fetus have been described.

Decongestants

Pseudoephedrine, phenylephrine, phenylpropanolamine and oxymetazoline, intranasal spray for rhinosinusitis can be used in pregnancy. No adverse effect has been seen in the fetus during pregnancy and lactation in usual doses with these medicines.

Antihistaminics

Chlorphenaramine,bromphenaramine,triprolidine can be safely used in pregnancy. Diphenhydramine is safe in pregnancy but may exert oxytocic action. Terfenadine is also not associated with increased risk to fetus.

Non sedative antihistaminics

Studies on loratidine, cetrizine, fexofenadine, astemizole, cromolyn sodium have shown that risk of congenital anomalies in the fetus does not increase with the use of these drugs in pregnancy.

Expectorants

With use of guaiphenesin with or without dextromethorphan, no adverse effect has been seen in the fetus during pregnancy and lactation. Other mucolytics or expectorants containing potassium iodide should be avoided after ten weeks as iodide can cross the placenta and may cause fetal goiter.

Antitussives

Dextromethorphan is safe in pregnancy. Alcohol-containing preparations should be avoided for long term use.

GASTROINTESTINAL DRUGS

Antacids

Antacids containing aluminium, calcium, magnesium, magaldrate, sodium bicarbonate and combinations of these are associated with minimal risk to fetus when used in moderate doses.

Proton Pump Inhibitors

Omeprazole and pantoprazoe are used to treat hyperacidity during pregnancy has not shown to increase adverse effects on the fetus.

Ranitidine is a preferred after antacid. It is generally considered safe in pregnancy.

ANTIDOPAMINERGIC DRUGS IN PREGNANCY

Issues surrounding the treatment of hyperprolactinemia in pregnancy are mainly concerned with the effects of dopamine agonists on the fetus and the possible stimulatory effect of the increased estrogen levels of pregnancy on tumor size.

The safety of bromocriptine exposure in utero has been evaluated by extensive monitoring including a multicentric study of 2587 pregnancies in 2437 women exposed to bromocriptine during part or all of gestation, with examinations of offspring up to the age of 9 years. The drug does not appear to be associated with any increase in the risk of spontaneous abortion, congenital abnormalities, multiple pregnancies and no adverse effects on postnatal development have been detected. However, it is advised that fetal exposure to bromocriptine should be limited to as short a period as possible by discontinuing the drug as soon as pregnancy is confirmed.

Data on the safety of use in pregnancy of cabergoline and quinagolide is limited compared with bromocriptine. Over 300 pregnancies have been recorded in women taking cabergoline and almost 200 in women taking quinagolide and no apparent adverse effects on the pregnancy or fetal development have been detected.[19,20]

For women with microadenomas, the subsequent risk of adenoma growth during pregnancy appears to be 1% after discontinuing the drug and symptomatic follow-up in each trimester appears to be reasonable in such patients. For women with macroadenomas, prepregnancy debulking of the tumor may be undertaken with appropriate follow-up (2.8% risk of tumor enlargement).

Dose

Bromocriptine is started at 1.25 mg orally at bedtime for a week after which it is gradually increased upto 5 mg 12 hourly.

Cabergoline is started at 0. 25 mg twice a week for 4 weeks. The dose can be increased stepwise in 0.5 mg increments until reaching lowest maximally effective and tolerated dose. Consensus has not been reached regarding maximum safe dose during pregnancy. For suppressing lactation, 0.25 mg is given 12 hourly for two days or 1 mg stat may be given.

ANTIEPILEPTICS IN PREGNANCY[1-6]

Approximately 0.5-2% of pregnant women are on antiepileptic medication. A benefit risk assessment is important for the mother and child and usually there is more risk for the both mother and the child if the mother's seizures are not controlled during pregnancy. It is best that women with epilepsy who are wishing to get pregnant should have their epilepsy properly controlled before conceiving and have higher doses of folic acid supplements. Pregnancy seems to affect different epileptic women in different ways. There is no change in the status of 50%, about 40% show improvement and remaining 10% get worse.

Single drug therapy at the lowest effective dose should be aimed for. Women should be offered a detailed level II ultrasound examination and their levels of maternal serum alpha-fetoproteins should be monitored. With proper prenatal and postpartum management, up to 95 percent of pregnancies in which women took antiepileptics are reported to have favorable outcome.

Although most first-line antiepileptic drugs have been associated with some degree of fetal risk, the vast majority of exposed fetuses are not affected. Dose of antiepileptic drug may have to be increased with advancing period of gestation especially if other high risk factors like hypertension, hyponatremia, and hypoalbuminemia are associated (Table 29.5).

All three first-line drugs for treating epilepsy—carbamazepine (Tegretol), valproic acid (Depakote), and phenytoin (Dilantin)—have been associated with some fetal risks[21-26] (Table 29.5).

Patients on carbamazepine, valproic acid, and phenytoin can breastfeed their infants because a very small amount of these drugs is excreted into breast milk. These have no apparent effect on the baby. Phenobarbital, however, is excreted in large amounts into breast milk and is not compatible with breast-feeding, because it may cause sedation and CNS depression in the baby.

The babies of women treated with enzyme inducing anticonvulsants (carbamazepine, phenytoin, primidone, phenobarbitone) are at increased risk of hemorrhagic disease of the newborn caused by deficiency of vitamin K-dependent clotting factors. Women on these drugs should be treated prophylactically with vitamin K daily from 36 weeks gestation at a dose of 10 mg/day oral × 1 month prepartum until delivery and their babies should receive vitamin K 1 mg IM at birth.

29

Drugs in Pregnancy

Drug	Foetal risk	Effect on fetus	Acts by
Phenytoin 100 mg. 12 hourly to a maximum of 400 mgm/day	10% (highest risk)	Fetal hydantoin syndrome	Prolonged inactivation of sodium channels, increasing GABA.
Valproic acid 200 mg TDS, maximum of 800 mg, 8 hourly.	5-9% risk	Neural tube and limb defect	As above
Carbamazepine 200-400 mg, TDS	1%, lowest risk	Neural tube and limb defect	Prolonged inactivation of sodium channels
Phenobarbital 60 mg, 1-3 times a day	Risk not high	Studies claim that it lowers IQ	GABA receptor mediated synaptic inhibition
Newer antiepileptics Lamotrigine, Gabapentin, Topiramate Oxcarbazepine	0-2.4%	Neural tube defects	

Table 29.5: Antiepileptics in pregnancy

Hypertensive disorders during pregnancy are classified into 4 categories, as recommended by the National High Blood Pressure Education Program Working Group on High Blood Pressure in Pregnancy: chronic hypertension, preeclampsia-eclampsia, preeclampsia superimposed on chronic hypertension and gestational hypertension (transient hypertension of pregnancy or chronic hypertension identified in the later half of pregnancy). This terminology is preferred over the older but widely used term PIH (pregnancy-induced hypertension) because it is more precise.

Antihypertensive drugs should be used in pregnancy only if conservative therapy including optimum bedrest, diet control and sedation fails and blood pressure is higher than 160/100 m.[27-33] The purpose of giving treatment is to prevent maternal complications and if possible to prolong pregnancy till the fetal maturity is achieved.

The commonly used drugs can be classified as:

I. *Sympatholytics*
   Central sympatholytics → Methyldopa, Clonidine
   Beta Adrenergic Blockers → Propranolol, Metoprolol, Atenolol
   Alpha Adrenergic Blockers → Prazosin, Phentolamine
   Alpha and beta adrenergic blockers →Labetalol

II. *Vasodilators*
   Arteriolar → Hydralazine, diazoxide
   Arteriolar + Venous → Sodium nitroprusside

III. *Diuretics* → Not used in pregnancy as antihypertensives but is used selectively in some patients with pulmonary edema or congestive heart failure.

IV. *Calcium channel blockers* → Nifedipine, Verapamil

V. *ACE inhibitors* → Contraindicated in pregnancy.

Alphamethyldopa (Aldomet)

Safe, first line antihypertensive drug, reduces maternal and perinatal morbidity and mortality. Act on central alpha 2 receptors to decrease efferent sympathetic activity. It reduces the peripheral vascular resistance with minimal effect on cardiac output. Aldomet leads to dilatation of both arteries and veins which increases intravascular volume. It also maintains renal blood flow. After oral administration, less than one third of the dose is absorbed. It is partly metabolized and is partly excreted in urine. The onset of its antihypertensive effect is over 4-6 hours and lasts for 12-24 hours. Aldomet crosses the placenta and is excreted at low concentration in human breast milk, but no neonatal side effect has been associated with its use. Side effects associated with this drug occur in about 22% of patients who may suffer from mild depression, sedation, postural hypotension, hepatitis. It might lead to a problem during cross matching of blood, as methyldopa treatment causes a positive direct coomb's test. Dose: 250 mg BD or TDS, gradually increasing as required over a period of 2 days to a maximum of 3 gm/day. Contraindications to methyldopa are hepatic disorders, psychiatric patients and congestive cardiac failure.

Labetalol

Reasonably safe first-line medication Combined alpha and beta adrenergic blocking agent widely used in treating hypertension during pregnancy. Unlike some other beta-blockers, it is not associated with fetal growth restriction. Intravenous and oral forms are used as an alternative to hydralazine in severe preeclampsia/eclampsia. It is contraindicated in patients with hypersensitivity, cardiogenic shock, pulmonary edema, bradycardia, atrioventricular block, uncompensated congestive heart failure and reactive airway disease. Dose: Labetalol – 400 to 800 mg/day in divided doses to a maximum of 2400 mg/day. If BP $\geq$ 160/110 mm Hg: 20 mg IV bolus; subsequent doses of 40 mg followed by 80 mg IV may be administered at 10 min intervals to achieve BP controlor up to a total of 300 mg has been injected. It may also be administered as continuous infusion of 1 mg/kg/hour.

Atenolol

Not safe for use in pregnancy. Associated with intrauterine growth restriction when used in randomized trials focusing on the treatment of chronic hypertension during pregnancy. Selectively blocks beta-1 receptors with little or no effect on beta-2 receptors. Concern exists that beta-blockers prescribed during pregnancy, particularly atenolol, may be associated with intrauterine growth restriction. Beta-adrenergic blockade may reduce symptoms of acute hypoglycemia and mask signs of hyperthyroidism; abrupt withdrawal may exacerbate symptoms of hyperthyroidism and cause thyroid storm; so the patient must be monitored closely and drug is withdrawn slowly. Contraindications include hypersensitivity; congestive heart failure, cardiogenic shock, AV conduction abnormalities, heart block (without a pacemaker) and pulmonary edema. Dose is 50-100 mg PO od.

Vasodilators

Nitroprusside

Reduces peripheral resistance by acting directly on arteriolar and venous smooth muscle. This is a rapid-acting parenteral antihypertensive of short duration of action. Its use is restricted to cases of severe hypertension not responsive to other drugs. Its safety for use during pregnancy has not been established.Contraindicated in documented hypersensitivity; subaortic stenosis, idiopathic hypertrophic cardiomyopathy and atrial fibrillation or flutter. If BP $\geq$ 160/110 mm Hg it is given in the dose of 0.25 mcg/kg/min continuous I/V infusion, titrate to BP with maximum dose of 5 mcg/kg/min. Infusion rates >10 mcg/kg/min IV may lead to cyanide toxicity.

Hydralazine

It acts on the smooth muscles of arterial vasculature leading to vasodilatation. Hydralazine increases cardiac output by vasodilatation. It also increases plasma volume by reflex stimulation of the renin angiotensin system. If administered orally, peak action occurs by 3 to 4 hours. Action of hydralazine lasts for 6 to 12 hours. Its side effects include headache, anxiety, nausea, flushing epigastric pain and lupus like syndrome. Dose is 40-200 mg twice a day.

Calcium Channel Blockers

Nifedipine

Acts by decreasing peripheral resistance without compromising cardiac output. Their onset of action is fast without any sedative effect. These agents prevent influx of calcium in vascular smooth muscle cells leading to vascular relaxation. They also relax the uterus and can be used for tocolysis. It causes no major side effect on the mother or the fetus. It can also be used in cases of fulminating preeclampsia by oral route to obtain a quick reduction in blood pressure levels. Sublingual administration should be avoided as it may lead to unpredictable absorption resulting in sudden fall in maternal blood pressure which might compromise the maternal cerebral circulation and decrease the uteroplacental blood flow with consequent fetal distress. Avoid concurrent use with magnesium sulphate because of risk of profound hypotension. Side effects are mild in the form of flushes, headache, GI upset, and ischemic pain. Dose: Nifedipine 5 to 30 mg 2 to 3 times/day, maximum dose 80-120 mg/ day.

Diuretics

Hypertension in pregnancy is accompanied by depletion of the central intravascular volume which is worsened by diuretics. So diuretic use in PIH should be avoided. However it may be used with caution in cases of pregnancy induced hypertensive disorder with pulmonary edema or with congestive heart failure. Diuretics causes hyperuricemia and hinders the use of serum uric acid as a sensitive indicator of disease process in PIH. It increases excretion of water by interfering with chloride-binding cotransport system, which in turn inhibits sodium and chloride reabsorption in ascending loop of Henle and distal renal tubule. Dose: 10 mg IV initial dose of furosemide increased to 20-80 mg/d PO/IV/IM.

Angiotensin Converting Enzyme Inhibitor

These agents are strictly contraindicated in pregnancy as they might cause renal failure in the fetus. Skeletal abnormalities like deficient skull ossification and limb reduction defects are drugs specific abnormalities.

ANTICONVULSANTS

Convulsions in a pregnant patient may endanger life of both mother and fetus.

Magnesium Sulfate

$MgSO_4$ is the drug of choice for prophylaxis and treatment of eclamptic fits. Compared with the traditional drugs used to terminate seizures (e.g. diazepam, dilantin), magnesium sulfate has a lower risk of recurrent seizures with lower perinatal morbidity and mortality. Seizures usually terminate after the loading dose of magnesium. Once the seizures terminate, most patients have an improved blood pressure control. Benzodiazepine or phenytoin (Dilantin) can be used for seizures that are not responsive to magnesium sulfate. After the initial loading dose of magnesium, significant hypertension continues in approximately 10-15% of eclamptic patients. Maintaining a diastolic BP of 90 mm Hg is the goal of antihypertensive therapy. Magnesium ions block neuromuscular transmission by blocking release of acetylcholine from the nerve endings. $MgSO_4$ may also have some central action. It can be given by IV/IM route for seizure prophylaxis in preeclampsia but for treating true eclampsia, IV route is preferred for a quicker action. **Pritchard Regime:** On admission 4 gm (8 ml-50% weight per volume ampoules) is diluted with 12 ml of distilled water (20% solution) and injected IV over 5-10 min followed by 10 ml of 50% solution (5 gm) IM in each buttock. Subsequent dose of 10 ml 50% solution (5 gm) of magnesium sulfate IM is given in alternate buttock every four hours. In cases of eclampsia, $MgSO_4$ is continued for 24 hours after delivery. **Zuspan Regimen:** Loading dose of magnesium sulfate for an active/recent seizure is 4-6 g IV over 20 minutes (dilute the 50% solution with normal saline and administer the 20% solution using an infusion pump) followed by a maintenance dose of magnesium sulfate 1-2 g/hour as IV infusion. Concurrent use of magnesium sulfate with nifedipine may cause hypotension and neuromuscular blockade. $MgSO_4$ may cause hyporeflexia, respiratory depression and bradycardia. Patient's reflexes should be monitored and infusion should be discontinued if reflexes are absent or if serum magnesium level exceeds 7 mEq/L. Levels of 8-12 mEq/dL may cause loss of reflexes, diplopia, flushing or slurring of speech; levels >12 mEq/dL may cause muscular paralysis, ventilatory failure and circulatory collapse; patients should have

29

Drugs in Pregnancy

frequent neurological evaluation. Presence of patellar reflex, adequate respiratory function RR > 14/min and urinary output > 25 ml/hr is ensured before administering each dose. Loss of deep tendon reflex indicates that the magnesium level may be toxic; some clinicians follow serum magnesium levels 6 hourly along with neurological examination; magnesium may alter cardiac conduction, leading to heart block in digitalized patients. Calcium gluconate 10% solution 10-20 ml slow IV can be given as an antidote for clinically significant hypermagnesemia.

Phenytoin

It is used if the patient has recurrent seizures despite optimum magnesium sulfate therapy. May also be used in cases of renal failure, serious magnesium-related toxicity or when seizures occur due to causes other than eclampsia. Phenytoin acts on motor cortex where it inhibits spread of seizure activity. Activity of brain stem centers responsible for tonic phase of grand mal seizures also may be inhibited. Dose of phenytoin is 20 mg/kg loading by infusion at a maximum rate of 50 mg/min IV followed by maintenance dose of 200 mg 8 hourly.

Diazepam

Useful for treatment of seizures resistant to magnesium sulfate. Depresses all levels of CNS, possibly by increasing activity of gamma amino butyric acid (GABA). Dose is 10 mg slow I/Vat a rate of 1 mg/min.

ANTITHROMBOTIC THERAPY

Use of antithrombotic drugs is required during pregnancy for prevention of venous thromboembolism (VTE) in high-risk patients, treatment of VTE and prevention of arterial emboli in patients with mechanical heart valve prostheses.[34,35] However, there are several problems with use of anti-thrombotic drugs during pregnancy.

Warfarin

Warfarin, as well as the other coumarin compounds, cross the placenta and have the potential to cause both bleeding in the fetus and teratogenicity. Warfarin embryopathy may occur in 4-10% of patients if it is given during the first trimester. The daily maintenance dose of warfarin differs greatly between individuals, commonly between 0.5 mg/day and 15 mg/day, and often fluctuates.

The drug is rapidly and completely absorbed and immediately blocks further hepatic synthesis of the functional vitamin K-dependent procoagulants (II, VII, IX, X). However, its impact on the INR (international normalized ratio) is delayed until preformed coagulation factors are removed, so dose adjustment must allow for these delayed effects. INR is a good indicator of effectiveness and risk of bleeding during warfarin therapy and is best kept at about 2.5, with a target range of 2.0-3.0

Maternal effects of warfarin sodium can be reversed by giving fresh frozen plasma but the fetus requires 1-2 weeks after discontinuation of treatment to reverse anticoagulant effect. A pregnant woman on warfarin therapy is switched over to heparin during the first twelve weeks to avoid teratogenic effects and last 4 weeks of pregnancy to avoid fetal maternal complications during delivery.

Unfractionated Heparin (UFH) and Low Molecular Weight Heparin (LMWH)

These do not cross the placenta and are safe for the fetus, but long-term treatment with UFH is problematic because of it's inconvenient route of administration, need to continuously monitor anticoagulant activity and its potential side effects, such as heparin-induced thrombocytopenia and osteoporosis.

LMWH is the drug of choice in the prevention and treatment of VTE during pregnancy because of the ease of administration, monitoring and lower risk of side effects.

Patients with mechanical heart valve prostheses represent a major clinical challenge. Warfarin, the drug of choice in nonpregnant women, can be administered between the 12th and 36th week. Full-dose UFH is recommended in the first trimester and after week 36. The patient on heparin will have normal clotting 4-6 hours after discontinuing the medication.

ANTITUBERCULAR DRUGS IN PREGNANCY

Pregnancy with tuberculosis presents a therapeutic challenge. Snider et al[36] reviewed all available literature on pregnant women treated with isoniazid (INH), ethambutol (EMB), rifampicin (RMP) or streptomycin (SM) and reported on the relative safety of these drugs and whether risk of teratogenesis justifies abortion on medical grounds. Other than the ototoxicity of SM, none of these drugs in normal dosages are proved teratogens to human fetuses. The use of INH in combination with EMB for a pregnant woman with tuberculosis is recommended, if the disease is not extensive. If a third drug is warranted, then RMP could be added. Because of its ototoxicity, SM should not be used, unless RMP is contraindicated or proves unsatisfactory. Routine therapeutic abortion is not indicated for a pregnant woman who is taking first-line antituberculosis drugs.

VACCINES

Vaccination of a pregnant woman with inactivated vaccines has not been shown to cause an increase risk to the fetus. Live vaccines are usually

29

Drugs in Pregnancy

contraindicated in pregnancy because pregnancy is an immunocompromised state and there is a potential risk of causing the disease in the mother and the fetus.

Vaccines that should be Avoided during Pregnancy

- Live, attenuated influenza vaccine. While a woman is recommended to receive the influenza vaccine while pregnant, she should not receive the live version of the vaccine.
- MMR. Women who are pregnant should not receive live, weakened viral vaccines, including the ones for measles, mumps and rubella (MMR). A woman should avoid becoming pregnant for four weeks after receiving this vaccine.
- Varicella. As with MMR, this vaccine contains a live, weakened virus and should not be given to a pregnant women. Additionally, women should avoid becoming pregnant for at least one month after receiving this vaccine.
- Rabies vaccine contains inactivated rabies virus and can be given to pregnant woman in case of exposure.

ANTIDEPRESSANT DRUGS

- Selective serotonin reuptake inhibitors tricyclic antidepressants are good therapeutic choices during pregnancy.
- Lithium salts should be discontinued till 8 weeks as it may cause Ebstein anomaly.
- MAO inhibitors should be avoided as threatening hyperthermic crisis may be precipitated.

ANALGESICS DURING PREGNANCY

- Salicylates[37]: Other than aspirin and acetaminophen pose theoretical risk of closure of ductus arteriosis and associated cardiac and pulmonary abnormality.
- No adverse outcome with low dose aspirin, paracetamol intake.
- Ketorolac, pentazocin should be used cautiously during pregnancy and safety has not been established during lactation.
- Tramadol: Safety has not been established during pregnancy or lactation.
- Analgin, nimuselide are contraindicated during pregnancy.
- Indomethacin: Its effects are reversible as long as drug is not given after 34 weeks. It causes oligoamnios, constriction of ductus arteriosus, intraventricular hemorrhage and necrotising enterocolitis.
- Narcotic analgesis (Meperidine, morphine): It cause neonatal withdrawal syndrome.

IMMUNOSUPPRESSIVE DRUGS

- Used in patients with organ transplants.
- Corticosteroids therapy is associated with cleft lip and cleft palate in animal studies.
- Azathioprine is safe for use in human pregnancy.
- Cyclosporin has significant maternal toxicity especially nephrotoxicity and should be given only if benefits outweigh risks.
- Cyclophosphamide is a suspected teratogen and should be avoided in early pregnancy.

ANTINEOPLASTICS

The use of antineoplastic agents in pregnant women poses obvious risks to both the woman and the developing fetus, particularly during organogenesis.

Antimetabolites

Folate antagonists (aminopterin,methotrexate) cause fetal aminopterin syndrome and should be avoided during pregnancy.

Alkylating Agents

Busulfan causes fetal growth retardation, cleft palate and eye defects in the fetus. Use of cyclophosphamide during pregnancy is associated with major congenital anomalies in 14% while 86% fetuses were normal. It causes cleft palate, absence of digits, imperforate anus and fetal growth retardation. It should be avoided during first trimester but can be given later.

Plant Alkaloids

Vincristine and vinblastine have shown to slightly increase the risk of developing congenital anomalies during first trimester but can be given to treat life threatening malignancies like acute leukemias.

Antibiotics

Use of daunorubicin, doxorubicin, bleomycin should be guarded especially during the first trimester but they may be administered later in pregnancy. No reports linking the use of bleomycin with congenital defects in humans have been seen. These drugs may be used during first trimester to treat acute leukemias or lymphomas as life saving therapy, although adverse effects on the fetus cannot be ruled out.

Alcohol

- Threshold value: 15 ml/day.
- Causes growth restriction and behavioral disturbances in the fetus.

- Brain, cardiac and spinal defects in the baby have been noted.
- Craniofacial abnormalities are associated.
- Even low levels of alcohol cannot be recommended during pregnancy.

ANTI-INFECTIVE AGENTS (TABLE 29.6)

Table 29.6: Anti-infective agents[3,4]

Category A	Category B	Category C	Category D
Nystatin vaginal tablets	Amoxicillin, Ampicillin, amoxicillin-clavulanate, Nitrofurantoin Metronidazole (although there is some controversy about oral intake in the first trimester), Cephalosporins Clindamycin, Erythromycin, Azithromycin, Sulfa drugs (except near term), Famciclovir Valacyclovir, Clotrimazole-vaginal	Septran, Trimethoprim, Clarithromycin, Ciprofloxacin, Fluconazole, Miconazole, Isoniazid, Rifampin, Mebendazole, Albendazole Ziduvidine, Chloroquine, Acyclovir, Pyrantel Ganciclovir Oseltamivir (Tamiflu)	Tetracycline derivatives, which can cause discoloration of teeth: tetracycline, doxycycline, minocycline, Sulfa drugs - if near delivery (because they can increase the chance of serious newborn jaundice), Quinine, Aminoglycosides (cause ototoxicity in 1-2%), chloramphenicol (grey baby syndrome).

ANESTHETIC DRUGS

General Anesthesia

No report of teratogenecity in humans has been associated with the use of thiopental, curare and succinylcholine.

Inhalational anesthesia including nitrous oxide and halothane have not been reported to increase risk to fetus.

Local Anesthesia

Use of lidocaine and bupivacaine is not associated with any major or minor malformations of the fetus.

ORAL CONTRACEPTIVES

Accidental use of oral contraceptives during pregnancy has not been reported to be associated with congenital anomalies.

ESTABLISHING PREGNANCY EXPOSURE REGISTRIES [38]

In spite of the lack of data on the safety of drug use in human pregnancies, pregnant women are exposed to drugs either as prescribed therapy or inadvertently before pregnancy is known (over one-half of pregnancies are unplanned). Because little is known about the teratogenic potential of a drug in humans before marketing, epidemiologically sound,written study protocols for post-marketing surveillance of drug use in pregnancy is critical for the detection of drug-induced fetal effects.

FDA defines a pregnancy exposure registry as a prospective observational study that collects information on women who take medicines and vaccines during pregnancy.

Enrollment requires that the health of the baby be unknown to reduce bias. Data collected on babies born to women taking a particular medicine are compared with babies of women not taking the medicine. Thus these studies are being increasingly used to proactively monitor for major fetal effects and to describe margins of safety associated with drug exposure during pregnancy. These will provide vital information to the clinicians regarding counseling of a patient on medication as to the actual risk involved to the fetus at different periods of gestation.

While sufficient data is not available to give definitive recommendations regarding the ideal therapy for most of the disorders during pregnancy, this chapter attempts to outline the broadly acceptable clinical therapeutic guidelines and other suitable options available. This chapter is not exhaustive and the reader is encouraged to refer to package inserts and evolving management options appearing from time to time in recent journals.

29

REFERENCES

1. Young LY, Koda-Kimble MA. Applied Therapeutics: The Clinical Use of Drugs. 6th edn. Vancouver, WA: Applied Therapeutics, Inc.; 1995.
2. DiPiro JT, Talbert RL, Yee GC, Matzke GR, Wells BG, Posey LM. Pharmacotherapy: A Pathophysiologic Approach. 3rd edn. Stamford, CT: Appleton & Lange; 1997:1565-84.
3. Berkow R. The Merck Manual of Diagnosis and Therapy. 16th edn. Rahway, NJ: Merck Research Laboratories; 1992:1857-62.
4. Finasteride for benign prostatic hypertrophy. Drug Ther Bull 1995;33:19
5. FDA. Federal Register 1980;44:37434.
6. Briggs GG, et al. Drugs in Pregnancy and Lactation. A Reference Guide to Fetal and Neonatal Risk. 4th edn. Baltimore, MD: Williams & Wilkins; 1994.
7. McQueen, KD. Drugs in Pregnancy and Lactation. In: Textbook of Therapeutics: Drug and Disease Management. 6th edn. Herfindal T, Gourley DR, (Eds.) Williams & Wilkins: Baltimore MD. 1996.
8. Koren G, Pastuszak A, Itso S. Drugs in pregnancy. N Engl J Med 1998;338:1128-36.
9. Koren G, Bologa M, Long D, et al. Perception of teratogenic risk by pregnant women exposed to drugs and chemicals during the first trimester. Am J Obstet Gynecol 1989;160:1190-94.
10. Pikee Saxena, Sudha Salhan, Nivedita Sarda, Deoki Nandan. A randomized comparison between sublingual, oral and vaginal route of misoprostol for preabortion cervical ripening in first-trimester pregnancy termination in Australian New Zealand Journal of Obstet Gynecol 2008;48:101-6
11. King JF, Grant A, Keirse MJ, Chalmers, I. Beta-mimetics in preterm labour: An overview of the randomized controlled trials. Br J Obstet Gynaecol 1988;95:211-22.
12. Goodwin TM, Zografyan A. Oxtocin receptor antagonists. Update. Clin Perinatol 1998; 25:859-71.
13. Slattery MM, Morrison JJ. Preterm Delivery. Lancet 2002;360:1489-97.
14. King J, Flenady V. Prophylactic antibiotics for inhibiting preterm labor with intact membranes. Cochrane Database Systemic Rev 2002;(4):CD000246.
15. NIH Consensus Development Panel on the effects of cortiocosteroids for fetal maturation on perinatal outcomes. JAMA 1995;273:413-18.

Antiemetic drugs used in pregnancy 550
Antiemetics 550
Antiepileptics in pregnancy 554, 555
Antiglobulin 259
Antihistamines 551
Antihistaminics 553
Antihypertensive drugs 307
Anti-infective agents 564
Antimetabolites 563
Antineoplastics 563
Antiretroviral drugs 478
Antiretroviral therapy 480
Antithrombotic therapy 560
Antithyroid drugs (ATD) 414
Antitubercular drugs in pregnancy 561
Antituberculosis treatment 443
Antitussives 553
Anxiolytics 528
Aortic regurgitation 382
Aortic stenosis 382
Arterial blood gases (ABG) 394, 524
Arterial flow 185
Arteriography 394
ARV in different situations 481
Assessment of
    general fetal anatomy 28
    response to therapy 284
    thyroid function in pregnancy 407
Assisted reproductive technique (ART) 152, 155
Asymmetrical growth restriction 177
Asymptomatic bacteriuria (ASBU) 431
Atenolol 557
Atosiban 549
Atrial flutter 35
Atrial septal defect (ASD) 36, 376
Augmentation of labor 247
Autoimmune thyroid disorders and miscarriages 419
Autonomic dysfunction 332
Autosomal dominant polycystic kidney disease 435

B

Basic biology of energy balance 488
Behavioral alteration 78
Betamimetics 82
Biguanides 335

Biochemical
    markers 7, 77
    screening 30
    serum markers 8
    studies 184
Biophysical profile 58, 62, 69, 116, 189
Biophysical tests 301
Biparietal diameter 182
Birth after cesarean 249
Birth asphyxia 219
Bladder 29
Blood glucose levels for initiating insulin therapy 336
Blunt dissection 248
Bone length abnormalities 48
Bone marrow activity 278
Borderline ventriculomegaly 40
Bradycardia 35
Brain 300
Breastfeeding 475
Breech extraction 218
Breech presentation 201
Brow presentation 226
Burns and Marshall technique 214

C

Calcium channel antagonists 89
Calcium channel blockers 549, 558
Carbamazepine 546, 555
Carbohydrate metabolism in diabetic pregnancy 324, 325
Cardiac arrhythmias 385
Cardiac defects 10, 34
Cardiac disease 369
Cardiac involvement 318
Cardiopulmonary resuscitation (CPR) 539, 540
Cardiovascular disease 327
Cardiovascular system 332, 517
Care of neonate at birth 483
Care of newborn 450
Causes of
    anemia 278
    antepartum hemorrhage 132, 149
    jaundice in pregnancy 350
    maternal alloimmunization 258
Centers for disease control (CDC) 476
Central nervous system malformations 10

Central venous pressure (CVP) 520, 523
Cerebroplacental ratio 185
Cervical assessment 75
Cervical cancer in pregnancy 503
Cervical cerclage 78
Cervicovaginal fibronectin 76
Cesarean delivery 502
Cesarean scar pregnancy 232
Cesarean section (CS) 230
    for breech 219
    in placenta previa 142
    surgical techniques 250
Changes in
    myomas during pregnancy 500
    thyroid physiology during pregnancy
        406
Characteristic clinical features of TORCH
        infection 461
Chest radiograph 445
Chest X-ray 394
Chlamydia trachomatis 99, 479
Chorionic villus sampling 4, 5, 19, 258
Choroid plexus cyst 12
Chromosomal abnormalities 2
Chromosomal study 52
Chronic asthma during pregnancy 552
Chronic hypertension 57, 298, 317
Chronic polyhydramnios 121
Classification of
    diabetes in pregnancy 323
    hypertension in pregnancy 298
    IUGR 177
    preeclampsia 299
Clinical course in PROM 103
Clinical examination in pregnant woman
        277
Clinical features of anemia in pregnancy
        276
CMV infection 466
Coarctation of aorta 36, 379
Cocaine 546
Collagen vascular disorders 57
Colloid 259
Colposcopy in pregnancy 505
Combination tocolytic therapy 92
Combined first and second trimester
        screening 9
Combined first trimester screening 7
Complete breech 201

Complications
    associated with hydramnios 122
    in adult life 180
    of ECV 205
Components of expectant management
        106
Compound presentation 226
Concurrent RTI and STI 473
Condition specific antepartum fetal
        testing 68
Conduct of breech delivery 209
Confined placental mosaicism (CPM) 18
Congenital
    anomalies 135, 184
    diaphragmatic hernia 46
    heart disease (CHD) 376
    hyperbilirubinemia 364
    infection 460
    malformations 160, 219
    tuberculosis 444
Conjoined twins 160
Connective tissue disorders 318
Conotruncal malformation 37
Conservative surgery 248
Contingent screening 4
Continuous intravenous infusion 314
Continuous positive airway pressure
        (CPAP) 525
Contraception 341, 451, 457, 484
Contraception in anemic women 293
Contraction stress test 58, 59, 189
Contraindications to VBAC 242
Control of
    hypertension 531
    seizures 458, 531
Coombs test 259
Corticosteroids 80, 549
Corticotropin releasing hormone (CRH) 73
Cost implications 493
Criteria for
    advising pregnancy post-transplanta-
        tion 438
    defining anemia 274
    diagnosis of HELLP syndrome 315
Crown-rump length (CRL) 6
CT and MRI 392
CT pulmonary angiography (CTPA) 395
Cushing's syndrome 318

Index

Cyanotic heart lesions 378
Cyclooxygenase inhibitors 89
Cystic hygroma 42
Cytomegalovirus 468

D

Dandy-Walker malformation 41
Decidual hemorrhage 74
Decongestants 553
Deep vein thrombosis 391
Definition of perinatal transmission 472
Delivery 309, 320
Delivery 41, 214, 309, 320, 375, 413
Delivery-related perinatal death 240
Detection of
    fetal DNA and fetal cells in maternal 15
    Rh alloimmunization 261
Diabetes mellitus 57, 331
Diabetic ketoacidosis 327
Diabetic nephropathy 331, 434
Diabetic retinopathy 331
Diagnosis of
    hyperthyroidism 411
    IUGR 180
    maternal infection 462
    megaloblastic anemia 285
    preterm labor 78
Diagnostic criteria for diabetes during
        pregnancy 331
Diagnostic tests 392, 394
Diazepam 560
Dietary therapy 334
Diethylstilbestrol 546
Differential diagnosis of HELLP syndrome
        316
Difficulty in delivery of
    buttocks 211
    legs 211
Disorders of amniotic fluid 121
Dizygotic twins 155
Dopaminergic antagonists 551
Doppler
    blood flow velocimetry 184
    sonography 4, 5
    study 124
    ultrasonography 66
    velocimetry 58
    venous ultrasound 392

Down syndrome 5
Drug treatment 107, 282
Drugs for bronchial asthma 551
Ductus venosus sonography 7
Duodenal atresia 47
Duration of exposure to maternal secre-
        tions 475
Dye dilution method 124
Dysfunctional labor 502

E

Early delivery and glucocorticoids 270
Echocardiography 394
Echogenic bowel 11
Echogenic intracardiac focus 11, 34
Eclampsia 298, 312
Ectopic pregnancy 231, 258
Edema 298
Education of nursing personnel 77
Edward syndrome 5
Effect of
    diabetes mellitus on pregnancy 325
    epilepsy on pregnancy 455
    future fertility 231
    HIV on pregnancy 484
    hyperthyroidism on pregnancy 410
    myoma on pregnancy 500
    pregnancy on
        diabetes mellitus 325
        epilepsy 454
        HIV disease progression 484
        renal structure and function 426
        tuberculosis 442
    renal disease on pregnancy 427
    tuberculosis on pregnancy 443
Ehlers–Danlos syndrome 99
Elective cesarean section 206
Emergency cardiac care for parturients
        540
Encephalocele 38
End organ damage 318
Endocrine disorders 318
Endotracheal intubation 526
Epilepsy 454
Equivocal-hyperstimulation 60
Equivocal-suspicious 60
Esophageal atresia 47
Estimated date of delivery (EDD) 112

Estimated fetal weight 182, 183
Ethambutol 447
Ethanol 546
Etiology of chronic hypertension 318
Etiopathogenesis of
    anemia in pregnancy 274
    megaloblastic anemia 284
Etretinate 546
Examination of placenta and cord 53
Expectant 248
Expectant management 105, 106, 139, 304
Expectorants 553
Extended breech 201
External cephalic version (ECV) 167, 204
Extrahepatic biliary obstruction 364
Extrapulmonary tuberculosis 444
Eye involvement 318
Eyes 300

F

Face 32
Face presentation 223
Facial anomalies 11
Facial cleft 41
Factors affecting MTCT of HIV 472
Factors predicting success rates 235
Factors predisposing to PROM 99
Femur length (FL) 182
Fern test 101
Fertility 488
Fetal
    anomalies 489, 501
    Fetal arterial Doppler 66
    Fetal autopsy 52
    Fetal benefits 241
    Fetal blood sampling 4, 20, 269
    Fetal cardiac arrhythmia 34
    Fetal cardiac sampling 21
    Fetal complications 123, 179
    Fetal concerns 417
    Fetal distress 205
    Fetal ductus venosus 67
    effects 328
        hyperthyroidism 415
        maternal antithyroid drugs 414
    evaluation 304
    extremity 34
    factors 475

fibronectin assay 79
imaging 4, 10
indications 310
intrahepatic vessel sampling 21
kick count 58
macrosomia 114
monitoring 116, 524
movement assessment 58
nasal bone 30
nonstress test (NST) 338
Rh determination 264
risks 158, 240
side effects 84, 549
surveillance 306, 429
thyroid physiology 408
tissue biopsy 4, 21
venous Doppler 67
Fetomaternal outcome 115
Fetoplacental factors 113
Fetoscopy 4, 22
First line anti-TB drugs used in pregnancy 448
First line drugs 447
First trimester screening 4, 5, 27
Flexed breech 201
Fluorescent in situ hybridization technique 18
Footling breech 202
Frank breech 201
Fulminant viral hepatitis 353
Functional residual capacity (FRC) 517

G

Gamma amino butyric acid (GABA) 560
Gardnerella vaginalis 99
Gastrointestinal drugs 553
Gastrointestinal malformations 10
Gastrointestinal system 45, 519
Gastroschisis 46
General principles of antepartum management 428
Genetic disorders 2
Genetic sonography 13
Genitourinary system 43
Genitourinary tract 34
German measles 462
Gestational diabetes 323, 490
Gestational hypertension 298

Gestational hyperthyroidism 409
Glomerular filtration rate (GFR) 426
Glomerulonephritis 431
Glyburide 334
Glycemic control during labor 339
Glycemic management of diabetes 340
Graves' disease 410
Guidelines for managing abnormal Pap
    smear 504

H

H_2 receptor antagonist 554
Hashimoto's thyroiditis 416
Hb Bart's disease 288
HbH disease 288, 290
Head 37
    circumference (HC) 182
    injury 219
Heart 29, 32, 301
HELLP syndrome 310, 315, 532, 353
Hemodynamic changes 370
Hemolytic disease of fetus and newborn
    (HDFN) 255
Hemolytic jaundice 363
Hepatitis
    A 362
    B 362
    C 363
    E 363
Hepatorenal syndrome 434
Herpes virus 468
Hingorani's sign 511
HIV in children 472
Holoprosencephaly 40
Home uterine activity monitoring 75
Human immunodeficiency virus (HIV) 470
Hydralazine 558
Hydramnios 156
Hydrocephalous 39
Hydronephrosis 45
Hydrops fetalis 49
Hypercoagulability 390
Hyperemesis gravidarum 360
Hypertension 157, 297
Hypertensive disease 489, 516
Hypertensive disorders of pregnancy 57,
    530
Hyperthyroidism 409

Hypertrophic cardiomyopathy 384
Hypoplastic left ventricle 36
Hypothyroidism 416
Hypoxic ischemic encephalopathy 241
Hysterectomy 248

I

Identification of viable pregnancy 28
Idiopathic thrombocytopenic purpura
    (ITP) 359
Imaging studies 14
Imaging techniques 203
Immunoglobulin G (IgG) antibodies 255
Immunological measures 478
Immunosuppressive drugs 563
Implications for
    fetus of obese mother 493
    offspring 342
In utero treatment 39, 40
In vitro fertilization (IVF) 153
Incomplete breech 202
Indeterminate bleeding 150
Indication of parenteral therapy 283
Indications for
    delivery in severe preeclampsia 310
    maternal TORCH screen 462
    cesarean in multifetal pregnancy 168
    fetal surveillance 57
Indigo carmine test 102
Individual congenital malformations 34
Indomethacin 88, 125, 548 549
Induction 246
Infantile polycystic kidney disease (IPKD)
    44
Infection in postpartum period 502
Inferior vena cava 67
Inflammatory response syndrome (SIRS)
    534
INH prophylaxis in pregnant women 450
Inhaled beta agonists 552
Inhaled steroids 552
Initial laboratory tests 351
Initiate insulin therapy 336
Insulin therapy 335
Insulin treated diabetes 338
Integrated screening 4, 9
Intermittent intramuscular injections 314
Interpretation of
    biophysical profile and pregnancy 64

Management of High-Risk Pregnancy—A Practical Approach

OGTT 330
results 60
Interventions aimed at decreasing MTCT of HIV 477
Intracranial anatomy 31
Intracytoplasmic sperm injection (ICSI) 153
Intrahepatic cholestasis of pregnancy 354
Intrapartum
considerations 339
issues 491
management 166, 311, 402, 457
period 221
Intrauterine
death 258
growth restriction (IUGR) 176, 512
transfusion (IUT) 269
Intraventricular hemorrhage (IVH) 104
Invasive
amnioreduction 125
cervical cancer 506
diagnostic procedures 4
evaluation 265
monitoring 523
prenatal diagnostic procedures 16
prenatal testing for aneuploidy 22
Iodide 546
Iodine nutrition in pregnancy 408
Iron
content of different salts 282
deficiency anemia 279
prophylaxis 281
supplementation 281
Irregular heart rate 35
Irregular treatment 444
Isoniazid 447, 561
Isotretinoin 546
Isoxsuprine 548

K

Karyotyping 124, 187
Ketorolac 88
Kidney 29, 300
Kidney abnormalities 43

L

Labetalol 557

Labor 41, 375, 413
Lactation 493
Laparoscopy 512
Laparotomy 512
Last menstrual period (LMP) 112
Left to right shunts 376
Leiomyomas 499
Lifestyle modifications 319, 334
Liley's curve 17
Lithium 546
Liver 300
functions in pregnancy 349
involvement in drug reactions 364
Local anesthesia 564
Local lesions of cervix 149
Localization of placenta 184
Locked twins 169
Long chain hydroxylacylco-enzymea dehydrogenase 352
Lovset's maneuver 213
Low birth weight 158
Low molecular weight heparin (LMWH) 397, 561
Lower urinary tract obstruction 45, 128
Lower uterine segment 133
Lupus nephritis 430

M

Macrosomia 241
Magnesium sulfate 85, 549, 559
Magnetic resonance imaging 4, 14, 137
Magnitude of
disease 441
problem 470
Maintenance tocolytic therapy 93
Malpresentations 134, 157, 502
Management during pregnancy 333
Management in labor 225
Management of
asymptomatic placenta previa 138
breech in labor 207
coagulopathy 148
deep vein thrombosis 398
hyperthyroidism in pregnancy 415
hypothyroidism in pregnancy 418
IUGR 187
labor 245, 292

life-threatening hepatic failure 365
obesity in pregnancy 495
pregnancy 115, 290, 331
preterm labor 340
preterm PROM 105
PROM 104
pulmonary embolism 400
renal failure 149
Rh negative
    immunized pregnant women 262
    nonimmunized women 260
    symptomatic placenta previa 139
term PROM 105
    third stage of labor 247
Manning's score BPS 189
Manual exploration of scar after cesarean
        section 249
Marfan's syndrome 372
Maternal age and parity 155
Maternal and fetal
    benefits 240
    complications 278
    risks 156, 319
Maternal
    benefits 240
    CD4 and lymphocyte count 473
    complications 122
    concerns 417
    demographic factors 113
    effects 325
    evaluation 304
    fetal monitoring 106
    hemoglobin disorders 57
    hemorrhage 516, 532
    indications 310
    morbidity and mortality 238
    neutralizing antibody status 473
    risks 156, 240
    serum alpha fetoprotein 8, 30
    serum assay in second trimester 8
    serum screening 4
    side effects 86, 88, 549
    surveillance 305, 428
    thyrotoxicosis 57
    uterine circulation 67
    weight gain 181
Matrix metalloproteinases (MMP) 98

Maturity 475
Mauriceau-Smellie-Veit maneuver 217
Measles 562
Measurement of
    blood pressure 297
    symphysiofundal height (SFH) 181
Mechanical ventilation 526
Mechanism of
    action 82
    labor 203, 225
    teratogenicity 546
Mediators of inflammation and infection
        77
Medical amnioreduction 125
Medical complications 326
Megaloblastic anemia 284
Metformin 335
Methods of delivery 212
Microbiological methods 446
Middle cerebral artery 66, 265
Mild diet treated gestational diabetes 339
Mild polyhydramnios 124
Mild preeclampsia 299
Minor blood group antigens 270
Miscarriages 489
Mitral regurgitation 381
Mitral stenosis 380
Mitral valve prolapse 380
Mode of delivery 40, 108, 194, 311, 339, 474,
        482, 507
Moderate to severe polyhydramnios 124
Modified biophysical profile 58, 65
Monitoring in antenatal period 244
Monitoring progress of labor 208
Monoamniotic twins 160
Monozygotic pregnancy 153
Mortality probability models 521
MR angiography 395
Multicystic dysplasia 43
Multi-drug resistant tuberculosis (MDR-TB)
        444
Multiple pregnancy 258
Mumps 562
Mycoplasma hominis 74
Myocardial infarction 385
Myomectomy 502
Myomectomy during cesarean section 503

N

Naegle's formula 113
Nasal bone sonography 7
Nasal bones 12
National Tuberculosis Control Program 39
446
Neck 37
Neisseria gonorrhea 99, 479
Neonatal complications 179, 461
Neonatal effects 328
Neonatal management 342
Neonatal outcome 94
Neonatal side effects 549
Neonatal side effects 88
Nephropathy 326
Neural tube defect (NTD) 54
Neurological development of fetus 417
Neuromuscular blocking agents 529
Neuropathy 326
Newborn immune response 475
Newer tests 102
NICU admissions 494
Nifedipine 558
Nipple stimulation 117
Nitrazine test 101
Nitric oxide donors 92
Nitroprusside 557
Nonsedative antihistaminics 553
Non-Doppler flow test 68
Noninvasive diagnostic method 15
Noninvasive diagnostic procedure 4
Noninvasive screening procedures 4
Nonprostaglandin induction 247
Nonstress test (NST) 58, 60, 188
Nuchal displacement of arm 214
Nuchal fold 11, 31
Nuchal translucency 5, 6, 29
Nutrition 527
Nutritional status of mother 474
Nutritional supplement 551

O

Obesity 487, 493
Obesity related adverse outcomes in
pregnancy 489
Objectives of
fetal surveillance 57
first trimester screening 28

Obstetric cases requiring critical care 515
Obstetric complications 325
Obstetric measures 478
Obstructed labor 502
Obstructive uropathies 45
Oligohydramnios 125
Omphalocele 45
One step approach 330
Open neural tube defect 37
Operative intervention 496
Operative procedures 474
Oral
anticoagulants 398
contraceptives 564
hypoglycemic agents 334
iron therapy 282
steroids 552
Outflow tract obstruction 36
Outpatient management 305
Ovarian tumor 510
Overcoming difficulties in breech delivery
211
Overt enlargement 40
Ovulation induction drugs 155
Oxygen therapy 525
Oxytocin antagonists 91
Oxytocin challenge test (OCT) 58, 59, 189

P

Palpation of abdomen 202
Para-aminosalicylic acid (PAS) 448
Parental counseling 40
Parenteral iron therapy 283
Patau syndrome 5, 13
Paternal Rh phenotype and genotype 262
Pathologic uterine overdistention 73
Pathophysiology of placental insufficiency
178
Patient education 77
Patients on dialysis 436
Peak systolic velocity 265
Pending relevant trials 249
Per speculum examination 100
Per vaginal examination in OT 141
Percentage reverse flow 185
Percutaneous umbilical blood sampling 21
Perinatal outcome in breech delivery 219
Perinatal torch transmission 462

Index

Peripartum cardiomyopathy 383, 516
Pervaginum findings 202
Phenobarbital 555
Phenytoin 546, 555, 560
Physiological changes in pregnancy 407
Placenta
    accreta 232
    previa 133, 232, 501, 533
Placental
    abruption 232, 501
    barrier 474
    dysfunction 114
    growth factor (PLGF) 157
    size 134
Planned vaginal delivery 207
Planned VBAC in special circumstances
    241
Plant alkaloids 563
Polycystic kidney disease 55
Polyhydramnios 121
Ponderal index 183
Poor maternal nutrition 444
Postmaturity syndrome 114
Postnatal
    advice 496
    care 293
    examination 49
    visit 249
Postpartum
    care and advice 341
    hemorrhage 158, 492, 502, 533
    issues 492
    management 168, 457
    thyroiditis 410, 420
Post-transplant patient 437
Preconception 456
Preconception counseling 331, 371
Preeclampsia 298, 430, 501
Preeclamptic liver disease 358
Pregestational diabetes 323
Pregnancy and hyperthyroidism 410
Pregnancy loss 500
Pregnant women at high risk
    for TORCH infection 464
    of anemia 276
Preimplantation diagnosis 4, 23
Preinvasive cancer 504
Prelabor rupture of membrane (PROM) 98

Preload index 185
Premature atrial contractions 35
Premature rupture of membranes 98, 501
Premature ventricular contractions 35
Prenatal diagnosis of fetal infection 464
Prenatal screening 27
Pre-pregnancy 495
Prepregnancy initiative 77
Preterm birth 241
Preterm labor 157, 500
Prevalence of
    anemia 273
    diabetes mellitus 322
Prevention of
    intrauterine growth restriction 194
    iron deficiency anemia 281
    post-term pregnancy 117
    preterm labor 77
    Rh alloimmunization 261
Previous cesarean section 234
Previous history of placenta previa 134
Primary and recurrent HSV infection 463
Primary maternal CMV 463
Primary prevention 477
Pritchard regime 559
Problems in babies with IUGR at birth 179
Prophylactic antibiotic therapy 108
Prophylactic measures 395
Prostaglandin induction 246
Prostaglandin synthetase inhibitors 87
Prosthetic heart valves 382
Proteinuria 297
Prothrombin time (PT) 349
Protocol for diagnosis of TB in pregancy
    446
Proton pump inhibitors 553
Pulmonary artery hypertension (PAH) 377
Pulmonary artery occlusion pressure
    (PAOP) 523
Pulmonary edema 532, 538
Pulmonary embolism 392, 537
Pulmonary stenosis 37
Pulsatility index 66, 185
Pyelectasis 12, 45
Pyrazinamide 448

Q

Quadruple test 4, 9

R

Race 155
Radiation exposure 530
Radiation treatment 508
Reasons of failure to respond 284
Recommendations for
  induction of labor 115
  screening for thalassemia 289
Recurrence risk 40
Reflux nephropathy 432
Renal
  agenesis 43
  calculi 435
  cortical necrosis 433
  disease 57
  disorders 318
  malformations 11
  plasma flow (RPF) 426
  system 519
Resistance index 66, 185
Respiratory
  care in pregnancy 525
  complications 491
  distress syndrome (RDS) 104,550
  problems 240
  system 517
Response to therapy 287
Retinopathy 326
Retroversion of gravid uterus 508
Rheumatic heart disease 380
Rifampicin 447
Risk associated with failed VBAC 239
Risk factors for preeclampsia 301
Risk of uterine rupture 238
Risk scoring 74
Risks and benefits of ercs 240
Risks and benefits of VBAC 238
Ritodrine 82, 548
Role of
  conization in pregnancy 505
  USG 244
Routine noninvasive monitoring 522
Rubella 462, 467, 562

S

Safety in pregnancy 552
Salbutamol 548
Saline 259

Scar thickness 245
Screening
  diagnostic procedures 4
  for fetal chromosomal abnormalities 14
  for thyroid dysfunction during pregnancy 421
  methods 2, 5
  protocols 464
  recommendations and prevention 467
Second line drugs 448
Second trimester
  screening 8, 30
  trimester USG scan 31
Secondary prevention 477
Selective reduction and termination 170
Sepsis 516, 534
Septal defects 36
Sequential and contingent screening 9
Sequential screening 4
Serologic tests 463
Serological studies 124
Severe anemia 57
Severe disease 310
Severe preeclampsia 299
Severity of anemia 277
Short humerus and femur 11
Short interdelivery interval 242
Sickle cell anemia 291
Single fetal demise 169
Skeletal malformations 11
Skeletal system 48
Skeleton 29
Skin incision and wound infection 492
Smoking 134
Sonographic detection of major fetal structural ma 10
Sonographic evaluation of minor markers 11
Sonographic findings reported in congenital infect 465
Specific renal pathology in pregnancy 429
Spina bifida 38
Spine 32, 37
Status epilepticus 457
Status of fetal membranes 474
Steroids 306
Stillbirth 233
Stomach 29

Index

Stopping ARV drugs 483
Streptomycin 448
Structural cardiac defects 36
Subcapsular liver hematoma 317
Subclinical hyperthyroidism 409
Subclinical hypothyroidism (SCH) 418
Sulindac 88, 125
Sulphonylureas 334
Superimposed preeclampsia-eclampsia 298
Supportive measures during antitubercular therapy 449
Supraventricular tachycardia 35
Sweeping (or stripping) of membranes 117
Symmetrical IUGR 177
Symptoms of tuberculosis in pregnancy 442
Systemic vascular resistance (SVR) 517

T

Tachycardia 35
Technique of contraction stress test 59
Teratogenic drugs 546
Teratogenicity 545
Terbutaline 83, 548
Termination of pregnancy 358
Tetracycline 546
Tetralogy of Fallot 37, 372, 378
Thalassemia 287
Thalidomide 546
Theophylline 553
Thiazolidenediones 335
Three dimensional USG 30
Thromboembolic complications 490
Thrombotic thrombocytopenic purpura (TTP) 359
Thyroid nodules and thyroid carcinoma 419
Timing and mode of delivery 193
Timing of
    delivery 108, 338
    ECV 204
    vertical transmission 476
Tissue inhibitor of metalloproteinase (TIMP) 77
    te insulin 337
    sis 81
    ic therapy 80

Tocolytics 108, 547
Total parenteral nutrition (TPN) 527
Toxemia of pregnancy 353
Toxoplasmosis 467
Tracheal intubation and mechanical ventilation 526
Transabdominal chorionic villus sampling 19
Transcerebellar view 31
Transcervical chorionic villus sampling 19
Transport of a critically ill obstetric patient 519
Transposition of
    great arteries 379
    great vessels 37
Transthalamic view 31
Transverse lie 220
Treatment for iugr 192
Treatment modalities 270
Treatment of
    acute severe hypertension 308
    diabetic ketoacidosis 328
    infection 78
    tuberculosis in
        lactating women 449
        pregnant women 446
Trichomonas vaginalis 99
Triple test 4, 8
Truncus arteriosus 37
Tuberculin skin test 445
Tuberculosis (TB) 441
Tumor markers 512
Twin
    birth study 249
    gestation 241
    pregnancy 153
    reversed arterial perfusion (TRAP) sequence 161
Twin-to-twin transfusion syndrome (TTTS) 162
Two step approach 330
Types of
    anemia 277
    virus 474
    breech 201
    inherited thrombophilias 390
    insulin 335
    viral hepatitis in pregnancy 362